Essentials

of Obstetrics
and Gynecology

D0565313

Essentials of Obstetrics and Gynecology

4th Edition

NEVILLE F. HACKER, MD
Associate Professor of Obstetrics and Gynaecology
Director, Gynaecological Cancer Center
Royal Hospital for Women
Randwick, New South Wales
Australia

J. GEORGE MOORE, MD[†]
Professor and Chairman Emeritus
Department of Obstetrics and Gynecology
David Geffen School of Medicine at UCLA
Los Angeles, California

JOSEPH C. GAMBONE, DO, MPH
Professor of Obstetrics and Gynecology
Department of Obstetrics and Gynecology
David Geffen School of Medicine at UCLA
Los Angeles, California

[†]Deceased.

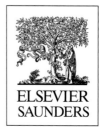

ELSEVIER
SAUNDERS

ELSEVIER
SAUNDERS

170 S. Independence Mall W 300 E
Philadelphia, Pennsylvania 19106-3399

ESSENTIALS OF OBSTETRICS AND GYNECOLOGY

Copyright © 2004, 1998, 1992, 1986 by Elsevier Inc.

All rights reserved. No part of this publication may be reproduced or transmitted in any form or by any means, electronic or mechanical, including photocopying, recording, or any information storage and retrieval system, without permission in writing from the publisher.

Permissions may be sought directly from Elsevier's Health Sciences Rights Department in Philadelphia, PA, USA: phone: (+1) 215 239 3804, fax: (+1) 215 239 3805, e-mail: healthpermissions@elsevier.com. You may also complete your request on-line via the Elsevier homepage (http://www.elsevier.com), by selecting 'Customer Support' and then 'Obtaining Permissions'.

NOTICE

Obstetrics and gynecology is an ever-changing field. Standard safety precautions must be followed, but as new research and clinical experience broaden our knowledge, changes in treatment and drug therapy become necessary or appropriate. Readers are advised to check the product information currently provided by the manufacturer of each drug to be administered to verify the recommended dose, the method and duration of administration, and the contraindications. It is the responsibility of the treating physician, relying on experience and knowledge of the patient, to determine dosages and the best treatment for the patient. Neither the publisher nor the editor assumes any responsibility for any injury and/or damage to persons or property.

The Publisher

ISBN-13: 978–0–7216–0179–3
ISBN-10: 0–7216–0179–0

IE ISBN-13: 978–0–8089–2058–8
IE ISBN-10: 0–8089–2058–8

Publishing Director: William Schmitt
Managing Editor: Rebecca Gruliow
Design Manager: Ellen Zanolle

Printed in China

Last digit is the print number: 9 8 7 6 5 4

Contributors

EDITORS

Neville F. Hacker, MD
Associate Professor of Obstetrics and Gynaecology;
Director, Gynaecological Cancer Center, Royal
Hospital for Women, Randwick, New South Wales,
Australia
  Breast Disease; Principles of Cancer Therapy;
  Cervical Dysplasia and Cancer; Vulvar and
  Vaginal Cancer; Uterine Corpus Cancer

J. George Moore, MD[†]
Professor and Chairman Emeritus, Department of
Obstetrics and Gynecology, David Geffen School of
Medicine at UCLA, Los Angeles, California
  Clinical Approach to the Patient; Female
  Reproductive Anatomy and Embryology;
  Maternal Physiologic and Immunologic
  Adaptation to Pregnancy; Common Medical
  and Surgical Conditions Complicating
  Pregnancy; Congenital Anomalies and Benign
  Conditions of the Uterine Corpus and Cervix;
  Congenital Anomalies and Benign Conditions of
  the Ovaries and Fallopian Tubes; Endometriosis
  and Adenomyosis; Dysfunctional Uterine
  Bleeding

Joseph C. Gambone, DO, MPH
Professor of Obstetrics and Gynecology,
Department of Obstetrics and Gynecology, David
Geffen School of Medicine at UCLA, Los Angeles,
California
  Practice Management and Ethics in Obstetrics
  and Gynecology; Clinical Approach to the
  Patient; Female Reproductive Anatomy and
  Embryology; Obstetric Hemorrhage and
  Puerperal Sepsis; Common Medical and Surgical
  Conditions Complicating Pregnancy; Congenital
  Anomalies and Benign Conditions of the Vulva
  and Vagina; Dysmenorrhea and Chronic Pelvic
  Pain; Ectopic Pregnancy; Endometriosis and
  Adenomyosis; Gynecologic Procedures;
  Dysfunctional Uterine Bleeding; Climacteric;
  Menstrual Cycle–Influenced Disorders; PDA
  Companion Co-editor

PART EDITORS

Grace Elizabeth Kong
Medical Student, Class of 2004, David Geffen
School of Medicine at UCLA, Los Angeles,
California
  PDA Companion Co-editor

Brian J. Koos, MD, DPhil
Professor and Vice Chair, Department of Obstetrics
and Gynecology, David Geffen School of Medicine
at UCLA, Los Angeles, California
  Maternal Physiologic and Immunologic
  Adaptation to Pregnancy; Common Medical
  and Surgical Conditions Complicating
  Pregnancy

Larry R. Laufer, MD
Head, Division of Reproductive Endocrinology and
Infertility, Department of Obstetrics and
Gynecology, Naval Medical Center, San Diego,
California
  Puberty and Disorders of Pubertal Development;
  Amenorrhea, Oligomenorrhea, and
  Hyperandrogenic Disorders; Climacteric;
  Menstrual Cycle–Influenced Disorders

[†]Deceased.

Anita L. Nelson, MD
Professor of Obstetrics and Gynecology, David
Geffen School of Medicine at UCLA; Chief,
Women's Health Care Programs, Research and
Education Institute at Harbor-UCLA Medical
Center, Los Angeles, California
  Congenital Anomalies and Benign Conditions of
  the Vulva and Vagina; Congenital Anomalies and
  Benign Conditions of the Uterine Corpus and
  Cervix; Congenital Anomalies and Benign
  Conditions of the Ovaries and Fallopian Tubes;
  Ectopic Pregnancy; Family Planning

OTHER CONTRIBUTORS

Martha J. Baird, CNM, MP, MSN
Director of Education, Women's Health Care Nurse
Practitioner Program, Department of Obstetrics and
Gynecology, Harbor-UCLA, Los Angeles, California
  Human Sexuality

Richard A. Bashore, MD
Professor Emeritus, Department of Obstetrics and
Gynecology, David Geffen School of Medicine at
UCLA, Los Angeles, California
  Fetal Surveillance During Labor; Uterine
  Contractility and Dystocia

Jonathan S. Berek, MD, MMSc
Professor and Chair, College of Applied Anatomy;
Executive Vice Chair, Department of Obstetrics and
Gynecology; Chief, Division of Gynecologic
Oncology and Gynecology Service; Director, UCLA
Women's Reproductive Cancer Program, David
Geffen School of Medicine at UCLA, Los Angeles,
California
  Ovarian Cancer; Gestational Trophoblastic
  Neoplasia

Narender N. Bhatia, MD
Chief, Gynecologic Urology, Department of
Obstetrics and Gynecology, Harbor-UCLA Medical
Center, Los Angeles, California
  Genitourinary Dysfunction

Michael S. Broder, MD, MSHS
Vice President, Zynx Health, Beverly Hills,
California; Assistant Clinical Professor, Department
of Obstetrics and Gynecology, David Geffen School
of Medicine at UCLA, Los Angeles, California
  Gynecologic Procedures

Richard P. Buyalos, Jr, MD
Co-Director, Fertility and Surgical Associates of
California; Associate Clinical Professor, David
Geffen School of Medicine at UCLA, Los Angeles,
California
  Puberty and Disorders of Pubertal Development

Mary E. Carsten, PhD
Professor Emeritus of Obstetrics/Gynecology, David
Geffen School of Medicine at UCLA, Los Angeles,
California
  Endocrinology of Pregnancy and Parturition

Lony C. Castro, MD
Professor and Chair, Department of Obstetrics and
Gynecology, Western University of Health Sciences,
College of Osteopathic Medicine of the Pacific,
Pomona, California; Director, High Risk Obstetrical
Clinics, Riverside County Regional Medical Center,
Riverside, California
  Hypertensive Disorders of Pregnancy

Anita Backus Chang, MD
Director of Obstetric Anesthesia, UCLA Medical
Center; Associate Clinical Professor, David Geffen
School of Medicine at UCLA, Los Angeles,
California
  Normal Labor, Delivery, and Postpartum Care

Ramen H. Chmait, MD
Florida Institute for Fetal Diagnosis and Therapy,
Tampa, Florida
  Obstetric Procedures

Catherine Marin DeUgarte, MD
Fellow, Reproductive Endocrinology and Infertility,
Department of Obstetrics and Gynecology,
Harbor-UCLA Medical Center, Los Angeles,
California
  Ectopic Pregnancy; Human Sexuality; Domestic
  Violence and Sexual Assault; Puberty and
  Disorders of Pubertal Development

Janice I. French, CNM, MS
Project Coordinator, Los Angeles Best Babies
Collaborative, Department of Obstetrics and
Gynecology, Cedars-Sinai Medical Center, Los
Angeles, California
  Pelvic Infections

Paul A. Gluck, MD
Associate Clinical Professor, Department of Obstetrics and Gynecology, University of Miami School of Medicine, Miami, Florida
  Clinical Performance Improvement

Robert H. Hayashi, MD
J. Robert Willson Professor of Obstetrics; Fellowship Director, Division of Maternal-Fetal Medicine, Department of Obstetrics & Gynecology, University of Michigan Medical School, Ann Arbor, Michigan
  Obstetric Hemorrhage and Puerperal Sepsis; Uterine Contractility and Dystocia

Calvin J. Hobel, MD
Vice Chair, Department of Obstetrics and Gynecology, Miriam Jacobs Chair in Maternal-Fetal Medicine, Cedars–Sinai Medical Center; Professor of Obstetrics and Gynecology, Professor of Pediatrics, David Geffen School of Medicine at UCLA, Los Angeles, California
  Antepartum Care; Normal Labor, Delivery, and Postpartum Care; Obstetric Complications

Joel B. Lench, MD
Director, Nurse Midwife Program, Department of Obstetrics and Gynecology, Naval Medical Center, San Diego, California
  Pelvic Infections

John K.H. Lu, PhD
Professor, Departments of Obstetrics and Gynecology and Neurobiology, David Geffen School of Medicine at UCLA, Los Angeles, California
  Female Reproductive Physiology

Michael C. Lu, MD, MS, MPH
Assistant Professor, Department of Obstetrics and Gynecology, David Geffen School of Medicine at UCLA; Department of Community Health Sciences, UCLA School of Public Health, Los Angeles, California
  Endocrinology of Pregnancy and Parturition; Antepartum Care

Donald E. Marsden, BMedSc(Hon), MBBS, FRCOG, FRACOG, CGO
Professor, Gynaecological Cancer Center, Royal Hospital for Women, Barker Street, Randwick, New South Wales, Australia
  Practice Management and Ethics in Obstetrics and Gynecology

James A. McGregor, MD CM
Visiting Professor, Obstetrics and Gynecology, David Geffen School of Medicine at UCLA, Los Angeles, California; Assistant Head, Perinatology, Obstetrix, Tucson, Arizona
  Pelvic Infections

David R. Meldrum, MD
Clinical Professor of Obstetrics and Gynecology, Department of Obstetrics and Gynecology, David Geffen School of Medicine at UCLA; Department of Reproductive Medicine, University of California at San Diego; Reproductive Partners Medical Group, Los Angeles, California
  Infertility and Assisted Reproductive Technologies

Thomas R. Moore, MD
Professor and Chairman, Department of Reproductive Medicine, University of California San Diego School of Medicine, San Diego, California
  Multifetal Gestation and Malpresentation; Obstetric Procedures

Sathima Natarajan, MD
Clinical Assistant Professor, Department of Pathology, David Geffen School of Medicine at UCLA, Los Angeles, California
  Pathology Module: PDA Companion

Bahij S. Nuwayhid, MD, PhD
Regional Chairman, Department of Obstetrics and Gynecology, Texas Tech University HSC-El Paso, El Paso, Texas
  Maternal Physiologic and Immunologic Adaptation to Pregnancy

Ketan S. Patel, MD
Senior Associate Consultant, Division of Reproductive Endocrine and Infertility, Mayo Clinic in Scottsdale, Arizona
  Amenorrhea, Oligomenorrhea, and Hyperandrogenic Disorders

Andrea J. Rapkin, MD
Professor, Department of Obstetrics and Gynecology, David Geffen School of Medicine at UCLA, Los Angeles, California
  Dysmenorrhea and Chronic Pelvic Pain

Robert C. Reiter, MD
Vice President, Quality and Clinical Performance
Improvement; Patient Safety Medical Officer,
ProMedica Health System, Toledo, Ohio
　Clinical Performance Improvement

Klaus J. Staisch, MD
Professor Emeritus, Department of Obstetrics and
Gynecology, Washington University School of
Medicine, St. Louis, Missouri
　Fetal Surveillance During Labor

Khalil Tabsh, MD
Professor, Department of Obstetrics and
Gynecology, David Geffen School of Medicine at
UCLA, Los Angeles, California
　Rhesus Isoimmunization

Nancy Theroux, RN, PhD
Clinical Administrator, UCLA Perinatal Group,
David Geffen School of Medicine at UCLA;
Assistant Clinical Professor, UCLA School of
Nursing, Los Angeles, California
　Rhesus Isoimmunization

Paul J. Toot, MD
Professor, Department of Obstetrics and
Gynecology, David Geffen School of Medicine at
UCLA, Los Angeles, California; Physician
Specialist—Obstetrics and Gynecology, Los Angeles
County/Olive View-UCLA Medical Center, Sylmar,
California
　Female Reproductive Physiology

Linda Yielding, RN, MBA
Corporate Director, Quality; Corporate Patient
Safety Officer, Clinical Outcomes and Resource
Management Department, ProMedica Health
System, Toledo, Ohio
　Clinical Performance Improvement

This edition of Essentials of Obstetrics and Gynecology *is dedicated to Dr. J. George "Jerry" Moore, an inspiring teacher, a great mentor, and a dear friend to both of us.*

Neville F. Hacker
Joseph C. Gambone

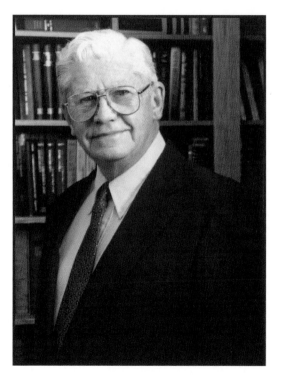

J. George Moore, MD
1917–2003

Preface to the Fourth Edition

The development and completion of the fourth edition of *Essentials of Obstetrics and Gynecology* was associated with great challenge, the need to make important choices, and profound sadness. First, was the sadness of losing a colleague and fellow editor, Dr. J. George (Jerry) Moore, who died on October 30th, 2003, at the age of 86. Jerry was for both of us a wonderful friend, an inspiring mentor, and most of all a tireless teacher. We do take great joy in the fact that he will continue to be a teacher because of the publication of this work, which he contributed to until his final days. We dedicate this edition of the book to him.

The great challenge today in medical education is to keep up with the ever-advancing technology that medical students and residents in training in obstetrics and gynecology have available to them. The recent digital electronics revolution allows for rapid access to current essential information for learning and practice. This edition of *Essentials of Obstetrics and Gynecology* has a companion electronic component designed to be used in a hand-held personal digital appliance (PDA) that includes an outline version of each of the forty-three chapters in the book. Students and residents should find this easily accessed information helpful to them as they move about the clinics and hospitals during their years of training. The PDA component also contains a set of electronic calculators that will be useful to students and residents for learning the practice of obstetrics and gynecology. The latest obstetric statistics, a glossary of obstetric terms, and a learning module of interesting pathologic cases in gynecology and obstetrics are contained in the PDA.

It was our intention to keep to the "essentials" of obstetrics and gynecology in this edition of the book. We, therefore, had to make choices about the breadth and depth of information to include in a textbook intended for students in the field. A few of the chapters in the last edition have been eliminated, and some have been combined into new updated chapters. This edition contains forty-three chapters, all in color, with revised tables and illustrations and new color photographs. Every attempt has been made to include material consistent with the medical student educational objectives set forth by the Association of Professors in Gynecology and Obstetrics (APGO). These learning objectives are listed on their website at www.apgo.org.

This edition includes some new chapter authors, each one an authority on the chapter topic. Several new Part Editors, Brian J. Koos, Larry R. Laufer, and Anita L. Nelson, have contributed to the content and editing of this edition and have made a significant impact on the quality of the book. In addition to the authors and editors of this edition, we wish to acknowledge all those who have contributed to this textbook in previous editions.* Their knowledge and their words formed the foundation of this work and continue to enlighten students in obstetrics and gynecology.

We wish to acknowledge the secretarial assistance of Helen McGilligan at the Gynecologic Cancer Center at the Royal Hospital for Women in Sydney, Australia and Sergio Huidor at the David Geffen School of Medicine at UCLA. We have appreciated the vision and friendly professionalism of William R. Schmitt at Elsevier and Saunders. Finally, we thank our wives and soul mates, Estelle and Marge, for their support and patience during this project.

Joseph C. Gambone
Neville F. Hacker

Contributors from previous editions
John Marshall, Juan J. Arce, Carol L. Archie, A. David Barnes, Michael J. Bennett, Jennifer Blake, Clifford Bochner, J. Robert Bragonier, Charles R. Brinkman III, Philip G. Brooks, John E. Buster, Maria Bustillo, R. Jeffrey Chang, George Chapman, Gautam Chaudhuri, Kenneth A. Conklin, Irvin M. Cushner (deceased), Alan H. DeCherney, William J. Dignam, John A. Eden, Robin Farias-Eisner, Larry C. Ford (deceased), Michelle Fox, Ann Garber, Anne D.M. Graham, William A. Growdon, John Gunning (deceased), Lewis A. Hamilton, Hunter A. Hammill, George S. Harris, James M. Heaps, Howard L. Judd, Samir Khalife, Ali Khraibi, Oscar A. Kletzky (deceased), Thomas B. Lebherz (deceased), Ronald S. Leuchter, Arnold L. Medearis, Rober Monoson, John Morris, Suha H. N. Murad, Lauren Nathan, John Newnham, Tuan Nguyen, Gary Oakes, Aldo Palmieri, Groesbeck P. Parham, Anthony E. Reading, Jean M. Ricci (Goodman), Michael G. Ross, Edward W. Savage, James R. Shields, William D. Schlaff, Eric Surrey, Maclyn E. Wade, Mathan Wasserstrum, and Barry G. Wren.

Preface to the First Edition

A generation ago most schools of medicine in the United States presented courses in theoretical obstetrics and gynecology extending over a period of 18 months, supplemented by practical clerkships of 8 to 16 weeks in the third and fourth years. Most students procured as source textbooks a fairly complete compendium of obstetrics and another in gynecology. These tests not only served the students in medical school but were of great value during their housestaff training and were added to their reference library as they entered practice.

During the decade of the 1960s, theoretical obstetrics and gynecology in many institutions were condensed into a general course known as "An Introduction to Clinical Medicine" or "The Pathophysiology of Disease." Practical work in the clinics and wards was condensed into core clerkships, and in obstetrics and gynecology the "core" was generally restricted to 6 or 8 weeks, with electives available in subspecialty areas (high-risk obstetrics, gynecology oncology, reproductive endocrinology, acting internships, and outpatient gynecology). This condensation of experience into the "core" of obstetrics and gynecology during the clinical years left students with a difficult choice in selecting a textbook that would not overwhelm them with information yet would still stimulate their interest in the subject. Understandably it became increasingly difficult to hold the student responsible for a critical body of knowledge.

Textbooks prescribed for the core clerkships often do not have sufficient depth and sometimes do not possess key references or practical information. On the other hand, the classic texts of obstetrics and gynecology or gynecologic surgery are generally considered by students to be too expensive or too comprehensive for them to absorb during the clerkship. This book is a response to their dilemma. The chapters have all been written by members of the Obstetrics and Gynecology Faculty at the University of California, Los Angeles (UCLA) Medical Center and its affiliated hospitals—Harbor (LA County) General Hospital, Cedars-Sinai Medical Center, Martin Luther King, Jr. General Hospital, and Kern County Medical Center. Some authors have changed their institutional affiliations prior to the publication of the book. It is hoped that the book will serve the needs of the student, be useful during housestaff training, and be a helpful text in the medical practitioner's library. Fundamental principles and practice of obstetrics and gynecology are presented succinctly, but we have endeavored to cover all important aspects of the subject in sufficient detail to allow a reasonable understanding of the pathophysiology and a safe approach to clinical management.

The text is divided into five sections: an introductory section, obstetrics, reproductive endocrinology, gynecology, and gynecologic oncology. Special emphasis is given to family planning and important aspects of women's health. The basic operations of obstetrics and gynecology are included to allow a reasonable understanding of the technical procedures. Neville F. Hacker and J. George Moore have been responsible for the overall organization of the book. The most difficult tasks have been to maintain uniformity of style and to keep the text within 550 pages without sacrificing essential information. Calvin Hobel, John Marshall, J. George Moore, and Jonathan Berek have organized their particular sections. Neville F. Hacker has been largely responsible for the final editing of all sections.

This book would not have been possible without the special help of the following individuals, to whom we are most grateful: Gwynne Gloege, the very talented principal medical illustrator at UCLA, who was responsible for the overall uniformity and high quality of the illustrations; Yao-shi Fu, M.D., and Robert Nieberg, M.D., from the Department of Pathology, who provided illustrations and advice regarding gynecologic pathology; Normal Chang, who was responsible for the photography; and Linda Olt, who provided invaluable editorial assistance and also prepared the index. At W.B. Saunders, we are particularly grateful to Dana Dreibelbis, the Executive Editor who provided the initial inspiration and subsequent guidance for this project. Finally, this project would never have been completed without the untiring efforts, skill, and ever-cheerful countenance of Cheri Buonaguidi, the Obstetrics and Gynecology student coordinator at UCLA. She carefully read and accurately typed each version of the manuscript and worked with each of the contributors until all chapters were completed.

J. George Moore
Neville F. Hacker

Contents

PART ONE

Introduction

Joseph C. Gambone

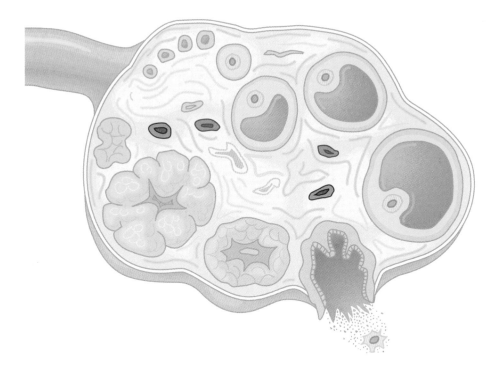

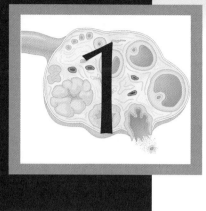

Practice Management and Ethics in Obstetrics and Gynecology

Joseph C. Gambone and Donald E. Marsden

PRACTICE MANAGEMENT

The practice of medicine, including obstetrics and gynecology, has become more complex and "business-like" in recent years. Changing methods of reimbursement for health services, prompted by escalating health care costs, have led to significant management challenges for obstetricians and gynecologists and other health care professionals. They must now understand and deal with a vast number of insurance plans, assisting their office staff and patients with claim forms and other paperwork. At the same time, employers and patients are asking for improvements in health care quality and evidence of value for their premium payments, with an increased emphasis on patient safety.

In most Western countries prior to the mid-1940s, medical services were reimbursed almost entirely on a self-pay, fee-for-service basis with little or no insurance coverage. Although costs were comparatively low, patients without funds were generally managed in municipal emergency rooms. The quality of care was highly variable and generally self-regulated.

In the United States, the concept of specialty board certification blossomed in the 1930s, but once a specialist was certified, only the American Medical Association (AMA), state medical boards, and/or hospital committees formally evaluated the quality of care provided, and then only in instances of repeated poor-quality care. Continuing medical education (CME) was poorly developed and in large part confined to hospital grand rounds and clinical and pathologic conferences (CPCs), which were usually sporadically attended. CME credits were not required for state medical license renewal.

Prior to World War II, health maintenance organizations (HMOs) were introduced, notably by Henry J. Kaiser. Medical care was jointly supported by the employer and employee on the basis of a capitated payment system (per member, per month) to the medical care provider. The provider (HMO) was not generally paid additional fees for needed services. Kaiser-Permanente survives today as one of the most successful prepaid health care systems.

During the ensuing years (late 1940s), federal wage and price controls limited salary negotiation in private industry and induced many employers to offer health benefits in order to attract employees. Much of the expense of these benefits was tax-free in the United States, and this tended to alter the relationship between the value of health services and their cost. Such economic trends allowed for guaranteed low cost fee-for-service medical care to those who were employed. Not all employers could provide health care insurance, however, and the self-employed often opted out of or could not afford reasonable coverage. Unfortunately, the indigent and the recently un-employed had no guaranteed medical care.

In the mid-1960s, federal health care programs were introduced in the United States in the form of Medicare (for those disabled or older than 65 years) and Medicaid (for the indigent). Medicare was linked to social security, and copayments were required for physician's outpatient care or office visits (part B) and hospital care (part A). A portion of the cost of Medicaid was assigned to the state. Obviously, this provided health care for the disabled, the elderly, and the indigent, but many were not indigent enough to qualify yet were unable to afford fee-for-service medical care or commercial health insurance. Hence, these persons fell, and continue to fall, through the medical "safety net."

The cost of Medicare, Medicaid, fee-for-service payments, and commercial health insurance has escalated enormously, due in part to newer, more expensive technology and the unrestricted use of clinical resources such as magnetic resonance imaging (MRI) or the routine use of unproven methods of fetal monitoring during labor. In 1965, when Medicare and Medicaid were initiated, it was estimated that the annual cost of these programs in 1990 would be $9 billion. The actual cost was closer to $75 billion.

At present, over 45 million beneficiaries are enrolled in Medicare, and this figure is projected to double by the year 2030. The annual per capita cost of health care has risen sixfold since 1970 (from $950 in 1970 to an estimated $5775 in 2003 in constant dollars). **The United States annually spends more on health care than on education and defense combined, and total health care expenditures (estimated at over $1.6 trillion in 2003) now exceed those for food. Government spending (Federal and State) amounts to nearly half (46%) of total expenditures at about $730 billion.**

During the 1990s, large employers in the United States organized negotiating groups such as the Pacific Business Group on Health in California for the purchase of health services. Their efforts were highly successful at controlling the rapid increase in health care premium costs for over 8 years. Using incentives, such as pharmacy benefits for their employees, they were able to shift large numbers of consumers into less costly "managed" health plans. The annual increase in premium costs to employers decreased dramatically from 1990 until 1998 (Table 1-1). Over time, however, a consumer and provider "backlash" against managed care led to the abandonment of this method as the primary means of cost containment for health services. Health care costs are now rising dramatically again (estimated at 6 times the rate of general inflation for 2003), and employers are now shifting a greater proportion of health care premium costs to their employees.

The cost of obstetric and gynecologic care has increased greatly during the 30 years from 1970 to 2000. Many possible causes have been identified and discussed. Three of the major causes identified are

Table 1-1. Health care premium increase (%) in the US from 1990 to 2001			
Year	%	Year	%
1990	17	1996	2
1991	18	1997	4
1992	12	1998	3.7
1993	10	1999	7.8
1994	6.5	2000	9.4
1995	−1	2001	10.2

(1) the rapid development of expensive technology that often improves outcomes only slightly but substantially increases cost, (2) the acknowledged over-utilization of new technology because of a lack of general agreement on the indications for its use, and (3) an extremely costly medical malpractice system, which has led to "defensive" practice and needless use of tests and procedures because of the fear of a lawsuit.

In some areas of the United States, obstetricians are paying over $100,000 annually for malpractice insurance. Efforts to bring about tort reform to reduce this expense and the large cost of defensive practice have thus far been unsuccessful. Obstetricians and gynecologists will need to become more involved in ensuring that medical malpractice insurance is reasonable and fair. They also will need to focus more efforts on improving care and reducing medical errors (see Chapter 5). **Society, with the help of involved practitioners, will need to decide who will be treated and how health care resources should be allocated in the future.**

THE ETHICAL PRACTICE OF OBSTETRICS AND GYNECOLOGY

Obstetrics and gynecology encompasses many high-profile areas of ethical concern such as in vitro fertilization (IVF) and other assisted reproductive technologies (ART), abortion, the use of aborted tissue for research or treatment, surrogacy, contraception for minors, and sterilization of the mentally retarded. Nevertheless, most ethical problems in the practice of medicine arise in cases in which the medical condition or desired procedure itself presents no moral problem. **In the past, the main areas of ethical concern have related to the competence and**

beneficence of the physician. Current areas of ethical concern should include the goals, values, ambitions, and preferences of the patient, as well as those of the community at large. Consideration of such issues enriches the study of obstetrics and gynecology by emphasizing that scientific knowledge and technical skills are most meaningful in a social and moral context.

WHAT IS ETHICS?

The term *ethics* is derived from a Greek word meaning "pertaining to custom or habit," and *morality* was the Latin equivalent. Now, morality often refers to concepts of right and wrong and ethics or moral philosophy to the systematic study of moral behavior. Obstetricians and gynecologists cannot be expected to be trained ethicists, and many institutions are setting up committees to help with the more difficult decisions, but as the President's Commission for the Study of Ethical Problems in Medicine has stated, "the primary responsibility for ensuring that morally justified decisions are made lies with the physician."

ETHICAL PRINCIPLES

During the day-to-day consideration of ethical dilemmas in health care, a number of principles or ideals and the concepts derived from them are commonly accepted and taken into account. Four such principles or ideals are **nonmaleficence, beneficence, autonomy, and justice;** these are generally accepted as the major ethical concepts that apply to health care.

Nonmaleficence

The principle of *primum non nocere* or "first, do no harm" originated from the Hippocratic school, and although few would dispute the basic concept, in day-to-day medical practice, physicians and their patients may need to accept the infliction of varying degrees of harm in order to achieve a desired outcome. Although the performance of radical hysterectomy and lymphadenectomy for invasive cervical cancer may be associated with significant morbidity and a small risk of mortality, all would consider that the risks and adverse consequences of the operation are more than outweighed by the potential benefits. Too stringent an application of the principle of nonmaleficence could prevent doctors from

offering treatments that may be in the patient's best interest, such as palliative surgery for the terminally ill. On the other hand, there is an ethical obligation to be certain that recommended medical treatment, surgery, or diagnostic testing is not likely to cause more harm than benefit.

Beneficence

An ancient belief held that all individuals have a duty to promote the welfare of others when in a position to do so. The duty of beneficence is an important part of the Hippocratic Oath, though most would see its strict application as an ideal rather than a duty. One could save many starving people in a Third World country by giving a large portion of one's income in aid, but few would consider it a moral duty to do so. On the other hand, when the concept of beneficence involves a specific patient encounter, the duty applies. A physician prevented by conscience from participating in an abortion, for example, would generally be expected to provide lifesaving care for a woman suffering complications after such a procedure.

Autonomy

The right of self-determination is a basic concept of biomedical ethics. **To exercise autonomy, an individual must be capable of effective deliberation and be neither coerced into a particular course of action nor limited in her or his choices by external constraints.** Being capable of effective deliberation implies a level of intellectual capacity and the ability to exercise that capacity.

There are a number of situations in which it may be reasonable to limit autonomy: (1) to prevent harm to others, (2) to prevent self-harm, (3) to prevent immoral acts, (4) to benefit others, and (5) to prevent offense to others. Most would accept limiting autonomy to prevent murder, rape, or theft, but to what extent it would be appropriate in order to avoid offending others is more difficult to determine.

The exercise of autonomy may put considerable stress and conflict on those providing health care, as in the case of a woman with a ruptured ectopic pregnancy who refuses a lifesaving blood transfusion for religious reasons and dies despite the best efforts of the medical team. More complex questions are raised by court-ordered cesarean deliveries for the benefit of the fetus.

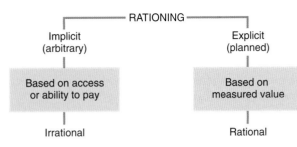

Figure 1-1. Representation of arbitrary rationing commonly based on access or ability to pay vs. planned clinical resource management based on measured value. *Explicit* rationing is objectionable to many despite the fact that *implicit* rationing still occurs.

Table 1-2. The PREPARED system: A checklist to assist patient and provider in the process of informed consent	
P rocedure	The course of action being considered
R eason	The indication or rationale
E xpectation	The chances of benefit and failure
P references	Patient-centered priorities (utilities) affecting choice
A lternatives	Other reasonable options
R isks	The potential for harm from procedures
E xpenses	All direct and indirect costs
D ecision	Fully informed collaborative choice

Reproduced with permission from Reiter RC, Lench JB, Gambone JC: Consumer advocacy, elective surgery, and the "Golden Era of Medicine." Obstet Gynecol 74:815, 1989.

Justice

Justice relates to the way in which the benefits and burdens of society are distributed. The general principle that equals should be treated equally was espoused by Aristotle and is widely accepted today, but it does require that one be able to define the relevant differences between individuals and groups. Some believe all rational persons to have equal rights; others emphasize need, effort, contribution, and merit; still others seek criteria that maximize both individual and social utility. **In most Western societies, race, sex, and religion are not considered morally legitimate criteria for the distribution of benefits, although they too may be taken into account to right what are perceived to be historic wrongs, in programs of affirmative action.** When resources are scarce, issues of justice become even more acute, as there are often competing claims from parties who appear equal by all relevant criteria, and the selection criteria themselves become a moral issue. Most modern societies find the *rational* rationing of health care resources to be appropriate and acceptable (Figure 1-1).

Informed Consent

The concept of informed consent may be derived from both respect for the principle of autonomy and from a desire to protect patients and research subjects from harm. **There is general agreement that consent must be genuinely voluntary and made after adequate disclosure of information.** As a minimum, when a patient consents to a procedure in health care, she should be informed about the expectation of benefit as well as the other reasonable alternatives and possible risks that are known. Table 1-2 provides a useful checklist (PREPARED) that expands on the minimum information to include the reason or rationale for the procedure, any appropriate patient preferences (e.g., avoiding surgery or a long course of medication), and the expenses involved in having the procedure.

Confidentiality

Confidentiality is a cornerstone of the relationship between doctor and patient. This duty arises from considerations of autonomy but also helps promote beneficence, as is the case with honesty. In obstetrics and gynecology, such conflicts can arise as in the case of a woman with a sexually transmitted disease who refuses to have a sexual partner informed, or a school-aged child seeking contraceptive advice or an abortion.

There are many other situations in which conflicting responsibilities make confidentiality a difficult issue. The Health Insurance Portability and Privacy Act (HIPPA) provides strict rules that physician practices and health care organizations must adhere to regarding the confidentiality and security of patient health care records. Some are concerned that these regulations could restrict the flow of information about patient care and may hinder efforts to improve overall performance.

Maternal-Fetal Relationships

Caring for a pregnant woman creates a unique relationship because the management of the mother inevitably affects her baby. Until recently, the only way by which an obstetrician could produce a healthy baby was by maintaining optimal maternal health, but as the fetus becomes more accessible to diagnostic and therapeutic interventions, new problems emerge. **Procedures performed on the fetus may violate the personal integrity and autonomy of the mother.** The obstetrician with a dual responsibility to mother and fetus faces a potential conflict of interest. **Most conflicts will be resolved due to the willingness of most women to undergo considerable self-sacrifice to benefit their fetus.** When a woman refuses consent for a procedure that presents her with significant risk, her autonomy will generally be respected. However, there may be cases in which an intervention that is likely to be efficacious carries little risk to the mother and can reasonably be expected to prevent substantial harm to the fetus. These have occasionally ended in a court-ordered intervention.

In surrogacy, where a woman voluntarily carries a fetus for others, a totally different relationship exists between the mother, her fetus, and third parties. The pregnant woman has no intention of keeping the child, and others have a strong vested interest in the "quality" of what may easily be seen as a "product." The mother may be under threat of liability for damages if the baby is harmed as a result of her actions, or she may be forced to behave in a way prescribed by contract. Legal questions aside, the ethical implications of these relationships are immense.

Relationships with Other Health Professionals

Health care is a multidisciplinary activity, and although the doctor has traditionally been the final arbiter and decision maker, this has often caused concern among other health care professionals. **Rejection of the "Nuremberg defense" of obedience to the orders of a superior and increasing recognition of professional rights have led to a situation in which all those involved in health care claim a right to participate in decision making.** Physicians have not been as aware of the sensitivities of the nursing profession and other allied health professionals as they should have been. For example, the decision, no matter how it is made, to either operate or not on a newborn with severe spina bifida inevitably leaves nurses with responsibilities to the infant, the parents, and the doctor that may be in direct conflict with their personal values. They may rightly request to be party to the decision-making process, and

although the exact models whereby such a goal may be achieved are debatable, physicians must be aware of the legitimate moral concerns of nurses and others involved.

Relationships with Other Parties

Health care takes place in an increasingly complex environment. Hospitals, health insurance companies, and governments all claim an interest in what services are made available or paid for, and this may prevent individual patients from receiving what their physician may consider optimal care. This poses moral problems not only for physicians on a case-by-case basis but also for insurance companies and society as a whole.

The interface of medicine and the law raises major ethical issues because legality and morality are not always synonymous. Professional liability insurance premiums for obstetricians are testimony to the relevance of legal issues to obstetric practice. Professional liability is affecting every major decision that is made by the practicing obstetrician and gynecologist, and under these conditions, the "tunnel vision" that ensues may obscure the ability to see clear answers to ethical questions.

CONCLUSIONS

The long-term future of obstetric and gynecologic practice is promising, but there are a number of challenges that lie ahead. Physicians and other health care professionals must ensure that all changes in practice management, prompted by the need to be efficient, also maintain or increase quality. They will need to demonstrate to patients and employers the value for the care that they deliver. Patient safety and the reduction of medical error should be stressed. Consumers will need to understand that optimal value may involve denial of ineffective or relatively ineffective but expensive procedures and treatments. Improving the quality of women's health care efficiently is particularly important.

All branches of medicine, but especially obstetrics and gynecology, will face an increasing number of ethical problems in the future. It is essential that practicing obstetricians and gynecologists prepare themselves to deal with these problems, partly because managing practices in an ethical manner transforms them from mere dispensers of health care to caring, responsive, and trustworthy physicians. Also, if health care providers do not respond to this challenge, other potentially less-qualified elements of society (e.g., legislators and special interest groups) will respond for them, to the possible detriment of both patients and physicians.

Suggested Reading

American College of Obstetricians and Gynecologists: Ethical decision making in obstetrics and gynecology. ACOG Technical Bulletin 136, Nov 1989.

American College of Obstetricians and Gynecologists: Ethical guidance for patient testing (ACOG Committee Opinion 159). Washington, DC, ACOG, 1995.

American College of Obstetricians and Gynecologists: Informed refusal (ACOG Committee Opinion 166). Washington, DC, ACOG, 1995.

American College of Obstetricians and Gynecologists: Patient choice: Maternal fetal conflict (ACOG Committee Opinion 55). Washington, DC, ACOG, 1987.

Institute of Medicine report: To err is human. Washington, DC, Institute of Medicine, 2000.

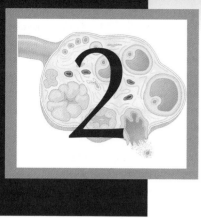

Clinical Approach to the Patient

Joseph C. Gambone and J. George Moore

As in most areas of medicine, a careful history and physical examination form the basis for patient evaluation and clinical management in obstetrics and gynecology. This chapter outlines the essential details of the clinical approach to, and evaluation of, the obstetric and gynecologic patient, as well as patients with special needs. Because many women, during their reproductive years in particular, are cared for exclusively by an obstetrician/gynecologist, this chapter concludes with general information about immunizations and current screening recommendations for both reproductive and general health preventive care.

OBSTETRIC AND GYNECOLOGIC EVALUATION

In few areas of medicine is it necessary to be more sensitive to the emotional and psychological needs of the patient than in obstetrics and gynecology. By their very nature, the history and physical examination may cause embarrassment to some patients. The members of the medical care team are individually and collectively responsible for ensuring that each patient's privacy and modesty are respected while providing the highest level of medical care. Box 2-1 lists the appropriate steps for the clinical approach to the patient.

While a casual and familiar approach may be acceptable to many younger patients, it may offend others and be quite inappropriate for many older patients. Different circumstances with the same patient may dictate different levels of formality. Entrance to the patient's room should be announced by a knock and spoken identification. A personal introduction with the stated reason for the visit should occur before any questions are asked or an examina-

tion is begun. The placement of the examination table should always be in a position that maximizes privacy for the patient as other health care professionals enter the room.

OBSTETRIC HISTORY

A complete history must be recorded at the time of the prepregnancy evaluation or at the initial antenatal visit. Several detailed standardized forms are available, but this should not negate the need for a detailed chronologic history taken personally by the physician who will be caring for the patient throughout her pregnancy. While taking the history, major opportunities will usually arise to provide counseling and explanations that serve to establish rapport and a supportive patient/physician encounter.

Box 2-1. Approach to the patient

The doctor should always:
- Knock before entering the patient's room.
- Identify himself/herself.
- Meet the patient initially when she is fully dressed, if possible.
- Address the patient courteously and respectfully.
- Respect the patient's privacy and modesty during the interview and examination.
- Ensure cleanliness, good grooming, and good manners in all patient encounters.
- Beware that a casual and familiar approach is not acceptable to all patients; it is generally best to avoid addressing an adult patient by her first name.
- Maintain the privacy of the patient's medical information and records.

PREVIOUS PREGNANCIES

Each prior pregnancy should be reviewed in chronologic order and the following information recorded:

1. **Date of delivery** (or pregnancy termination).
2. **Location of delivery** (or pregnancy termination).
3. **Duration of gestation** (recorded in weeks). When correlated with birth weight, this information allows an assessment of fetal growth patterns. The gestational age of any spontaneous abortion is of importance in any subsequent pregnancy.
4. **Type of delivery** (or method of terminating pregnancy). This information is important for planning the method of delivery in the present pregnancy. A difficult forceps delivery or a cesarean section may require a personal review of the labor and delivery records.
5. **Duration of labor** (recorded in hours). This may alert the physician to the possibility of an unusually long or short labor.
6. **Type of anesthesia.** Any complications of anesthesia should be noted.
7. **Maternal complications.** Urinary tract infections, vaginal bleeding, hypertension, and postpartum complications may be repetitive; such knowledge is helpful in anticipating and preventing problems with the present pregnancy.
8. **Newborn weight** (in grams or pounds and ounces). This information may give indications of gestational diabetes, fetal growth problems, shoulder dystocia, or cephalopelvic disproportion.
9. **Newborn gender.** This may provide insight into patient and family expectations and may indicate certain genetic risk factors.
10. **Fetal and neonatal complications.** Certain questions should be asked to elicit any problems and to determine the need to obtain further information. Inquiry should be made as to whether the baby had any problems after it was born, whether the baby breathed and cried right away, and whether the baby left the hospital with the mother.

MENSTRUAL HISTORY

A good menstrual history is essential because it is the determinant for establishing the expected date of confinement (EDC). A modification of **Nägele's rule** for establishing the EDC is to add 9 months and 7 days to the first day of the last normal menstrual period (LMP). For example:

LMP: July 20, 2002
EDC: April 27, 2003

This calculation depends on a normal 28-day cycle, and adjustments must be made for longer or shorter cycles. Any bleeding or spotting since the last normal menstrual period should be reviewed in detail and taken into account when calculating an EDC. The PDA contains a calculator based upon Nägele's rule for estimating obstetric due dates.

CONTRACEPTIVE HISTORY

This information is important for risk assessment. Oral contraceptives taken during early pregnancy have been associated with birth defects, and retained intrauterine devices (IUDs) can cause early pregnancy loss, infection, and premature delivery.

MEDICAL HISTORY

The importance of a good medical history cannot be overemphasized. In addition to common disorders, such as diabetes mellitus, hypertension, and renal disease, which are known to affect pregnancy outcome, all serious medical conditions should be recorded.

SURGICAL HISTORY

Each surgical procedure should be recorded chronologically, including date, hospital, surgeon, and complications. Trauma must also be listed (e.g., a fractured pelvis may result in diminished pelvic capacity).

SOCIAL HISTORY

Habits such as smoking, alcohol use, and drug abuse are important factors that must be recorded and managed appropriately. The patient's contact or exposure to domesticated animals, particularly cats (which carry a risk of toxoplasmosis), is important.

The patient's type of work and lifestyle may affect the pregnancy. Exposure to solvents (carbon tetrachloride) or insulators (polychlorobromine compounds) in the workplace may lead to teratogenesis or hepatic toxicity.

OBSTETRIC PHYSICAL EXAMINATION
GENERAL PHYSICAL EXAMINATION

This procedure must be systematic and thorough and performed as early as possible in the prenatal period. A complete physical examination provides an opportunity to detect previously unrecognized abnormalities. Normal baseline levels must also be established, particularly those of weight, blood pressure, funduscopic (retina) appearance, and cardiac status.

PELVIC EXAMINATION

The initial pelvic examination should be done early in the prenatal period and should include the following: (1) inspection of the external genitalia, vagina, and cervix; (2) collection of cytologic specimens from the ectocervix and superficial endocervical canal; and (3) palpation of the cervix, uterus, and adnexa. The initial estimate of gestational age by uterine size becomes less accurate as pregnancy progresses. Rectal and rectovaginal examinations are also important aspects of this initial pelvic evaluation.

CLINICAL PELVIMETRY

This assessment is carried out following the bimanual pelvic examination and before the rectal examination. It is important that clinical pelvimetry be carried out systematically. The details of clinical pelvimetry are described in Chapter 9.

DIAGNOSIS OF PREGNANCY

The diagnosis of pregnancy and its location, based on physical signs and examination alone, may be quite challenging during the early weeks of amenorrhea. Urine pregnancy tests in the office are reliable a few days after the first missed period, and office ultrasonography is used increasingly as a routine.

SYMPTOMS OF PREGNANCY

The most common symptoms in the early months of pregnancy are amenorrhea, urinary frequency, breast engorgement, nausea, tiredness, and easy fatigability. Amenorrhea in a previously normally menstruating, sexually active woman should be considered to be caused by pregnancy until proven otherwise. Urinary frequency is most likely caused by the pressure of the enlarged uterus on the bladder.

SIGNS OF PREGNANCY

The signs of pregnancy may be divided into presumptive, probable, and positive.

Presumptive Signs. The presumptive signs are primarily those associated with skin and mucous membrane changes. Discoloration and cyanosis of the vulva, vagina, and cervix are related to the generalized engorgement of the pelvic organs and are, therefore, nonspecific. The dark discoloration of the vulva and vaginal walls is known as **Chadwick's sign.** Pigmentation of the skin and abdominal striae are nonspecific and unreliable signs. The most common sites for pigmentation are the midline of the lower abdomen (linea nigra), over the bridge of the nose, and under the eyes. The latter is called chloasma or the mask of pregnancy. Chloasma is also an occasional side effect of oral contraceptives.

Probable Signs. The probable signs of pregnancy are those mainly related to the detectable physical changes in the uterus. During early pregnancy, the uterus changes in size, shape, and consistency. Early uterine enlargement tends to be in the anteroposterior diameter so that the uterus becomes globular. In addition, because of asymmetric implantation of the ovum, one cornua of the uterus may enlarge slightly (**Piskaçek's sign**). Uterine consistency becomes softer, and it may be possible to palpate or to compress the connection between the cervix and fundus. This change is referred to as **Hegar's sign.** The cervix also begins to soften early in pregnancy.

Positive Signs. The positive signs of pregnancy include the detection of a fetal heartbeat and the recognition of fetal movements. Modern Doppler techniques for detecting the fetal heartbeat may be successful as early as 9 weeks and are nearly always positive by 12 weeks. Fetal heart tones can usually be detected with a stethoscope between 16 and 20 weeks. The multiparous woman generally recognizes fetal movements between 15 and 17 weeks, whereas the primigravida usually does not recognize fetal movements until 18 to 20 weeks.

LABORATORY TESTS FOR PREGNANCY

Pregnancy Tests. Tests to detect pregnancy have revolutionized early diagnosis. Although they are considered a probable sign of pregnancy, the accuracy of these tests is good. All commonly used methods depend on the detection of human chorionic gonadotropin (hCG) or its β subunit. Depending on the specific sensitivity of the test, pregnancy may be suspected even prior to a missed period.

Diagnostic Ultrasonography. The imaging technique of ultrasonography has made a significant contribution to the diagnosis and evaluation of pregnancy. Using real-time ultrasonography, an intrauterine gestational sac can be identified at 5 menstrual weeks (21st postovulatory day) and a fetal image can be detected by 6 to 7 weeks. A beating heart is noted at 8 weeks. Radiographic imaging, usually avoided in early pregnancy, depends on detection of the fetal skeleton, which is usually not seen until 16 weeks.

GYNECOLOGIC HISTORY

A full history is equally as important in evaluating the gynecologic patient as in evaluating a patient in general medicine or surgery. The history-taking must be systematic to avoid omissions, and it should be conducted with sensitivity and without haste.

PRESENT ILLNESS

The patient is asked to state her main complaint and to relate her present illness, sequentially, in her own words. Pertinent negative information should be recorded, and, as much as possible, questions should be reserved until after the patient has described the course of her illness. Generally, the history provides substantial clues to the diagnosis, so it is important to evaluate fully the more common symptoms encountered in gynecologic patients.

Abnormal Vaginal Bleeding. Vaginal bleeding before the age of 9 years and after the age of 52 years is cause for concern and requires investigation. These are the limits of normal menstruation, and although the occasional woman may menstruate regularly and normally up to the age of 57 or 58 years, it is important to ensure that she is not bleeding from uterine cancer or from exogenous estrogens. Prolongation of menses beyond 7 days or bleeding between menses, except for a brief *kleine regnen* at ovulation, may connote abnormal ovarian function, uterine myomata, or endometriosis.

Abdominal Pain. Many gynecologic problems are associated with abdominal pain. The common gyne-cologic causes of acute lower abdominal pain are salpingo-oophoritis with peritoneal inflammation, torsion and infarction of an ovarian cyst, endometriosis, or rupture of an ectopic pregnancy. Patterns of pain radiation should be recorded and may provide an important diagnostic clue. Chronic lower abdominal pain is generally associated with endometriosis, chronic pelvic inflammatory disease, or large pelvic tumors.

Amenorrhea. The most common causes of amenorrhea are pregnancy and the normal menopause. It is abnormal for a young woman to reach the age of 16 without menstruating (primary amenorrhea). Pregnancy should be suspected in a woman between 15 and 45 years of age who fails to menstruate within 35 days from the first day of her last menstruation. In a patient with amenorrhea who is not pregnant, inquiry should be made about menopausal or climacteric symptoms such as hot flashes, vaginal dryness, or mild depression.

Other Symptoms. Other pertinent symptoms of concern include dysmenorrhea, premenstrual tension, fluid retention, leukorrhea, constipation, dyschezia, dyspareunia, and abdominal distention. Lower back and sacral pain may indicate uterine prolapse, enterocele, or rectocele.

MENSTRUAL HISTORY

The menstrual history should include the age at menarche (average is 12 to 13 years), interval between periods (21 to 35 days with a median of 28 days), duration of menses (average is 5 days), and character of the flow (scant, normal, heavy, usually without clots). Any intermenstrual bleeding (metrorrhagia) should be noted. The date of onset of the LMP and the date of the previous menstrual period should be recorded. Inquiry should be made regarding menstrual cramps (dysmenorrhea); if present, the age at onset, severity, and character of the cramps should be recorded, together with an estimate of the disability incurred. Midcycle pain (*mittelschmerz*) and a midcycle increase in vaginal secretions are indicative of ovulatory cycles.

CONTRACEPTIVE HISTORY

The type and duration of each contraceptive method must be recorded, along with any attendant complications. These may include amenorrhea or thromboembolic disease with oral contraceptives; dysmenorrhea, heavy bleeding (menorrhagia), or pelvic infection with the intrauterine device; or contraceptive failure with the diaphragm, contraceptive sponge, or contraceptive cream.

OBSTETRIC HISTORY

Each pregnancy, delivery, and any associated complications are listed sequentially with relevant dates.

SEXUAL HISTORY

The health of, and current relationship with, the husband or partner(s) may provide insight into the present complaints. Inquiry should be made regarding any pain (dyspareunia), bleeding, or dysuria associated with sexual intercourse. Sexual satisfaction should be discussed tactfully.

PAST HISTORY

As in the obstetric history, any significant past medical or surgical history should be recorded, as should the patient's family history. A list of current medications is important.

SYSTEMIC REVIEW

A review of all other organ systems should be undertaken. Habits (tobacco, alcohol, drug abuse), medications, usual weight with recent changes, and loss of height (osteoporosis) are important parts of the systemic review.

GYNECOLOGIC PHYSICAL EXAMINATION
GENERAL PHYSICAL EXAMINATION

A complete physical examination should be performed on each new patient and repeated at least annually. The initial examination should include the patient's height, weight, and arm span (in adolescent patients or those with endocrine problems) and should be carried out with the patient completely disrobed but suitably draped. The examination should be systematic and should include the following points.

Vital Signs. Temperature, pulse rate, respiratory rate, and blood pressure should be recorded.

General Appearance. The patient's body build, posture, state of nutrition, demeanor, and state of well-being should be recorded.

Head and Neck. Evidence of supraclavicular lymphadenopathy, oral lesions, webbing of the neck, or goiter may be pertinent to the gynecologic assessment.

Breasts. The breast examination is particularly important in gynecologic patients (see Chapters 30 and 32).

Heart and Lungs. Examination of the heart and lungs is of importance, particularly in a patient who requires surgery. The presence of a pleural effusion may be indicative of a disseminated malignancy, particularly ovarian cancer.

Abdomen. Examination of the abdomen is critical in the evaluation of the gynecologic patient. The contour, whether flat, scaphoid, or protuberant, should be noted. The latter appearance may suggest ascites. The presence and distribution of hair, especially in the area of the escutcheon, should be recorded, as should the presence of striae or operative scars.

Abdominal tenderness must be determined by placing one hand flat against the abdomen in the non-painful areas initially, then gently and gradually exerting pressure with the fingers of the other hand (Figure 2-1). Rebound tenderness (a sign of peritoneal irritation), muscle guarding, and abdominal rigidity should be gently elicited, again first in the nontender areas. A

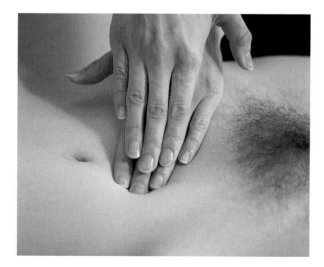

Figure 2-1. The abdomen is palpated by placing the left palm flat against the abdominal wall and then gently exerting pressure with the fingers of the right hand.

"doughy" abdomen, in which the guarding increases gradually as the pressure of palpation is increased, is often seen with a hemoperitoneum.

It is important to palpate any abdominal mass. The size should be specifically noted. Other characteristics may be even more important, however, in suggesting the diagnosis, such as whether the mass is cystic or solid, smooth or nodular, fixed or mobile, and whether it is associated with ascites. In determining the reason for abdominal distention (tumor, ascites, or distended bowel), it is important to percuss carefully the areas of tympany (gaseous distention) and dullness. A large tumor is generally dull on top with loops of bowel displaced to the flanks. Dullness that shifts as the patient turns onto her side (shifting dullness) is suggestive of ascites.

Back. Abnormal curvature of the vertebral column (dorsal kyphosis or scoliosis) is an important observation in evaluating osteoporosis in a postmenopausal woman. Costovertebral angle tenderness suggests pyelonephritis, whereas psoas muscle spasm may occur with gynecologic infections or acute appendicitis.

Extremities. The presence or absence of varicosities, edema, pedal pulsations, and cutaneous lesions may suggest pathologic conditions within the pelvis. The height of pitting edema should be noted (e.g., ankle, shin, to the knee or above).

PELVIC EXAMINATION

The pelvic examination must be conducted systematically and with careful sensitivity. The procedure should be performed with smooth and gentle movements and accompanied by reasonable explanations.

Vulva. The character and distribution of hair, the degree of development or atrophy of the labia, and the character of the hymen (imperforate or cribriform) and introitus (virginal, nulliparous, or multiparous) should be noted. Any clitorimegaly should be noted, as should the presence of cysts, tumors, or inflammation of **Bartholin's gland**. The urethra and **Skene's glands** should be inspected for any purulent exudates. The labia should be inspected for any inflammatory, dystrophic, or neoplastic lesions. Perineal relaxation and scarring should be noted because they may cause dyspareunia and defects in rectal sphincter tone. The urethra should be "milked" for any inflammatory

exudates, which if found should be cultured for pathologic organisms.

Speculum Examination. The vagina and cervix should be inspected with an appropriately sized bivalve speculum (Figure 2-2), which should be warmed and lubricated with warm water only, so as not to interfere with the examination of cervical cytology or any vaginal exudate. After gently spreading the labia to expose the introitus, the speculum should be inserted with the blades entering the introitus transversely, then directed posteriorly in the axis of the vagina with pressure exerted against the relatively insensitive perineum to avoid contacting the sensitive urethra. As the anterior blade reaches the cervix, the speculum is opened to bring the cervix into view. As the vaginal epithelium is inspected, it is important to rotate the speculum through 90 degrees, so that lesions on the anterior or posterior walls of the vagina ordinarily covered by the blades of the speculum are not over-

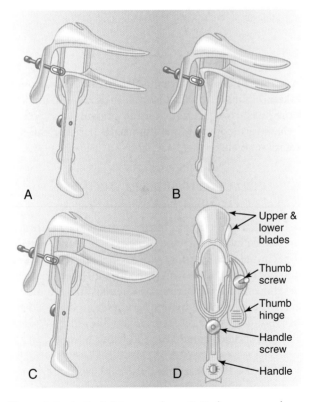

Figure 2-2. *A,* Pediatric speculum. *B,* Pederson speculum. *C,* Graves speculum. The Pederson speculum has narrower blades and is more appropriate for examining a nulliparous patient. *D,* Parts of a speculum.

looked. Vaginal wall relaxation should be evaluated using either a Sims' speculum or the posterior blade of a bivalve speculum. The patient is asked to bear down (Valsalva's maneuver) or to cough to demonstrate any stress incontinence. If the patient's complaint involves urinary stress or urgency, this portion of the examination should be carried out before the bladder is emptied.

The cervix should be inspected to determine its size, shape, and color. The nulliparous patient generally has a conical, unscarred cervix with a circular, centrally placed os; the multiparous cervix is generally bulbous and the os has a transverse configuration (Figure 2-3). Any purulent cervical discharge should be cultured. Plugged, distended cervical glands (nabothian follicles) may be seen on the ectocervix. In premenopausal women, the squamocolumnar junction of the cervix is usually visible around the cervical os, particularly in patients of low parity. Postmenopausally, the junction is invariably retracted within the endocervical canal. A cervical cytologic smear (Papanicolaou, or Pap, smear) should be taken before the speculum is withdrawn. The exocervix is gently scraped with a wooden spatulum, and the endocervical tissue gently sampled with a cytobrush.

Bimanual Examination. The bimanual pelvic examination provides information about the uterus and adnexa (fallopian tubes and ovaries). During this portion of the examination, the urinary bladder should be empty; if it is not, the internal genitalia will be difficult to delineate, and the procedure is more apt to be uncomfortable for the patient. The labia are separated, and the gloved, lubricated index finger is inserted into the vagina, avoiding the sensitive urethral meatus. Pressure is exerted posteriorly against the perineum and puborectalis muscle, which causes the introitus to gape somewhat, thereby usually allowing the middle finger to be inserted as well. Intromission of the two fingers into the depth of the vagina may be facilitated by having the patient bear down slightly.

The cervix is palpated for consistency, contour, size, and tenderness to motion. **If the vaginal fornices are absent, as may occur in postmenopausal women, it is not possible to appreciate the size of the cervix on bimanual examination. This can be determined only on rectovaginal or rectal examination.**

The uterus is evaluated by placing the abdominal hand flat on the abdomen with the fingers pressing gently just above the symphysis pubis. With the vaginal fingers supinated in either the anterior or the posterior vaginal fornix, the uterine corpus is pressed gently against the abdominal hand (Figure 2-4). As the uterus is felt between the examining fingers of both hands, the size, configuration, consistency, and mobility of the organ are appreciated. If the muscles of the abdominal wall are not compliant or if the uterus is retroverted, the outline, consistency, and mobility must be determined by ballottement with the vaginal fingers in the fornices; in these circumstances, however, it is impossible to discern uterine size accurately.

By shifting the abdominal hand to either side of the midline and gently elevating the lateral fornix up to the abdominal hand, it may be possible to outline a right adnexal mass (Figure 2-5). The left adnexa are best appreciated with the fingers of the left hand in the vagina (Figure 2-6). The examiner should stand sideways, facing the patient's left, with the left hip maintaining pressure against the left elbow, thereby providing better tactile sensation because of the relaxed musculature in the forearm and examining hand. The **pouch of Douglas** is also carefully assessed for nodularity or tenderness, as may occur with endometriosis, pelvic inflammatory disease, or metastatic carcinoma.

It is usually impossible to feel the normal tube, and conditions must be optimal to appreciate the normal ovary. The ovary has the size and consistency of a shelled oyster and may be felt with the vaginal fingers as they are passed across the undersurface of the abdominal hand. The ovaries are very tender to compression, and the patient is uncomfortably aware

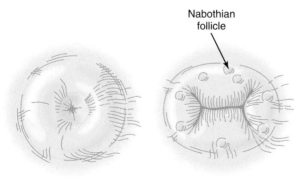

Nabothian
follicle

A   NULLIPAROUS   B   MULTIPAROUS

Figure 2-3. Cervix of a nulliparous patient *(A)* and a multiparous patient *(B)*. Note the circular os in the nulliparous cervix and the transverse os, owing to lacerations at childbirth, in the multiparous cervix.

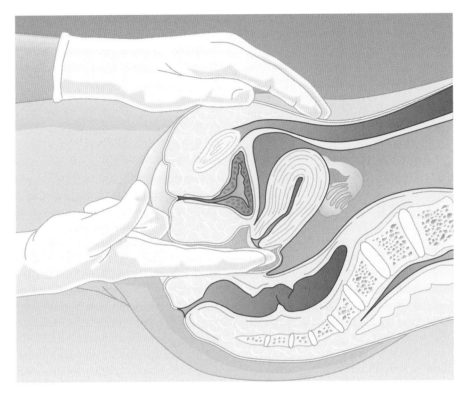

Figure 2-4. Bimanual evaluation of the uterus by exerting gentle pressure on the uterus with the vaginal fingers against the abdominal hand.

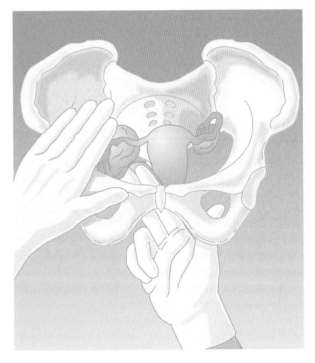

Figure 2-5. Bimanual examination of the right adnexa. Note that fingers of the right hand are in the vagina.

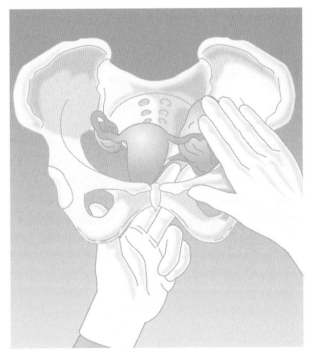

Figure 2-6. Bimanual examination of the left adnexa. Note that fingers of the left hand are in the vagina.

of any ovarian compression or movement during the examination.

It may be impossible to differentiate between an ovarian or tubal mass or even a lateral uterine mass. Generally, left adnexal masses are more difficult to evaluate than those on the right because of the position of the sigmoid colon on the left side of the pelvis. An ultrasonic examination should be helpful for delineating these features.

RECTAL EXAMINATION

The anus should be inspected for lesions, hemorrhoids, or inflammation. Rectal sphincter tone should be recorded and any mucosal lesions noted. A guaiac test should be performed to determine the presence of occult blood.

A rectovaginal examination is helpful in evaluating masses in the cul-de-sac, the rectovaginal septum, or adnexa. It is essential in evaluating the parametrium in patients with cervical cancer. Rectal examination may also be essential in differentiating between a rectocele and an enterocele (Figure 2-7).

LABORATORY EVALUATION

Appropriate laboratory tests normally include a urinalysis, complete blood count, erythrocyte sedimentation rate, and blood chemistry analyses. Special tests, such as tumor marker and hormone assays, are performed when indicated.

ASSESSMENT

A reasonable differential diagnosis should be possible with the information gleaned from the history, physi-

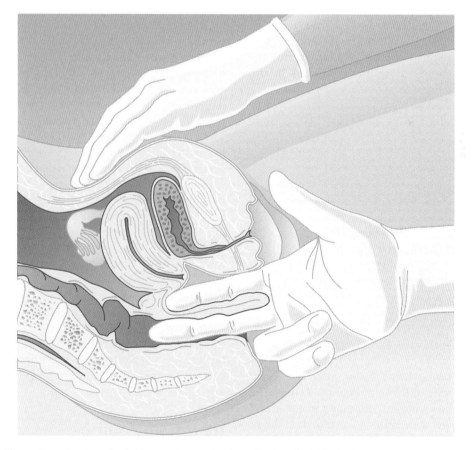

Figure 2-7. Rectovaginal bimanual examination. During the Valsalva's maneuver, an enterocele will separate the two fingers.

cal examination, and laboratory tests. The plan of management should aim toward a chemical or histologic confirmation of the presumptive diagnosis, and the appropriate therapeutic options, along with the rationale for each option, should be recorded.

PATIENTS WITH SPECIAL NEEDS
THE PEDIATRIC AND ADOLESCENT PATIENT

Girls experience fewer gynecologic problems than do adult women, but their concerns need to be met effectively and skillfully in a way that will allay anxiety and create a positive attitude toward their gynecologic health. Unique complaints fall generally into a handful of categories: congenital anomalies, genital injuries, inflammation of the unestrogenized genital tract, pubertal problems, and psychosexual concerns. Genital ambiguity, trauma and vaginal bleeding in the prepubertal child are covered briefly in this chapter.

GENITAL AMBIGUITY

Dealing with genital ambiguity in the newborn requires a coordinated and timely response. **The family's psychological well-being must be addressed because they must feel confident in the gender identity of their child.** Ambiguity can result from masculinization of a female child due to exogenous hormone ingestion or maternal or fetal overproduction of androgen. It may also result from incomplete virilization of a male infant, hormonal insensitivity, gonadal dysgenesis, or chromosomal anomalies (see Chapters 32 and 33). **In assessing an infant with ambiguous genitals, fluid and electrolyte balance should be monitored and blood drawn for 17-hydroxyprogesterone and cortisol to rule out 21-hydroxylase deficiency.** Life-threatening illness may be missed in children with the salt-losing form of congenital adrenal hyperplasia.

TRAUMA

Straddle injuries are the most common cause of trauma to the genitalia of a young girl, and the injuries have a seasonal peak when bicycles come out in the spring. The majority of these injuries are to the labia. Penetrating vaginal injuries can cause major intra-abdominal damage with minimal external findings. **Sexual assault must always be considered.** After a life-threatening condition is ruled out, an ice pack, chilled bag of intravenous solution, or cool compress may be applied to the injured area and the child

allowed to rest quietly for 20 minutes before being assessed further. Extensive injuries usually require examination under anesthesia and surgical repair.

In any case of trauma, concurrent damage to the rectum or urinary tract should be considered. **If there is any reason to suspect sexual or physical abuse, the child protection authorities must be notified, and the examination should include the collection of medicolegal evidence.**

VAGINAL BLEEDING IN THE PREPUBERTAL CHILD

Vaginal bleeding is a frequent and distressing complaint in childhood. Although it will most often be of benign etiology, more serious pathology must always be ruled out. Vaginal bleeding in the newborn is most often physiologic as a result of maternal estrogen withdrawal. In such cases, there should be supportive evidence of a hormonal effect, such as the presence of breast tissue and pale, engorged vaginal epithelium. Bleeding disorders are uncommon in this age group but should be considered. Vitamin K is routinely given to the newborn, but some patients refuse the medication.

Precocious puberty (see Chapter 32) may present with vaginal bleeding, although most commonly other evidence of maturation will have preceded the bleeding and will be evident on examination. At the very least, a pale, estrogenized vaginal epithelium will be seen, and cytology from the vagina will confirm the hormonal effect. Transient precocious puberty may occur in response to a **functional ovarian cyst,** and vaginal bleeding may be triggered by the spontaneous resolution of the cyst. **Exogenous hormonal exposure** should be considered, because children have been known to ingest birth control pills. **Ovarian tumors** resulting in pseudoprecocious puberty should be ruled out.

Vulvovaginitis is common but is a diagnosis of exclusion. When bleeding is present, it is necessary to assess the vagina and to rule out a foreign body or vaginal tumor.

Vaginal tumors are the most serious possibility to be considered. **Sarcoma botryoides** classically presents with vaginal bleeding and grape-like vesicles. Fortunately, this is a rare tumor.

THE GERIATRIC PATIENT

The gynecologic assessment of the elderly woman may present a special challenge. Many older patients tend to underreport their symptoms, possibly because of a

Table 2-1. Recommended preventive health screening for women

Intervention/Procedure	Risk
Pap smear annually from age 18 or sexual activity; after 3 consecutive normal smears, every 2 to 3 years in low-risk women until age 70	Cervical dysplasia/cancer
Mammography every other year from age 40 and then annually age 50 to 70	Breast cancer
Smoking cessation counseling, warning second-hand smoke exposure	Lung cancer, heart disease, other health risks associated with smoking
Regular blood pressure screening (every 2 years)	Hypertension and stroke
Cholesterol/lipid profile every 5 years until age 65	Heart disease
Total skin inspection and selective biopsies	Skin cancer (sun exposure)
Diet and exercise counseling	Osteoporosis, fracture, and deformity
Blood sugar study with family history, obesity, or history of gestational diabetes	Diabetes mellitus; other comorbidities associated with obesity
Sigmoidoscopy or colonoscopy every 3 to 5 years after age 50	Colorectal cancer
Cervical sampling for *chlamydia*, *N. gonorrhoeae*, syphilis, and HIV based on history	Sexually transmitted infections
PPD of tuberculin for high-risk women	Tuberculosis

Pap, Papanicolaou test; HIV, human immunodeficiency virus; PPD, purified protein derivative

belief that any new physical problems are due to the normal aging process. Also, a fear of loss of their independence may contribute to this denial and this may lead to a delay of diagnosis and perhaps a worse prognosis. In addition to the routine gynecologic history and physical examination, these patients should be evaluated for any sensory impairments, such as visual or hearing loss, any impaired mobility, malnutrition, urinary incontinence, or confusion, which may be due to polypharmacy. Appropriate referral, when improvement can be reasonably expected, should be considered for these problems once identified.

Gynecologic conditions such as atrophic vaginitis, uterine and vaginal prolapse, and genital tract malignancies are among the more common problems encountered in the geriatric patient.

PATIENTS WITH DISABILITIES

Women with developmental or acquired disabilities should receive the same high quality obstetric and gynecologic care as anyone else, with a goal of sustaining their best level of functioning. Assisting families of mentally or physically disabled individuals with obstetric or gynecologic problems or attending for them in special institutions can be quite challenging. The woman with a disability is a person with special and unique needs, and communicating to her a sense of caring and respect is paramount.

IMMUNIZATIONS AND PREVENTIVE HEALTH SCREENING

Because public health recommendations for immunizations may change, it is best to check a reliable source periodically (e.g., www.cdc.gov) for the latest information before counseling patients. General recommendations include: a **rubella titer** obtained on all women of childbearing age in the absence of proof of immunity and then **measles, mumps and rubella (MMR)** vaccine should be given to nonpregnant women who are not immune; **influenza vaccine** annually for all women older than age 64 and women aged 19 to 64 who are health care workers or who have chronic illnesses such as heart disease or diabetes mellitus; **tetanus-diphtheria booster** between ages 14 and 16; **hepatitis B vaccine** for women who are intravenous drug users or have other high-risk behaviors such as exposure to blood products or recent multiple sexual partners; and **pneumococcal vaccine** every 10 years from ages 19 to 64 for women with chronic illnesses, alcoholism, or who are immunosuppressed.

Table 2-1 contains recommended preventive health screening procedures for women.

Suggested Reading

Cope Z: The Early Diagnosis of the Acute Abdomen. London, Oxford Medical Publications, 2001.

Lewis MA, Mickman JL: Approach to the patient with developmental disabilities. *In* Pregler JP, DeCherney AH (eds): Women's Health: Principles and Clinical Practice. Hamilton, Ontario, B.C. Decker, 2002.

Pham T: Approach to the geriatric patient. *In* Pregler JP, DeCherney AH (eds): Women's Health: Principles and Clinical Practice. Hamilton, Ontario, B.C. Decker, 2002.

Wilkes MS, Anderson M: Approach to the adolescent patent. *In* Pregler JP, DeCherney AH (eds): Women's Health: Principles and Clinical Practice. Hamilton, Ontario, B.C. Decker, 2002.

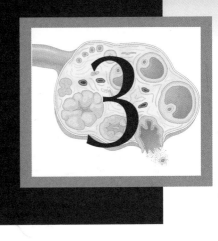

3

Female Reproductive Anatomy and Embryology

Joseph C. Gambone and J. George Moore

The scope of obstetrics and gynecology assumes a reasonable background in reproductive anatomy, embryology, physiology (see Chapter 4), and endocrinology (see Chapter 6 and Part Four). A physician cannot effectively practice obstetrics and gynecology without understanding the physiologic processes that transpire in a woman's life as she passes through infancy, adolescence, reproductive maturity, and the climacteric. As the various clinical problems are addressed, it is important to consider those anatomic, developmental, and physiologic changes that normally take place at key points in a woman's life cycle.

Most of this text deals with the disruptive deviations from normal female anatomy and physiology, whether they be congenital, functional, traumatic, inflammatory, neoplastic, or even iatrogenic. As the etiology and pathogenesis of clinical problems are considered, each should be studied in the context of normal anatomy, development, and physiology.

DEVELOPMENT OF THE EXTERNAL GENITALIA

Prior to the 7th week of development, the appearance of the external genital area is the same in males and females. Elongation of the genital tubercle into a phallus with a clearly defined terminal glans portion is noted in the 7th week, and gross inspection at this time may lead to faulty sexual identification. Ventrally and caudally, the urogenital membrane, made up of both endodermal and ectodermal cells, further differentiates into the genital folds laterally and the urogenital folds medially. **The lateral genital folds develop into the labia majora, whereas the urogenital folds develop**

subsequently into the labia minora and prepuce of the clitoris.

The external genitalia of the fetus are readily distinguishable as female at approximately 12 weeks (Figure 3-1). In the male, the urethral ostium is located conspicuously on the elongated phallus by this time and is smaller, owing to urogenital fold fusion dorsally, which produces a prominent raphe from the anus to the urethral ostium. In the female, the hymen is usually perforated by the time delivery occurs.

ANATOMY OF THE EXTERNAL GENITALIA

The perineum represents the inferior boundary of the pelvis. It is bounded superiorly by the levator ani muscles and inferiorly by the skin between the thighs (Figure 3-2). Anteriorly, the perineum extends to the symphysis pubis and the inferior borders of the pubic bones. Posteriorly, it is limited by the ischial tuberosities, the sacrotuberous ligaments, and the coccyx. **The superficial and deep transverse perineal muscles cross the pelvic outlet between the two ischial tuberosities and come together at the perineal body. They divide the space into the urogenital triangle anteriorly and the anal triangle posteriorly.**

The urogenital diaphragm is a fibromuscular sheet that stretches across the pubic arch. It is pierced by the vagina, the urethra, the artery of the bulb, the internal pudendal vessels, and the dorsal nerve of the clitoris. Its inferior surface is covered by the crura of the clitoris, the vestibular bulbs, the greater vestibular (Bartholin's) glands, and the superficial perineal muscles. Bartholin's glands are situated just posterior

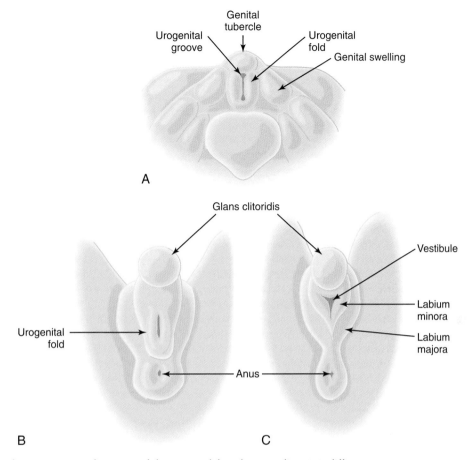

Figure 3-1. Development of the external female genitalia. *A,* Indifferent stage (approximately 7 weeks). *B,* Approximately 10 weeks. *C,* Approximately 12 weeks.

to the vestibular bulbs, and their ducts empty into the introitus just below the labia minora. They are often the site of gonococcal infections and painful abscesses.

VULVA

The external genitalia are referred to collectively as the vulva. As shown in Figure 3-3, **the vulva includes the mons veneris, labia majora, labia minora, clitoris, vulvovaginal (Bartholin's) glands, fourchette, and perineum.** The most prominent features of the vulva, the labia majora, are large, hair-covered folds of skin that contain sebaceous glands and subcutaneous fat and lie on either side of the introitus. The labia minora lie medially and contain no hair but have a rich supply of venous sinuses, sebaceous glands, and nerves. The labia minora may vary from scarcely noticeable structures to leaf-like flaps measuring up to 3 cm in length. Anteriorly, each splits into two folds. The posterior pair of folds attach to the inferior surface of the clitoris, at which point they unite to form the frenulum of the clitoris. The anterior pair are united in a hoodlike configuration over the clitoris, forming the prepuce. Posteriorly, the labia minora may extend almost to the fourchette.

The clitoris lies just in front of the urethra and consists of the glans, the body, and the crura. Only the glans clitoridis is visible externally. The body, composed of a pair of corpora cavernosa, extends superiorly for a distance of several centimeters and divides into two crura, which are attached to the undersurface of either pubic ramus. Each crus is covered by the corresponding ischiocavernosus muscle. Each vestibular bulb (equivalent to the corpus spongiosum of the penis) extends posteriorly from the glans on either side of the lower vagina. Each bulb is

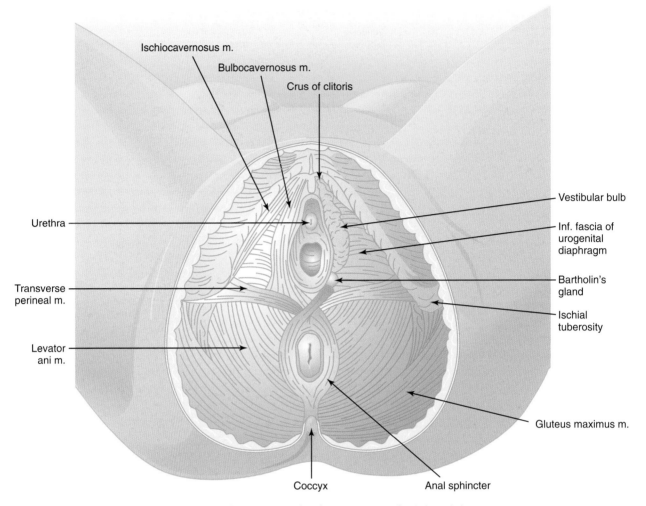

Figure 3-2. The perineum, showing superficial structures on the left and deeper structures on the right.

attached to the inferior surface of the perineal membrane and covered by the bulbocavernosus muscle. These muscles aid in constricting the venous supply to the erectile vestibular bulbs and also act as the sphincter vaginae.

As the labia minora are spread, the vaginal introitus, guarded by the hymenal ring, is seen. Usually, the hymen is represented only by a circle of carunculae myrtiformes around the vaginal introitus. The hymen may take many forms, however, such as a cribriform plate with many small openings or a completely imperforate diaphragm.

The vestibule of the vagina is that portion of the introitus extending inferiorly from the hymenal ring between the labia minora. The fourchette represents the posterior portion of the vestibule just above the perineal body. **Most of the vulva is innervated by the branches of the pudendal nerve. Anterior to the urethra, the vulva is innervated by the ilioinguinal and genitofemoral nerves.** This area is not anesthetized adequately by a pudendal block, and repair of paraurethral tears should be supplemented by additional subcutaneous anesthesia.

INTERNAL GENITAL DEVELOPMENT

The upper vagina, cervix, uterus, and fallopian tubes are formed from the paramesonephric (müllerian) ducts. Although human embryos, whether male or female, possess both paired paramesonephric

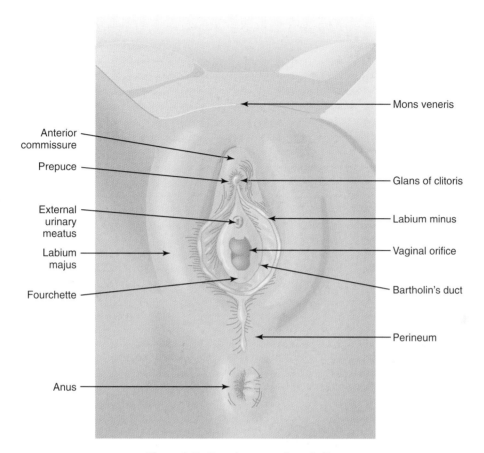

Mons veneris

Anterior commissure

Prepuce

Glans of clitoris

External urinary meatus

Labium minus

Labium majus

Vaginal orifice

Fourchette

Bartholin's duct

Perineum

Anus

Figure 3-3. Female external genitalia.

and mesonephric (wolffian) ducts, **the absence of Y chromosomal influence leads to the development of the paramesonephric system** with virtual total regression of the mesonephric system. With a Y chromosome present, a testis is formed and müllerian-inhibiting substance is produced, creating the reverse situation.

Mesonephric duct development occurs in each urogenital ridge between weeks 2 and 4 and is thought to influence the growth and development of the paramesonephric ducts. **The mesonephric ducts terminate caudally by opening into the urogenital sinus.** First evidence of each paramesonephric duct is seen at 6 weeks' gestation as a groove in the coelomic epithelium of the paired urogenital ridges, lateral to the cranial pole of the mesonephric duct. **Each paramesonephric duct opens into the coelomic cavity cranially** at a point destined to become a tubal ostium. Coursing caudally at first, parallel to the developing

mesonephric duct, the blind distal end of each paramesonephric duct eventually crosses dorsal to the mesonephric duct, and the two ducts approximate in the midline. **The two paramesonephric ducts fuse terminally at the urogenital septum, forming the uterovaginal primordium.** The distal point of fusion is known as the **müllerian tubercle (Müller's tubercle)** and can be seen protruding into the urogenital sinus dorsally in embryos at 9 to 10 weeks' gestation (Figure 3-4). **Later dissolution of the septum between the fused paramesonephric ducts leads to the development of a single uterine fundus, cervix, and, according to some investigators, the upper vagina.**

Degeneration of the mesonephric ducts is progressive from 10 to 16 weeks in the female fetus, although vestigial remnants of the latter may be noted in the adult (Gartner's duct cyst, paroöphoron, epoöphoron) (Figure 3-5). The myometrium and endometrial stroma are derived from adjacent mesenchyme; the

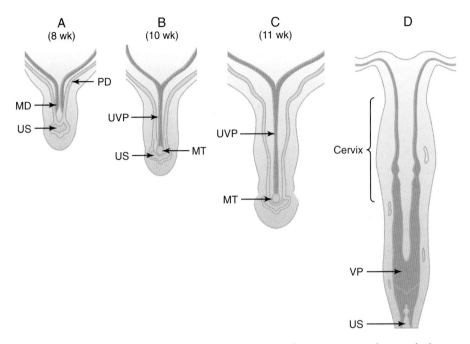

Figure 3-4. Early embryologic development of the genital tract *(A–C)* and vaginal plate *(D)*. PD, paramesonephric duct; MD, mesonephric duct; US, urogenital sinus; MT, müllerian tubercle; UVP, uterovaginal primordium; VP, vaginal plate. *(Redrawn from Didusch JF, Koff AK: Contrib Embryol Carnegie Inst 24:61, 1933.)*

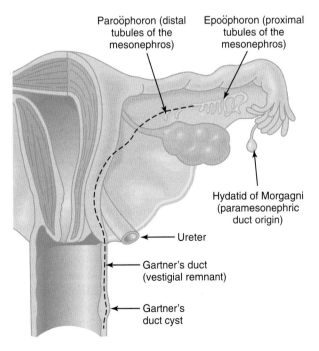

Figure 3-5. Remnants of the mesonephric (wolffian) ducts that may persist in the anterolateral vagina or adjacent to the uterus within the broad ligament or mesosalpinx.

glandular epithelium of the fallopian tubes, uterus, and cervix is derived from the paramesonephric duct.

Solid vaginal plate formation and lengthening occur from the 12th through the 20th weeks, followed by caudad to cephalad canalization, which is usually completed in utero. Controversy surrounds the relative contribution of the urogenital sinus and paramesonephric ducts to the development of the vagina, and it is uncertain whether the whole of the vaginal plate is formed secondary to growth of the endoderm of the urogenital sinus or whether the upper vagina is formed from the paramesonephric ducts.

VAGINA

The vagina is a flattened tube extending posterosuperiorly from the hymenal ring at the introitus up to the fornices that surround the cervix (Figure 3-6). Its epithelium, which is stratified squamous in type, is normally **devoid of mucous glands** and hair follicles and is nonkeratinized. Gestational exposure to diethylstilbestrol (taken by the mother) may result in columnar glands interspersed with the squamous epithelium of the upper two-thirds of the vagina

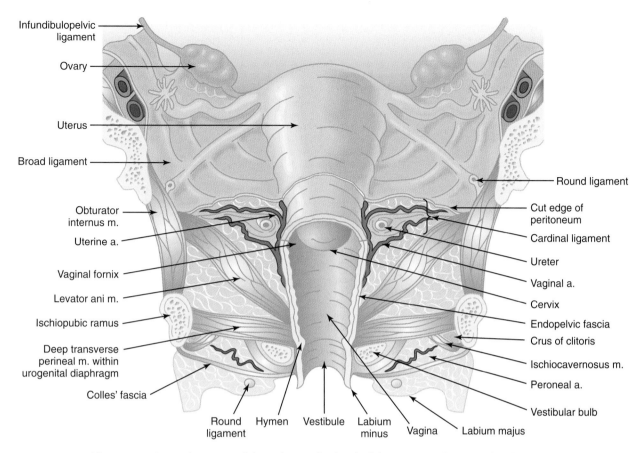

Figure 3-6. Coronal section of the pelvis at the level of the uterine isthmus and ischial spines, showing the ligaments supporting the uterus.

(vaginal adenosis). Deep to the vaginal epithelium are the muscular coats of the vagina, which consist of an inner circular and an outer longitudinal smooth muscle layer. Remnants of the mesonephric ducts may sometimes be demonstrated along the vaginal wall in the subepithelial layers and may give rise to **Gartner's duct cysts.** The adult vagina averages about 8 cm in length, although its size varies considerably with age, parity, and the status of ovarian function. An important anatomic feature is the immediate proximity of the posterior fornix of the vagina to the pouch of Douglas, which allows easy access to the peritoneal cavity from the vagina, by either culdocentesis or colpotomy.

UTERUS

The uterus consists of the cervix and the uterine corpus, which are joined by the isthmus. The uterine isthmus represents a transitional area wherein the endocervical epithelium gradually changes into the endometrial lining. In late pregnancy, this area elongates and is referred to as the lower uterine segment.

The cervix is generally 2 to 3 cm in length. In infants and children, the cervix is proportionately longer than the uterine corpus (Figure 3-7). The portion that protrudes into the vagina and is surrounded by the fornices is covered with a nonkeratinizing squamous epithelium. **At about the external cervical os, the squamous epithelium covering the ectocervix changes to simple columnar epithelium, the site of transition being referred to as the squamocolumnar junction.** The cervical canal is lined by irregular, arborized, simple columnar epithelium, which extends into the stroma as cervical "glands" or crypts.

The uterine corpus is a thick, pear-shaped organ, somewhat flattened anteroposteriorly, that consists of

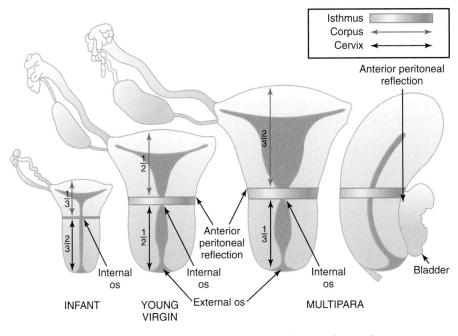

Figure 3-7. Changing proportion of the uterine cervix and corpus from infancy to adulthood. *Modified from Cunningham FG, MacDonald PC, Gant NF, et al (eds): Williams Obstetrics, 20th ed. East Norwalk, CT, Appleton & Lange, 1997.*

largely interlacing smooth muscle fibers. The endometrial lining of the uterine corpus may vary from 2 to 10 mm in thickness (which may be measured by ultrasonic imaging), depending on the stage of the menstrual cycle. Most of the surface of the uterus is covered by the peritoneal mesothelium.

Four paired sets of ligaments are attached to the uterus (Figure 3-8). Each round ligament inserts on the anterior surface of the uterus just in front of the fallopian tube, passes to the pelvic side wall in a fold of the broad ligament, traverses the inguinal canal, and ends in the labium majus. **The round ligaments are of little supportive value in preventing uterine prolapse** but help to keep the uterus anteverted. **The uterosacral ligaments** are condensations of the endopelvic fascia that arise from the sacral fascia and insert into the posteroinferior portion of the uterus at about the level of the isthmus. These ligaments contain sympathetic and parasympathetic nerve fibers that supply the uterus. They provide important support for the uterus and are also significant in precluding the development of an enterocele. **The cardinal ligaments (Mackenrodt's)** are the other important supporting structures of the uterus that prevent prolapse. They extend from the pelvic fascia

on the lateral pelvic walls and insert into the lateral portion of the cervix and vagina, reaching superiorly to the level of the isthmus. **The pubocervical ligaments** pass anteriorly around the bladder to the posterior surface of the pubic symphysis.

In addition, there are four peritoneal folds. Anteriorly, **the vesicouterine fold** is reflected from the level of the uterine isthmus onto the bladder. Posteriorly, **the rectouterine fold** passes from the posterior wall of the uterus, to the upper fourth of the vagina, and thence onto the rectum. The pouch between the two folds forms a cul-de-sac, called the pouch of Douglas. Laterally, the **two broad ligaments** each pass from the side of the uterus to the lateral wall of the pelvis. Between the two leaves of each broad ligament are contained the fallopian tube, the round ligament, and the ovarian ligament, in addition to nerves, blood vessels, and lymphatics. **The fold of broad ligament containing the fallopian tube is called the mesosalpinx.** Between the end of the tube and ovary and the pelvic side wall, where the ureter passes over the common iliac vessels, is the infundibulopelvic ligament, which contains the vessels and nerves for the ovary. The ureter may be injured when this ligament is ligated during a salpingo-oophorectomy procedure.

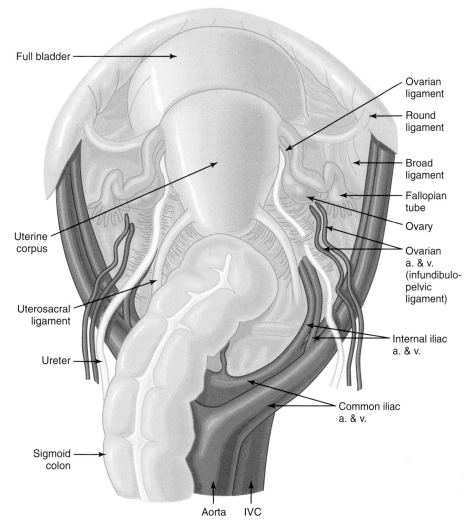

Figure 3-8. View of the internal genital organs in the female pelvis.

FALLOPIAN TUBES

The oviducts are bilateral muscular tubes (about 10 cm in length) with lumina that connect the uterine cavity with the peritoneal cavity. They are enclosed in the medial four-fifths of the superior aspect of the broad ligament. The tubes are lined by a ciliated, columnar epithelium that is thrown into branching folds. That segment of the tube within the wall of the uterus is referred to as the **interstitial portion.** The medial portion of each tube is superior to the round ligament, anterior to the ovarian ligament, and relatively fixed in position. This nonmobile portion of the tube has a fairly narrow lumen and is referred to as the **isthmus.** As the tube proceeds laterally, it is located anterior to

the ovary; it then passes around the lateral portion of the ovary and down toward the cul-de-sac. The **ampullary and fimbriated portions** of the tube are suspended from the broad ligament by the meso-salpinx and are quite mobile. The mobility of the fim-briated end of the tube plays an important role in fertility. The ampullary portion of the tube is the most common site of ectopic pregnancies.

NORMAL EMBRYOLOGIC DEVELOPMENT OF THE OVARY

The earliest anatomic event in gonadogenesis is noted at approximately 4 weeks gestational age (i.e., 4 weeks from conception), when a thickening of the peritoneal, or coelomic, epithelium on the ventromedial surface of the urogenital ridge occurs. A bulging **genital ridge** is subsequently produced by rapid proliferation of the coelomic epithelium in an area that is medial, but parallel, to the mesonephric ridge. Prior to the 5th week, this indifferent gonad consists of germinal epithelium surrounding the internal blastema, a primordial mesenchymal cellular mass designated to become the ovarian medulla. After 5 weeks, projections from the germinal epithelium extend like spokes into the mesenchymal blastema to form **primary sex cords**. Soon thereafter in the 7th week, a testis can be identified histologically if the embryo has a Y chromosome. In the absence of a Y chromosome, definitive ovarian characteristics do not appear until somewhere between the 12th and 16th weeks.

As early as 3 weeks' gestation, relatively large primordial germ cells appear intermixed with other cells in the endoderm of the yolk sac wall of the primitive hindgut. These germ-cell precursors migrate along the hindgut dorsal mesentery (Figure 3-9) and are all contained in the mesenchyme of the undifferentiated urogenital ridge by 8 weeks' gestation. Subsequent replication of these cells by mitotic division occurs, with maximal mitotic activity noted up to 20 weeks' gestation and cessation noted by term. These oogonia, the end result of this germ-cell proliferation, are incorporated into the cortical sex cords of the genital ridge.

Histologically, the first evidence of follicles is seen at about 20 weeks, with germ cells surrounded by flattened cells derived from the cortical sex cords. These flattened cells are recognizable as granulosa cells of coelomic epithelial origin and theca cells of mesenchymal origin. The oogonia enter the prophase of the first meiotic division and are then called **primary oocytes** (see Chapter 4). It has been estimated that more than 2 million primary oocytes, or their precursors, are present at 20 weeks' gestation, but only about 300,000 primordial follicles are present by 7 years of age.

Regression of the primary sex cords in the medulla produces the **rete ovarii,** which are found histologically in the hilus of the ovary along with another testicular analogue called **Leydig's cells,** which are thought to be derived from mesenchyme. Vestiges of the rete ovarii and of the degenerating mesonephros may also be noted at times in the mesovarium or mesosalpinx. Structural homologues in males and females are shown in Table 3-1.

ANATOMY OF THE OVARIES

The ovaries are oval, flattened, compressible organs, approximately $3 \times 2 \times 2$ cm in size. They are situated on the superior surface of the broad ligament and are suspended between the ovarian ligament medially and the suspensory ligament of the ovary or infundibulopelvic ligament laterally and superiorly. Each occupies a position in the ovarian fossa (of Waldeyer), which is a shallow depression on the lateral pelvic wall just posterior to the external iliac vessels and anterior to the ureter and hypogastric vessels. In endometriosis and salpingo-oophoritis, the ovaries may be densely adherent to the ureter. Generally, the serosal covering and the tunica albuginea of the ovary are quite thin, and developing follicles and corpora lutea are readily visible.

The blood supply to the ovaries is provided by the long ovarian arteries, which arise from the abdominal aorta immediately below the renal arteries. These vessels course downward and cross

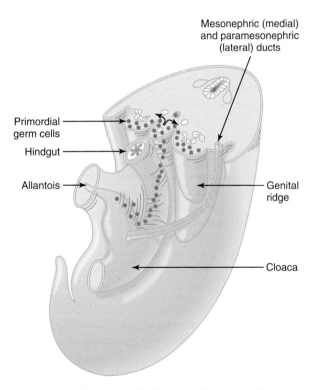

Mesonephric (medial) and paramesonephric (lateral) ducts

Primordial germ cells

Hindgut

Allantois

Genital ridge

Cloaca

Figure 3-9. Migratory path of primordial germ cells from the yolk sac, along the hindgut mesentery, to the urogenital ridge at approximately 5 weeks.

Table 3-1. Structural homologues in males and females

Primordia	Female	Male	Major Determining Factors
GONADAL			
Germ cells	Oogonia	Spermatogonia	Sex chromosomes
Coelomic epithelium	Granulosa cells	Sertoli's cells	
Mesenchyme	Theca cells	Leydig's cells	
Mesonephros	Rete ovarii	Rete testis	
DUCTAL			
Paramesonephric (müllerian) duct	Fallopian tubes Uterus Superior 2/3 of vagina	Hydatid testis	Absence of Y chromosome
Mesonephric (wolffian) duct	Gartner's duct	Vas deferens Seminal vesicles	Testosterone Müllerian inhibiting factor
Mesonephric tubules	Epoöphoron Paroöphoron	Epididymis Efferent ducts	
EXTERNAL GENITALIA			
Urogenital sinus	Vaginal contribution Skene's glands Bartholin's glands	Prostate Prostatic utricle Cowper's glands	Presence or absence of testosterone, dihydrotestosterone (DHT), and 5α-reductase enzyme
Genital tubercle	Clitoris	Penis	
Urogenital folds	Labia minora	Corpora spongiosa	
Genital folds	Labia majora	Scrotum	

laterally over the ureter at the level of the pelvic brim, passing branches to the ureter and the fallopian tube. The ovary also receives substantial blood supply from the uterine artery through the uterine-ovarian arterial anastomosis. **The venous drainage from the right ovary is directly into the inferior vena cava, whereas that from the left ovary is into the left renal vein** (Figure 3-10).

ANATOMY OF THE URETERS

The ureters extend 25 to 30 cm from the renal pelves to their insertion into the bladder at the trigone. Each descends immediately under the peritoneum, crossing the pelvic brim beneath the ovarian vessels just anterior to the bifurcation of the common iliac artery. In the true pelvis, the ureter initially courses inferiorly, just anterior to the hypogastric vessels, and stays closely attached to the peritoneum. It then passes forward along the side of the cervix and beneath the uterine artery toward the trigone of the bladder.

LYMPHATIC DRAINAGE

The lymphatic drainage of the vulva and lower vagina is principally to the inguinofemoral lymph nodes and then to the external iliac chains (Figure 3-10). The lymphatic drainage of the cervix takes place through the parametria (cardinal ligaments) to the pelvic nodes (the hypogastric, obturator, and external iliac groups) and then to the common iliac and para-aortic chains. The lymphatic drainage from the endometrium is through the broad ligament and infundibulopelvic ligament to the pelvic and para-aortic chains. The lymphatics of the ovaries pass via the infundibulopelvic ligaments to the pelvic and para-aortic nodes (Figure 3-10).

ANATOMY OF THE LOWER ABDOMINAL WALL

Because most intraabdominal gynecologic operations are performed through lower abdominal incisions, it is important to review the anatomy of the lower abdominal wall with special reference to the muscles and fasciae. After transecting the skin, subcutaneous fat, superficial fascia (Camper's), and deep fascia (Scarpa's) the anterior rectus sheath is encountered (Figure 3-11). **The rectus sheath is a strong fibrous compartment formed by the aponeuroses of the three lateral abdominal wall muscles.** The aponeuroses meet in the midline to form the linea alba and partially encase the two rectus abdominis muscles.

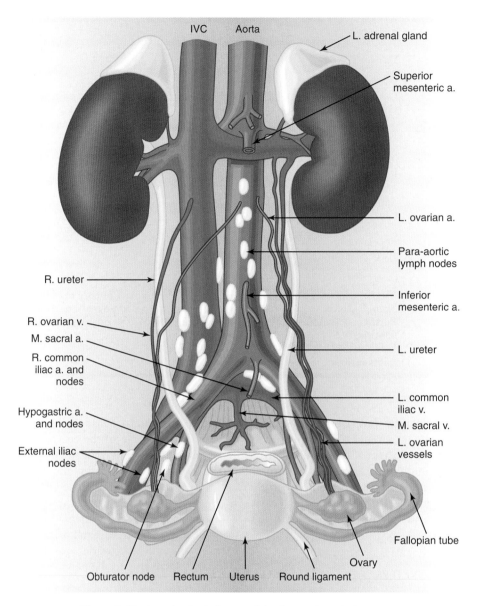

Figure 3-10. Lymphatic drainage of the internal genital organs.

The composition of the rectus sheath differs in its upper and lower portions. Above the midpoint between the umbilicus and the symphysis pubis, the rectus muscle is encased anteriorly by the aponeurosis of the external oblique and the anterior lamina of the internal oblique aponeurosis and posteriorly by the aponeurosis of the transversus abdominis and the posterior lamina of the internal oblique aponeurosis. **In the lower fourth of the abdomen, the posterior aponeurotic layer of the sheath terminates in a free crescentic margin, the semilunar fold of Douglas.**

Each rectus abdominis muscle, encased in the rectus sheath on either side of the midline, extends from the superior aspect of the symphysis pubis to the anterior surface of the fifth, sixth, and seventh costal cartilages. A variable number of tendinous intersections (three to five) crosses each muscle at irregular intervals, and any transverse rectus surgical incision forms a new fibrous intersection during healing. The muscle is not attached to the posterior sheath and, following separation from the anterior sheath, can be retracted laterally, as in the Pfannenstiel incision. **Each rectus muscle has a firm**

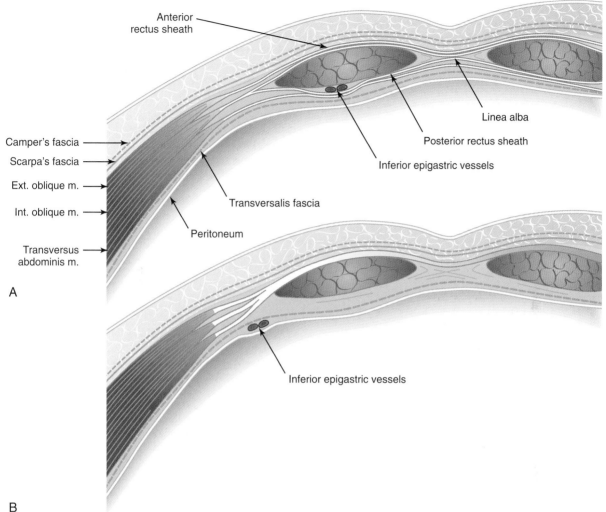

Figure 3-11. Transverse section through the anterior abdominal wall just below the umbilicus *(A)* and just above the pubic symphysis *(B)*. Note the absence of the posterior rectus sheath in *B*.

aponeurosis at its attachment to the symphysis pubis, and this tendinous aponeurosis can be transected if necessary to improve exposure, as in the Cherny incision, and resutured securely during closure of the abdominal wall.

The inferior epigastric arteries arise from the external iliac arteries and proceed superiorly just lateral to the rectus muscles between the transversalis fascia and the peritoneum. They enter the rectus sheaths at the level of the semilunar line and continue their course superiorly just posterior to the rectus muscles. In a transverse rectus muscle–cutting incision, the

epigastric arteries can be retracted laterally or ligated to allow a wide peritoneal incision.

ABDOMINAL WALL INCISIONS

The most commonly used lower abdominal incision in gynecologic surgery is the Pfannenstiel incision (Figure 3-12). Although it does not always give sufficient exposure for extensive operations, it has cosmetic advantages in that it is generally only 2 cm above the symphysis pubis, and the scar is later covered by the pubic hair. Because the rectus abdominis muscles

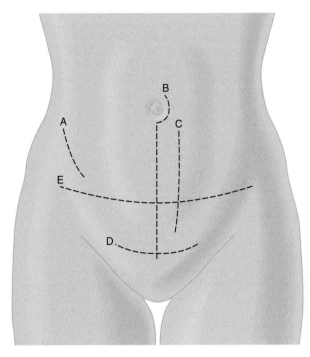

Figure 3-12. Abdominal wall incisions: McBurney's *(A)*, lower midline *(B)*, left lower paramedian *(C)*, Pfannenstiel or Cherny *(D)*, and transverse, Maylard or Bardenheuer *(E)*.

are not cut, eviscerations and wound hernias are extremely uncommon. **For extensive pelvic procedures (e.g., radical hysterectomy and pelvic lymphadenectomy), a transverse muscle–cutting incision (Bardenheuer or Maylard) at a slightly higher level in the lower abdomen gives sufficient exposure.** In addition, the skin incision falls within the lines of Langer, so a good cosmetic result can be expected. When it is anticipated that upper abdominal exploration will be necessary, such as in a patient with suspected ovarian cancer, a midline incision through the linea alba or a paramedian vertical incision is indicated.

Suggested Reading

Agur AMR (ed): Grant's Atlas of Anatomy, 9th ed. Baltimore, Williams & Wilkins, 1991.

Clemente CD: Anatomy: An Atlas of the Human Body, 4th ed. Baltimore, Williams & Wilkins, 1997.

Cunningham EG, MacDonald PC, Gant NF, et al (eds): Williams Obstetrics, 20th ed. Norwalk, CT, Appleton & Lange, 1997.

Smout CFV, Jacoby F, Lillie EW: Gynecological and Obstetrical Anatomy. Baltimore, Williams & Wilkins, 1969.

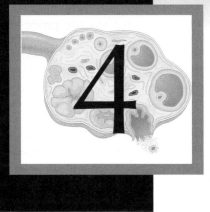

Female Reproductive Physiology

Paul J. Toot and John K.H. Lu

THE MENSTRUAL CYCLE

Each menstrual cycle represents a complex interaction between the hypothalamus, pituitary gland, ovaries, and endometrium. Cyclic changes in gonadotropin and steroid hormones induce functional as well as morphologic changes in the ovary, resulting in follicular maturation, ovulation, and corpus luteum formation. Similar changes at the level of the endometrium allow for successful implantation of the developing embryo.

The reproductive cycle can be viewed from the perspective of each of the aforementioned organ systems. The cyclic changes within the hypothalamic-pituitary axis, ovary, and endometrium are approached separately in this chapter, but these endocrinologic events occur in concert in a uniquely integrated fashion. In addition, fertilization, implantation, and placentation are discussed.

HYPOTHALAMIC-PITUITARY AXIS
PITUITARY GLAND

The pituitary gland lies below the hypothalamus at the base of the brain within a bony cavity (sella turcica) and is separated from the cranial cavity by a condensation of dura mater overlying the sella turcica (diaphragma sellae). The pituitary gland is divided into two major portions (Figure 4-1). **The neurohypophysis, which consists of the posterior lobe (pars nervosa), the neural stalk (infundibulum), and the median eminence, is derived from neural tissue and is in direct continuity with the hypothalamus and central nervous system. The adenohypophysis, which consists of the pars distalis (anterior lobe), pars intermedia (intermediate lobe), and pars tuberalis, which surrounds the neural stalk, is derived from ectoderm.**

The arterial blood supply to the median eminence and the neural stalk (pituitary portal system) represents a major avenue of transport for hypothalamic secretions to the anterior pituitary.

The neurohypophysis serves primarily to transport oxytocin and vasopressin (antidiuretic hormone) along neuronal projections from the supraoptic and paraventricular nuclei of the hypothalamus to their release into the circulation.

The anterior pituitary contains different cell types that produce six protein hormones: follicle-stimulating hormone (FSH), luteinizing hormone (LH), thyroid-stimulating hormone (TSH), prolactin, growth hormone (GH), and adrenocorticotropic hormone (ACTH).

The gonadotropins, FSH and LH, are synthesized and stored in cells called **gonadotrophs,** whereas TSH is produced by **thyrotrophs.** FSH, LH, and TSH are glycoproteins, consisting of α and β subunits. The α subunits of FSH, LH, and TSH are identical. The same α subunit is also present in human chorionic gonadotropin (hCG). The β subunits are individual for each hormone. The half-life for circulating LH is about 30 minutes, whereas that of FSH is several hours. The difference in half-lives may account, at least in part, for the differential secretion patterns of these two gonadotropins.

Prolactin is secreted by lactotrophs. Unlike the case with other peptide hormones produced by the adenohypophysis, pituitary release of prolactin is under tonic **inhibition** by the hypothalamus. The half-life for circulating prolactin is about 20 to 30 minutes. In

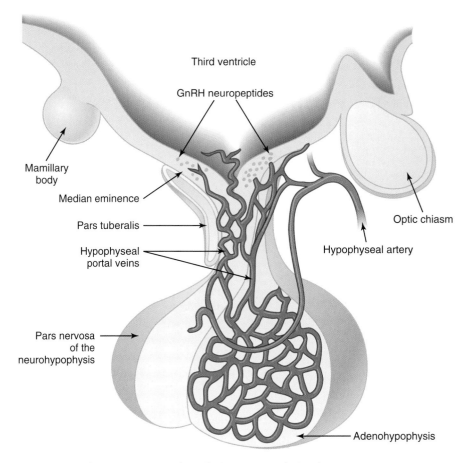

Figure 4-1. Hypophyseal-pituitary portal circulatory system.

addition to its lactogenic effect, prolactin may directly or indirectly influence hypothalamic, pituitary, and ovarian functions in relation to the ovulatory cycle, particularly in the pathologic state of chronic hyperprolactinemia (see Chapter 33).

GONADOTROPIN SECRETORY PATTERNS

A normal ovulatory cycle can be divided into a follicular and a luteal phase (Figure 4-2). The follicular phase begins with the onset of menses and culminates in the preovulatory surge of LH. The luteal phase begins with the onset of the preovulatory LH surge and ends with the first day of menses.

Decreasing levels of estradiol and progesterone from the regressing corpus luteum of the preceding cycle initiate a rise of FSH by a negative feedback mechanism, which stimulates follicular growth and estradiol secretion. At lower levels of estradiol there is a negative feedback effect on the ready-release form of LH from the pool of gonadotropins in the pituitary gonadotrophs. As estradiol levels rise later in the follicular phase, there is a positive feedback on the release of storage gonadotropins, resulting in the LH surge and ovulation. The latter occurs 36 to 44 hours after the onset of this mid-cycle LH surge. With pharmacologic doses of progestins contained in contraceptive pills, there is a profound negative feedback effect on gonadotropin-releasing hormone (GnRH) so that none of the gonadotropin pool (ready-release or storage) is released. Hence, ovulation is (generally) blocked (see Chapter 27).

During the luteal phase, both LH and FSH are significantly suppressed through the negative feedback effect of elevated circulating estradiol and progesterone. This inhibition persists until progesterone and estradiol levels decline near the end

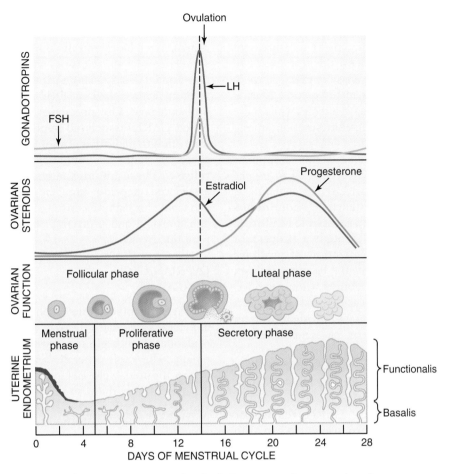

Figure 4-2. Hormone levels during a normal menstrual cycle.

of the luteal phase as a result of corpus luteal regression, should pregnancy fail to occur. The net effect is a slight rise in serum FSH, which initiates new follicular growth for the next cycle. The duration of the corpus luteum's functional regression is such that menstruation generally occurs 14 days after the LH surge in the absence of pregnancy.

HYPOTHALAMUS

Five different small peptides or biogenic amines that affect the reproductive cycle have been isolated from the hypothalamus. All exert specific effects on the hormonal secretion of the anterior pituitary gland. They are **GnRH, thyrotropin-releasing hormone (TRH), somatotropin release-inhibiting factor (SRIF) or somatostatin, corticotropin-releasing factor (CRF), and prolactin release-inhibiting**

factor (PIF). Only GnRH and PIF are discussed in this chapter.

GnRH is a decapeptide that is synthesized primarily in the arcuate nucleus. It is responsible for the synthesis and release of both LH and FSH. Because it usually causes the release of more LH than FSH, it is commonly called LH-releasing hormone (LH-RH) or LH-releasing factor (LRF). Both FSH and LH appear to be present in two different forms within the pituitary gonadotrophs. One is a releasable form and the other a storage form. GnRH reaches the anterior pituitary via the hypophyseal portal vessels and stimulates the synthesis of both FSH and LH, which are stored within gonadotrophs. Subsequently, GnRH activates and transforms these molecules into releasable forms. GnRH can also induce immediate release of both LH and FSH into the circulation. Some receptor data suggest that GnRH may have a direct effect on ovarian function as well.

GnRH is secreted in a pulsatile fashion throughout the menstrual cycle. The frequency of GnRH release, as assessed indirectly by measurement of LH pulses, varies from approximately every 90 minutes in the early follicular phase to every 60 to 70 minutes in the immediate preovulatory period. During the luteal phase, pulse frequency decreases while pulse amplitude increases. A considerable variation among individuals has been identified.

Intravenous and subcutaneous administration of exogenous pulsatile GnRH has been used to induce ovulation in selected women who are not ovulating as a result of hypothalamic dysfunction. **Continuous infusion of GnRH results in a reversible inhibition of gonadotropin secretion through a process of "downregulation" or desensitization of pituitary gonadotrophs.** This represents the basic mechanism of action for the GnRH agonists (nonapeptides, containing only nine amino acids) that have been successfully used in the therapy of such ovarian hormone-dependent disorders as endometriosis, leiomyomata, hirsutism, and precocious puberty.

Several mechanisms control the secretion of GnRH. **Estradiol appears to enhance hypothalamic release of GnRH and may help induce the midcycle LH surge by increasing GnRH release or by enhancing pituitary responsiveness to the decapeptide. Gonadotropins have an inhibitory effect on GnRH release.** Catecholamines may play a major regulatory role as well. Dopamine is synthesized in the arcuate and periventricular nuclei and may have a direct inhibitory effect on GnRH secretion via the tuberoinfundibular tract that projects onto the median eminence. Serotonin also appears to inhibit GnRH pulsatile release, whereas norepinephrine stimulates it. Endogenous opioids suppress release of GnRH from the hypothalamus in a manner that may be partially regulated by ovarian steroids.

The hypothalamus produces PIF, which exerts chronic inhibition of prolactin release from the lactotrophs. A number of pharmacologic agents (e.g., chlorpromazine) that affect dopaminergic mechanisms influence prolactin release. Dopamine itself is secreted by hypothalamic neurons into the hypophyseal portal vessels and inhibits prolactin release directly within the adenohypophysis. Based on these observations, it has been proposed that hypothalamic dopamine may be the major PIF. In addition to the regulation of prolactin release by PIF, the hypothalamus may also produce prolactin-releasing factors (PRF) that can elicit large and rapid increases in prolactin release under certain conditions, such as breast stimulation during nursing. Neither PIF nor PRF has been well characterized biochemically as of 2003. TRH serves to stimulate prolactin release as well. This phenomenon may explain the association between primary hypothyroidism (with secondary TRH elevation) and hyperprolactinemia. **The precursor protein for GnRH, called GnRH-associated peptide (GAP), has been identified to be both a potent inhibitor of prolactin secretion and an enhancer of gonadotropin release. These findings suggest that this GnRH-associated peptide may be a physiologic PIF** and could explain the inverse relationship between gonadotropin and prolactin secretions seen in many reproductive states.

OVARIAN CYCLE
ESTROGENS

During early follicular development, circulating estradiol levels are relatively low. About 1 week before ovulation, levels begin to increase, at first slowly, then rapidly. The levels generally reach a maximum 1 day before the mid-cycle LH peak. After this peak and before ovulation, there is a marked and precipitous fall. During the luteal phase, estradiol rises to a maximum 5 to 7 days after ovulation and returns to baseline shortly before menstruation. Estrone secretion by the ovary is considerably less than secretion of estradiol but follows a similar pattern. Most of the estrone is derived from the conversion of androstenedione through the action of the enzyme aromatase resulting in a process called aromatization (Figure 4-3).

PROGESTINS

During follicular development, the ovary secretes only very small amounts of progesterone and 17a-hydroxyprogesterone. The bulk of the progesterone comes from the peripheral conversion of adrenal pregnenolone and pregnenolone sulfate. Just before ovulation, the unruptured but luteinizing graafian follicle begins to produce increasing amounts of progesterone. At about this time, a marked increase also occurs in serum 17a-hydroxyprogesterone. The elevation of basal body temperature is temporally related to the central effect of progesterone. As with estradiol, secretion of progestins by the corpus luteum reaches a maximum 5 to 7 days after ovulation and returns to baseline shortly before menstruation. Should pregnancy occur, progesterone levels, and therefore basal body temperature, remain elevated.

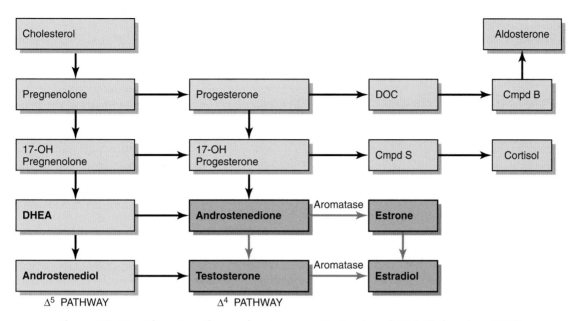

Figure 4-3. Steroidogenic pathways showing aromatization in red. OH, Hydroxylase; DOC, desoxycorticosterone; cmpd B, corticosterone; cmpd S, II-desoxycortisol.

ANDROGENS

Both the ovary and the adrenal glands secrete small amounts of testosterone, but most of the testosterone is derived from the metabolism of androstenedione, which is also secreted by both the ovary and the adrenal gland. Near mid-cycle, an increase occurs in plasma androstenedione, which reflects enhanced secretion from the follicle. During the luteal phase, a second rise occurs in androstenedione, which reflects enhanced secretion by the corpus luteum. The adrenal gland also secretes androstenedione in a diurnal pattern similar to that of cortisol. The ovary secretes small amounts of the very potent dihydrotestosterone (DHT), but the bulk of DHT is derived from the conversion of androstenedione and testosterone. The majority of dehydroepiandrosterone (DHEA) and virtually all DHEA sulfate (DHEA-S), which are extremely weak androgens, are secreted by the adrenal glands, although small amounts of DHEA are secreted by the ovary.

SERUM-BINDING PROTEINS

Circulating estrogens and androgens are mostly bound to specific sex hormone–binding globulins (SHBG) or to serum albumin. The remaining fraction of sex hormones is unbound (free), and this is the biologically active fraction. It is unclear whether steroids bound to serum proteins (e.g., albumin) are accessible for tissue uptake and utilization. The synthesis of SHBG in the liver is increased by estrogens and thyroid hormones but decreased by testosterone.

PROLACTIN

Serum prolactin levels do not change strikingly during the normal menstrual cycle. Both the serum level of prolactin and prolactin release in response to TRH are somewhat more elevated during the luteal phase than during the mid-follicular phase of the cycle. This suggests that high amounts of circulating estradiol and progesterone may enhance prolactin release. **Prolactin release varies in such a manner that the highest levels occur during sleep.**

Prolactin may participate in the control of ovarian steroidogenesis. Prolactin concentrations in follicular fluid change markedly during follicular growth. The highest prolactin concentrations are seen in small follicles during the early follicular phase. Prolactin concentrations in the follicular fluid may be inversely related to the production of progesterone. In addition, hyperprolactinemia may alter gonadotropin secretion. Despite these observations, the physiologic role of prolactin during the normal menstrual cycle has not been established.

FOLLICULAR DEVELOPMENT

Primordial follicles undergo sequential development, differentiation, and maturation until a mature graafian follicle is produced. The follicle then ruptures, releasing the ovum. Subsequent luteinization of the ruptured follicle produces the corpus luteum.

At approximately 8 to 10 weeks of fetal development, oocytes become progressively surrounded by precursor granulosa cells, which then separate themselves from the underlying stroma and oocyte by a basal lamina. This oocyte-complex is called a **primordial follicle.** In response to gonadotropin and ovarian steroids, the follicular cells become cuboidal and the stromal cells around the follicle become prominent. This process, which takes place in utero (i.e., in the fetal ovary) at between 20 and 24 weeks' gestation, results in a primary follicle. As granulosa cells proliferate, a clear gelatinous material surrounds the ovum, forming the **zona pellucida.** This larger unit is called a secondary follicle.

In the adult ovary, a graafian follicle forms as the innermost three or four layers of rapidly multiplying granulosa cells become cuboidal and adherent to the ovum **(cumulus oophorus).** In addition, a fluid-filled antrum forms among the granulosa cells. As the liquor continues to accumulate, the antrum enlarges and the centrally located primary oocyte migrates eccentrically to the wall of the follicle. The innermost layer of granulosa cells of the cumulus, which are in close contact with the pellucida, become elongated and form the **corona radiata.** The corona radiata is released with the oocyte at ovulation. Covering the granulosa cells is a thin basement membrane, outside of which connective tissue cells organize themselves into two coats: the *theca interna* and *theca externa.*

During each cycle, a cohort of follicles is recruited for development. Among the many developing follicles, only one usually continues differentiation and maturation into a follicle that ovulates. The remaining follicles undergo atresia. On the basis of in vitro measurement of local steroid levels, growing follicles can be classified as either estrogen-predominant or androgen-predominant. Follicles greater than 10 mm in diameter are usually estrogen-predominant, whereas smaller follicles are usually androgen-predominant. Mature preovulatory follicles reach mean diameters of approximately 18 to 25 mm. Furthermore, in estrogen-predominant follicles, antral FSH concentrations continue to rise while serum FSH levels decline beginning at the mid-follicular phase. In smaller, androgen-predominant follicles, antral fluid FSH values decrease while serum FSH levels decline; thus, the intrafollicular steroid milieu appears to play an important role in determining whether a follicle undergoes maturation or atresia. Additional follicles may be "rescued" from atresia by administration of exogenous gonadotropins.

Follicular maturation is dependent on the local development of receptors for FSH and LH. FSH receptors are present on granulosa cells. Under FSH stimulation, granulosa cells proliferate and the number of FSH receptors per follicle increases proportionately. Thus, the growing primary follicle is increasingly more sensitive to stimulation by FSH; as a result, estradiol levels increase. Estrogens, particularly estradiol, enhance the induction of FSH receptors and act synergistically with FSH to increase LH receptors.

During early stages of folliculogenesis, LH receptors are present only on the theca interna layer. LH stimulation induces steroidogenesis and increases the synthesis of androgens by thecal cells. In nondominant follicles, high local androgen levels may enhance follicular atresia. However, in the follicle destined to reach ovulation, FSH induces aromatase enzyme and its receptor formation within the granulosa cells. As a result, androgens produced in the theca interna of the dominant follicle diffuse into the granulosa cells and are aromatized into estrogens. **FSH also enhances the induction of LH receptors on the granulosa cells of the follicle that is destined to ovulate.** These are essential for the appropriate response to the LH surge, leading to the final stages of maturation, ovulation, and the luteal phase production of progesterone. Thus, **the presence of greater numbers of FSH receptors and granulosa cells and increased induction of aromatase enzyme and its receptors may differentiate between the follicle of the initial cohort that will develop normally and those that will undergo atresia.**

Growth factors such as insulin, insulin-like growth factor (IGF), fibroblast growth factor (FGF), and epidermal growth factor (EGF) may also play significant mitogenic roles in folliculogenesis, including enhanced responsiveness to FSH.

OVULATION

The pre-ovulatory LH surge initiates a sequence of structural and biochemical changes that culminate in ovulation. Before ovulation, a general dissolution of the entire follicular wall occurs, particularly the portion that is on the surface of the ovary. Presumably this occurs as a result of the action of proteolytic enzymes. With degeneration of the cells on the surface, a stigma forms, and the follicular basement membrane finally bulges through the stigma. When this ruptures, the oocyte together with the corona radiata and some cumulus oophera cells are expelled into the peritoneal cavity, and ovulation takes place.

Ovulation is now known from ultrasonic studies to be a gradual phenomenon, with the collapse of the follicle taking from several minutes to as long as an hour or more. The oocyte adheres to the surface of the ovary, allowing an extended period during which the muscular contractions of the fallopian tube may bring it in contact with the tubal epithelium. Probably both muscular contractions and tubal ciliary movement contribute to the entry of the oocyte into, and the transportation along, the fallopian tube. Ciliary activity may not be essential, because some women with immotile cilia also become pregnant.

At birth, primary oocytes are in the prophase of the first meiotic division. They continue in this phase until the next maturation division occurs in conjunction with the mid-cycle LH surge. **A few hours preceding ovulation, the chromatin is resolved into distinct chromosomes, and meiotic division takes place with unequal distribution of the cytoplasm to form a secondary oocyte and the first polar body. Each element contains 23 chromosomes, each in the form of two monads.** The second maturation spindle forms immediately, and the oocyte remains at the surface of the ovary. No further development takes place until after ovulation and fertilization have occurred. At that time, and before the union of the male and female pronuclei, another division occurs to reduce the chromosomal component of the egg pronucleus to 23 single chromosomes (22 plus X or Y), each composed of the one monad. The ovum and a second polar body are thus formed. The first polar body may also divide.

LUTEINIZATION AND CORPUS LUTEUM FUNCTION

After ovulation and under the influence of LH, the granulosa cells of the ruptured follicle undergo luteinization. These luteinized granulosa cells, plus the surrounding theca cells, capillaries, and connective tissue, form the corpus luteum, which produces copious amounts of progesterone and some estradiol. **The normal functional life span of the corpus luteum is about 9 to 10 days.** After this time it regresses, and unless pregnancy occurs, menstruation ensues and the corpus luteum is gradually replaced by an avascular scar called a *corpus albicans*. The events occurring in the ovary during a complete cycle are shown in Figure 4-4.

HISTOPHYSIOLOGY OF THE ENDOMETRIUM

The endometrium is uniquely responsive to the circulating progestins, androgens, and estrogens. It is this responsiveness that gives rise to menstruation and makes implantation and pregnancy possible.

Functionally, the endometrium is divided into two zones: (1) the **outer portion,** or **functionalis,** that undergoes cyclic changes in morphology and function during the menstrual cycle and is sloughed off at menstruation; and (2) the **inner portion,** or **basalis,** that remains relatively unchanged during each menstrual cycle and, after menstruation, provides stem cells for the renewal of the functionalis. Basal arteries are regular blood vessels found in the basalis, whereas spiral arteries are specially coiled blood vessels seen in the functionalis.

The cyclic changes in histophysiology of the endometrium can be divided into three stages: the menstrual phase, the proliferative or estrogenic phase, and the secretory or progestational phase.

MENSTRUAL PHASE

Because it is the only portion of the cycle that is visible externally, the first day of menstruation is taken as day 1 of the menstrual cycle. The first 4 to 5 days of the cycle are defined as the menstrual phase. **During this phase, there is disruption and disintegration of the endometrial glands and stroma, leukocyte infiltration, and red blood cell extravasation.** In addition to this sloughing of the functionalis, there is a compression of the basalis due to the loss of ground substances. Despite these degenerative changes, early evidence of renewed tissue growth is usually present at this time within the basalis of the endometrium.

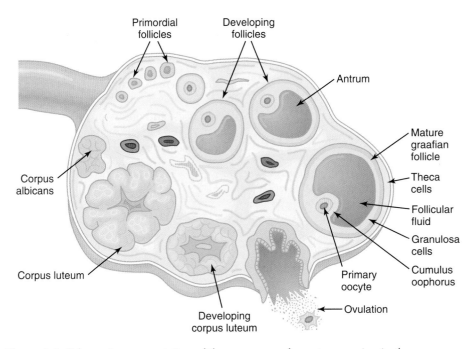

Figure 4-4. Schematic representation of the sequence of events occurring in the ovary during a complete follicular cycle. *Adapted from Yen SC, Jaffe R (eds): Reproductive Endocrinology. Philadelphia, WB Saunders, 1978.*

PROLIFERATIVE PHASE

The proliferative phase is characterized by endometrial proliferation or growth secondary to estrogenic stimulation. Because the bases of the endometrial glands lie deep within the basalis, these epithelial cells are not destroyed during menstruation. As menstruation ends each month, they provide the source of stem cells that divide and migrate through the stroma to form a new epithelial lining of the endometrium and new endometrial glands.

During this phase of the cycle, the large increase in estrogen secretion causes marked cellular proliferation of the epithelial lining, the endometrial glands, and the connective tissue of the stroma (Figure 4-5). Numerous mitoses are present in these tissues and there is an increase in the length of the spiral arteries, which traverse almost the entire thickness of the endometrium. By the end of the proliferative phase, cellular proliferation and endometrial growth have reached a maximum, the spiral arteries are elongated and convoluted, and the endometrial glands are straight, with narrow lumens containing some glycogen. True secretory function in the glands must await progesterone secretion by the corpus luteum.

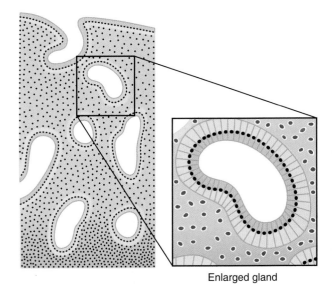

Enlarged gland

Early Proliferative Phase Endometrium

Figure 4-5. Early proliferative phase endometrium. Note the regular, tubular glands lined by pseudostratified columnar cells.

SECRETORY PHASE

Following ovulation, progesterone secretion by the corpus luteum stimulates the glandular cells to secrete glycogen, mucus, and other substances. The glands become tortuous and the lumens are dilated and filled with these substances. The stroma becomes edematous. Mitoses are rare. The spiral arteries continue to extend into the superficial layer of the endometrium and become convoluted (Figure 4-6).

The marked changes that occur in endometrial histology during the secretory phase permit relatively precise timing (dating) of secretory endometrium.

If pregnancy does not occur by day 23, the corpus luteum begins to regress, secretion of progesterone and estradiol declines, and the endometrium undergoes involution. About 1 day prior to the onset of menstruation, marked constriction of the spiral arterioles takes place, causing ischemia of the endometrium followed by leukocyte infiltration and red blood cell extravasation. It is thought that these events occur secondary to prostaglandin production by the endometrium. The resulting necrosis causes menstruation or sloughing of the endometrium. Thus, menstruation, which clinically marks the beginning of

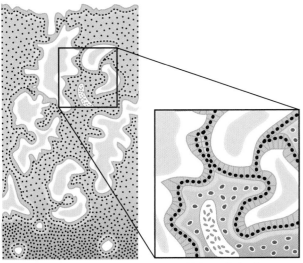

Enlarged glands

Late Secretory Phase Endometrium

Figure 4-6. Late secretory phase endometrium. Note the tortuous, saw-toothed appearance of the endometrial glands with secretions in the lumens. The stroma is edematous and necrotic during this stage leading to sloughing of the endometrium at the time of menstruation.

the menstrual cycle, is actually the terminal event of a physiologic process that enables the uterus to be prepared to receive another conceptus.

SPERMATOGENESIS, SPERM CAPACITATION, AND FERTILIZATION

Fertilization, or conception, is the union of male and female pronuclear elements. Conception normally takes place in the fallopian tube, after which the fertilized ovum continues to the uterus, where implantation occurs and development of the conceptus continues.

Spermatogenesis requires about 74 days. Together with transportation, a total of about 3 months elapses before sperm are ejaculated. The sperm achieve motility during their passage through the epididymis, but sperm capacitation, which renders them capable of fertilization in vivo, does not occur until they are removed from the seminal plasma after ejaculation. Interestingly, sperm aspirated from the epididymis and testis can be used to achieve fertilization in vitro employing intracytoplasmic injection techniques directly into the ooplasm.

Estrogen levels are high at the time of ovulation, resulting in an increased quantity, decreased viscosity, and favorable electrolyte content of the cervical mucus. These are the ideal characteristics for sperm penetration. **The average ejaculate contains 2 to 5 mL of semen; 40 to 300 million sperm may be deposited in the vagina, 50% to 90% of which are morphologically normal.** Fewer than 200 sperm achieve proximity to the egg. Only one sperm fertilizes a single egg released at ovulation.

The major loss of sperm occurs in the vagina following coitus, with expulsion of the semen from the introitus playing an important role. In addition, digestion of sperm by vaginal enzymes, destruction by vaginal acidity, phagocytosis of sperm along the reproductive tract, and further loss from passage through the fallopian tube into the peritoneal cavity all diminish the number of sperm capable of achieving fertilization.

Those sperm that do migrate from the alkaline environment of the semen to the alkaline environment of the cervical mucus exuding from the cervical os are directed along channels of lower-viscosity mucus into the cervical crypts where they are stored for later ascent. Two waves of passage to the tubes may occur. Uterine contractions, probably facilitated by prostaglandin in the seminal plasma, propel sperm to the tubes within 5 minutes. Some evidence indicates that these sperm may not be as capable of fertilization as those that arrive later largely under their own power. Sperm may be found within the peritoneal cavity for long periods, but it is not known whether they are capable of fertilization. **Ova are usually fertilized within 12 hours of ovulation.**

Capacitation is the physiologic change that sperm must undergo in the female reproductive tract before fertilization. Human sperm can also undergo capacitation after a short incubation in defined culture media without residence in the female reproductive tract, which allows for in vitro fertilization (Chapter 35).

The acrosome reaction is one of the principal components of capacitation. The acrosome, a modified lysosome, lies over the sperm head as a kind of "chemical drill-bit" designed to enable the sperm to burrow its way into the oocyte (Figure 4-7). The overlying plasma membrane becomes unstable and eventually breaks down, releasing hyaluronidase, a neuraminidase, and corona-dispersing enzyme. Acrosin, bound to the remaining inner acrosomal membrane, may play a role in the final penetration of the zona pellucida. The latter contains species-specific receptors for the plasma membrane. After traversing the zona, the postacrosomal region of the sperm head fuses with the oocyte membrane, and the sperm nucleus is incorporated into the ooplasm. This process triggers release of the contents of the cortical granules that lie at the periphery of the oocyte. This cortical reaction results in changes in the oocyte membrane and zona pellucida that prevent the entrance of further sperm into the oocyte.

The process of capacitation may be inhibited by a factor in the semen, thus preserving maximum release of enzyme to allow effective penetration of the corona and zona pellucida surrounding the oocyte. The cellular investments of the oocyte may further activate the sperm, thus facilitating penetration to the oocyte membrane. The corona is not required for normal fertilization to occur, as its removal has no effect on the rate or quality of fertilization in vitro. The major function of these surrounding granulosa cells and their intercellular matrix may be to serve as a sticky mass that causes adherence to the ovarian surface and to the mucosa of the tubal epithelium.

Following penetration of the oocyte, the sperm nucleus decondenses to form the male pronucleus, which approaches and finally fuses with the female pronucleus at syngamy to form the zygote. **Fertilization restores the diploid number of chromosomes and determines the sex of the zygote.** In couples with infertility resulting from severe sperm abnormalities, fertilization and subsequent pregnancy can be successfully achieved after the injection of a single sperm, with or without its tail, into the cytoplasm of the oocyte (Chapter 35).

CLEAVAGE, MORULA, BLASTOCYST

Following fertilization, cleavage occurs. This consists of a rapid succession of mitotic divisions that produce a mulberry-like mass known as a morula. **Fluid is secreted by the outer cells of the morula, and a single fluid-filled cavity develops, known as the blastocyst cavity.** An inner-cell mass can be defined, attached eccentrically to the outer layer of flattened cells; the latter becomes the trophoblast. The embryo at this stage of development is called a **blastocyst,** and the zona pellucida disappears at about this time. A blastocyst cell can be removed and tested for genetic imperfections without harming further development of the conceptus.

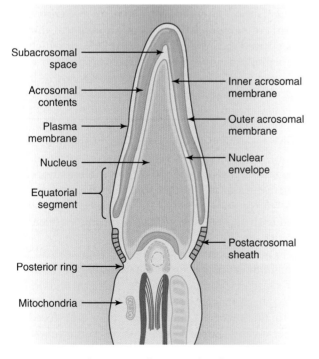

Figure 4-7. The sperm head.

Labels (left): Subacrosomal space, Acrosomal contents, Plasma membrane, Nucleus, Equatorial segment, Posterior ring, Mitochondria

Labels (right): Inner acrosomal membrane, Outer acrosomal membrane, Nuclear envelope, Postacrosomal sheath

IMPLANTATION

The fertilized ovum reaches the endometrial cavity about 3 days after ovulation.

Hormones influence egg transportation. Estrogen causes "locking" of the egg in the tube, and progesterone reverses this action. Prostaglandins have diverse effects. Prostaglandin E relaxes the tubal isthmus, whereas prostaglandin F stimulates tubal motility. It is unknown whether abnormalities of egg transportation play a role in infertility, but in animal studies, acceleration of ovum transportation causes a failure of implantation. Additional cytokines may be released by the tubal epithelium and embryo to enhance embryo transportation and development and to signal the impending implantation to the endometrium.

Initial embryonic development primarily occurs in the ampullary portion of the Fallopian tube with subsequent rapid transit through the isthmus. This process takes approximately 3 days. **On reaching the uterine cavity, the embryo undergoes further development for 2 to 3 days before implanting.** The zona is shed and the blastocyst adheres to the endometrium, a process that is probably dependent on the changes in the surface characteristics of the embryo, such as electrical charge and glycoprotein content. A variety of proteolytic enzymes may play a role in separating the endometrial cells and digesting the intercellular matrix.

Initially, the wall of the blastocyst facing the uterine lumen consists of a single layer of flattened cells. The thicker opposite wall has two zones: the trophoblast and the inner cell mass (embryonic disk). The latter differentiates at 7.5 days into a thick plate of primitive "dorsal" ectoderm and an underlying layer of "ventral" endoderm. **A group of small cells appears between the embryonic disk and trophoblast. A space develops within them, which becomes the amniotic cavity.**

Under the influence of progesterone, decidual changes occur in the endometrium of the pregnant uterus. The endometrial stromal cells enlarge and form polygonal or round decidual cells. The nuclei become round and vesicular, and the cytoplasm becomes clear, slightly basophilic, and surrounded by a translucent membrane. During pregnancy, the decidua thickens to a depth of 5 to 10 mm. The *decidua basalis* is the decidual layer directly beneath the site of implantation. Recent information suggests that integrins, a class of proteins involved in cell-to-cell adherence, peak within the endometrium at the time of implantation and may play a significant role. Additional growth factors act in a synergistic fashion to enhance the implantation process. The **decidua capsularis** is the layer overlying the developing ovum and separating it from the rest of the uterine cavity. The *decidua vera* (parietalis) is the remaining lining of the uterine cavity (Figure 4-8). The space between the decidua capsularis and decidua vera is obliterated by the 4th month with fusion of the capsularis and vera.

The decidua basalis enters into the formation of the basal plate of the placenta. The spongy zone of the decidua basalis consists mainly of arteries and dilated veins. The decidua basalis is invaded extensively by trophoblastic giant cells, which first appear as early as the time of implantation. Minute levels of human chorionic gonadotropin (hCG) appear in the maternal serum at this time. **Nitabuch's layer** is a zone of fibrinoid degeneration where the trophoblast meets the decidua. When the decidua is defective, as in placenta accreta, Nitabuch's layer is absent.

When the free blastocyst contacts the endometrium after 4 to 6 days, the syncytiotrophoblast, a syncytium

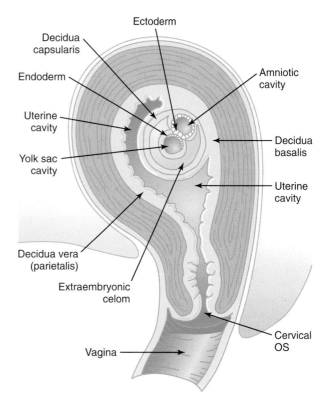

Figure 4-8. Early stage of implantation.

of cells, differentiates from the cytotrophoblast. **At about 9 days, lacunae, irregular fluid-filled spaces, appear within the thickened trophoblastic syncytium.** This is soon followed by the appearance of maternal blood within the lacunae, as maternal tissue is destroyed and the walls of the mother's capillaries are eroded.

PLACENTA

As the blastocyst burrows deeper into the endometrium, the trophoblastic strands branch to form the solid, primitive villi traversing the lacunae. The villi, which are first distinguished about the 12th day after fertilization, are the essential structures of the definitive placenta. Located originally over the entire surface of the ovum, the villi later disappear except over the most deeply implanted portion, the future placental site.

Embryonic mesenchyme first appears as isolated cells within the cavity of the blastocyst. When the cavity is completely lined with mesoderm, it is termed the **extraembryonic celom.** Its membrane, the **chorion,** is composed of trophoblast and mesenchyme. When the solid trophoblast is invaded by a mesenchymal core, presumably derived from cytotrophoblast, secondary villi are formed.

Maternal venous sinuses are tapped about 15 days after fertilization. By the 17th day, both fetal and maternal blood vessels are functional, and a placental circulation is established. The fetal circulation is completed when the blood vessels of the embryo are connected with chorionic blood vessels that are formed from cytotrophoblast. Proliferation of cellular trophoblasts at the tips of the villi produces cytotrophoblastic columns that progressively extend through the peripheral syncytium. Cytotrophoblastic extensions from columns of adjacent villi join together to form the cytotrophoblastic shell, which attaches the villi to the decidua. By the 19th day of development, the cytotrophoblastic shell is thick. Villi contain a central core of chorionic mesoderm, where blood vessels are developing, and an external covering of syncytiotrophoblasts or syncytium.

By 3 weeks, the relationship of the chorion to the decidua is evident. The greater part of the chorion, denuded of villi, is designated the chorion laeve (smooth chorion). Until near the end of the 3rd month, the chorion laeve remains separated from the amnion by the extraembryonic celomic cavity. Thereafter, amnion and chorion are in intimate contact. The villi adjacent to the decidua basalis enlarge and branch (*chorion frondosum*) and progressively assume the form of the fully developed human placenta (Figure 4-9). **By 16 to 20 weeks, the chorion laeve contacts and fuses with the decidua vera, thus obliterating most of the uterine cavity.**

AMNIOTIC FLUID

Throughout normal pregnancy, the amniotic fluid compartment allows the fetus room for growth, movement, and development. Without amniotic fluid, the uterus would contract and compress the fetus. **In cases of leakage of amniotic fluid early in the first trimester, the fetus may develop structural abnormalities including facial distortion, limb reduction, and abdominal wall defects secondary to uterine compression.**

Toward midpregnancy (20 weeks), the amniotic fluid becomes increasingly important for fetal pulmonary development. The latter requires a fluid-filled respiratory tract and the ability of the fetus to "breathe" in utero, moving amniotic fluid into and out of the lungs. **The absence of adequate amniotic fluid during midpregnancy is associated with pulmonary hypoplasia at birth, which is often incompatible with life.**

The amniotic fluid also has a protective role for the fetus. It contains antibacterial activity and acts to inhibit the growth of potentially pathogenic bacteria. During labor and delivery, the amniotic fluid continues to serve as a protective medium for the fetus, aiding dilatation of the cervix. The premature infant, with its fragile head, may benefit most from delivery with the amniotic membranes intact (en caul). In addition, the amniotic fluid may serve as a means of communication for the fetus. Fetal maturity and readiness for delivery may be signaled to the maternal uterus via fetal urinary hormones excreted into the amniotic fluid.

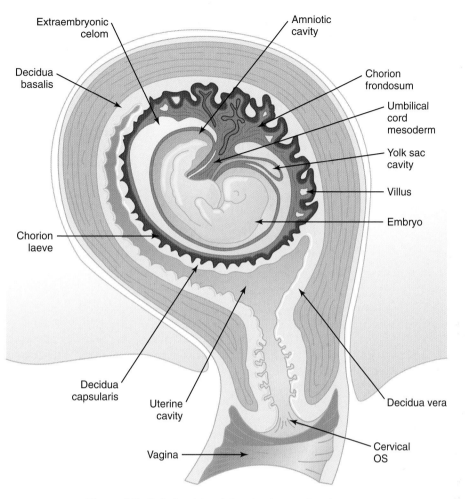

Figure 4-9. Relationship of the chorion to the placenta.

Suggested Reading

Adashi E: The ovarian cycle. *In* Yen SSC, Jaffe RB (eds): Reproductive Endocrinology, 4th ed. Philadelphia, WB Saunders, 1997.

Speroff L, Glass RH, Kase NG: Clinical Gynecologic Endocrinology and Fertility, 6th ed. Baltimore, Williams & Wilkins, 1999.

Strauss J, Gurpide E: The endometrium: Regulation and dysfunction. *In* Yen SSC, Jaffe RB (eds): Reproductive Endocrinology, 4th ed. Philadelphia, WB Saunders, 1997.

Thorner M, Vince M, Horvath E, et al: The anterior pituitary. *In* Wilson JD, Foster DW (eds): Williams Textbook of Endocrinology, 8th ed. Philadelphia, WB Saunders, 1992.

Yen SSC: The human menstrual cycle: Neuroendocrine regulation. *In* Yen SSC, Jaffe RB (eds): Reproductive Endocrinology, 4th ed. Philadelphia, WB Saunders, 1997.

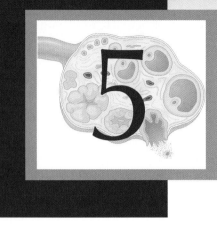

Clinical Performance Improvement: Assessing the Quality and Safety of Women's Health Care

Robert C. Reiter, Linda Yielding, and Paul A. Gluck

Beginning with the pioneering work of Ernest Codman to assess the "end results" of surgical interventions and medical errors, measurements of the quality of health care have been available to health care professionals since the early part of the 20th century. Mortality and morbidity conferences, tissue committees, and tumor boards are a few examples. Hospital accreditation groups, such as the American College of Surgeons, the Joint Commission for the Accreditation of Healthcare Organizations (JCAHO) and especially groups such as the American College of Obstetricians and Gynecologists (ACOG) have a long history of establishing standards and guidelines that are recommended to ensure appropriate medical care. **The effort to ensure compliance with accepted standards of medical practice and patient safety has been established as quality assurance (QA).**

QA traditionally has emphasized internal or self-imposed quality review. This method has generally used retrospective assessment of health care processes and short-term inpatient outcomes to identify substandard care by a small percentage of health care providers, and has been termed the *bad apple approach*. Improving quality by emphasizing the ongoing assessment of a greater portion of daily medical care is obviously a better way to improve performance. **This prospective process, referred to as continuous quality improvement (CQI), relies on a multidisciplinary team approach to identify opportunities for improvement within the health care organiza-**tion or system of care. **This newer process pays less attention to blaming individual doctors for low quality and puts more emphasis on improving the system of care.**

Quality assurance, continuous improvement, and clinical innovation are depicted graphically in Figure 5-1. Collectively, these three clinical improvement strategies, when appropriately applied, serve to optimize the probability of a successful health care outcome.

HEALTH CARE QUALITY ASSESSMENT

Quality assessment traditionally evaluates unintended and wasteful variation (differences in how and which diagnostic tests and procedures are performed). Analyses of variations in health care have been applied to virtually all major surgical procedures, including hysterectomy and cesarean delivery. **Substantial variation has been shown in the performance of many surgical procedures as well as in the management of medical conditions such as acute myocardial infarction and pneumonia.** Furthermore, these analyses have documented significant wasteful variation not only in the usage rates of selected health care procedures but also in their costs and outcomes. **Analysis of usage variation has helped to focus attention on the critical need for clinical practice guidelines that are based on measured outcomes of care (so-called "evidence-based practice").**

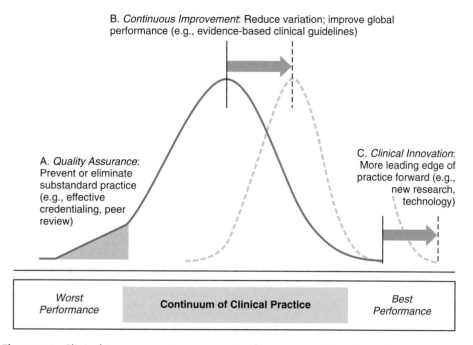

Figure 5-1. Clinical improvement strategies. Graphic representation of quality assurance (*A*); continuous improvement (*B*); and clinical innovation (*C*).

EFFICACY, EFFECTIVENESS, AND EFFICIENCY

Efficacy refers to the way medical and surgical procedures work in the best of hands under ideal conditions. By contrast, effectiveness refers to more realistic results in actual clinical practice. One of the goals of CQI (referred to as *performance improvement* by the JCAHO) is to reduce the difference between efficacy and effectiveness by adopting "best practice" protocols.

To assess the effectiveness of health care and health care procedures meaningfully, **the effectiveness of the care being assessed must be compared both to the outcome expected if no treatment were given, and to the expected outcome with optimal care or "best practice."** Much of the information that we currently have about the effectiveness of health care procedures does not consider either the natural course of a disease or what generally happens in common practice.

Efficiency or cost-effectiveness refers to effectiveness with the least waste in terms of complications and resources. The goal of CQI is optimal value, where value is defined as quality divided by its cost.

STRUCTURE, PROCESS, AND OUTCOME

Health care assessment is often based upon the evaluation of the structure, processes and outcomes of diagnostic and treatment services. **Structure** refers to the quality of resources, equipment, and health care providers. **Process** refers to the way a procedure or course of action is carried out, that is, how the mechanisms, procedures, and resources available are brought to bear on a particular health care problem. **Outcome** refers to the complications, costs, and short- and long-term results of a specific procedure, including the patient's health status and satisfaction after treatment.

Traditionally, QA has tended to focus on the assessment of the structure and process of care, and only on short-term outcomes, such as postoperative morbidity. Longer-term clinical outcomes, such as functional status, well-being, and other health-related quality of life measurements, have been evaluated less frequently. A clinical or health outcome is something that a patient can experience, value, and assess without professional interpretation. These endpoints are preferred for quality assessment. Table 5-1 lists some clinical or health outcomes with corre-

Table 5-1. Clinical or health outcomes (which are preferred for assessing quality) and their corresponding intermediate or surrogate end points	
Clinical or Health Outcomes and End Points (Preferred)	Intermediate or Surrogate Outcomes or End Points (Less Useful)
Longevity, angina, heart attack	Cholesterol level
Stroke	Blood pressure
Take healthy baby home	Positive pregnancy test
Mortality from flu	Percentage of patients receiving flu vaccine
Need for blood transfusion	Estimated blood loss

Modified from Gambone JC, Reiter RC: Quality assessment and improvement. *In* Berek JS, Adashi EY, Hilliard PA (eds): Novak's Gynecology, 12th ed. Baltimore, Williams & Wilkins, 1996, pp 33–49.

sponding intermediate outcomes. Frequently, intermediate outcomes are used as surrogates for success without actually ever measuring whether an impact has occurred on the more relevant clinical or health outcome.

NEWER MEASURES AND REPORTING FOR HEALTH CARE QUALITY

Health services researchers have validated and are using newer methods for the measurement of quality in health care. Short inventories for measuring health-related quality of life and functional status before, during, and after treatment, such as the SF-36 (short form with 36 items) and the newer SF-12 (short form with 12 items) are currently being utilized to measure longer-term health outcomes.

Over the past decade, **concerns regarding both costs and quality of health care have lead to calls for public reporting of hospital- and even physician-specific quality data.** Many states have subsequently mandated public reporting of so-called **"Quality Report Cards,"** usually consisting of hospital- and physician-specific crude mortality data. Unfortunately, most of these reports have been derived from publicly available billing data, which are easily accessed but were not designed for assessing quality of care. As a result **these reports have not significantly impacted consumer choice or quality of care.**

HEALTH CARE QUALITY IMPROVEMENT

The mandate from payers (government and employers) and the public to measure and improve health care services is clear. Unfortunately, change based on adoption of national standards derived from evidence-based practice and randomized controlled trials (RCTs) alone may be too expensive and slow to meet this mandate. Furthermore, the results from RCTs may not always establish how diagnostic and therapeutic procedures actually work in clinical practice. **For these reasons, health care organizations and physician groups must develop the tools to identify and adopt best practices and improve clinical outcomes locally.**

Paralleling the evolving science of outcomes assessment is the evolving science of outcomes improvement. Health care organizations have adapted successful models of continuous quality improvement from industry, as well as newer research or "evidence-based" models of care. Adoption of "best practice" models of care must be based on continuous reassessment of evolving practice, research, and innovation. **Methods such as the FOCUS-PDCA cycle (Figure 5-2), originally developed at Bell Laboratories to test small incremental changes, have been applied to health care processes and used successfully for CQI.** Use of such a standardized improvement process has been shown to improve the effectiveness of clinical improvement efforts and accelerate the pace of change. Several other key clinical improvement tools are highlighted below.

CLINICAL GUIDELINES

Unintended variation in health care processes generally connotes, and frequently results in, lower quality of care. Clinical guidelines, also referred to as protocols, practice parameters, algorithms, and clinical pathways, are tools that have been developed to reduce wasteful variation in the performance of medical

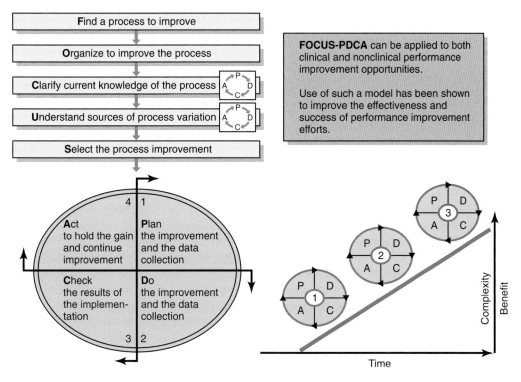

Figure 5-2. FOCUS-PDCA. A continuous improvement model to guide the process of making improvements now widely used in health care. *From Langley DJ, Nolan KM, Nolan TW: The Foundation of Improvement, Silver Springs, MD, API Publishing, 1992.*

and surgical procedures and to improve outcomes of care.

A guideline is a summary of optimal care processes for a medical condition stated in general terms so as to allow sufficient variation for patient differences and preferences. Previously, guidelines were derived largely by consensus and the opinion of experts. More recently, these "authority-based" guidelines have been replaced by so-called "evidence-based" guidelines, which are based on objective evaluation of outcomes and the available medical literature. Adoption of evidence-based guidelines, such as those produced by the US Agency for Health care Research and Quality, the US Preventive Services Task Force, and the international Cochrane Collaborative, has been shown to improve health care outcomes and reduce costs. However, their acceptance has not been widespread in the United States, in part because of the financial consequences of their adoption.

Clinical pathways (also known as critical paths or care maps) are broad, detailed multidisciplinary guidelines that organize, sequence, and time the best or ideal management strategy, usually for a specific condition or procedure. For example, a pathway for patients undergoing hysterectomy details diagnostic and therapeutic milestones that are expected on each day of the patient's hospital stay. About 80% to 90% of patients are expected to stay on the pathway during treatment.

Disease management protocols are comprehensive approaches to patient care for an entire episode of illness (inpatient and outpatient). A disease management model provides guidelines for the continuous tracking and modification of the care plan, facilitation of care across clinical services, confirmation of service delivery, and evaluation of variances in practice and outcomes.

PATIENT-FOCUSED CARE

Patients are the ultimate consumers of medical and surgical care, and meeting their expectations should be the goal of health care providers.

Involvement of patients in the actual decision-making process in elective medical and surgical care is essential for customer satisfaction, decreasing medical malpractice litigation and improving clinical outcomes. Because **more than 80% of health care decisions involve weighing benefits and risks**, better methods to inform and involve patients in their care should be developed and implemented.

A model of collaboration is recommended. This avoids the extremes of complete patient autonomy on the one hand and the more common patient abdication with total physician control on the other. **Research indicates that about 90% of patients want as much information as possible and prefer to be involved when there is a therapeutic or diagnostic choice.**

Newer high-technology approaches, such as computerized interactive video disk programs, have been developed to facilitate the process of collaborative decision making. These supplements, while helpful, should not take the place of a non-hurried conversation between the patient and the physician. **For most health care decisions, collaborative choice should eventually replace the far less interactive and less effective process of informed consent,** which was developed primarily to avoid litigation.

PATIENT SAFETY

Safety in health care is not a new concept. Facilities have had safety programs in place since the early 1900s, but these programs have traditionally focused on emergency preparedness, environmental safety, security, and infection control. The term **"patient safety,"** meaning avoidance of medical error, was first coined by the American Society of Anesthesiologists in 1984, when they inaugurated the Anesthesia Patient Safety Foundation to give assurance that the effects of anesthesia would not harm patients.

Medical errors now rank as the fifth leading cause of death in the United States. The Institute of Medicine (IOM) published an alarming report in 1999 called *To Err Is Human: Building a Safer Health System*. This report estimated that between 44,000 and 98,000 Americans die each year as a result of medical errors. Table 5-2 compares the risk of death from medical errors during hospital admissions to lifestyle-related risks and common women's health risks. **Error is defined as failure of a planned action to be completed as intended (e.g., failing to operate when obvious signs of appendicitis are present)** or the **use of a wrong plan to achieve an aim (e.g., wrong diagnosis, wrong medication administered).** Medication errors alone, occurring either in or out of the hospital, are estimated to account for over 7,000 deaths annually. According to the National Council on Patient Information and Education, "more than 2/3 of all physician visits end with a prescription." An estimated 39% to 49% of all medication errors occur at the stage of drug ordering. Patient noncompliance also contributes to medical errors.

In 2001, more than 100,000 medication errors were reported to the United States Pharmacopoeia (USP) MedMARx error tracking service. Because reporting was voluntary and limited to 368 facilities, the scope of the problem is likely to be much larger. A preventable Adverse Drug Event (ADE) is one type of medication error. Administering the incorrect drug, an incorrect dose, wrong frequency, or incorrect route may cause an ADE.

The drug that cures one patient's condition may be the cause of another patient's injury or death due to an adverse drug reaction (ADR). The latter may account for 1 out of 5 injuries or deaths for hospitalized patients. ADRs commonly occur from an overdose, a side effect, or an interaction among several concomitantly administered drugs. In order to minimize ADRs, health-care providers should avoid the following actions:

1. Prescribing unnecessary medications
2. Treating mild side effects of one drug with a second, more toxic drug
3. Misinterpreting a drug's side effect for a new medical problem and prescribing another medication
4. Prescribing a medication when there is any uncertainty about dosing

In the absence of automated systems, providers should strive to write legibly and use only approved abbreviations and dose expressions. Table 5-3 lists abbreviations and dose expressions identified by the IOM as more likely to lead to errors. Most organizations have adopted this list, either partially or in its entirety, as a means of reducing medication errors.

FUTURE AUTOMATION

Computerized Physician Order Entry (CPOE) has been found to decrease serious medical errors by 55% and reduce potential undetected ADEs by 84%. Properly designed computerized systems

Table 5-2. Risks in perspective	
Activity	Estimated Chance of Death in a Year
Risk of death from medical error during inpatient hospitalization	1 in 500
Risks for men and women of all ages who participate in	
Motorcycling	1 in 1,000
Automobile driving	1 in 6,000
Power boating	1 in 6,000
Rock climbing	1 in 7,500
Playing football	1 in 25,000
Canoeing	1 in 100,000
Risks for women aged 15–44 years	
Using tampons	1 in 350,000
Having sexual intercourse (PID)	1 in 50,000
Preventing pregnancy	
Using birth control pills	
Nonsmoker	1 in 63,000
Smoker	1 in 16,000
Using IUDs	1 in 100,000
Using diaphragm, condom, or spermicide	None
Using fertility awareness methods	None
Undergoing sterilization	
Laparoscopic tubal ligation	1 in 67,000
Hysterectomy	1 in 1,600
Vasectomy	1 in 300,000
Continuing pregnancy	1 in 11,000
Terminating pregnancy	
Legal abortion	
Before 9 weeks	1 in 260,000
Between 9 and 12 weeks	1 in 100,000
Between 13 and 15 weeks	1 in 34,000
After 15 weeks	1 in 10,200

Data from Hatcher RA, Trussell J, Stewart F, et al: Contraceptive Technology, 16th ed. New York, Irvington Publishers, 1992.

improve physician workflow by providing interactive real-time decision-making support, consent for protocols and guidelines, and on-line dosing information. Unfortunately, poorly designed CPOE systems have the potential to actually increase medication errors. Bar coding may become essential for the safe dispensing and administration of medications and for documentation of their usage. **Bar coding has demonstrated a 74% improvement in the rate of errors caused by administration of the wrong medication, 57% improvement in errors caused by incorrect doses, 91% improvement in wrong-patient errors, and a 92% improvement in wrong-time errors.**

The Leapfrog Group, a consortium of Fortune 500 companies and other large health care purchasers, **has recommended three interventions: the use of CPOE, staffing ICUs with critical care specialists,** **and referral to "centers of excellence"** as means of improving quality of care and patient safety nationwide. Their goal is to recognize and reward health care providers who meet these three standards, which in turn will improve patient outcomes and decrease health care costs.

MEDICAL ERROR REPORTING

According to the Agency for Healthcare Research & Quality (AHRQ), "Reporting is an important component of systems to improve patient safety." Incident reporting is an important and inexpensive method to detect medical error and prevent future adverse events. Unfortunately, this method may fail to effectively impact clinical outcomes, as most hospital reporting systems do not capture the majority of errors. Reporting should be considered a quality

Table 5-3. Examples of dangerous abbreviations/dose expressions

Abbreviation/Dose Expression	Intended Meaning	Misinterpretation
AU	aurio uterque (each ear)	Mistaken for OU (oculo uterque—each eye).
D/C	discharge, discontinue	Premature discontinuation of medications when D/C (intended to mean "discharge") has been misinterpreted as "discontinued" when followed by a list of drugs.
µg	microgram	Mistaken for "mg" when handwritten.
o.d. or OD	once daily	Misinterpreted as "right eye" (OD—oculus dexter) and administration of oral medications in the eye.
TIW or tiw	three times a week	Mistaken as "three times a day."
per os	orally	The "os" can be mistaken for "left eye."
q.d. or QD	every day	Mistaken as q.i.d., especially if the period after the "q" or the tail of the "q" is misunderstood as an "i."
qn	nightly or at bedtime	Misinterpreted as "qh" (every hour).
qhs	nightly at bedtime	Misread as every hour.
q6PM, etc.	every evening at 6 PM	Misread as every 6 hours.
q.o.d. or QOD	every other day	Misinterpreted as "q.d." (daily) or "q.i.d." (four times daily) if the "o" is poorly written.
sub q	subcutaneous	The "q" has been mistaken for "every" (e.g., one heparin dose ordered "sub q 2 hours before surgery" misunderstood as every 2 hours before surgery).
SC	subcutaneous	Mistaken for SL (sublingual).
U or u	unit	Read as a zero (0) or a four (4), causing a 10-fold overdose or greater (4U seen as "40" or 4u seen as 44").
IU	international unit	Misread as IV (intravenous).
cc	cubic centimeters	Misread as "U" (units).
x3d	for 3 days	Mistaken for "three doses."
BT	bedtime	Mistaken as "BID" (twice daily).
ss	sliding scale (insulin) or ½ (apothecary)	Mistaken for "55."
> and <	greater than and less than	Mistakenly used opposite of intended.
/ (slash mark)	separates two doses or indicates "per"	Misunderstood as the number 1 ("25 unit/10 units" read as "110" units.
Name letters and dose numbers run together (e.g., Inderal 40 mg)	Inderal 40 mg	Misread as Inderal 140 mg.
Zero after decimal point (1.0)	1 mg	Misread as 10 mg if the decimal point is not seen.
No zero before decimal dose (.5 mg)	0.5 mg	Misread as 5 mg.

improvement process rather than a performance evaluation method.

A founding member of The National Patient Safety Foundation and The National Patient Safety Partnership, JCAHO has formed a coalition with the USP, the AMA, and the AHA to create patient safety reporting principles. Recognizing that fear of liability discourages error reporting, JCAHO has advised Congress that federal statutory protection must be afforded to those who report medical error. **An anonymous nonpunitive environment will encourage reporting.** Many states have implemented mandatory reporting systems for selected medical errors to improve patient safety and reduce errors. Others consider incident reporting and analysis as peer review activities immune from liability. **The IOM report recommends that health care providers be required to report errors that result in serious harm. Information collected should be made available to the public.** AHRQ publishes case summaries of reported medical errors and near misses on their web site. An example of an Obstetrics and Gynecology case reported to AHRQ is summarized in Box 5-1. A more detailed commentary and other examples of specific cases can be found on the Internet at www.webmm.ahrq.gov/. Click on "OB/GYN" in the current case and commentaries box.

DISCLOSURE OF MEDICAL ERROR

The National Patient Safety Foundation (NPSF) was one of the first organizations to address the issue of disclosure. Their position, finalized in November 2000, states, **"When a health care injury occurs, the patient and the family or representative are entitled to a prompt explanation of how the injury occurred and its short- and long-term effects.** When an error contributed to the injury, the patient and the family or representative should receive a truthful and compassionate explanation about the error and

---

Box 5-1. Case history: Laparoscopy with complications

CASE SUMMARY

A 28-year-old multiparous obese female presented for laparoscopic tubal ligation. The patient had undesired fertility and was sure of her decision for permanent sterilization. She consented to a laparoscopy.

During the procedure, poor visualization and inadequate gas expansion led the team to believe that they had not yet entered the peritoneal cavity. Replacement of the trocar and laparoscope were performed. The anesthesiologist then noted a rapid decrease in the patient's blood pressure and increasing tachycardia, indicating a possible vascular injury. Conversion to open laparotomy revealed bleeding due to a laceration of the right common iliac artery. Pressure was applied, and vascular surgery was consulted. End-to-end anastomosis of the artery was successfully performed, followed by the planned bilateral tubal ligation. The patient had an uncomplicated postoperative course. Serial Dopplers of distal arterial pulses were normal, and the patient was discharged home in stable condition.

The main operator was a trainee, supervised by a senior attending. The trainee was relatively inexperienced in the procedure. The patient was obese, which added somewhat to the complexity, but nevertheless the procedure was considered routine and the complication unexpected.

FINDINGS AND CONCLUSIONS

Major vascular injury, as occurred in this case, is not a rare complication of laparoscopic surgery. Prospective studies have reported that injury to the bowel or major vessels during laparoscopic procedures occurs in about 3 per 1000 cases. Vascular injury to the major vessels is second only to neglected bowel injuries as a cause of death in laparoscopic surgery. Such vascular injuries carry a reported mortality of 6% to 11%. There is probably a great degree of underreporting of vascular injury.

Laparoscopy is a procedure in which attention to technical details is especially important. While these details need not be enumerated here, several generalizations seem appropriate:

- Ensuring stabilization of the abdomen before trocar insertion is essential through adequate pneumoperitoneum and sufficient anesthetic paralysis or, if necessary, use of towel clips.
- Accepted procedures must be followed to ensure adequacy of the incision, angle of insertion, the amount of force used, and so on.
- If the initial attempt at trocar insertion fails, reestablish pneumoperitoneum before reinserting the trocar.
- Trainees should develop tactile and neuromuscular skills through practice on simulators, cadavers, or animals prior to initial human experience.

the remedies available to the patient. They should be informed that the factors involved in the injury will be investigated so that steps can be taken to reduce the likelihood of similar injury to other patients."

In 2001, JCAHO began requiring hospitals to disclose any serious harm caused by medical errors to the harmed parties. Disclosing error can be very difficult for physicians because they may struggle with intense feelings of incompetence, betrayal of the patient, and fear of litigation. **Studies suggest that physicians with good relationship skills are less likely to get sued. Furthermore, suits settle rapidly and for less money if errors are disclosed early. Simple rules for disclosing errors include: admit the mistake, acknowledge the listener's anger, speak slowly, and stop frequently to allow the listener to talk.** Tell the person that an error has occurred and apologize. Usually, the attending physician is the one who should disclose. Medical students should not disclose, because they may not be prepared to offer advice on necessary follow-up.

Regulatory, economic and public pressure makes the assessment and improvement of quality and safety essential in the delivery of women's health care. Optimal health outcomes can only be achieved when principles from continuous quality assessment are combined with the systems approach of safety science and guidelines from evidence-based medicine. **With advances in medical science, changes in the delivery of health care, new technology, and better understanding of the causes of medical errors, the quality process must be dynamic, continuous, and patient centered.**

Suggested Reading

American College of Obstetricians and Gynecologists (ACOG) Committee Opinion: Physician responsibility under managed care, No. 170. Washington, DC, ACOG, April 1996.

Berwick DM: Continuous improvement as an ideal in health care. N Engl J Med 310:53, 1989.

Committee on Quality of Health Care in America. Institute of Medicine: "To Err is Human: Building a Safer Health System." Washington, DC, National Academy Press, 1999.

Committee on Quality of Health Care in America. Institute of Medicine. "Crossing the Quality Chasm: A New Health System for the 21st Century." Washington, DC, National Academy Press, 2001.

Donabedian A: The quality of care: How can it be assessed? JAMA 260:1743, 1988.

PART TWO | Obstetrics

Brian J. Koos

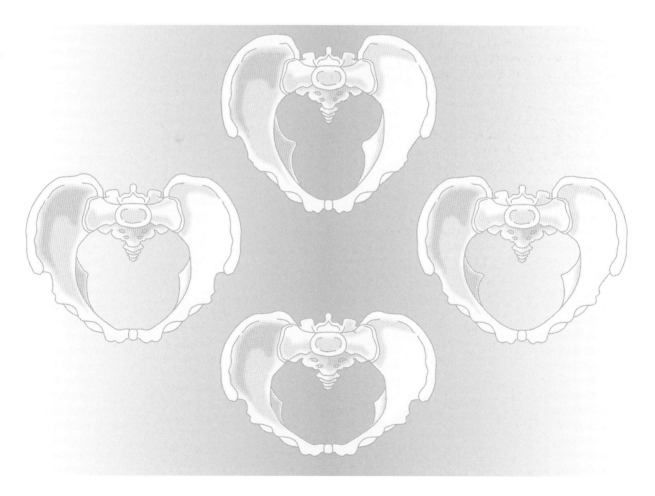

6

Endocrinology of Pregnancy and Parturition

Mary E. Carsten and Michael C. Lu

Women undergo major endocrinologic and metabolic changes that establish, maintain, and terminate pregnancy. The aim of these changes is the safe delivery of an infant that can survive outside of the uterus. The maturation of the fetus and the adaptation of the mother are regulated by a variety of hormones. This chapter deals with the properties, functions, and interactions of the most important of these hormones as they relate to pregnancy and parturition.

FETOPLACENTAL UNIT

The concept of the fetoplacental unit is based on observations of the interactions of hormones of fetal and maternal origin. **The fetoplacental unit largely controls the endocrine events of the pregnancy.** Although the fetus, the placenta, and the mother all provide input, the fetus appears to play the most active and controlling role of the three in its growth and maturation, and probably also in the events that lead to parturition.

FETUS

The adrenal gland is the major endocrine component of the fetus. In midpregnancy, it is larger than the fetal kidney. The fetal adrenal cortex consists of an outer definitive, or adult, zone and an inner, fetal, zone. The definitive zone later develops into the three components of the adult adrenal cortex: the zona fasciculata, the zona glomerulosa, and the zona reticularis. During fetal life, the definitive zone secretes primarily glucocorticoids and mineralocorticoids. **The fetal zone, at term, constitutes 80% of the fetal gland and primarily secretes androgens during fetal life.** It involutes following delivery and completely disappears by the end of the first year of life. The fetal adrenal medulla synthesizes and stores catecholamines. It is poorly developed, and its role during fetal growth and maturation is not known.

PLACENTA

The placenta produces both steroid and peptide hormones in amounts that vary with gestational age. Precursors for progesterone synthesis come from the maternal circulation. **Because of the lack of the enzyme 17α-hydroxylase, the human placenta cannot directly convert progesterone to estrogen** but must use androgens, largely from the fetal adrenal gland, as its source of precursor for estrogen production.

MOTHER

The mother adapts to pregnancy through major endocrinologic and metabolic changes. **The ovaries produce progesterone in early pregnancy** until its production shifts to the placenta. **The maternal hypothalamus and posterior pituitary produces and releases oxytocin,** which causes uterine contractions and milk letdown. **The anterior pituitary produces prolactin,** which stimulates milk production. Several important changes in maternal metabolism are described later in the chapter.

HORMONES

The fetoplacental unit produces a variety of hormones to support the maturation of the fetus and the adaptation of the mother. Some of the major peptide and steroid hormones, as well as other transmitters involved in pregnancy and parturition, are described later.

PEPTIDE HORMONES
Human Chorionic Gonadotropin

Human chorionic gonadotropin (hCG) is secreted by trophoblastic cells of the placenta and maintains pregnancy. This hormone is a glycoprotein with a molecular weight of 40,000 to 45,000 and **consists of two subunits: alpha (α) and beta (β).** The α subunit is shared with luteinizing hormone (LH) and thyroid-stimulating hormone (TSH). **The specificity of hCG is related to its β subunit (β-hCG),** and a radioimmunoassay that is specific for the β subunit allows positive identification of hCG. The presence of hCG at times other than pregnancy signals the presence of an hCG-producing tumor, usually a hydatidiform mole, choriocarcinoma, or embryonal carcinoma (a germ cell tumor).

During pregnancy, hCG begins to rise 8 days after ovulation (9 days after the mid-cycle LH peak). This provides the basis for virtually all immunologic or chemical pregnancy tests. With continuing pregnancy, hCG values peak at 60 to 90 days and then decline to a moderate, more constant level. **For the first 6 to 8 weeks of pregnancy, hCG maintains the corpus luteum and thereby ensures continued progesterone output until progesterone production shifts to the placenta.** Titers of hCG are usually abnormally low in patients with an ectopic pregnancy or threatened abortion and abnormally high in those with trophoblastic disease (e.g., moles or choriocarcinoma). This hormone may also regulate steroid biosynthesis in the placenta and the fetal adrenal gland and stimulate testosterone production in the fetal testicle. Although immune suppression has been ascribed to hCG, this effect has not been verified.

Human Placental Lactogen

Human placental lactogen (hPL) originates in the placenta. It is a single-chain polypeptide with a molecular weight of 22,300, and it resembles pituitary growth hormone and human prolactin in structure. Maternal serum concentrations parallel placental weight, rising

throughout gestation to maximum levels in the last 4 weeks. At term, hPL accounts for 10% of all placental protein production. Low values are found with threatened abortion and intrauterine fetal growth restriction. **Human placental lactogen antagonizes the cellular action of insulin and decreases maternal glucose utilization, which increases glucose availability to the fetus.** This may play a role in the pathogenesis of gestational diabetes.

Corticotropin-Releasing Hormone

Corticotropin-releasing hormone (CRH) originates in the fetal hypothalamus and also in the placenta towards the end of pregnancy. This 41-amino acid peptide stimulates adrenocorticotropic hormone (ACTH) secretion, which in turn stimulates the fetal adrenal to secrete cortisol and dehydroepiandrosterone sulfate (DHEA-S). Fetal cortisol, in turn, stimulates placental CRH release, which then stimulates fetal ACTH secretion, completing a positive feedback loop that **plays an important role in the activation of labor.** Elevated levels of CRH in midgestation have been found to be associated with an increased risk for subsequent preterm labor.

Prolactin

Prolactin is a peptide from the anterior pituitary with a molecular weight of about 20,000. Normal nonpregnant levels are approximately 10 ng/mL. **During pregnancy, maternal prolactin levels rise in response to increasing maternal estrogen output that stimulates the anterior pituitary lactotrophs.** Although the decidua is a secondary source of prolactin production, this source contributes little to the plasma pool. **The main effect of prolactin is stimulation of postpartum milk production.** In the second half of pregnancy, prolactin secreted by the fetal pituitary may be an important stimulus of fetal adrenal growth. Prolactin may also play a role in fluid and electrolyte shifts across the fetal membranes.

STEROID HORMONES
Progesterone

Progesterone is the most important human progestogen. In the luteal phase, it induces secretory changes in the endometrium and in pregnancy, higher levels induce decidual changes. Up to the 6th or 7th week of pregnancy, the major source of progesterone is the ovary. Thereafter, the placenta begins to play the major role. **If the corpus luteum of pregnancy is removed before 7 weeks and continuation of the pregnancy is desired, progesterone should be given to prevent spontaneous abortion.** Circulating progesterone is mostly bound to carrier proteins and less than 10% is free and physiologically active.

The myometrium receives progesterone directly from the venous blood draining the placenta. Progesterone prevents uterine contractions and may also be involved in establishing an immune tolerance for the products of conception.

The fetus inactivates progesterone by transformation to corticosteroids or by hydroxylation or conjugation to inert excretory products. However, the placenta can convert these inert materials back to progesterone. Steroid biochemical pathways are shown in Figure 6-1.

Estrogens

Both fetus and placenta are involved in the biosynthesis of estrone, estradiol, and estriol. Cholesterol is converted to pregnenolone and pregnenolone sulfate in the placenta. These precursors are converted to dehydroepiandrosterone sulfate (DHEA-S) largely in the fetal, and to a lesser extent the maternal, adrenals. The

DHEA-S is further metabolized by the placenta to estrone (E1) and, via testosterone, to estradiol (E2). **Estriol (E3), the most abundant estrogen in human pregnancy, is synthesized in the placenta from 16α-hydroxy-DHEA-S, which is produced in the fetal liver from adrenal DHEA-S.** Placental sulfatase is required to deconjugate 16α-hydroxy-DHEA-S prior to conversion to E3 (Figure 6-2). Steroid sulfatase activity in the placenta is high except in rare cases of sulfatase deficiency.

A sudden decline of estriol in the maternal circulation may indicate fetal compromise in neurologically intact fetuses. Anencephalic fetuses lack a hypothalamus and have hypoplastic anterior pituitary and adrenal glands; thus, estriol production is only about 10% of normal. Although estriol determinations have been used as a means of monitoring fetal well-being, present use is limited, and estriol measurements have generally been replaced by biophysical assessments (see Chapter 8).

Androgens

During pregnancy, androgens originate mainly in the fetal zone of the fetal adrenal cortex. Androgen secretion is stimulated by ACTH and hCG, the latter being effective primarily in the first half of

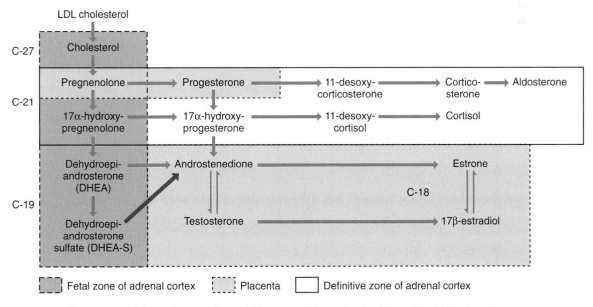

Figure 6-1. Main pathways of steroid hormone biosynthesis. Adrenal DHEA is largely transported as its sulfate, DHEA-S, which can also be formed from steroid sulfates starting with cholesterol sulfate.

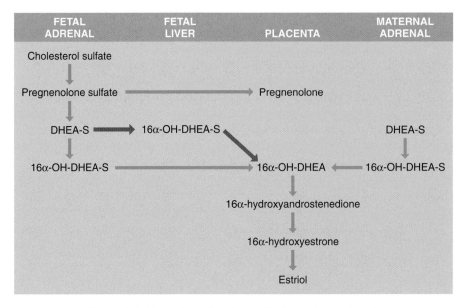

Figure 6-2. Formation of estriol in the fetal-placental unit.

pregnancy, when it is present in high concentration. The fetal adrenal favors production of DHEA over testosterone and andro-stenedione. **Fetal androgens enter the umbilical and placental circulation and serve as precursors for estradiol and estriol** (see Figure 6-1).

The fetal testis also secretes androgens, particularly testosterone, which is converted within target cells to dihydrotestosterone (DHT), which is required for the development of male external genitalia. The main trophic stimulus appears to be hCG.

Glucocorticoids

Cortisol is derived from circulating cholesterol (see Figure 6-1). Maternal plasma cortisol concentrations rise throughout pregnancy, and the diurnal rhythm of cortisol secretion persists. The plasma level of transcortin rises in pregnancy, probably stimulated by estrogen, and the plasma-free cortisol concentration doubles. **Both the fetal adrenal and the placenta participate in cortisol metabolism.** The fetal adrenal is stimulated by ACTH, originating from the fetal pituitary, to produce both cortisol and DHEA-S. In contrast to DHEA-S, which is produced in the fetal zone, cortisol originates in the definitive zone (see Figure 6-1). **Cortisol plays an important role in the maturation of the lungs.** It promotes differentiation of

type II alveolar cells and the biosynthesis and release of surfactant into the alveoli. Surfactant decreases the force required to inflate the lungs. Insufficiency of surfactant leads to respiratory distress in the premature infant, which can cause death. **Cortisol also plays an important role in the activation of labor,** increasing the release of placental CRH and prostaglandins.

OTHER HORMONES AND TRANSMITTERS
Oxytocin

The oxytocic prohormone which originates in the supraoptic and paraventricular nuclei of the hypothalamus, migrates down the nerve fibers, and oxytocin accumulates at the nerve endings in the posterior pituitary. Oxytocin is a nonapeptide which is released from the posterior pituitary by various stimuli, such as distention of the birth canal and mammary stimulation. **Oxytocin causes uterine contractions, but impairment of oxytocin production, as in diabetes insipidus, does not interfere with normal labor.** Fluctuations in circulating oxytocin levels before the onset of labor do not correspond to changes in uterine activity. Maternal serum oxytocin levels rise only during the first stage of labor. Oxytocin can be administered to induce labor, especially in term pregnancies, or to increase the frequency and strength of contractions during spontaneous labor.

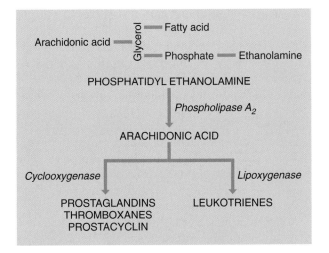

ARACHIDONIC ACID

Cyclooxygenase | Lipoxygenase

PROSTAGLANDINS
THROMBOXANES
PROSTACYCLIN | LEUKOTRIENES

Figure 6-3. Diagram of prostaglandin and leukotriene biosynthesis.

Relaxin

Relaxin is a peptide hormone that originates mostly from the ovary. In the human, it reaches its peak concentration in the maternal circulation at the 10th week of pregnancy and then declines. **Its primary function appears to be in promoting implantation of the embryo.** Although human relaxin shows no effect on relaxation of the cervix, it may be involved in inhibiting myometrial activity during pregnancy.

Prostaglandins and Leukotrienes

Prostaglandins are a family of ubiquitous, biologically active lipids that are involved in a broad range of physiologic and pathophysiologic responses. **They are not true hormones** in that they are not synthesized in one gland and transported via the circulating blood to a target organ. Rather, they are synthesized at or near their site of action. **Prostaglandin E_2 (PGE_2) and prostaglandin $F_{2\alpha}$ ($PGF_{2\alpha}$), prostacyclin, and thromboxane A_2 are synthesized in the endometrium, myometrium, the fetal membranes, decidua, and placenta. PGE_2 and $PGF_{2\alpha}$ cause contraction of the uterus.** Their receptors in the myometrium are downregulated during pregnancy. Prostaglandins can also cause contraction of other smooth muscles, such as those of the intestinal tract. Hence, when used pharmacologically, prostaglandins may give rise to undesirable side effects such as nausea,

vomiting, and diarrhea. The amniotic fluid concentrations of PGE_2 and $PGF_{2\alpha}$ rise throughout pregnancy and increase further during spontaneous labor. Levels are lower in women who require oxytocin for induction of labor than in women going into spontaneous labor. Administration of PGE_2 or $PGF_{2\alpha}$ by various routes induces labor or abortion at any stage of gestation. **Various synthetic prostaglandin derivatives are currently in use to terminate pregnancy at any stage and to induce labor at term.**

Prostaglandins are thought to play a major role in the initiation and control of labor. **Prostaglandin synthesis begins with the formation of arachidonic acid, an obligatory precursor of the prostaglandins of the "2" series (i.e., PGE_2, $PGF_{2\alpha}$).** Arachidonic acid is stored in esterified form as glycerophospholipid in the trophoblastic membranes. The initial step is the hydrolysis of glycerophospholipids, which is catalyzed by phospholipase A_2 or C. **Phospholipase A_2 preferentially acts on chorionic phosphatidyl ethanolamine to release arachidonic acid** (Figure 6-3). Free arachidonic acid does not accumulate. Labor appears to be accompanied by a cascade of events in the chorion, amnion, and decidua that releases arachidonic acid from its stored form and converts it to active prostaglandins. 17β-Estradiol stimulates several enzymes active in the synthesis of prostaglandins from arachidonic acid.

There are two cyclooxygenase isoenzymes referred to as COX-1 or PGHS-1 and COX-2 or PGHS-2. These isoenzymes originate from separate genes. COX-1 is expressed in quiescent cells, whereas COX-2 is inducible and is expressed at sites of inflammation upon cell activation and potentiates the inflammatory process. COX-1 mRNA expression is low in fetal membranes and does not change with gestational age, whereas COX-2 mRNA expression in the amnion increases with gestational age.

Increased phospholipase A_2 activity may lead to premature labor. Endocervical, intrauterine, or urinary tract infections are often associated with premature labor. Many of the organisms producing these infections have phospholipase A_2 activity, which could produce free arachidonic acid, followed by prostaglandin synthesis, which could trigger labor.

Prostaglandin synthetase inhibitors can prolong gestation. Nonsteroidal antiinflammatory drugs (NSAIDs) inhibit phospholipase A_2, whereas aspirin-like drugs inhibit cyclooxygenase. Because PGE_2 keeps the ductus arteriosus open, premature closure of the ductus may occur after ingestion of

NSAIDs or aspirin in large amounts or for a prolonged period of time, resulting in fetal pulmonary hypertension and death.

An additional pathway for arachidonic acid metabolism is the conversion of arachidonic acid to leukotrienes (see Figure 6-3). Both prostaglandins and leukotrienes induce decidualization, which means that they initiate changes in the endometrium to facilitate implantation of the fertilized ovum.

Although $PGF_{2\alpha}$ is more potent in producing uterine contractile activity, **PGE_2 is the most potent prostaglandin for ripening the cervix** by inducing changes in the connective tissue. Hence, PGE_2 and its synthetic derivatives are clinically useful for cervical ripening before the induction of labor or abortion.

CHANGES IN MATERNAL METABOLISM

Maternal metabolism adapts to pregnancy through endocrinologic regulation as described below.

ANGIOTENSIN-ALDOSTERONE

Aldosterone is a mineralocorticoid synthesized in the zona glomerulosa of the adrenal cortex. The main source in pregnancy is the maternal adrenal. The fetal adrenal and the placenta do not participate significantly in aldosterone production, although the fetal adrenal is capable of synthesizing it. **Aldosterone secretion is regulated by the renin-angiotensin system.** Increased renin formed in the kidney converts angiotensinogen (renin-substrate) to angiotensin I, which is further metabolized to angiotensin II, which in turn stimulates aldosterone secretion. **Aldosterone stimulates the absorption of sodium and the secretion of potassium in the distal tubule of the kidney, thereby maintaining sodium and potassium balance.** Renin-substrate (a plasma protein) concentration rises in pregnancy. It is thought that the high concentrations of progesterone and estrogen present during pregnancy stimulate renin and renin-substrate formation, thus giving rise to increased levels of angiotensin II and greater aldosterone production. **Aldosterone secretion rates decline in pregnancy-induced hypertension and, in some cases, may fall below nonpregnant levels.**

CALCIUM METABOLISM

Although calcium absorption is increased in pregnancy, total maternal serum calcium declines. The fall in total calcium parallels that of serum albumin, since approximately half of the total calcium is bound to albumin. **Ionic calcium, the physiologically important calcium fraction, remains essentially constant throughout pregnancy because of increased maternal production of parathyroid hormone.** In late pregnancy, coinciding with maximal calcification of the fetal skeleton, increased serum parathyroid hormone enhances both maternal intestinal absorption of calcium and bone resorption. The latter counteracts the inhibition of bone resorption caused by increased circulating estrogen. Urinary calcium excretion is decreased.

Calcium ions are actively transported across the placenta, and fetal serum levels of total as well as ionized calcium are higher than maternal levels in late pregnancy. High fetal ionic calcium suppresses fetal parathyroid hormone production and parathyroid hormone does not cross the placenta. Furthermore, calcitonin production is stimulated, thus providing the fetus with ample calcium for calcification of the skeleton. In the first 24 to 48 hours postpartum, the total serum calcium concentration in the neonate usually falls, while the phosphorus concentration rises. Both adjust to adult levels within 1 week.

PARTURITION

Labor is the physiologic process by which a fetus is expelled from the uterus to the outside world. The biochemical basis of uterine contractions, the hormonal control of gestational length, and the initiation of labor are described below.

BIOCHEMICAL BASIS OF CONTRACTION

Muscle contraction is brought about by the sliding of actin and myosin filaments fueled by adenosine triphosphate (ATP) and calcium. **While skeletal muscle requires innervation, contraction of smooth muscles such as the myometrium is triggered primarily by hormonal stimuli.** Hormone receptors have been found in the myometrial cell membrane.

The binding of oxytocin and prostaglandins to their respective receptors activates a phospholipase C, which hydrolyzes phosphatidylinositol 4,5-bisphosphate, a lipid present in the cell membrane, to inositol trisphosphate and diacylglycerol (Figure 6-4). Inositol trisphosphate induces release of calcium from the sarcoplasmic reticulum, an intracelluar calcium storage

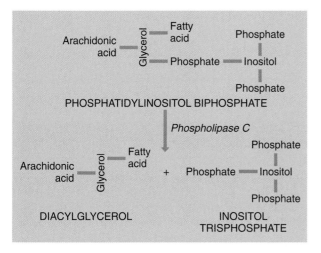

Figure 6-4. Diagram of inositol trisphosphate formation.

area. The resulting high intracellular free calcium concentration enables the myofibrils of the myometrium to contract. Subsequently, the calcium is pumped back into the sarcoplasmic reticulum with the help of ATP, and more calcium may enter from the extracellular fluid through both voltage-operated and receptor-operated channels that open briefly.

Unlike the heart, in which the bundle of His is present, no anatomic structures for synchronization of contractions have been found in the uterus. Instead, contraction spreads as current flows from cell to cell through areas of low resistance. Such areas are associated with gap junctions, which become especially prominent at parturition. Estradiol and prostaglandins promote the appearance of gap junctions, whereas progesterone opposes this action of estradiol.

HORMONAL CONTROL OF GESTATIONAL LENGTH AND INITIATION OF LABOR

Gestational length is under hormonal control and in most species, under the hormonal control of the fetus. Each species, however, has not only a unique gestational length but also unique mechanisms for controlling the length of gestation. Thus, although animal models provide important insight, they do not provide specific information concerning the control of the human gestational length or the mechanisms controlling initiation of labor. Nevertheless, animal models are well worth examining.

Animal Models

Most studies have been conducted in the sheep, **where the fetus appears to control the onset of labor.** The fetal hypothalamus stimulates the fetal pituitary to secrete ACTH, which brings about a surge of cortisol from the fetal adrenal. The cortisol surge induces the placental enzyme 17α-hydroxylase and formation of androgens, which are estrogen precursors (see Figure 6-1), simultaneously decreasing progesterone formation. The rise in the estrogen-to-progesterone ratio leads to (1) greater secretion of prostaglandins; (2) formation of myometrial gap junctions, which provide areas of low resistance to current flow and increase coordinated uterine contractions; (3) cervical ripening; and (4) the onset of labor. Administered ACTH, glucocorticoids, or dexamethasone can also initiate parturition. Removal of the fetal pituitary or adrenal, both of which are required for the cortisol surge, results in prolonged pregnancy.

In a breed of Guernsey cows with a genetic defect resulting in fetal pituitary and adrenal dysfunction, pregnancy is prolonged, and normal vaginal delivery does not occur. **In the rabbit, parturition directly follows a decline in progesterone production secondary to a decline in corpus luteum function.** Abortion can be prevented by administration of progesterone.

The Human

Fetal-maternal interaction occurs throughout pregnancy. **Hormonal effects determine getstational length and the onset of labor.** The human myometrium is exposed to elevated levels of progesterone and estrogens during pregnancy. Some clinical experience supports a hypothesis for the onset of labor similar to that postulated in the sheep, whereas other experience does not. Fetal anencephaly and adrenal hypoplasia frequently cause prolonged pregnancy. However, infusion of ACTH, glucocorticoids, or dexamethasone does not cause premature labor in the human. Progesterone injection has not been found helpful in the treatment of premature labor and administration of estradiol will not induce labor. **In most mammalian species, parturition occurs with an increase in the ratio of circulating estrogen to progesterone, whereas in humans and higher primates, parturition occurs without an increase in estrogen or apparent progesterone withdrawal.** Thus the changes in the human may be caused by changes in the responsiveness of the myometrium to these hormones.

There is evidence emerging now that a change in hormone receptors is responsible for the initiation of human parturition. **There are two progesterone receptors (PRA and PRB) in the human myometrium.** In contrast to PRB, which increases progesterone action, **PRA inhibits progesterone action.** The PRA and the ratio of PRA to PRB in myometria in labor are increased. **Progesterone is known to inhibit estrogen receptor α (ERα).** ERα was found to significantly increase in the laboring myometrium, while that of ERβ was unchanged. Thus, **there appears to be a positive correlation between PRA/PRB and ERα, and progesterone withdrawal occurs through increased PRA.** As a result, the responsiveness of the human term-pregnant myometrium to progesterone decreases with the onset of labor. However, these conclusions were reached by the experimental determination of mRNA levels.

ERα levels correlate positively with COX-2 and oxytocin receptor levels in the non-laboring myometrium. Changes in prostaglandin receptors occur with advancing gestation, and prostaglandin receptors are markedly elevated at term. Estrogen is also known to stimulate prostaglandin biosynthesis in the fetal membranes and the decidua. **The concentration of COX-2 increases throughout pregnancy** and is up-regulated in the fetal membranes and the myometrium in association with labor.

Furthermore, estrogen activates the formation of gap junctions and the synthesis of oxytocin receptors in the myometrium. Oxytocin receptor concentration determines the sensitivity of the myometrium to oxytocin. The concentration of circulating oxytocin does not rise before the onset of labor.

Other factors may facilitate the onset of labor. Multiple peptides, found in the nerve endings, play a role in controlling uterine blood flow and affect the mechanical activity of myometrial smooth muscle cells. Examples are **vasoactive intestinal peptide (VIP)** and **neuropeptide Y.** While the complete physiologic action of many peptides is still unknown, hormone-like effects of systemic (endocrine) and local (paracrine) action have been observed.

It may also be necessary to look more for hormonal changes in pregnancy-related tissues, such as the decidua and the fetal membranes. **Leukotrienes and platelet-activating factor (PAF) have been found in human fetal membranes.** PAF is a glycerophospholipid. Its concentration in the maternal plasma rises in late gestation. Like prostaglandins, PAF can initiate uterine contractions.

The fetal lung may be another source of prostaglandins and PAF. As the fetal lung matures, increasing amounts of prostaglandins and PAF along with surfactant are synthesized. The concept of a role for the fetal lung in the initiation of parturition is particularly attractive because the fetal lung is the last major organ to mature.

To summarize, labor is a release from the state of functional quiescence maintained during pregnancy by various putative inhibitors, including progesterone and relaxin. Labor is activated, in part, through decreased myometrial responsiveness to progesterone resulting from increased PRA, and increased responsiveness to estrogen resulting from increased ERα. **In addition, activation of the fetal hypothalamic-pituitary-adrenal (HPA) axis results in increased release of cortisol. These changes lead to an increase in the synthesis and release of prostaglandins, an increase in the formation of myometrial gap junctions, and the activation of myometrial oxytocin receptors, all of which stimulate the uterus to contract.** Other factors, such as leukotrienes and PAF, may also play an important role in stimulating uterine contractions. Cortisol also increases placental CRH gene expression, which positively feeds back on the fetal HPA axis to produce more cortisol. Ultimately, studies on the initiation of parturition should lead to solving the riddle of preterm labor. It is hoped that future research in this important area will further our knowledge and improve our ability to prevent premature labor and delivery, currently the leading cause of perinatal mortality.

Suggested Reading

Carsten ME, Miller JD: Calcium control mechanisms in the myometrial cell and the role of the phosphoinositide cycle. *In* Carsten ME, Miller JD (eds): Uterine Function: Molecular and Cellular Aspects. New York, Plenum Press, 1990, pp 121–167.

Mesiano S, Chan EC, Fitter JT, Kwek K, Yeo G, Smith R: Progesterone withdrawal and estrogen activation in human parturition are coordinated by progesterone receptor A expression in the myometrium. J Clin Endocrin Metabolism 87:2924–2930, 2002.

Norwitz ER, Robinson JN, Challis JRG: The control of labor. N Eng J Med 341:660–666, 1999.

Zakar T, Hertelendy F: Regulation of prostaglandin synthesis in the human uterus. J Matern Fetal Med 10:223–235, 2001.

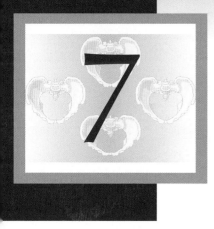

Maternal Physiologic and Immunologic Adaptation to Pregnancy

Brian J. Koos, Bahij S. Nuwayhid, and J. George Moore

Maternal physiologic adjustments to pregnancy are designed to support the requirements of fetal homeostasis and growth without unduly jeopardizing maternal well-being. This is accomplished by remodeling maternal systems to deliver energy and growth substrates to the fetus and to remove inappropriate heat and waste products. There appears to be a privileged immunologic sanctuary for the fetus and placenta during pregnancy.

NORMAL VALUES IN PREGNANCY

The normal values for several hematologic, biochemical, and physiologic indices during pregnancy differ markedly from those in the nonpregnant range and may also vary according to the duration of pregnancy. These alterations are shown in Table 7-1.

CARDIOVASCULAR SYSTEM
CARDIAC OUTPUT

The hemodynamic changes associated with pregnancy are summarized in Table 7-2. Retention of sodium and water during pregnancy accounts for a total body water increase of 6 to 8 L, two thirds of which is located in the extravascular space. The total sodium accumulation averages 500 to 900 mEq by the time of delivery. **The total blood volume increases by about 40% above nonpregnant levels, with wide individual variations.** The plasma volume rises as early as the 6th week of pregnancy and reaches a plateau by about 32 to 34 weeks' gestation, after which

little further change occurs. The increase averages 50% in singleton pregnancies and approaches 70% with a twin gestation. The red blood cell mass begins to increase at the start of the second trimester and continues to rise throughout pregnancy. By the time of delivery it is 20% to 35% above nonpregnant levels. **The disproportionate increase in plasma volume compared to the red cell volume results in hemodilution with a decreased hematocrit reading, sometimes referred to as physiologic anemia of pregnancy.** If iron stores are adequate, the hematocrit tends to rise from the 2nd to the 3rd trimester.

Cardiac output rises by the 10th week of gestation; it reaches about 40% above nonpregnant levels by 20 to 24 weeks, after which there is little change. The rise in cardiac output, which peaks while blood volume is still rising, reflects increases mainly in stroke volume and, to a lesser extent, in heart rate. As pregnancy advances, heart rate continues to increase, and at or near term, stroke volume falls to values close to normal nonpregnant levels. With twin and triplet pregnancies, the changes in cardiac output are greater than those seen with singleton pregnancies.

The cardiovascular responses to exercise are altered during pregnancy. **For any given level of exercise, oxygen consumption is higher in pregnant than in nonpregnant women.** Similarly, the cardiac output for any level of exercise is also increased during pregnancy compared to that seen in a nonpregnant state, and the maximum cardiac output is reached at lower levels of exercise. It is not clear that any of the changes in hemodynamic responses to exercise are detrimental

Table 7-1. Common laboratory values in pregnancy

Test	Normal Range (Nonpregnant)	Change in Pregnancy	Timing
SERUM CHEMISTRIES			
Albumin	3.5–4.8 g/dL	↓ 1 g/dL	Most by 20 wk, then gradual
Calcium (total)	9–10.3 mg/dL	↓ 10%	Gradual fall
Chloride	95–105 mEq/L	No significant change	Gradual rise
Creatinine (female)	0.6–1.1 mg/dL	↓ 0.3 mg/dL	Most by 20 wk
Fibrinogen	1.5–3.6 g/L	↑ 1–2 g/L	Progressive
Glucose, fasting (plasma)	65–105 mg/dL	↓ 10%	Gradual fall
Potassium (plasma)	3.5–4.5 mEq/L	↓ 0.2–0.3 mEq/L	By 20 wk
Protein (total)	6.5–8.5 g/dL	↓ 1 g/dL	By 20 wk, then stable
Sodium	135–145 mEq/L	↓ 2–4 mEq/L	By 20 wk, then stable
Urea nitrogen	12–30 mg/dL	↓ 50%	1st trimester
Uric acid	3.5–8 mg/dL	↓ 33%	1st trimester, rise at term
URINE CHEMISTRIES			
Creatinine	15–25 mg/kg/day (1–1.4 g/day)	No significant change	
Protein	Up to 150 mg/day	Up to 250–300 mg/day	By 20 wk
Creatinine clearance	90–130 mL/min/ 1.73 m²	↑ 40%–50%	By 16 wk
SERUM ENZYMATIC ACTIVITIES			
Amylase	23–84 IU/L	↑ 50%–100%	
Transaminase			
Glutamic pyruvic (SGPT)	5–35 mU/mL	No significant change	
Glutamic oxaloacetic (SGOT)	5–40 mU/mL	No significant change	
Hematocrit (female)	36%–46%	↓ 4%–7%	Bottoms at 30–34 wk
Hemoglobin (female)	12–16 g/dL	↓ 1.5–2 g/dL	Bottoms at 30–34 wk
Leukocyte count	4.8–10.8 × 10³/mm³	↑ 3.5 × 10³/mm³	Gradual
Platelet count	150–400 × 10³/mm³	Slight decrease	
SERUM HORMONE VALUES			
Cortisol (plasma)	8–21 g/dL	↑ 20 g/dL	
Prolactin (female)	25 ng/mL	↑ 50–400 ng/mL	Gradual, peaks at term
Thyroxine (T₄), total	5–11 g/dL	↑ 5 g/dL	Early sustained
Triiodothyronine (T₃), total	125–245 ng/dL	↑ 50%	Early sustained

Data from Main DM, Main EK: Obstetrics and Gynecology: A Pocket Reference. Chicago, Year Book, 1984, p 7.

Table 7-2. Cardiovascular changes in pregnancy

Parameter	Amount of Change	Timing
Arterial blood pressures		
Systolic	↓ 4–6 mm Hg	All bottom at 20–24 wk, then rise gradually to prepregnancy
Diastolic	↓ 8–15 mm Hg	values at term
Mean	↓ 6–10 mm Hg	
Heart rate	↑ 12–18 beats/min	Early 2nd trimester, then stable
Stroke volume	↑ 10%–30%	Early 2nd trimester, then stable
Cardiac output	↑ 33%–45%	Peaks in early 2nd trimester, then stable until term

Data from Main DM, Main EK: Obstetrics and Gynecology: A Pocket Reference. Chicago, Year Book, 1984, p 18.

to mother and fetus, but it suggests that maternal cardiac reserves are lowered during pregnancy and that shunting of blood away from the uterus might occur during or after exercise.

INTRAVASCULAR PRESSURES

Systolic pressure falls only slightly during pregnancy, whereas diastolic pressure decreases more markedly; this decrease begins in the first trimester, reaches its nadir in midpregnancy, and returns toward nonpregnant levels by term. These changes reflect the elevated cardiac output and reduced peripheral resistance that characterize pregnancy. Toward the end of pregnancy, vasoconstrictor tone, and with it blood pressure, normally increase. The normal rise of blood pressure toward prepregnant levels as term approaches has important implications for the diagnosis of preeclampsia.

Blood pressure, as measured with a sphygmomanometer cuff around the brachial artery, varies with posture. In late pregnancy, it is probably highest when the gravid woman is sitting and somewhat lower when she is lying down (a minority show a dramatic fall due to vena caval compression).

When elevations in blood pressure are clinically detected during pregnancy, it is customary to repeat the measurement with the patient lying on her side. This practice usually introduces a systematic error. In the lateral position, the blood pressure cuff around the brachial artery is raised about 10 cm above the heart. This leads to a hydrostatic fall in measured pressure, yielding a reading about 7 mm Hg lower than if the cuff were at heart level, as occurs during sitting or supine measurements.

MECHANICAL CIRCULATORY EFFECTS OF THE GRAVID UTERUS

As pregnancy progresses, the enlarging uterus displaces and compresses various abdominal structures, including the iliac veins and inferior vena cava (and probably also the aorta), with marked effects. The supine position accentuates this venous compression, producing a fall in venous return and hence cardiac output. In most gravid women, a compensatory rise in peripheral resistance minimizes the fall in blood pressure. In up to 10% of gravid women, however, a significant fall occurs in blood pressure accompanied by symptoms of nausea, dizziness, and even syncope. This **supine hypotensive syndrome** is relieved by

changing position to the side. The expected baroreflexive tachycardia, which normally occurs in response to other maneuvers that reduce cardiac output and blood pressure, does not accompany caval compression. In fact, bradycardia is often associated with the syndrome.

The venous compression by the gravid uterus elevates pressure in veins that drain the legs and pelvic organs, thereby exacerbating varicose veins in the legs and vulva and causing hemorrhoids. The rise in venous pressure is the major cause of the lower extremity edema that characterizes pregnancy. The hypoalbuminemia associated with pregnancy also shifts the balance of the other major factor in the Starling equation (colloid osmotic pressure) in favor of fluid transfer from the intravascular to the extracellular space. **Because of venous compression, the rate of blood flow in the lower veins is also markedly reduced, causing a predisposition to thrombosis.** The various effects of caval compression are somewhat mitigated by the development of a paravertebral collateral circulation that permits blood from the lower body to bypass the occluded inferior vena cava.

During late pregnancy, the uterus can also partially compress the aorta and its branches. This is thought to account for the observation in some patients of lower pressure in the femoral artery compared with that in the brachial artery. This aortic compression can be accentuated during uterine contractions and may be a cause of fetal distress when a patient is in the supine position. This phenomenon has been referred to as the **Poseiro effect.** Clinically, it can be suspected when the femoral pulse is not palpable.

REGIONAL BLOOD FLOW

Blood flow to most regions of the body increases and reaches a plateau relatively early in pregnancy. Notable exceptions occur in the uterus, kidney, breasts, and skin, in each of which blood flow increases with gestational age. **Two of the major increases (those to the kidney and to the skin) serve purposes of elimination: the kidney of waste material and the skin of heat.** Both processes require plasma rather than whole blood, which gives point to the disproportionate increase of plasma over red blood cells in the blood expansion.

Early in pregnancy, renal blood flow increases to levels approximately 30% above nonpregnant levels and remains unchanged as pregnancy advances. This change accounts for the increased creatinine clearance and lower serum creatine level. Engorgement of the breasts begins early, and mammary blood flow increases two to three times toward the end of pregnancy. The skin blood flow increases slightly during the third trimester, reaching 12% of cardiac output.

There is little available information on the distribution of blood flow to other organ systems during pregnancy. The uterine blood flow increases from about 100 mL/min in the nonpregnant state (2% of cardiac output) to approximately 1200 mL/min (17% of cardiac output) at term. Uterine blood flow, and thus gas and nutrient transfer, to the fetus is vulnerable. **When maternal cardiac output falls, blood flow to the brain, kidneys, and heart is supported by a redistribution of cardiac output, which shunts blood away from the uteroplacental circulation.** Similarly, changes in perfusion pressure can lead to decreases in uterine blood flow. Because the uterine vessels are maximally dilated during pregnancy, little autoregulation can occur to improve uterine blood flow.

CONTROL OF CARDIOVASCULAR CHANGES

The precise mechanisms accounting for the cardiovascular changes in pregnancy have not been fully elucidated. The rise in cardiac output and fall in peripheral resistance during pregnancy may be explained in terms of the circulatory response to an arteriovenous shunt, represented by the uteroplacental circulation. The elevations in cardiac output and uterine blood flow follow different time courses in pregnancy, however, with the former reaching its maximum in the 2nd trimester and the latter increasing to term. Neither can the augmented cardiac output be accounted for by an increase in blood volume, because the filling pressures of the heart are not elevated during pregnancy.

A unifying hypothesis suggests that the changes in circulating steroid hormones in combination with changes in production of vasodilatory prostaglandins, atrial natriuretic peptide, nitric oxide, and aldosterone affect venous distensibility and arterial tone. The venous vascular capacitance and arterial compliance are increased, both of which lead to an increase in blood volume and cardiac output. Similarly, the same hormonal changes cause relaxation in the cytoskeleton of the maternal heart. These changes allow the end diastolic volume to increase without any changes in the filling pressures, thus producing a 25% augmentation of stroke volume.

OXYGEN-CARRYING CAPACITY OF BLOOD

Plasma volume expands proportionately more than red blood cell volume, leading to a fall in hematocrit. Optimal pregnancy outcomes are generally achieved with a maternal hematocrit of 33% to 35%. Hematocrit readings below 27 to 29, or above 39 to 41, are associated with progressively less favorable outcomes. **Despite the relatively low "optimal" hematocrit, the arteriovenous oxygen difference in pregnancy is below nonpregnant levels.** This supports the concept that the hemoglobin concentration in pregnancy is more than sufficient to meet oxygen-carrying requirements.

A high proportion of women in the reproductive age group enter pregnancy without sufficient stores of iron to meet the increased needs of pregnancy.

RESPIRATORY SYSTEM

The major respiratory changes in pregnancy involve three factors: the mechanical effects of the enlarging uterus, the increased total body oxygen consumption, and the respiratory stimulant effects of progesterone.

RESPIRATORY MECHANICS IN PREGNANCY

The changes in lung volume and capacities associated with pregnancy are detailed in Table 7-3. Assessment of mechanical changes during pregnancy reveals that the diaphragm at rest rises to a level of 4 cm above its usual resting position. The chest enlarges in transverse diameter by about 2.1 cm. Simultaneously, the subcostal angle increases from an average of 68.5 degrees to 103.5 degrees during the latter part of gestation. The increase in uterine size cannot completely explain the changes in chest configuration, as these mechanical changes occur early in gestation.

As pregnancy progresses, the enlarging uterus elevates the resting position of the diaphragm. This results in less negative intrathoracic pressure and a decreased resting lung volume, that is, a decrease in functional residual capacity (FRC). The enlarging uterus produces no impairment in diaphragmatic or thoracic muscle motion. Hence, the vital capacity (VC) remains unchanged. **These characteristics— reduced FRC with unimpaired VC—are analogous to those seen in a pneumoperitoneum** and contrast with those seen in severe obesity or abdominal binding, where the elevation of the diaphragm is accompanied by decreased excursion of the respiratory

Table 7-3. Lung volumes and capacities in pregnancy

Test	Definition	Change in Pregnancy
Respiratory rate	Breaths/minute	No significant change
Tidal volume	The volume of air inspired and expired at each breath	Progressive rise throughout pregnancy of 0.1–0.2 L
Expiratory reserve volume	The maximum volume of air that can be additionally expired after a normal expiration	Lowered by about 15% (0.55 L in late pregnancy compared with 0.65 L postpartum)
Residual volume	The volume of air remaining in the lungs after a maximum expiration	Falls considerably (0.77 L in late pregnancy compared with 0.96 L postpartum)
Vital capacity	The maximum volume of air that can be forcibly inspired after a maximum expiration	Unchanged, except for possibly a small terminal diminution
Inspiratory capacity	The maximum volume of air that can be inspired from resting expiratory level	Increased by about 5%
Functional residual capacity	The volume of air in lungs at resting expiratory level	Lowered by about 18%
Minute ventilation	The volume of air inspired or expired in 1 min	Increased by about 40% as a result of the increased tidal volume and unchanged respiratory rate

Data from Main DM, Main EK: Obstetrics and Gynecology: A Pocket Reference. Chicago, Year Book, 1984, p 14.

muscles. Reductions in both the expiratory reserve volume and the residual volume contribute to the reduced FRC.

OXYGEN CONSUMPTION AND VENTILATION

Total body oxygen consumption increases about 15% to 20% in pregnancy. Approximately half of this increase is accounted for by the uterus and its contents. The remainder is accounted for mainly by increased maternal renal and cardiac work. Smaller increments are due to greater breast tissue mass and to increased work of the respiratory muscles.

In general, a rise in oxygen consumption is accompanied by cardiorespiratory responses that facilitate oxygen delivery (i.e., by increases in cardiac output and alveolar ventilation). To the extent that elevations in cardiac output and alveolar ventilation keep pace with the rise in oxygen consumption, the arteriovenous oxygen difference and the arterial partial pressure of carbon dioxide (P_{CO_2}), respectively, remain unchanged. **In pregnancy, the elevations in both cardiac output and alveolar ventilation are greater than those required to meet the increased oxygen consumption.** Hence, despite the rise in total body oxygen consumption, the arteriovenous oxygen difference and arterial P_{CO_2} both fall. The fall in P_{CO_2}, by definition, indicates hyperventilation.

The rise in minute ventilation reflects an approximate 40% increase in tidal volume at term; the respiratory rate does not change during pregnancy. During exercise, pregnant subjects show a 38% increase in minute ventilation and a 15% increase in oxygen consumption above comparable levels for postpartum subjects.

When injected into normal nonpregnant subjects, progesterone increases ventilation. The central chemoreceptors become more sensitive to CO_2 (i.e., the curve describing the ventilatory response to increasing CO_2 has a steeper slope). **Such increased respiratory sensitivity to CO_2 is characteristic of pregnancy and probably accounts for the hyperventilation of pregnancy.**

In summary, both at rest and with exercise, minute ventilation and, to a lesser extent, oxygen consumption are increased during pregnancy over the nonpregnant control values. The respiratory stimulating effect of progesterone is probably responsible for the disproportionate increase in minute ventilation over oxygen consumption.

ALVEOLAR-ARTERIAL GRADIENT AND ARTERIAL BLOOD GAS MEASUREMENTS

Pregnancy is characterized by hyperventilation (the arterial P_{CO_2} falls to a level of 27 to 32 mm

Hg) and associated respiratory alkalosis. Renal compensatory bicarbonate excretion leads to a final maternal blood pH of between 7.40 and 7.45. During labor (without conduction anesthesia), the hyperventilation associated with each contraction produces a further transient fall in Pco_2. By the end of the first stage of labor, when cervical dilation is complete, a decrease in arterial Pco_2 persists, even between contractions.

In general, when alveolar Pco_2 falls during hyperventilation, alveolar partial pressure of oxygen (Po_2) shows a corresponding rise, leading to a rise in arterial Po_2. In the 1st trimester, the mean arterial Po_2 may be 106 to 108 mm Hg. There is a slight downward trend in arterial Po_2 as pregnancy proceeds. This reflects, at least in part, an increased alveolar-arterial gradient, possibly resulting from the decrease in FRC discussed previously, which leads to a ventilation-perfusion mismatch.

DYSPNEA OF PREGNANCY

In general, airway resistance is unchanged or even decreased in pregnancy. **Despite the absence of obstructive or restrictive effects, dyspnea is a common symptom in pregnancy. Some studies have suggested that dyspnea may be experienced at some time during pregnancy by as many as 60% to 70% of women.**

The underlying pathophysiology remains unclear. The frequent onset during the 1st or 2nd trimester excludes mechanical factors. The marked change in Pco_2 to unusually low levels may result in the sensation of dyspnea.

RENAL PHYSIOLOGY
ANATOMIC CHANGES IN THE URINARY TRACT

The urinary collecting system, including the calyces, renal pelves, and ureters, undergoes marked dilation in pregnancy, as is readily seen on intravenous urograms. It begins in the 1st trimester, is present in 90% of women at term, and may persist until the 12th to 16th postpartum week. Progesterone appears to produce smooth muscle relaxation in various organs, including the ureter. **As the uterus enlarges, partial obstruction of the ureter occurs at the pelvic brim in both the supine and the upright positions.** Because of the relatively greater effect on the right side, some have ascribed a role to the dilated ovarian venous plexus. Ovarian venous drainage is asymmetric, with the right vein emptying into the inferior vena cava and the left into the left renal vein.

RENAL BLOOD FLOW AND GLOMERULAR FILTRATION RATE

Renal plasma flow and the glomerular filtration rate (GFR) increase early in pregnancy, achieve a plateau at about 40% above nonpregnant levels by midgestation, and then remain unchanged to term. As was true for cardiac output, renal blood flow and GFR (clinically measured as the creatinine clearance) reach their peak relatively early in pregnancy, before the greatest increase in intravascular and extracellular volume occurs. **The elevated GFR is reflected in lower serum levels of creatinine and urea nitrogen,** as noted in Table 7-1.

The mechanism for the decrease in renal vascular resistance is not clear.

RENAL TUBULAR FUNCTION

Although 500 to 900 mEq of sodium are retained during pregnancy, sodium balance is maintained with exquisite precision. Despite the large amounts of sodium consumed daily (100 to 300 mEq), only 20 to 30 mEq of sodium is retained every week. Pregnant women given high or low sodium diets are able to demonstrate decreases or increases in sodium tubular reabsorption, respectively, which maintain sodium and fluid balance.

Pregnant women also maintain fluid balance with no change in the concentrating or diluting ability of the kidney. Plasma osmolarity is reduced by approximately 10 mOsm/kg of water. Potassium metabolism during pregnancy is unchanged, although about 350 mEq of potassium are retained during pregnancy for fetoplacental development and expansion of maternal red cell mass.

Pregnancy causes compensated respiratory alkalosis with chronic losses of renal bicarbonate. These reductions in the renal buffering capacity predispose pregnant women to severe metabolic acidosis (either ketoacidosis or lactic acidosis).

FLUID VOLUMES

The maternal extracellular volume, which consists of intravascular and interstitial components, increases throughout pregnancy, leading, in effect, to a state of physiologic extracellular hypervolemia.

The intravascular volume, which consists of plasma and red cell components, increases approximately 50% during pregnancy. Maternal interstitial volume shows its greatest increase in the last trimester.

The magnitude of the rise in maternal plasma volume correlates with the size of the fetus; it is particularly marked in cases of multiple gestation. Multiparous women with poor reproductive histories show smaller increments in plasma volume and GFR when compared with those with a history of normal pregnancies and normal-sized babies.

Volume regulation in pregnancy is poorly understood.

RENIN-ANGIOTENSIN SYSTEM IN PREGNANCY

The elements of the renin-angiotensin system are markedly altered in pregnancy. Plasma concentrations of renin, renin substrate, and angiotensin I and II are increased. **Renin levels remain elevated throughout pregnancy.** It is possible that at least a portion of the elevated renin measured in the peripheral blood of pregnant women may represent a different, high-molecular-weight form.

The uterus, like the kidney, can produce renin, and extremely high concentrations of renin occur in the amniotic fluid. The role played by renin is not clear.

HOMEOSTASIS OF MATERNAL ENERGY SUBSTRATES

The metabolic regulation of energy substrates, including glucose, amino acids, fatty acids, and ketone bodies, is complex and interrelated.

INSULIN EFFECTS AND GLUCOSE METABOLISM

In pregnancy, the insulin response to glucose stimulation is augmented. By the 10th week of normal pregnancy and continuing to term, fasting concentrations of insulin are elevated and those of glucose reduced. Until midgestation, these changes are accompanied by enhanced intravenous glucose tolerance (although oral glucose tolerance remains unchanged). **Glycogen synthesis and storage by the liver increases, and gluconeogenesis is inhibited.** Thus, during the first half of pregnancy, the anabolic actions of insulin are potentiated.

After early pregnancy, insulin resistance emerges, so glucose tolerance is impaired. The fall in serum glucose for a given dose of insulin is reduced compared with the response in earlier pregnancy. Elevation of circulating glucose is prolonged after meals, although fasting glucose remains reduced, as in early pregnancy.

A variety of humoral factors have been suggested to account for the anti-insulin environment of the latter part of pregnancy. Perhaps the most important is human placental lactogen (hPL), which antagonizes the peripheral effects of insulin. It is secreted by the placenta into the maternal circulation in amounts parallel to placental growth. Levels of **unbound cortisol** are also increased. In addition, **progesterone** may exert some anti-insulin effects. Although basal levels of **glucagon** are elevated in pregnancy, secretion of glucagon is suppressed normally by a glucose challenge. **Growth hormone** is not elevated, and the pituitary response to hypoglycemia is diminished.

LIPID METABOLISM

The potentiated anabolic effects of insulin that characterize early pregnancy lead to the inhibition of lipolysis. **During the second half of pregnancy, however, probably as a result of rising hPL levels, lipolysis is augmented, and the plasma concentration of free fatty acids after an overnight fast is elevated.** Teleologically, the free fatty acids act as substrates for maternal energy metabolism, whereas glucose and amino acids cross the placenta to the fetus. In the humoral milieu of the second half of the pregnancy, the increased free fatty acids lead to ketone body (β-hydroxybutyrate and acetoacetate) formation. Pregnancy is thus associated with an increased risk of ketoacidosis, especially after prolonged fasting.

In the context of maternal lipid metabolism, the most dramatic lipid change in pregnancy is the rise in fasting triglyceride concentration.

PLACENTAL TRANSFER OF NUTRIENTS

The transfer of substances across the placenta occurs by several mechanisms, including simple diffusion, facilitated diffusion, and active transport. **Several physiochemical factors, such as molecular size, degree of ionization, and lipid solubility, affect the rate of diffusion.** Substances with molecular weights greater than 1000 Daltons, such as polypeptides and proteins, cross the placenta slowly, if at all.

Amino acids are actively transported across the placenta, making fetal levels higher than maternal levels.

Table 7-4. Maternal-fetal transfer during pregnancy		
Function	Substance	Placental Transfer
Glucose homeostasis	Glucose	Excellent—"facilitated diffusion"
	Amino acids	Excellent—active transport
	Free fatty acids (FFA)	Very limited—essential FFA only
	Ketones	Excellent—diffusion
	Insulin	No transfer
	Glucagon	No transfer
Thyroid function	Thyroxine (T_4)	Very poor—diffusion
	Triiodothyronine (T_3)	Poor—diffusion
	Thyrotropin-releasing hormone (TRH)	Good
	Thyroid-stimulating immunoglobulin (TSI)	Good
	Thyroid-stimulating hormone (TSH)	Negligible transfer
	Propylthiouracil	Excellent
Adrenal hormones	Cortisol	Excellent transfer and active placental conversion of cortisol to cortisone
	ACTH	No transfer
Parathyroid function	Calcium	Active transfer against gradient
	Magnesium	Active transfer against gradient
	Phosphorus	Active transfer against gradient
	Parathyroid hormone	Not transferred
Immunoglobulins	IgA	Minimal passive transfer
	IgG	Good—both passive and active transport from 7 wk gestation
	IgM	No transfer

Data from Main DM, Main EK: Obstetrics and Gynecology: A Pocket Reference. Chicago, Year Book, 1984, p 37.

Glucose is transported by facilitated diffusion, leading to rapid equilibrium with only a small maternal-fetal gradient. **Glucose is the main energy substrate of the fetus** although amino acids and lactate may contribute up to 25% of fetal oxygen consumption. The degree and mechanism of placental transfer of these and other substances are summarized in Table 7-4.

OTHER ENDOCRINE CHANGES
THYROID

The thyroid gland undergoes moderate enlargement during pregnancy. This is not due to elevation of thyroid-stimulating hormone, which remains unchanged.

Circulating thyroid hormone exists in two primary active forms: thyroxine (T_4) and triiodothyronine (T_3). The former circulates in higher concentrations, is more highly protein-bound, and is less metabolically potent than T_3, for which it may serve as a prohormone. Circulating T_4 is bound to carrier proteins, approximately 85% to thyroxine-binding globulin

(TBG) and most of the remainder to another protein, thyroxine-binding prealbumin. It is believed that only the unbound fraction of the circulating hormone is biologically active. **TBG is increased during pregnancy because the high estrogen levels induce increased hepatic synthesis.** The body responds by raising total circulating levels of T_4 and T_3. The net effect is that the free, biologically active concentration of each hormone is unchanged from that in the nonpregnant state. Therefore, clinically, the free T_4 index, which corrects the total circulating T_4 for the amount of binding protein, is an appropriate measure of thyroid function, with the same normal range as in the nonpregnant state. **Thyroid hormones do not cross the placenta.**

ADRENAL

Adrenocorticotropic hormone (ACTH) and plasma cortisol levels are both elevated from 3 months' gestation to delivery. Although less so than thyroid hormones, circulating cortisol is also primar-

Table 7-5. Analysis of weight gain in pregnancy

Tissues and Fluids	INCREASE IN WEIGHT (GRAMS) UP TO:			
	10 wk	20 wk	30 wk	40 wk
Fetus	5	300	1500	3400
Placenta	20	170	430	650
Amniotic fluid	30	350	750	800
Uterus	140	320	600	970
Mammary gland	45	180	360	405
Blood	100	600	1300	1250
Interstitial fluid (no edema or leg edema)	0	30	80	1680
Maternal stores	310	2050	3480	3345
Total weight gained	650	4000	8500	12,500

Data from Hytten F, Chamberlain G (eds): Clinical Physiology in Obstetrics. Oxford, Blackwell Scientific, 1980, p 221.

ily bound to a specific plasma protein, corticosteroid-binding globulin (CBG) or transcortin. **Unlike the level of thyroid hormones, the mean unbound level of cortisol is elevated in pregnancy;** there is also some loss of the diurnal variation that characterizes its concentration in nonpregnant women.

WEIGHT GAIN IN PREGNANCY

The average weight gain in pregnancy uncomplicated by generalized edema is 12.5 kg (28 lb). The components of this weight gain are indicated in Table 7-5. The products of conception constitute only about 40% of the total maternal weight gain.

PLACENTAL TRANSFER OF OXYGEN AND CARBON DIOXIDE
FETAL OXYGENATION

The placenta receives 60% of the combined ventricular output, whereas the postnatal lung receives 100% of the cardiac output. Unlike the lung, which consumes little of the oxygen it transfers, **a significant percentage of the oxygen derived from maternal blood at term is consumed by placental tissue.** The degree of functional shunting of placental blood past exchange sites is approximately tenfold greater than in the lung. The major cause of this functional shunting is probably a mismatch between maternal and fetal blood flow at the exchange sites, analogous to the ventilation-perfusion inequalities that occur in the lung.

The uteroplacental circulation subserves fetal gas exchange. Oxygen, carbon dioxide, and inert gases cross the placenta by simple diffusion according to Fick's diffusion equation. For oxygen, transfer is described by the following formula:

$$VO_2 = K/PO_2 \times A/L \times \Delta P$$

where K/PO_2 is the placental diffusion coefficient for O_2, A refers to the surface area of the placenta, and L is the diffusion distance between maternal and fetal blood. The ΔP is the partial pressure difference for oxygen across the placental membrane.

Figure 7-1 depicts the anatomic distribution of uterine and umbilical blood flow and O_2 transfer across the placenta. A **maternal shunt,** which describes the fraction of blood shunted to the myoendometrium and is estimated to constitute 20% of uterine blood flow, is depicted. Similarly, a **fetal shunt,** which supplies blood to the placenta and fetal membranes and accounts for 19% of umbilical blood flow, is shown. The **maternal-to-fetal** PO_2 and PCO_2 gradients are calculated from measurements of gas tensions in the uterine and umbilical arteries and veins. Using the measurements depicted in Figure 7-1 and the Fick equation, a placental gas exchange for O_2 and CO_2 may be calculated as follows: for oxygen, 3.5 to 5.0 mL/min/kg of fetal body weight, and for CO_2, 3.6 to 4.0 mL/min/kg. **The umbilical vein of the fetus, like the pulmonary vein of the adult, carries the circulation's most highly oxygenated blood.** The umbilical venous PO_2 of about 28 mm Hg is relatively low by adult standards. This relatively low fetal tension is essential for survival in utero, because a high PO_2 initiates physiologic adjustments (e.g., closure of the ductus arteriosus and vasodilation of the

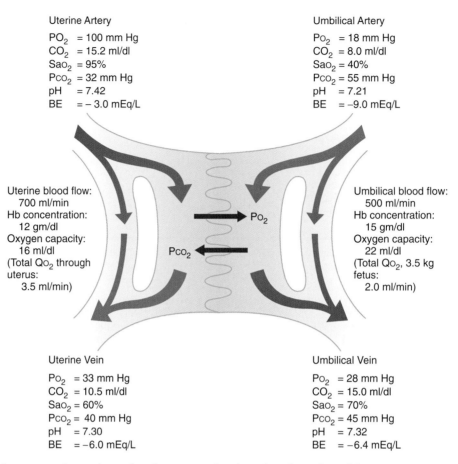

Uterine Artery

PO_2 = 100 mm Hg
CO_2 = 15.2 ml/dl
Sao_2 = 95%
Pco_2 = 32 mm Hg
pH = 7.42
BE = − 3.0 mEq/L

Umbilical Artery

Po_2 = 18 mm Hg
CO_2 = 8.0 ml/dl
Sao_2 = 40%
Pco_2 = 55 mm Hg
pH = 7.21
BE = −9.0 mEq/L

Uterine blood flow:
700 ml/min
Hb concentration:
12 gm/dl
Oxygen capacity:
16 ml/dl
(Total Qo_2 through uterus:
3.5 ml/min)

Po_2

Pco_2

Umbilical blood flow:
500 ml/min
Hb concentration:
15 gm/dl
Oxygen capacity:
22 ml/dl
(Total Qo_2, 3.5 kg fetus:
2.0 ml/min)

Uterine Vein

Po_2 = 33 mm Hg
CO_2 = 10.5 ml/dl
Sao_2 = 60%
Pco_2 = 40 mm Hg
pH = 7.30
BE = −6.0 mEq/L

Umbilical Vein

Po_2 = 28 mm Hg
CO_2 = 15.0 ml/dl
Sao_2 = 70%
Pco_2 = 45 mm Hg
pH = 7.32
BE = −6.4 mEq/L

Figure 7-1. Placental transfer of oxygen and carbon dioxide. *Adapted from Bonica JJ: Obstetric Analgesia and Anesthesia, 2nd ed. Amsterdam, World Federation of Societies of Anesthesiologists, 1980, p 29.*

pulmonary vessels) that normally occur in the neonate but would be harmful in utero.

FETAL AND MATERNAL HEMOGLOBIN DISSOCIATION CURVES

Most of the oxygen in blood is carried by hemoglobin in red blood cells. The maximum amount of oxygen carried per gram of hemoglobin, that is, the amount carried at 100% saturation, is fixed at 1.34 mL. The hemoglobin flow rates depend on blood flow rates and hemoglobin concentration. The uterine blood flow at term has been estimated at 700 to 1200 mL/min, with about 75% to 88% of this entering the intervillus space. The umbilical blood flow has been estimated at 350 to 500 mL/min, with more than 50% going to the placenta (Figure 7-1).

The hemoglobin concentration of the blood determines its oxygen-carrying capacity, which is expressed in milliliters of oxygen per 100 mL of blood. In the fetus at or near term, the hemoglobin concentration is about 18 g/dL and oxygen-carrying capacity is 20 to 22 mL/dL. Maternal oxygen-carrying capacity of blood, which is generally proportional to hemoglobin concentration, is lower than that of the fetus.

The affinity of hemoglobin for oxygen, which is reflected as the percent saturation at a given oxygen tension, depends on chemical conditions. As is illustrated in Figure 7-2, **when compared with that in nonpregnant adults, the binding of oxygen by hemoglobin is much greater in the fetus under standard conditions of Pco_2, pH, and temperature.** In contrast, maternal affinity is lower. **The shape of the fetal oxygen dissociation curve**

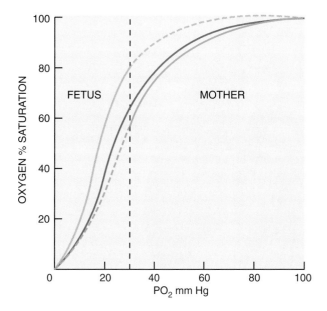

Figure 7-2. The oxygen dissociation curve for fetal blood compared with maternal blood. The central continuous curve is for normal adult blood under standard conditions. A vertical line at an oxygen partial pressure of 30 mm Hg divides the curves. The fetal curve normally operates below that level and the maternal curve above it. *Adapted from Hytten F, Chamberlain G (eds): Clinical Physiology in Obstetrics, 2nd ed. Oxford, Blackwell, 1991, p 418.*

permits larger amounts of oxygen to be transported per unit of blood at relatively low oxygen tensions. Furthermore, the difference between maternal and fetal hemoglobin dissociation curves permits transplacental transfer of large volumes of oxygen. Thus, transplacental equilibration of maternal blood with a Po_2 of 30 mm Hg and saturation of 55% will result in fetal blood with a Po_2 of 30 mm Hg but a saturation of almost 80%.

The decrease in the affinity of hemoglobin for oxygen produced by a fall in pH is referred to as the Bohr effect. Because of the unique situation in the placenta, a double Bohr effect facilitates oxygen transfer from mother to fetus. When CO_2 and fixed acids are transferred from fetus to mother, the associated rise in fetal pH increases the fetal red blood cell's affinity for oxygen uptake. The concomitant reduction in maternal blood pH decreases oxygen affinity and promotes its unloading of oxygen from maternal red cells.

FETAL CIRCULATION

Several anatomic and physiologic factors must be noted in considering the fetal circulation (Table 7-6 and Figure 7-3).

The normal adult circulation is a series circuit with blood flowing through the right heart, the lungs, the left heart, the systemic circulation, and finally the right heart. In the fetus, the circulation is a parallel system with the cardiac outputs from the right and left ventricles directed primarily to different vascular beds. For example, the right ventricle, which contributes about 65% of the combined output, pumps blood primarily through the pulmonary artery, ductus arteriosis, and descending aorta. Only a small fraction of right ventricular output flows through the pulmonary circulation. The left ventricle supplies blood mainly to the tissues supplied by the aortic arch, such as the brain. **The fetal circulation is a parallel circuit characterized by channels (ductus venosus, foramen ovale, and ductus arteriosus) and preferential streaming, which function to maximize the delivery of more highly oxygenated blood to the upper body and brain, less highly oxygenated blood to the lower body, and very low blood flow to the nonfunctional lungs.**

Table 7-6. **Components of the fetal circulation**		
Fetal Structure	From/To	Adult Remnant
Umbilical vein	Umbilicus/ductus venosus	Ligamentum teres hepatis
Ductus venosus	Umbilical vein/inferior vena cava (bypasses liver)	Ligamentum venosum
Foramen ovale	Right atrium/left atrium	Closed atrial wall
Ductus arteriosus	Pulmonary artery/descending aorta	Ligamentum arteriosum
Umbilical artery	Common iliac artery/umbilicus	Superior vesical arteries; lateral vesicoumbilical ligaments

Data from Main DM, Main EK: Obstetrics and Gynecology: A Pocket Reference. Chicago, Year Book, 1984, p 34.

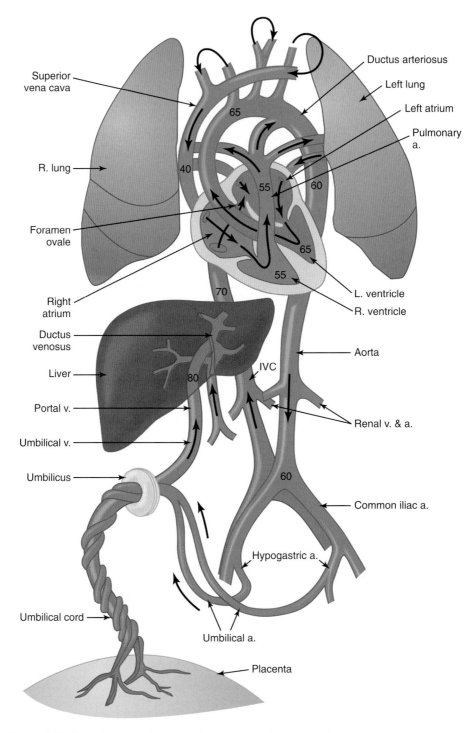

Figure 7-3. The fetal circulation. Numbers represent approximate values of percent saturation of blood with oxygen in utero. *Adapted from Parer JJ: Fetal circulation. In Sciarra JJ (ed): Obstetrics and Gynecology, vol 3: Maternal and Fetal Medicine. Hagerstown, MD, Harper & Row, 1984, p 2.*

The umbilical vein, carrying oxygenated (80% saturated) blood from the placenta to the fetal body, enters the portal system. A portion of this umbilical-portal blood passes through the hepatic microcirculation, where oxygen is extracted, and thence through the hepatic veins into the inferior vena cava. The majority of the blood bypasses the liver through the ductus venosus, which directly enters the inferior vena cava, which also receives the unsaturated (25% saturated) venous return from the lower body. Blood reaching the heart via the inferior vena cava has an oxygen saturation of about 70%, which represents the most highly oxygenated blood in the heart. Approximately one-third of blood returning to the heart from the inferior vena cava preferentially streams across the foramen ovale into the left atrium, where it mixes with the relatively meager pulmonary venous return. Blood flows from the left atrium into the left ventricle, and then to the ascending aorta.

The proximal aorta, carrying the most highly saturated blood leaving the heart (65%) gives off branches to supply the brain and upper body. Most of the blood returning via the inferior vena cava enters the right atrium, where it mixes with the unsaturated blood returning via the superior vena cava (25% saturated). Right ventricular outfow (O_2 saturation of 55%) enters the aorta via the ductus arteriosus, and the descending aorta supplies the lower body with blood having less O_2 saturation (about 60%) than that flowing to the brain and the upper body.

The role of the ductus arteriosus must be emphasized. Right ventricular output enters the pulmonary trunk, from which its major portion bypasses the lungs by flowing through the ductus arteriosus to the descending aorta. Although the descending aorta supplies branches to the lower fetal body, the major portion of descending aortic flow goes to the umbilical arteries, which carry deoxygenated blood to the placenta.

CHANGES IN THE ANATOMY OF THE CARDIOVASCULAR SYSTEM AFTER BIRTH

The following changes occur after birth (Table 7-6):
1. Elimination of the placental circulation, with interruption and eventual obliteration of the umbilical vessels
2. Closure of the ductus venosus
3. Closure of the foramen ovale
4. Gradual constriction and eventual obliteration of the ductus arteriosus
5. Dilatation of the pulmonary vessels and establishment of the pulmonary circulation

The elimination of the umbilical circulation, closure of the vascular shunts, and establishment of the pulmonary circulation will change the vascular circuitry of the neonate from an "in parallel" system to an "in series" system.

IMMUNOLOGY OF PREGNANCY

The fascinating growth and development of a semiallogeneic conceptus within an immunologically competent mother depends on the manner in which pregnancy alters the immune factors that govern tissue rejection. The concept of the fetus living in an isolated, sterile environment might give rise to the theory that the fetus does not require a highly effective immune system to ward off offensive antigens and antibodies. However, the fetus develops the framework of an immune system that becomes fully effective only after the neonatal period.

INNATE AND ADAPTIVE IMMUNITY

The human immune system is basically described in terms of two responses, innate and adaptive, which are interactive and complementary. In both systems, the effector cells exert their effect by secreting cytokines, or small proteins, which can be categorized as inflammatory cytokines, chemokines, T-cell derived lymphokines, and growth factors (Table 7-7).

The innate immune system, the first line of defense, involves a response that depends only on the foreign nature of the inciting antigen. The effector cells of this system are phagocytes (monocytes and tissue macrophages), granulocytes, and natural killer (NK) cells. NK cells are nonphagocytic lymphocytes that do not require a specific antigen. The antigen need only be foreign. **Interferons are one of the primary cytokine groups that activate NK cells and induce resistance to viral infectors.** NK cells and macrophages can either lyse invading infected or neoplastic cells or phagocytize and destroy the offending organisms (Figure 7-4). **Acute-phase proteins and complement have the ability to lyse some bacteria without cellular participation. Circulating factors such as complement and acute phase proteins are also part of the innate immune system.** The complement system is composed of multiple proteins that can be activated through either a classic or alternative pathway. Each pathway converges onto a final common cascade of reactions leading to the

Table 7-7. Cellular sources, target cells, and principal activities of cytokines

Cytokine	Cellular Sources	Target Cells	Principal Activities
INFLAMMATORY CYTOKINES			
Interleukin-1α	Macrophages	T and B cells	Lymphocyte activation, prostaglandin production
Interleukin-1β	Monocytes, B cells, fibroblasts, endothelial cells	Macrophages, endothelial cells, fibroblasts	Macrophage stimulation, pyrexia, enhanced leukocyte-endothelial interaction, tissue regeneration, enhanced MHC expression
Tumor necrosis factor	Macrophages, cytotoxic T cells, NK cells	Macrophages, neutrophils, fibroblasts	Cachexia, enhanced leukocyte-endothelial interaction, macrophage activation, enhanced cytotoxicity
Interleukin-6	Macrophages, fibroblasts	Macrophages, endothelial cells, hepatocytes	Acute phase response, T-cell activation, B-cell antibody production, prostaglandin production
CHEMOKINES			
Interleukin-8	Macrophages, monocytes, endothelial cells, keratinocytes, fibroblasts	Neutrophils, T cells, basophils	Neutrophil activation and degranulation, chemotactic for neutrophils and T cells
T-CELL–DERIVED LYMPHOKINES			
Interleukin-2	Activated $CD4^+$ T cells, NK cells	$CD4^-$ and $CD8^+$ T cells	T-cell growth and proliferation
Interleukin-3	Activated $CD4^+$ T cells	Hematopoietic precursors, stem cells, mast cells	Promotes growth and differentiation of myeloid progenitor cells
Interleukin-4	Activated $CD4^-$ T cells	B cells, eosinophils	B-cell growth and differentiation, IgE production, eosinophilia
Interleukin-5	Activated $CD4^-$ T cells	B cells	B-cell differentiation, antibody isotype switching
Interferon γ	Activated $CD4^-$ T cells, NK cells	$CD4^+$ and $CD8^+$ T cells, macrophages	Enhanced MHC class II expression, macrophage activation, enhanced endothelial-leukocyte interaction
Interferon-α	Mononuclear phagocytes	Virus-infected cells, NK cells	Inhibits viral replication, inhibits cell proliferation, increases MHC expression, activates NK cells
COLONY-STIMULATING FACTORS (CSFs)			
Granulocyte-CSF	Mononuclear phagocytes, endothelial cells, fibroblasts	Glanulocyte progenitors	Maturation of progenitors into glanulocytes
Granulocyte-macrophage CSF	T cells, mononuclear phagocytes, endothelial cells, fibroblasts	Granulocyte and macrophage progenitors	Maturation of progenitors into granulocytes and macrophages
Macrophage CSF	Mononuclear phagocytes, endothelial cells, fibroblasts	Macrophage progenitors	Maturation of progenitors into macrophages
PEPTIDE GROWTH FACTORS			
Transforming growth factor-β	T cells, mononuclear phagocytes	T cells, mononuclear phagocytes, other cells	Inhibits the activation of mononuclear phagocytes, inhibits activation and proliferation of T cells

Data from Branch DW, Scott JR: Immunology of pregnancy. *In* Creasy RK, Resnick R (eds): Maternal-Fetal Medicine. Philadelphia, WB Saunders, 1994.

INNATE IMMUNITY

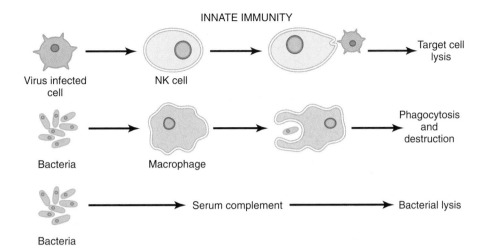

Figure 7-4. Summary of innate immunity. Surface antigens of viruses, bacteria, and tumors induce innate immune system function. In this system, natural killer (NK) cells and phagocytes, such as macrophages, can recognize certain antigens in a nonspecific fashion and either lyse the offending infected cells or tumor cells or ingest and destroy the offending organisms. Note that only the foreign nature of the antigen is required; antigen processing and major histocompatibility antigen participation are not necessary. *Reproduced with permission from Silver R, Branch DW: Immunology of Pregnancy. In Creasy RK, Resnick R (eds): Maternal-Fetal Medicine. Philadelphia, WB Saunders, 1999.*

destruction of microbial pathogens. The complement cascade can bind to foreign organisms, lyse bacteria, facilitate phagocytosis and attract circulating phagocytes.

The adaptive immune system involves both cellular and humoral responses to a specific antigen. The phagocytic cells in this system must first process the ingested antigen, which is recognized by T cells that are activated by this process. The recognition process occurs largely in the context of the major histocompatibility complex (MHC) (i.e., ABO self-antigens). **In this process, the T cells develop surface receptors for specific foreign antigens and undergo clonal proliferation** as noted in Figure 7-5.

ADAPTIVE IMMUNITY

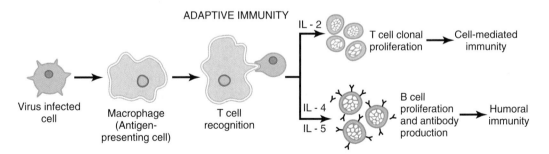

Figure 7-5. Summary of adaptive immunity. Adaptive immune responses initially require antigen processing and subsequent presentation to T cells. A T cell with a receptor specific for an inciting antigen will be activated and undergo clonal proliferation. In part, the type of cytokine produced by the activated T cell dictates the nature of the subsequent response. Interleukin-2 is the primary growth factor required for clonal proliferation of T cells and stimulates the proliferation of cytotoxic and memory T cells. Interleukin-4 and -5 stimulate B-cell proliferation, differentiation and antibody production. *Reproduced with permission from Silver R, Branch DW: Immunology of Pregnancy. In Creasy RK, Resnick R (eds): Maternal-Fetal Medicine. Philadelphia, WB Saunders, 1999.*

Cytotoxic (activated) T cells kill target cells. They also stimulate antibody production by B lymphocytes. Interleukin-2 is the primary growth factor required for clonal proliferation of T cells, and it stimulates the production of cytotoxic and memory T cells. Interleukin-4 and -5 stimulate B-cell proliferation and differentiation for immunoglobulin (antibody) production. The specificity of the B-cell response is governed by a process of gene rearrangement that creates a virtually limitless variety of immunoglobulin antigen-recognition sites, and a large menu of specific immunoglobulins is therefore possible.

Under certain conditions (e.g., pregnancy), T-suppressor cells may be activated and specifically suppress the activity of macrophages, B-cells, and T helper cells. Generally, viruses and parasites tend to elicit a T-cell adaptive immune response, whereas bacteria tend to elicit a B-cell antibody response.

DEVELOPMENT OF FETAL IMMUNITY

The innate immune effector cells first arise from hematopoietic progenitors noted in the blood islands of the yolk sac. By 8 embryonic weeks, the fetal liver becomes the source of these cells, and by 20 weeks the fetal bone marrow takes over. By 18 weeks, the various protein components of the innate immune system appear, but complement levels remain low. Complement levels begin to rise by the third trimester and reach normal levels by one year of age.

The cellular component of the adaptive immunity, T cells, are also derived from hematopoietic progenitors that are first seen in the blood islands of the yolk sac by 8 weeks. To differentiate into activated T cells, they must first migrate to the thymus gland, a relatively large organ in the fetus, the sole function of which appears to be nurturing and developing T cells. After maturation, T cells develop into either CD4 or CD8 types according to the surface receptor expressed. By 16 weeks, the thymus contains T cells in proportion to those found in the adult.

As previously noted, the requirement of mature T cells to recognize only antigens phagocytized in host cells is known as the MHC restriction. There are two types of MHC antigens. Class I MHC antigens (HLA-A, -B, and -C) are present in most cells of the body and are recognized by CD8 surface adhesive molecules. CD8-positive T cells act as cytotoxic or suppressor cells. Class II MHC molecules are expressed in far fewer cells, largely macrophages. Antigens presented in class II MHC molecules are recognized by T cells with the CD4 surface molecule. In the newborn, the proportion of CD4 T cells and CD8 T cells is similar to that in the adult.

Fetal B cells secrete IgG or IgA during the second trimester, but IgM antibodies are not secreted until the third trimester. Cord IgM levels greater than 20 mg/dL suggest an intrauterine infection. Maternal IgG crosses the placenta as early as the late 1st trimester, but the efficiency of the transport is poor until 30 weeks. For this reason premature infants are not as well protected by maternal antibodies.

IMMUNOBIOLOGY OF THE MATERNAL-FETAL INTERACTION

The maintenance of the antigenically dissimilar fetus in the uterus of the mother is of primary importance in obstetrics. Most of the attention in this field has come from the study of organ transplantation. The presence of the fetus is analogous to the grafting of tissues or organs between two individuals of the same species who are genetically dissimilar. Because all humans (except identical twins) are considered to be genetically dissimilar (allogeneic), such transplants are referred to as allografts. A number of mechanisms have been proposed to account for the tolerance and subsequent success of the fetal allograft.

The primary sites of modulation (suppression) of the maternal response to the fetus are the uterus, regional lymphatics, and placental surface. The uterus has been considered to be an immunologically privileged site, similar to the anterior chamber of the eye or the adrenal gland. These sites appear to possess decreased or altered afferent lymphatic systems that allow them to modify the host response to an allograft, and it appears that a similar mechanism may apply in the uterus during pregnancy.

The T cells, which primarily mediate the cellular response to foreign tissue by acting either to help or to suppress the immune response, are also locally altered in pregnancy. Cytotoxic T lymphocytes at the maternal-fetal interface have limited ability to mount an immune response to the trophoblast antigens. Pregnancy-related suppressor T cells capable of decreasing the maternal lymphocytic response have been described. These cells, in conjunction with placental interventions, can lead to an altered local immunologic environment.

The separate vascular compartments found in the hemo-monochorionic placentation of the human effectively remove the fetus from direct contact with the maternal immunologic defense system. This allows the placenta to function as an interface between two distinct systems. Tight trophoblastic intercellular junctions and a fibrinous covering of the trophoblast lead to control of the cellular and molecular fetomaternal transport. **Although the trophoblast has been shown to possess class I HLA antigens, the placenta lacks the class II MHC antigens that are necessary for the maternal lymphocytes to initiate an effective immunologic response.**

The placenta produces a number of pregnancy-associated plasma proteins and steroids that may alter the maternal immune response. These include **pregnancy-specific α_2-globulins, 1-glycoprotein, human placental lactogen (hPL), and human chorionic gonadotropin (hCG), as well as the sex steroids estrogen and progesterone. All of these substances have been shown to suppress nonspecifically the local immune response in pregnancy.**

In addition, the placenta functions as an immunoabsorbent to decrease the response against the fetus. Antibodies that are generated by the maternal immune response against paternal antigens in the placental surface (masking antibodies) and local immune complexes (blocking antibodies) may be trapped in the placenta. These complexes can either modify or block the immune response, or both, by facilitating enhancing antibodies and cellular suppression.

These mechanisms, which are summarized in Table 7-8, are thought to account for the maternal tolerance and the lack of host rejection seen in the majority of pregnancies.

IMMUNOLOGIC RESPONSE DURING NORMAL PREGNANCY

The mother's immunologic defense system remains intact during pregnancy. While allowing the fetal allograft to exist, the mother must still be able to protect herself and her fetus from infection and antigenically foreign substances. **The nonspecific (innate) mechanisms of the immunologic system (including phagocytosis and the inflammatory response) are not affected by pregnancy. The specific (adaptive) mechanisms of the immune response (humoral and cellular) are also not significantly affected.** No significant change occurs in the leukocyte count. The percentage of B or T lymphocytes is not appreciably altered, nor is there any consistent alteration in their performance during pregnancy.

Immunoglobulin levels do not change in pregnancy. **Maternal IgG is the major component of fetal immunoglobulin in utero and in the early neonatal period. IgG is the only immunoglobulin that is transported across the placenta.** Significant passive immunity can be transferred to the fetus in this manner, and aids in protecting it from infection during the perinatal period. IgM, because of its larger molecular size, is unable to cross the placenta. The other

Table 7-8. Proposed mechanisms for the success of the fetal allograft

Maternal Systemic	Uterus and Local Lymphatic System	Fetal	
		Placenta	Systemic
None (normal cell-mediated immunity)	Privileged immunologic site Localized, nonspecific suppression induces tolerance and generates suppressor T cells	Separation of the maternal-fetal circulations, including tight local barriers Lack of expression of the class II major histocompatibility antigen (HLA) at the maternal-fetal interface Limited immune response of cytotoxic T lymphocytes to trophoblast	Unidentified humoral and cellular immunosuppressive elements

immunoglobulins (IgA, IgD, and IgE) are also confined to the maternal compartment.

The fetal immune system develops early (8 to 20 weeks). Lymphocytes are present by the 7th week, and antigen recognition is demonstrable by the 12th week. In all of the immunoglobulin classes except IgA, fetal components are present by week 12. Production of the various immunoglobulins is progressive throughout gestation. **The newborn fetus at term has developed a sufficient defense system to combat bacterial and viral challenges.**

ROLE OF IMMUNOLOGY IN PREGNANCY-ASSOCIATED CONDITIONS

The major pregnancy-associated immunologic disease process is hemolytic disease of the newborn. Rh factor incompatibility, which is the most important of these conditions, is discussed in Chapter 16.

Hemolytic disease secondary to non-Rh sensitization and the destruction of lymphocytes or platelets secondary to sensitization against specific surface antigens have the same pathogenesis. Fetal cellular antigens leak into the maternal circulation, primarily at birth, and initiate an immune response. The reaction to these foreign antigens is by the humoral component (B cells) of the immune system. Antibody production is initiated, and IgM immunoglobulins, IgG immunoglobulins, or both are produced. Oftentimes no response, or only a weak response, can be measured.

An exception to the abovementioned mechanism is found in ABO incompatibility, in which naturally occurring antibodies can be found prior to any fetal cellular leakage. These antibodies are generally IgM and are not clinically significant. In group O individuals, however, both IgG and IgM antibodies may occur naturally, and the IgG antibodies may cross the placenta. **ABO incompatibility occurs largely in mothers with blood group O whose infants are of blood group A or B.** The hemolytic effect is less severe than Rh hemolytic disease, and hydrops fetalis does not occur.

Blood transfusions can also sensitize the mother to fetal red cell antigens. If the patient has a history of receiving a red cell transfusion and is sensitized to one of the irregular antigens, it is important to confirm the antigen status of the father, if possible, to determine whether the fetus is at risk for hemolytic disease. For example, **if the patient has antibodies to the potent and potentially lethal Kell antibody and the father is Kell-negative, the fetus could not inherit the Kell antigen and would therefore not be at risk.**

Suggested Reading

Burrow G, Ferris T (eds): Medical Complications During Pregnancy, 4th ed. Philadelphia, WB Saunders, 1995.

Heymann MA: Fetal cardiovascular physiology. *In* Creasy RK, Resnick R (eds): Maternal-Fetal Medicine, 3rd ed. Philadelphia, WB Saunders, 1994, p 276.

Nuwayhid B: Fetal homeostasis. *In* Iffy L, Komnitzky HA (eds): Principles and Practice of Obstetrics and Perinatology, vol 1. New York, Wiley, 1981.

Silver R, Branch DW: Immunology of pregnancy. *In* Creasy RK, Resnick R (eds): Maternal-Fetal Medicine. Philadelphia, WB Saunders, 1998.

Wegmann TG, Gill TJ: Immunology of Reproduction. London, Oxford University Press, 1983.

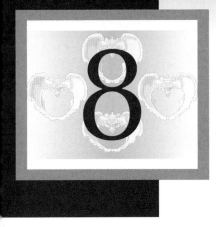

8

Antepartum Care: Preconception and Prenatal Care, Genetic Evaluation and Teratology, and Antenatal Fetal Assessment

Michael C. Lu and Calvin J. Hobel

PRECONCEPTION CARE

Because approximately half of all pregnancies in the United States are unplanned, preconception counseling is recommended for every woman of reproductive age. Preconception counseling and care provides an important opportunity for health promotion, risk reduction, and disease prevention. The elements of preconception counseling and care are listed in Table 8-1.

One example of how preconception care can improve obstetric outcomes is the opportunity to counsel and appropriately change dietary behavior. Women who are underweight (Body Mass Index [BMI] <19) have a greater risk of having a low birthweight or premature infant and women who are obese (BMI >29) are at significantly greater risk for obstetric complications, including pregnancy-induced hypertension, diabetes mellitus (DM), and fetal macrosomia (the PDA contains an electronic calculator for BMI). It is important that nutrition be balanced for at least 3 months before conception. Attempts at weight loss too soon before conception may have deleterious effects on fetal development.

PRENATAL CARE

The three basic components of prenatal care are (1) early and continuing risk assessment, (2) health promotion, and (3) medical and psychosocial interventions and follow-up. Risk assessment includes a complete history, a physical examination, laboratory tests, and assessment of fetal growth and well-being. Health promotion consists of providing information on proposed care, enhancing general knowledge of pregnancy and parenting, and promoting and supporting healthful behaviors. Interventions include treatment of any existing illness, provision of social and financial resources, and referral to and consultation with other specialized providers.

THE FIRST PRENATAL VISIT

The first prenatal visit provides an opportunity to assess or review medical, reproductive, family, genetic, nutritional, and psychosocial histories. Women whose health may be seriously jeopardized by the pregnancy, such as those with Eisenmenger syndrome or a history of peripartum cardiomyopathy, should be counseled about the option of terminating the pregnancy. Such reproductive histories as preterm birth, low birth weight, preeclampsia, stillbirth, congenital anomalies, or gestational diabetes are important to obtain because of the substantial risk of recurrence. Women with prior cesarean delivery should be asked about the circumstances of the delivery, and discussion about options for the mode of delivery for the current pregnancy should be initiated. Additionally, **the importance of screening women for domestic violence cannot be over-emphasized.** As many as 20% of women are physically abused during pregnancy (most studies report prevalence that clusters around 4% to 8%), making abuse more common than preeclampsia, diabetes, and other conditions that are routinely screened for during prenatal care.

Standardized forms have been developed to facilitate overall prenatal risk assessment. One such system

Table 8-1. Elements of preconception counseling and care	
Recommended Activities	**Intervention**
Medical and social history and physical examination	Review current medications for impact on fertility and pregnancy
	Review family and genetic history (e.g., diabetes, age risk, and risk for cystic fibrosis) • Nutritional assessment • Social situation assessment (e.g., risk of domestic violence) • Update Pap smear status
Laboratory assessment (based on physical examination and historic information)	• Hematocrit/hemoglobin • Urinalysis and culture • Serum folate level • Glucose testing • Lipids • Blood grouping and D (Rh) typing • Antibody screening
Special testing and counseling (based up historic information)	• PPD skin test for tuberculosis • Glycosolated hemoglobin • Offer HIV testing/counseling • STI testing—syphilis (VDRL or RPR) and others (chlamydia, gonorrhea) if indicated by history • Hepatitis B risk/testing • Rubella titer/vaccine (contraindicated during pregnancy) • Other immunity screening (e.g., varicella, toxoplasmosis, cytomegalic virus) • Folic acid Rx: All women 0.4 mg daily; previous history of neural tube defect, 4 mg daily unless contraindicated by pernicious anemia.

STI, sexually transmitted infections; PPD, purified protein derivative; HIV, human immunodeficiency virus; VDRL, venereal disease research laboratory; RPR, rapid plasma reagin.

is the Problem Oriented Prenatal Risk Assessment System or POPRAS (www.POPRAS.com).

A complete physical examination should be performed. Clinicians should be familiar with physical findings associated with normal pregnancy, such as systolic murmurs, exaggerated splitting, and S_3 during cardiac auscultation, or spider angiomata, palmar erythema, linea nigra, and striae gravidarum on inspection of the skin. During the breast examination, clinicians should initiate discussion about breastfeeding. A pelvic examination should be performed, and Pap smear status documented or obtained.

Prenatal laboratory testing should be undertaken as outlined in Table 8-1, if not done during preconception care. Screening for and treating asymptomatic bacteriuria significantly reduces the risk of pyelonephritis and preterm delivery.

Women who are **Rh negative** should receive Rh_0 (D) immune globulin (Rh_O-GAM) at 28 weeks of gestation and postpartum, and at any time when sensitization may occur (e.g., threatened abortion or

amniocentesis). **Rubella** vaccination is contraindicated during pregnancy, and pregnant women who are found to be seronegative should be vaccinated immediately postpartum. **Syphilis testing** is mandated by law in virtually all states. Early diagnosis and treatment of syphilis can reduce perinatal morbidity. Women who test negative for **hepatitis B surface antigen** and are at high risk for hepatitis B infection (e.g., health care workers) are candidates for vaccination before and during pregnancy. Infants born to women who test positive for hepatitis B surface antigen should receive both hepatitis B immune globulins (HBIG) and hepatitis B vaccine within 12 hours of birth, followed by 2 more injections of hepatitis B vaccine in the first 6 months of life.

Voluntary and confidential **HIV counseling and testing** should be offered and documented in the medical record. Diagnosis and treatment significantly reduce the risk of vertical transmission. Other tests may be obtained based on risk factors, such as testing for **gonorrhea and chlamydia.** All pregnant women at high risk for **tuberculosis** should be screened with a purified protein derivative (PPD) skin test when they begin prenatal care.

Additionally, the clinician should use the first prenatal visit to confirm pregnancy and determine viability, estimate gestational age and due date, diagnose and deal with early pregnancy loss, provide genetic counseling and information about teratology, and provide advice on alleviating unpleasant symptoms during pregnancy. Information about nutrition, behavioral changes to expect, and the benefits of breastfeeding should be provided as prenatal care progresses. Clinical pelvimetry should be performed sometime before labor begins (see Chapter 9).

CONFIRMING PREGNANCY AND DETERMINING VIABILITY

Women most commonly present to the clinician after missed menses. **About 30% to 40% of all pregnant women will have some bleeding during early pregnancy (e.g., implantation bleeding),** which may be mistaken for a period. Therefore, a pregnancy test should be performed in all women of reproductive age who present with abnormal vaginal bleeding.

The pregnancy test detects human chorionic gonadotropin (hCG) in the serum or the urine. **The most widely used standard is the First International Reference Preparation (1st IRP). The hCG molecule is first detectable 6 to 8 days after ovulation.** A titer of less than 5 IU/L is considered negative, and a level above 25 IU/L is a positive result. Values between 6 and 24 IU/L are considered equivocal, and the test should be repeated in 2 days. **A concentration of about 100 IU/L is reached about the date of expected menses.** Most qualitative urine pregnancy tests can detect hCG above 25 IU/L.

It is important to differentiate a normal pregnancy from a nonviable or ectopic gestation. In the first 30 days of a normal gestation, the level of hCG doubles every 2.2 days. In patients whose pregnancies are destined to abort, the level of hCG rises more slowly, plateaus, or declines.

The use of transvaginal ultrasonography has improved the accuracy of **predicting viability in early pregnancies.** Using transvaginal ultrasonography, the gestational sac should be seen at 5 weeks of gestation or a mean hCG level of about 1500 IU/L (1st IRP). The fetal pole should be seen at 6 weeks or a mean hCG level of about 5200 IU/L. Fetal cardiac motion should be seen at 7 weeks or a mean hCG level of about 17,500 IU/L. **The presence of a gestational sac of 8 mm (mean sac diameter) without a demonstrable yolk sac, 16 mm without a demonstrable embryo, or the absence of fetal cardiac motion in an embryo with a crown-rump length of greater than 5 mm indicates probable embryonic demise.** When there is any doubt about these measurements, it is best to repeat the evaluation in 1 week before terminating the pregnancy.

INCIDENCE OF EARLY PREGNANCY LOSS

Because the incidence of conception is unknown, the incidence of spontaneous abortion (miscarriage) cannot be determined with certainty. **Spontaneous abortion occurs in 10% to 15% of clinically recognizable pregnancies.** The term *biochemical pregnancy* refers to the presence of hCG in the blood of a woman 7 to 10 days after ovulation but in whom menstruation occurs when expected. In other words, conception has occurred, but spontaneous loss of the gestation takes place without prolongation of the menstrual cycle. When both clinical and biochemical pregnancies are considered, evidence would suggest that more than 50% of all conceptions are lost, the majority in the 14 days following conception.

Real-time ultrasonography has been extensively used to monitor the intrauterine events of the first trimester of pregnancy. **If a live, appropriately grown fetus is present at 8 weeks gestation, the fetal loss rate over the next 20 weeks (up to 28 weeks) is on the order of 3%.**

TYPES OF SPONTANEOUS ABORTION

The terms and definitions in the remainder of this chapter refer only to clinically recognizable pregnancies.

Threatened Abortion

The term *threatened abortion* is used **when a pregnancy is complicated by vaginal bleeding before the 20th week.** Pain may not be a prominent feature of threatened abortion, although a lower abdominal dull ache sometimes accompanies the bleeding. Vaginal examination at this stage usually reveals a closed cervix. Approximately one-third of pregnant women have some degree of vaginal bleeding during the first trimester, **and 25% to 50% of threatened abortions eventually result in loss of the pregnancy.**

Inevitable Abortion

In a case of inevitable abortion, **a clinical pregnancy is complicated by both vaginal bleeding and cramp-like lower abdominal pain.** The cervix is frequently partially dilated, contributing to the inevitability of the process.

Incomplete Abortion

In addition to vaginal bleeding, cramp-like pain, and cervical dilatation, an incomplete abortion involves **the passage of products of conception,** often described by the woman as looking like pieces of skin or liver.

Complete Abortion

In complete abortion, after **passage of all the products of conception,** the uterine contractions and bleeding abate, the cervix closes, and the uterus is smaller than the period of amenorrhea would suggest. In addition, the symptoms of pregnancy are no longer present, and the pregnancy test becomes negative.

Missed Abortion

The term *missed abortion* is used when **the fetus has died but is retained in the uterus,** usually for more than 6 weeks. Because **coagulation problems may develop,** fibrinogen levels should be checked weekly until the fetus and placenta are expelled (spontaneously) or removed surgically.

Recurrent Abortion

Three successive spontaneous abortions usually occur before a patient is considered as a recurrent aborter. Many clinicians feel that two successive 1st-trimester losses or a single 2nd-trimester spontaneous abortion is justification for an evaluation of a couple for the cause(s) of the pregnancy losses (see genetic evaluation section).

ETIOLOGY

Although many factors may result in the loss of a single pregnancy, relatively few factors are present consistently in couples who abort recurrently. Cause and effect relationships in individual patients are frequently difficult to determine.

General Maternal Factors

Infection with *Mycoplasma, Listeria,* or *Toxoplasma* should be specifically sought in women with recurrent abortions because despite being found infrequently, they are all treatable with antibiotics. Epidemiologic evidence of a causal link between exposure to potentially mutagenic or teratogenic agents and subsequent spontaneous abortion is scarce. Such exposures are likely to be uncommon and are not an important cause of reproductive loss in the general population. Exceptions to this are **maternal smoking and alcohol consumption,** for which there is **evidence of an increased incidence of chromosomally normal abortions.** Women who smoke 20 or more cigarettes daily and consume more than seven standard alcoholic drinks per week have a fourfold increase in their risk of spontaneous abortion. It has also been reported that there is a doubling of the risk of spontaneous abortion with as little as two drinks a week.

There is very little evidence that a sudden physical or emotional shock can cause the subsequent loss of a pregnancy. Psychodynamic factors may contribute, however, to the etiology of recurrent abortion in a few cases and may even be the major factor on rare occasions.

Three medical disorders are commonly linked to spontaneous abortion: **(1) diabetes mellitus, (2) hypothyroidism,** and **(3) systemic lupus erythematosus (SLE).** Although the evidence linking diabetes mellitus with spontaneous abortion is not conclusive, it is reasonable to test for this disease because treatment is appropriate regardless of any pregnancy loss. Severe hypothyroidism is more often associated with disordered ovulation than spontaneous abortion, but it should be specifically tested for if other clinical features suggest the condition is present. SLE is a widespread autoimmune disease with effects on a number of organs and systems. Up to 40% of clinical pregnancies are lost in women with this condition, and such patients have an increased risk of pregnancy loss prior to developing the clinical stigmata of SLE (see Chapter 17).

The risk of abortion increases with maternal age. If a live fetus is demonstrated by ultrasonography at 8 weeks' gestational age, fewer than 2% will abort spontaneously when the mother is younger than 30 years of age. If, however, she is older than 40 years, the risk exceeds 10%, and it may be as high as 50% at age 45 years. **The probable explanation is the increased incidence of chromosomally abnormal conceptuses in older women** (Table 8-2).

Table 8-2. Number of pregnancies, spontaneous abortions, and spontaneous abortion rates by maternal age at first pregnancy

Age at LMP (yr)	Pregnancies	Spontaneous Abortions	Spontaneous Abortion Rate (%)
<30	1856	208	11.2
30–35	590	85	14.4
35–40	82	15	18.3
>40	25	14	56.0

LMP, Last menstrual period.
Combined data from Alberman E: Maternal age and spontaneous abortion. *In* Bennett MJ, Edmonds DK (eds): Spontaneous and Recurrent Abortion. Oxford, Blackwell Scientific Publications, 1987.

Local Maternal Factors

No prospective study has been able to demonstrate unequivocally that a normal pregnancy can be lost as a result of abnormal hormone production by either the corpus luteum or the placenta. In addition to this, no controlled trial of exogenous hormones has been able to demonstrate any benefit, and there is some evidence that exogenous sex steroids may indeed be teratogenic. Until the existence of a "hormone deficiency" can be clearly demonstrated, it is best to avoid prescribing progestogens or other hormones to women who are pregnant.

Uterine abnormalities are known to be associated with pregnancy loss. Abnormalities include cervical incompetence, congenital abnormalities of the uterine fundus (as may result from gestational exposure to diethylstilbestrol) and acquired abnormalities of the uterine fundus.

Cervical incompetence occurs under a number of circumstances. The incompetence may be anatomic and is usually the result of trauma. This occurs most frequently as a result of mechanical dilatation at the time of termination of pregnancy by aspiration, but it may also occur at the time of curettage. **The diagnosis of cervical incompetence is usually made when a mid-trimester pregnancy is lost with a clinical picture of sudden unexpected rupture of the membranes, followed by painless expulsion of the products of conception.**

When cervical incompetence is suspected during pregnancy (e.g., history of cervical incompetence in a previous pregnancy or of cone biopsy of the cervix), sequential ultrasonography of the cervix and lower uterine segment may identify the problem before a pregnancy loss occurs.

A **congenitally abnormal uterus** may be associated with pregnancy loss in both the 1st and the 2nd trimester. Surgical correction of the abnormality, particularly with a history of second trimester loss, is frequently successful. The diagnosis of these abnormalities is made by either hysterography or hysteroscopy. Complete evaluation of the congenitally abnormal uterus usually requires laparoscopic, hysteroscopic, and hysterographic examination before any management plan for therapy can be made.

The most common acquired abnormalities of the uterus with the potential to affect fecundity are **submucous fibroids.** Although these tend to occur more frequently in women in their late 30s, they should be considered when investigating pregnancy loss in all women. Removal of submucous fibroids and large (>6 cm) intramural ones is associated with improved fecundity. Subserous fibroids do not appear to affect fecundity.

Intrauterine adhesions result from trauma to the basal layer of the endometrium from previous surgery or infection. When most of the uterine cavity has been obliterated (Asherman's syndrome), amenorrhea results but much more frequently, fewer intrauterine adhesions (synechiae) are present with reasonably normal menses and these lesions are not even suspected until a pregnancy is attempted and lost. Surgical correction of these intrauterine adhesions is recommended to improve fecundity.

Fetal Factors

The most common cause of spontaneous abortion is a significant genetic abnormality of the conceptus. In spontaneous 1st-trimester abortions, approximately two-thirds of fetuses have significant chromosomal anomalies, with approximately half of these being autosomal trisomies and the majority of the remainder being triploids, tetraploids, or 45 X monosomies. Fortunately, the majority of these are not inherited from either mother or father and are single nonrecurring events. **When seen on ultrasonography before spontaneous abortion occurs, many such pregnancies appear to consist of empty amniotic sacs.** When a fetus is present in many late 1st-trimester and early 2nd-trimester abortions, it is often significantly abnormal, either genetically or morphologically. It seems that nature has a way of identifying some of its major mistakes and causing them to be aborted.

Chromosomal Factors

Occasionally, chromosomal abnormalities occur as a result of some form of chromosomal anomaly in either of the parents, and **karyotyping is an important investigation** of couples suffering from recurrent abortion.

Immunologic Factors

A successful pregnancy depends on a number of immunologic factors that allow the host (mother) to retain an antigenically foreign product (fetus) without rejection taking place (see Chapter 7). The precise mechanism of this immunologic anomaly is not yet fully understood, but the immunologic functioning of some women, particularly those who abort recurrently, is different from that of women who carry pregnancies to term. The immunologic relationship between male and female in such a couple may be regarded as abnormal, and in some instances, treatment of this condition may result in a successful pregnancy.

MANAGEMENT
Threatened Abortion

A threatened abortion is best managed by an ultrasonic examination to determine whether the fetus is present and, if so, whether it is alive. Of those in whom a live fetus is present, 94% will produce a live baby, although the incidence of preterm delivery in these cases may be somewhat higher than in those who do not bleed in the 1st trimester. **Once a live fetus has been demonstrated to the couple on ultrasonography, management consists essentially of reassurance.** There is no need for admission to hospital nor is there any evidence that bed rest improves the prognosis.

Incomplete Abortion

Until bleeding has stopped or is minimal, it is best to insert an intravenous line and take blood for cross-matching and blood grouping, as shock may occur from hemorrhage or sepsis. **Once the patient's condition is stable, the remaining products of conception should be evacuated from the uterus under appropriate pain control.** These tissues should be sent for pathologic evaluation. An incomplete abortion that is infected must be managed vigorously. Delay in treatment may result in overwhelming sepsis that may lead to renal and hepatic failure, disseminated intravascular coagulation (DIC), and even death.

Missed Abortion

Suspected missed abortion (arrested increase in uterine size and/or inability to detect fetal heart sounds) should be confirmed by ultrasound. **Once the diagnosis has been made, it is appropriate to evacuate the retained products of conception surgically** to minimize the risk of sepsis and DIC and to reduce the extent of hemorrhage and the degree of pain that accompanies the spontaneous expulsive process.

General Management Considerations

When the patient is Rh negative and does not have Rh antibodies, **prophylactic $Rh_o(D)$ immune-globulin (Rh_o-GAM)** should be administered. All couples who have had a pregnancy loss should be seen and counseled some weeks after the event. At this time, questions that the couple may have can be answered, the findings of any pathologic studies discussed, and reassurance given about their chances of reproductive success in the future. There may be a need for more than one session, and, indeed, professional counseling may be appropriate.

Recurrent Abortion

As far as the mother is concerned, it is appropriate to rule out the presence of systemic disorders such as diabetes mellitus, SLE, and thyroid disease, and it is also necessary to test for the presence of a lupus anticoagulant. **Paternal and maternal chromosomes** should be evaluated, and **hysteroscopy or hysterography** should be performed to evaluate the uterine cavity. Given the possibility of the pregnancy losses being caused by infectious agents, it is also appropriate to rule out the presence of *Mycoplasma, Listeria, Toxoplasma, Treponema,* cytomegalovirus, and *Brucella.*

Over half of couples with recurrent losses will have normal findings during an evaluation. When a specific etiologic factor is found, appropriate management

Box 8-1. Indications for genetic counseling and prenatal diagnosis other than age

1. A previous child with or a family history of birth defects, chromosomal abnormality, or known genetic disorder
2. A previous child with undiagnosed mental retardation
3. A previous baby who died in the neonatal period
4. Multiple fetal losses
5. Abnormal serum marker screening results
6. Consanguinity
7. Maternal conditions predisposing the fetus to congenital abnormalities
8. A current pregnancy history of teratogenic exposure
9. A fetus with suspected abnormal ultrasonic findings
10. A parent who is a known carrier of a genetic disorder

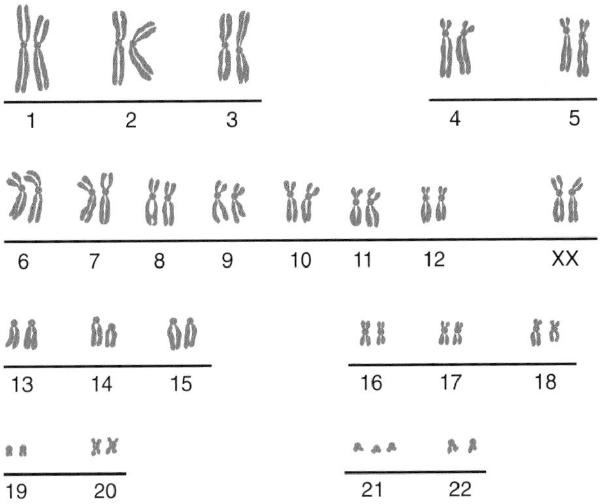

Figure 8-1. Karyotype of a patient with Down syndrome (47 XX + 21).

often leads to reproductive success. Many of the congenital abnormalities of the uterus can now be diagnosed using pelvic ultrasonography and may no longer require laparotomy for repair. Cervical incompetence is managed by the placement of a cervical suture (cerclage) at the level of the internal os, and this suture is best placed in the 1st trimester, once a live fetus has been demonstrated on ultrasonography.

ESTIMATING GESTATIONAL AGE AND DATE OF CONFINEMENT

Gestational age should be determined during the first prenatal visit. Accurate determination of gestational age may become important later in pregnancy for the management of obstetric conditions such as preterm labor, intrauterine growth restriction, and postdate pregnancy. Clinical assessment to determine gestational age is usually appropriate for the woman with regular menstrual cycles and a known last menstrual period that was confirmed by an early examination. Estimated date of confinement (EDC) or "due date" may be determined by adding 9 months and 7 days to the first day of the last menstrual period. The PDA contains an electronic calculator for EDC. This calculation presupposes a 28-day menstrual cycle and may be subject to error, especially in those with longer or shorter menstrual cycles.

Ultrasonography may also be used to estimate gestational age. Measurement of **fetal crown-rump length between 6 and 11 weeks of gestation** can define gestational age to within 7 days, or within 10 days by the average of multiple measurements **(e.g., biparietal diameter, femur length, abdominal and head circumferences)** obtained at 12 to 20 weeks. Thereafter, measurements become less reliable with advancing gestation (±3 weeks in the 3rd trimester).

PATIENTS WHO REQUIRE GENETIC COUNSELING

Ideally, couples should receive preconception counseling before they decide to have children, so that genetic disease in the couple or their families may be identified before pregnancy. The major reason couples are referred for prenatal diagnosis is age. Women older than 34 years have an increased risk of having children with chromosomal abnormalities. Other indications for genetic counseling and prenatal diagnosis are listed in Box 8-1.

CONGENITAL AND HEREDITARY DISORDERS
Chromosomal Disorders

Chromosomal abnormalities occur in 0.5% of live births, but the incidence associated with sponta-

neous abortions is much higher and is estimated to be approximately 50%. The most common chromosomal abnormalities among liveborn infants are sex chromosomal aneuploidies (e.g., Turner syndrome, Klinefelter syndrome), balanced robertsonian translocations (translocations within group D or between groups D and G), and autosomal trisomies (e.g., Down syndrome Figure 8-1).

Women older than 34 years are at increased risk of giving birth to children with autosomal trisomies (e.g., trisomy 21, 13, or 18) or sex chromosomal abnormalities (e.g., Turner syndrome [45 XO], Klinefelter syndrome [47 XXY]. The overall risk of Down syndrome (trisomy 21) is 1 per 800 live births. It increases to about 1 per 300 live births for women who are 35 to 39 years of age and to about 1 in 80 for those 40 to 45 years of age (Table 8-3). The incidence of Down syndrome diagnosed at the time of amniocentesis is considerably higher. In women 35 to 39 years of age, the rate is about 1 in 125; in those 40 to 45, it is about 1 in 20. The discrepancy between the rate of occurrence at delivery and that at amniocentesis is believed to be due in part to fetal loss in the late 2nd and 3rd trimester.

Ninety-five percent of cases of Down syndrome are due to meiotic nondisjunctional events leading to 47 chromosomes with an extra copy of chromosome number 21, whereas 4% of Down syndrome cases are due to an unbalanced translocation. Parents of a child with translocation Down syndrome have rearrangements between chromosome 21 and chromosomes 14, 15, 21, or 22. The remaining 1% of individuals with Down syndrome have the mosaic type, which consists of two populations of cells, one with 46 chromosomes (a normal karyotype) and one with 47 chromosomes.

A couple who has previously had a child with trisomy 21 (Down syndrome) or with a meiotic nondisjunctional type of chromosomal abnormality is believed to be at a small but definite increased risk (about 1%) of giving birth to another child with a chromosomal abnormality and should be referred for prenatal diagnosis.

Approximately 1 in 500 individuals carries a balanced translocation. Blood chromosomal studies should be performed on a couple after three or more spontaneous abortions because in approximately 3% to 5% of such couples, one member is a balanced translocation carrier. The recurrence risk for sponta-

Table 8-3. Risk table for chromosome abnormalities by maternal age at term

Age at Term (yr)	Risk for Trisomy 21*	Risk for Any Chromosome Abnormality[†,‡]
15	1:1,578	1:454
16	1:1,572	1:475
17	1:1,565	1:499
18	1:1,556	1:525
19	1:1,544	1:555
20	1:1,528	1:525
21	1:1,507	1:525
22	1:1,481	1:499
23	1:1,447	1:499
24	1:1,404	1:475
25	1:1,351	1:475
26	1:1,286	1:475
27	1:1,208	1:454
28	1:1,119	1:434
29	1:1,018	1:416
30	1:909	1:384
31	1:796	1:384
32	1:683	1:322
33	1:574	1:285
34	1:474	1:243
35	1:384	1:178
36	1:307	1:148
37	1:242	1:122
38	1:189	1:104
39	1:146	1:80
40	1:112	1:62
41	1:85	1:48
42	1:65	1:38
43	1:49	1:30
44	1:37	1:23
45	1:28	1:18
46	1:21	1:14
47	1:15	1:10
48	1:11	1:8
49	1:8	1:6
50	1:6	Data not available

*Data from Chuckle HA, Wald NJ, Thompson SC: Estimating a woman's risk of having a pregnancy associated with Down's syndrome using her age and serum alpha-fetoprotein level. Br J Obstet Gynaecol 94:387, 1987.
[†]Adapted from Hook EB: Rates of chromosomal abnormalities at different maternal ages. Obstet Gynecol 58:282-285, 1981.
[‡]Risk for any chromosome abnormality includes the risk for trisomy 21 and 18 in addition to trisomy 13, 47 XXY, 47 XYY, Turner syndrome genotype, and other clinically significant abnormalities. 47 XXX is not included.

neous abortions, abnormal offspring, or both is greatly increased among translocation carriers, and it can be estimated according to the translocation present. **These couples should be alerted to the advisability of prenatal diagnosis because of their increased risk for having liveborn children with unbalanced translocations.**

Using **fluorescence in situ hybridization** (FISH), a labeled chromosome-specific DNA segment or probe is hybridized to metaphase, prophase, or interphase chromosomes and visualized with fluorescent microscopy. FISH analysis has led to the identification of a number of genetic syndromes that could not previously be detected because the chromosomal deletion in these syndromes is beyond the resolution of banded chromosomal analysis. Syndromes identified by FISH analysis include Prader-Willi, Angelman-DiGeorge, and Williams' syndromes. Trisomies can also be identified in interphase cells with FISH probes.

Single Gene Disorders

Single gene disorders are relatively uncommon, but they can result in significant medical and psychosocial problems. These disorders follow the laws of mendelian inheritance. They may be passed from generation to generation, as with autosomal dominant disorders, or affect siblings without a family history of other affected family members, as in autosomal recessive disorders. Males may be affected with healthy females transmitting the abnormal gene, as in X-linked recessive disorders.

Autosomal Dominant Disorders

In autosomal dominant disorders, only one abnormal gene is necessary for disease manifestation. **The affected individual has a 50% chance of passing the gene and the disorder on to offspring.** The unaffected offspring cannot pass on the gene or the disorder. The occurrence and transmission of the genes are not influenced by gender. A spontaneous mutation of genetic material in the germ cells of clinically normal parents can also result in an affected offspring.

The hallmark of autosomal dominant disease is the variable expressivity. It is important to determine whether a child is affected by a spontaneous mutation or is the product of a parent with minimal expression of the same gene. A careful history and physical examination of family members, in addition to biochemical, radiologic, or histologic testing, may be necessary to determine the parents' genetic status.

Some of the common autosomal dominant disorders include tuberous sclerosis, neurofibromatosis, achondroplasia, craniofacial synostosis, adult-onset polycystic kidney disease, and several types of muscular dystrophy.

AUTOSOMAL RECESSIVE DISORDERS

With autosomal recessive disorders, two affected genes must be present for manifestation of the disease. Usually there is no family history, but if a family history exists, siblings of either sex are equally likely to be affected. Consanguineous couples are at an increased risk for having a child who is homozygous for a deleterious recessive gene, with subsequent pregnancies being at 25% risk for producing a similarly affected child.

Many autosomal recessive disorders may be diagnosed prenatally. Biochemical genetic disorders (e.g., Tay-Sachs disease) can be diagnosed by enzymatic assay, whereas others (e.g., sickle cell anemia, beta-thalassemia, and cystic fibrosis) can be diagnosed by DNA analysis from amniocytes or chorionic villi.

GENETIC SCREENING FOR AUTOSOMAL RECESSIVE DISORDERS

Carrier screening programs for autosomal recessive disorders have traditionally focused on high-risk populations, in which the frequency of heterozygotes is greater than in the general population. Screening for Tay-Sachs disease among Eastern European Jewish and French Canadian populations has proved to be particularly successful in the recognition of couples at 25% risk for having offspring affected with this fatal disease. Table 8-4 lists selected autosomal recessive disorders for which genetic screening has been initiated.

The most common gene carried by North American whites is the cystic fibrosis (CF) gene (carrier frequency, 1/25). With the use of recombinant DNA technology, the CF gene has been mapped to chromosome 7, and a gene deletion (AF508) has been found in approximately 70% of carriers. More than 400 mutations have been identified in the CF gene. **Genetic counseling is essential in offering**

CF carrier detection because 15% of carriers (and maybe more depending on ethnic group) remain undetected, and the limitations of the testing must be explained. At present, carrier detection is offered to individuals with a family history of CF, partners of identified CF carriers, parents of a fetus with ultrasonic findings of an echogenic bowel, and those who donate sperm.

SEX-LINKED DISORDERS

Sex-linked disorders, caused by recessive genes located on the X chromosome, primarily affect males, whereas unaffected (or mildly affected) females carry the deleterious gene. There is no male-to-male transmission of X-linked disorders. Using gene mapping technology, many sex-linked disorders such as **Duchenne muscular dystrophy (DMD) or fragile X syndrome** can now be diagnosed by chorionic villus sampling (CVS) or amniocentesis. X-linked disorders can occur because of new mutations of genetic material as a sporadic event or from the inheritance of the X-linked recessive gene from the carrier mother.

Fragile X syndrome is an X-linked disorder that is the second most common form of mental retardation after Down syndrome and the most common form of inherited mental retardation. It has an incidence of 1 per 1500 males and 1 per 2500 females. Mental impairment is variable in heterozygous females. The fragile X syndrome is caused by triplet repeat expansion in the long arm of the X chromosome. Using molecular genetic techniques, the number of triplet repeats can be measured in affected individuals to confirm a suspected diagnosis of fragile X or fragile X carrier status. In women who have a family history of mental retardation, genetic counseling is recommended for consideration of fragile X testing in the patient or family member.

MULTIFACTORIAL DISORDERS

Most birth defects are inherited in a multifactorial fashion, which means that both genes and the environment play a role. Common multifactorial disorders include cleft lip or palate, neural tube defects (spina bifida or anencephaly), congenital heart defects, and pyloric stenosis.

Neural tube defects occur in about 1 per 1000 births in the United States. In Northern Ireland, Wales, and Scotland, the incidence of neural tube defects is 6 to 8 per 1000 births. Both anecephaly (congenital absence of the forebrain) and spina bifida (open spine) are believed to occur prior to 30 days' gestation because of failure of the neural tube to close. Newborns with anencephaly are stillborn or die within the first few days of life. Newborns with spina bifida have a variable course, depending on the site of the lesion and whether it is a **meningocele** (herniation of the meninges through an open spinal defect with cord remaining in its usual position) or a **myelocele** (herniation of the spinal cord). **Folic acid has been shown to lower the risk of neural tube defects, and women who have had an infant with a neural tube defect should take vitamins plus 4 mg of folic acid daily prior to conception.**

With multifactorial disorders in general, and with neural tube defects in particular, a couple who has had one affected child has an increased risk of approximately 3% of having another similarly affected child.

Table 8-4. Selected autosomal recessive diseases in defined ethnic groups

Disease	Ethnic Group	Carrier Frequency
Sickle cell disease	Blacks	1/10
Cystic fibrosis	Whites	1/25
Tay-Sachs disease	Jews, French Canadians	1/30
Thalassemia	Mediterraneans, Southeast Asians	1/25

MATERNAL SERUM TRIPLE MARKER SCREENING

Current recommendations are to offer a woman the serum triple screening test that measures **alpha fetoprotein (AFP), hCG,** and **unconjugated estriol (UE3) at 16 to 18 weeks of gestation.** Amniotic fluid α-fetoprotein (AFP) levels are frequently elevated in blood samples of women carrying fetuses affected with neural tube defects. **Approximately 80% to 85% of all open neural tube defects can be detected by maternal serum AFP (MSAFP).** In addition to open neural tube defects, ventral wall defects (gastroschisis or omphalocele) can cause elevations of MSAFP.

If the MSAFP level is elevated, an ultrasound is done to rule out multiple gestation, fetal demise, or inaccurate gestational age (all of which can give false-positive results). If none of these factors are present, amniocentesis is recommended to determine the amniotic fluid AFP level and to measure acetylcholinesterase (AChE). **Acetylcholinesterase is a protein that is present only if there is an open neural tube defect.**

An association between low maternal serum AFP and Down syndrome has been noted. Prior to MSAFP screening, only maternal age was used to screen for Down syndrome. The sensitivity of MSAFP screening for trisomy 21 is improved further when maternal serum hCG and UE3 concentrations are also considered. The combination of low MSAFP, elevated hCG, and low UE3 levels will detect 60% of Down syndrome pregnancies. **Low MSAFP, low hCG, and low UE3 levels can also be used to screen for trisomy 18.**

The first step following an abnormal screening result is to perform ultrasonography to rule out a dating discrepancy or fetal demise. Following ultrasonography, amniocentesis is performed to establish the fetal karyotype. **Prenatal screening using all three chemical markers has the potential for replacing maternal age as the primary variable for determining which women should undergo amniocentesis.**

Genetic counseling is an essential component of screening programs. It provides education and alleviates anxiety in patients with abnormal test results. Patients must be informed of the differences between screening results and diagnostic testing.

DIAGNOSTIC PROCEDURES

Recombinant DNA technology coupled with first-trimester fetal tissue sampling has enhanced the growth and development of prenatal diagnosis. Obstetric procedures, such as ultrasonography, amniocentesis, chorionic villus sampling and cordocentesis (percutaneous umbilical blood sampling [PUBS]) are currently used during prenatal diagnosis. These procedures are described and discussed in Chapter 18.

TERATOLOGY

A teratogen is any agent or factor that can cause abnormalities of form or function (birth defects) in an exposed fetus. Such abnormalities include fetal wastage and intrauterine fetal growth restriction, malformations due to abnormal growth and morphogenesis, and abnormal central nervous system performance.

It was not until the teratogenic effects of rubella infection were demonstrated in 1941 that any notable consideration was given to environmental factors and their potentially deleterious effects on human pregnancy. In the succeeding decades, the susceptibility of the fetus to many environmental factors has been appreciated.

Probably the best known teratogen is **thalidomide,** which was shown to cause phocomelia and other malformations in the offspring of mothers who had been given the drug during pregnancy. It is the only example of a teratogen that, when introduced to the pregnant population, led to a dramatic epidemic of a specific malformation; withdrawal of the drug led to a virtual disappearance of the malformation.

Although drugs are the most obvious source for teratogenic exposure, chemical waste disposals, alcohol, tobacco, cosmetics, and occupational agents contain substances that individuals are exposed to daily. Some of these agents are known teratogens, whereas the fetal effects of others are not known.

EXPOSURE

Results of the Collaborative Perinatal Project indicate that more than 900 different drugs are taken by pregnant women in the United States and that **40% of women take medication during the first trimester, when organogenesis occurs.** During the first trimester alone, as many as 32% of pregnant women are exposed to analgesics (mostly aspirin), 18% to immunizing agents, 16% to antimicrobial and antiparasitic agents, and 6% to sedatives, tranquilizers, and antidepressants. The great majority of agents, including radiation and drugs, are readily avoidable.

PRINCIPLES OF TERATOLOGY
Fetal Susceptibility

The efficacy of a particular teratogen is, in part, dependent on the genetic makeup of both mother and fetus, as well as on a number of factors related to the maternal-fetal environment. For instance, many congenital abnormalities, such as oral clefts, congenital heart disease, and neural tube defects, are inherited through multifactorial inheritance.

Dose

Depending on the particular teratogen, there may be (1) no apparent effect at a low dose, (2) an organ-specific malformation at an intermediate dose, or (3) a spontaneous abortion at a high dose. Additionally, smaller doses administered over several days may produce a different effect from a single large dose.

Timing

Three stages of teratogenic susceptibility may be identified on the basis of gestational age. Prior to implantation (1 week in humans), there is no demonstrable teratogenic insult. **The most vulnerable stage is between 3 and 8 weeks' gestation, during the period of organogenesis.** The timing determines which organ system or systems are affected. Unfortunately, most women do not realize they are pregnant until this critical period of development is well under way. From about the 4th month of pregnancy to the end of gestation, embryonic development consists primarily of increasing organ size. With the exception of a limited number of tissues (brain and gonads), teratogenic exposure after the 4th month usually causes decreased growth without malformation.

Nature of Teratogenic Agents

Although few agents are known to cause serious malformations in a large proportion of exposed individuals, there are probably hundreds of potentially teratogenic agents, given the right set of circumstances (susceptible fetus, embryologically vulnerable period, large teratogenic dose). Furthermore, certain drugs combined with other drugs may be capable of producing malformations, although neither agent would be teratogenic when taken alone.

TERATOGENIC AGENTS

Teratogens may be assigned to three broad categories: (1) drugs and chemical agents, (2) infectious agents, and (3) radiation. The list that follows is far from exhaustive.

Box 8-2. Clinical features of fetal alcohol syndrome

CRANIOFACIAL
Eyes: Short palpebral fissures, ptosis, strabismus, epicanthic folds, myopia, microphthalmia
Ears: Poorly formed concha, posterior rotation
Nose: Short, hypoplastic philtrum
Mouth: Prominent lateral palatine ridges, micrognathia, cleft lip or palate, faulty enamel
Maxilla: Hypoplastic

CARDIAC
Murmurs, atrial septal defect, ventricular septal defect, tetralogy of Fallot

CENTRAL NERVOUS SYSTEM
Mild-to-moderate mental retardation, microcephaly, poor coordination, hypotonia

GROWTH
Prenatal-onset growth deficiency

MUSCULAR
Hernias of diaphragm, umbilicus, or groin

SKELETAL
Pectus excavatum, abnormal palmar creases, nail hypoplasia, scoliosis

---

Alcohol

The adverse effects of ethyl alcohol on fetal development were not fully realized until the 1970s. The frequency of the **fetal alcohol syndrome** runs as high as 0.2%, whereas an additional 0.4% of newborns show less severe features of the disorder (Box 8-2).

Antianxiety Agents

Antianxiety agents are currently used by a significant number of pregnant women. Data regarding their teratogenicity are conflicting, although **exposure to meprobamate or chlordiazepoxide has been associated with a greater than fourfold increase in severe congenital anomalies. Fluoxetine is now the drug of choice for anxiety and depression during pregnancy** and is considered safe to continue even in women who breastfeed.

Antineoplastic Agents

Aminopterin and methotrexate, both of which are folic acid antagonists, **have been clearly established as teratogens**. Exposure prior to 40 days' gestation is lethal to the embryo; later exposure during the first trimester produces fetal effects, including intrauterine growth restriction, craniofacial anomalies, abnormal positioning of extremities, mental retardation, early miscarriage, stillbirth, and neonatal death.

Alkylating agents, including busulfan, chlorambucil, cyclophosphamide, and nitrogen mustard, have been associated with fetal anomalies such as severe intrauterine growth restriction, fetal death, cleft palate, microphthalmia, limb reduction anomalies, and poorly developed external genitalia. During the first trimester, the teratogenic risks may be as high as 30%.

Anticoagulants

Coumarin derivatives. Use of warfarin (Coumadin) during the 1st trimester is associated with an increased risk of spontaneous abortion, intrauterine growth restriction, central nervous system defects (including mental retardation), stillbirth, and a characteristic syndrome of craniofacial features known as the fetal warfarin syndrome. Embryologically, the most vulnerable time appears to be between 6 and 9 weeks after conception. As many as 30% of exposed fetuses suffer serious teratogenic consequences or loss of the pregnancy occurs. Warfarin easily crosses the placenta, causing bleeding problems in the fetus, and is excreted in breast milk.

Heparin. Heparin has major advantages over coumarin anticoagulants during pregnancy because it does not cross the placenta. **Reported risks include prematurity and fetal demise.** Since no specific malformation syndrome has been described, these abnormalities may be more closely related to the maternal disease necessitating the heparin use.

Anticonvulsants

Approximately 1 in 200 pregnant women is epileptic. Box 8-3 lists the etiologic factors that may play a role in the congenital abnormalities associated with in utero exposure to anticonvulsants. The complexity in providing genetic counseling for pregnant epileptic women is underscored when considering the interactive effects of these factors, the effect of combined anticonvulsant treatment, and the genetic aspects of the disease itself. The goals of counseling include providing the patient with the teratogenic risks of her medication, the risk of seizures during pregnancy, the effect of pregnancy on seizures, and the risk of development of epilepsy in her offspring. **From a medication standpoint, the benefits of seizure prevention need to be weighed against the teratogenicity of the drug.**

Diphenylhydantoin (Dilantin). A specific syndrome, known as the **fetal hydantoin syndrome**, has been described, the clinical features of which include **craniofacial abnormalities, limb reduction defects, prenatal-onset growth restriction, mental deficiency, and cardiovascular anomalies.** Approximately 10% of exposed fetuses demonstrate fetal hydantoin syndrome, whereas an additional 30% may have isolated features of the syndrome. Hydantoins may also have a prenatal carcinogenic effect because several exposed infants with signs of fetal hydantoin syndrome have subsequently developed neuroblastomas.

Diphenylhydantoin is metabolized to toxic oxidative metabolites. The epoxide metabolite, which is normally eliminated by epoxide hydrolase, is thought to be responsible for the increase in congenital abnormalities. Epoxide hydrolase activity is genetically regulated by a single gene with at least two allelic forms, thus providing the potential for determining which infants are at increased risk for anticonvulsant-induced teratogenesis.

Box 8-3. Etiologic factors that may play a role in anticonvulsant teratogenicity

ANTIEPILEPTIC DRUGS
Dose, serum levels, metabolism, teratogenicity, metabolic interactions

GENETIC PREDISPOSITION
Maternal, paternal, and fetal metabolism

MATERNAL DISEASE
Teratogenicity, underlying disease, seizures

Oxazolidinedione Anticonvulsants. Trimethadione (Tridione) and paramethadione (Paradione), used to treat petit mal epilepsy, have been associated with a characteristic malformation syndrome in exposed fetuses. **The clinical features include craniofacial abnormalities, prenatal-onset growth restriction, an increased frequency of mental retardation, and cardiovascular abnormalities.** Because of this serious teratogenic potential and because petit mal epilepsy is rare during reproductive years, **oxazolidinedione anticonvulsants are contraindicated during pregnancy.**

Valproic acid. Valproic acid use during pregnancy is associated with a 1% to 2% risk of open spina bifida. Other findings reported to be associated with valproic acid exposure include cardiac defects, skeletal defects, and craniofacial malformations.

Women exposed to valproic acid during pregnancy should have genetic counseling and should be offered prenatal diagnosis, including careful ultrasonography to check for skeletal or cranial abnormalities and an amniotic fluid AFP analysis to detect open neural tube defects.

Carbamazepine. As with valproic acid, carbamazepine (Tegretol) exposure during pregnancy is associated with an **increased risk for fetal spina bifida** and is an indication for amniotic fluid AFP analysis. Some studies have reported a specific malformation pattern that includes minor craniofacial defects, fingernail hypoplasia, and developmental delay, which are features that would be unlikely to be detected prenatally.

Phenobarbital. The true teratogenicity of phenobarbital is difficult to assess because other drugs are usually taken in combination with this agent, but the risk appears to be very low. **Potential complications of phenobarbital include neonatal withdrawal symptoms and neonatal hemorrhage.** Fetal addiction should not be a complication at the dosage levels required for seizure control.

Hormones

Estrogen/progestin combinations. A large number of pregnant women are exposed to progestins or progestin/estrogen combinations because they continue taking birth control pills, unaware that they are pregnant. Recent analyses have failed to confirm any

teratogenicity, and the Federal Drug Administration has removed the product insert warnings. **The main abnormality associated with the use of strongly androgenic progestins during pregnancy is masculinization of the external genitalia in female fetuses, with a risk of up to 2%.**

Diethylstilbestrol (DES). Diethylstilbestrol, which in the past was widely used in the treatment of "threatened abortion," has clearly been established as a fetal teratogen and carcinogen when used in human pregnancy. **DES exposure poses an increased risk for cervical abnormalities and uterine malformations (see Figure 20-2), as well as for vaginal adenocarcinoma in female offspring.** Exposed males may be at increased risk for testicular abnormalities, infertility, and testicular malignancy.

Miscellaneous Agents

Diuretics. Although there is evidence of diuretic teratogenicity in rodents, teratogenicity has not been clearly demonstrated in humans.

Retinoids. Isotretinoin (Accutane) is prescribed for cystic acne or for acne that has not responded to other forms of treatment. **Exposure during pregnancy is clearly associated with a specific malformation pattern that includes central nervous system, cardiovascular, and craniofacial defects (especially ear abnormalities).** The central nervous system findings include hydrocephaly, facial nerve palsies, and cortical blindness. Microcephaly with severe ear anomalies, microtia, and cleft palate are common findings. The risk of spontaneous abortion or congenital malformations is greater than 50% in patients who take isotretinoin throughout the first trimester.

Etretinate, used for severe psoriasis, has been similarly associated with a characteristic malformation pattern. However, unlike isotretinoin, which has a half-life of less than 1 day, etretinate has a half-life of months, leading to a longer risk period even after the agent has been discontinued.

Tobacco smoking. Maternal tobacco smoking interferes with prenatal growth, including birth weight, birth length, and head circumference. The teratogenic effects are related to the extent of maternal exposure to tobacco and include an increased risk for spontaneous abortion, fetal death, neonatal death, and prematurity. Pregnant women should be strongly encouraged to avoid smoking (or second-hand smoke). They should continue to abstain after delivery because second-hand smoke exposure is associated with an increased risk of respiratory diseases in infants and children.

Illicit drugs. The social, medical, and legal problems associated with illicit drug use during pregnancy have grown considerably over the past few years. Prenatal cocaine exposure has received particular attention as a potential teratogen, particularly among chronic abusers. **Evidence of fetal malformations, particularly genitourinary tract anomalies, and behavioral abnormalities has been documented in fetuses prenatally exposed to cocaine.** Polydrug abuse is at least as significant a public health problem, with many cocaine users additionally abusing marijuana, alcohol, and cigarettes.

Infectious agents. The exact frequency of significant infection during pregnancy is not known, but it is probably between 15% and 25%. **Viruses, bacteria, and parasites may have serious effects on the fetus, including fetal death, growth delay, congenital malformations, and mental deficiency.** In more recent years, the AIDS epidemic has had a significant impact on pregnancy management.

Radiation. Prenatal ionizing radiation exposure occurs frequently as a result of therapeutic or diagnostic medical and dental procedures. **The medical effects of ionizing radiation are dose-dependent and include teratogenesis, mutagenesis, and carcinogenesis.** The most critical period appears to be from about 2 to 6 weeks after conception. Exposures before 2 weeks either produce a lethal effect or produce no effect at all. Teratogenicity is still a possibility after 5 weeks, but the risk for deleterious consequences is relatively small.

Theoretically, any dose of ionizing radiation at a critical time could cause fetal damage. In most circumstances, diagnostic levels of radiation do not produce a teratogenic risk in the developing fetus.

ADVICE DURING PREGNANCY

One of the most important functions of prenatal care is to provide information and support to the woman for self-care. The Cochrane pregnancy and childbirth database (www.cochrane.org) has compiled systematic reviews on the effectiveness of advice and interven-

tions during pregnancy and can be a useful source of information for prenatal care providers. The following sections will examine advice given to alleviate unpleasant symptoms, nutrition, lifestyle, and breastfeeding.

ALLEVIATING UNPLEASANT SYMPTOMS DURING PREGNANCY

Nausea and vomiting complicate up to 70% of pregnancies. Eating small, frequent meals, and avoiding greasy or spicy foods may help. Also, having protein snacks at night, saltine crackers at the bedside, and room-temperature sodas are nonpharmacologic approaches that may provide some relief. **Where medication is deemed to be necessary, antihistamines appear to be the drug of choice,** though no single product has been satisfactorily tested for efficacy and safety. **Vitamin B_6 (pyridoxine) and accupressure ("sea sickness arm bands") may be effective.** Patients with dehydration and electrolyte abnormalities from vomiting (hyperemesis gravidarum) should be evaluated for possible secondary causes, and they may need hospitalization for rehydration and antiemetic therapy.

Heartburn affects about two-thirds of women at some stage of pregnancy, resulting from progesterone-induced relaxation of the esophageal sphincter. Avoiding lying down immediately after meals and elevating the head of the bed may help reduce heartburn. When these simple measures fail, antacids, such as calcium carbonate, should be used.

Constipation is a troublesome problem for many women in pregnancy, secondary to decreased colonic motility. Dietary modification, including increased fiber and water intake, can help lessen this problem. Stool softeners may be used in combination with bulking agents. Irritant laxatives should be reserved for short-term use in refractory cases.

Hemorrhoids are caused by increased venous pressure in the rectum. Increased rest, with elevation of the legs, and avoidance of constipation are recommended.

Leg cramps are experienced by almost half of all pregnant women, particularly at night and in the later months of pregnancy. Massage and stretching may afford some relief during an attack. Both calcium and sodium chloride appear to help reduce leg cramps in pregnancy.

Backaches are common during pregnancy and are lessened by avoiding excessive weight gain. Addition-

Table 8-5. Appropriate weight gain in pregnancy		
	BMI*	Recommended Weight Gain (pounds)
Underweight	<19	28–40
Normal	19–25	25–35
Overweight	>25	15–25

*The PDA contains an electronic calculator for body mass index (BMI).

ally, exercise, sensible shoes, and specially shaped pillows can offer relief. In cases of muscle spasm or strain, analgesics (such as acetaminophen), rest, and heat may lessen the symptoms.

NUTRITIONAL COUNSELING

While the nutritional care plan should be individualized, every woman can benefit from nutritional education that includes counseling on weight gain, dietary guidelines, physical activity, avoidance of harmful substances and unsafe foods, and breastfeeding. The appropriate weight gain during pregnancy is listed in Table 8-5. Recommended rates of weight gain per week during the 2nd and 3rd trimesters are 1.1 pound, 0.9 pound, and 0.66 pound for pregnant women who are underweight, normal weight, and overweight, respectively. **Inadequate weight gain has been associated with low birth weight, whereas excessive weight gain has been associated with fetal macrosomia.** Women should avoid fasting (>13 hours without food) or skipping meals. This behavior is associated with accelerated ketosis and a greater risk of preterm delivery. They should have five feedings per day (breakfast, lunch, afternoon snack, dinner, and bedtime snack). **Pregnant women should never skip breakfast.**

Weight gain is of secondary importance to nutrition; the clinician should emphasize the right amount of nutrition over the right amount of weight gain. Normal pregnancy requires an increase in daily caloric intake of 300 kcal.

LIFESTYLE ADVICE

Women should be advised to rest when tired and reassured that the **fatigue usually abates by the fourth month of pregnancy.** Normal prepregnancy activity levels are usually acceptable. Advice regarding work should be individualized to the nature of the work, the health status of the woman, and the condition of the pregnancy. Work that requires prolonged standing, shift or night work, and high cumulative occupational fatigue has been associated with an increased risk for low birth weight and prematurity. Where working conditions involve occupational fatigue or stress, a change in work during pregnancy should be recommended by the prenatal care provider.

Women should be advised to continue to exercise during pregnancy, unless there is pregnancy-induced hypertension, preterm labor or rupture of membranes, intrauterine growth restriction, incompetent cervix, persistent 2nd- or 3rd-trimester bleeding, or medical conditions that severely restrict physiologic adaptations to exercise during pregnancy. They should avoid exercise in the supine position after the first trimester and should be encouraged to modify the intensity of their exercise according to maternal symptoms. Any type of exercise involving the potential for loss of balance or even mild abdominal trauma should be avoided.

Travel is acceptable under most circumstances. Prolonged sitting increases the risk of thrombus formation and thromboembolism. Pregnant women should be encouraged to ambulate periodically when taking a long flight or car ride. Support stockings may help reduce lower limb edema and varicose veins. International travel that places the patient at a high risk of infectious disease (such as travel to areas with a high rate of transmission of malaria or typhoid fever) should be avoided, whenever possible. When such travel cannot be avoided, appropriate vaccinations should be administered. Live attenuated virus vaccinations are generally contraindicated in pregnancy, but inactivated virus vaccines may be acceptable.

Women should be reassured that increased, unchanged, and decreased levels of sexual activity can all be normal during pregnancy. Abstinence or condom use may be advisable if there is an increased risk of preterm labor or repeated pregnancy loss, or in women with a history of persistent 2nd- or 3rd-trimester bleeding.

BREASTFEEDING

Breastfeeding has been shown to significantly reduce morbidity and improve cognitive development during infancy and childhood. Providers should initiate discussion with the pregnant woman and her family regarding breastfeeding during the first visit, including possible barriers to breastfeeding, such as prior poor experiences, misinformation, or nonsupportive work environment. Partners, peers, and other family members or friends may also exert an important influence on a woman's decision to breastfeed. Referral to a childbirth preparation class or a lactation consultant may provide additional encouragement to breastfeeding.

FOLLOW-UP VISITS

Additional prenatal visits are routinely scheduled every 4 weeks until 28 weeks' gestation, every 2 to 3 weeks until 36 weeks' gestation, and then weekly until delivery. The schedule of these follow-up visits, however, should be tailored to the needs of individual patients. The regularity of scheduled prenatal visits should be sufficient to allow the clinician to monitor the progression of the pregnancy, provide education and recommended screening and interventions, assess the well-being of the fetus and mother, reassure the mother, and detect and treat medical and psychosocial complications.

During each regularly scheduled visit, the clinician should evaluate blood pressure, weight, urine protein and glucose, uterine size for progressive growth, and fetal heart rate. After the woman reports quickening (first sensation of fetal movement, on the average at 20 weeks' gestation) and at each subsequent visit, she should be asked about **fetal movement.** Women are often instructed to perform routine fetal movement counting, though the benefit of such practice remains unsupported by current evidence. Between 24 and 34 weeks, women should be **taught warning symptoms of preterm labor** (uterine contractions, leakage of fluid, vaginal bleeding, low pelvic pressure, or low back pain). Patients at risk may require additional visits to assess signs and symptoms of preterm labor. Beginning in the late 2nd trimester, they should also be **taught to recognize the warning symptoms of preeclampsia** (headache, visual changes, hand or facial swelling, or epigastric or right upper quadrant pain). Near term, they should be instructed on the symptoms of labor.

Beginning at 28 weeks, systematic examination of the abdomen is carried out at each prenatal visit to **identify the lie** (e.g., longitudinal, transverse, oblique), **presentation** (e.g., vertex, breech, shoulder),

or position (e.g., flexion, extension, or rotation of the occiput) of the fetus. This can be accomplished by the **maneuvers of Leopold.** The **first maneuver** involves palpating the fundus to determine which part of the fetus occupies the fundus. The head is round and hard, whereas the breech is irregular and soft. The **second maneuver** involves palpating either side of the abdomen to determine on which side the fetal back lies. The fetal back is linear and firm, whereas the extremities have multiple parts. The **third maneuver** involves grasping the presenting part between the thumb and third finger just above the pubic symphysis to determine the presenting part. The **fourth maneuver** involves palpating for the brow and the occiput of the fetus to determine fetal head position when the fetus is in a vertex presentation. This is best accomplished with the examiner facing the patient's feet and placing both hands on either side of the lower abdomen just above the inlet. By exerting pressure in the direction of the pelvic inlet, the hand running along the back will bump into the occiput if the head is extended, whereas the hand on the same side of the small parts will bump into the brow if the head is flexed.

Depending on the practice setting and population, either universal or selective **screening for gestational diabetes** should be performed between 24 and 28 weeks of gestation. Risk factors for selective screening include family history of diabetes; previous birth of a macrosomic, malformed, or stillborn baby; hypertension; glycosuria; maternal age of 30 years or older; or previous gestational diabetes. **The cost-effectiveness of diabetic screening during pregnancy remains highly controversial.** Repeat measurements of **hemoglobin or hematocrit levels** early in the third trimester have been recommended. Tests **for sexually transmitted infections** (e.g., syphilis) may also be repeated at 32 to 36 weeks of gestation if the woman has specific risk factors for these diseases. The Centers for Disease Control and Prevention recommend **universal screening for maternal colonization of Group B Streptococcus** at 35 to 37 weeks of gestation. The value of selective ultrasound for specific indications has been clearly established; the value of routine ultrasound in low-risk pregnancies remains undetermined. Ultrasonic examination during pregnancy is not harmful, but controlled trials have failed to demonstrate that routine ultrasonic examinations for dating in early pregnancy, anatomic survey in mid-pregnancy, or anthropometry in late pregnancy improve perinatal outcome.

ANTENATAL TESTING GUIDELINES

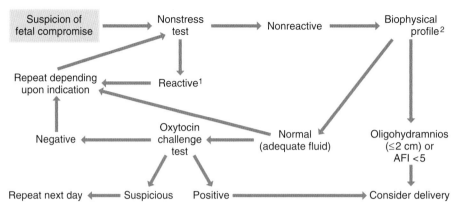

[1] All pregnancies complicated by IUGR or postdatism should have a complete biophysical profile that includes an ultrasonic evaluation.

[2] Ultrasonic assessment: (A) fetal movements, 3 per 10 minutes; (B) fetal breathing, 30 per 10 minutes; (C) amniotic fluid index (AFI) (N = 5-20). (D) fetal tone.

Figure 8-2. Algorithm for the antenatal evaluation of a high-risk pregnancy.

ASSESSMENT OF FETAL WELL-BEING

During the past 20 years, electronic advances have provided new technology that has made the fetus more accessible and has allowed visualization of the fetus and recording of intrauterine fetal events. A combination of the nonstress test, contraction stress test, and real-time ultrasonic assessment is used to assess fetal well-being. Figure 8-2 presents an algorithm that may be used to follow a high-risk pregnancy.

MATERNAL ASSESSMENT

A simple technique (kick counting) may be used to assess fetal well-being. The mother asseses fetal movement (kick counts) each evening on her left side. She should recognize 10 movements in 1 hour. She is told to contact her doctor or other health care provider if she does not perceive fetal movements at this rate or greater.

NONSTRESS TEST

The first assessment of fetal well-being is the nonstress test. With the mother resting in the left lateral supine position, a continuous fetal heart rate tracing is obtained using external Doppler equipment. The mother reports each fetal movement, and the effects of the fetal movements on heart rate are determined. **A normal fetus responds to fetal movement with an acceleration in fetal heart rate of 15 beats or more per minute above the baseline for at least 15 seconds** (Figure 8-3). If at least two such accelerations occur in a 20-minute interval, the fetus is regarded as being healthy, and the test is said to be reactive. A nonreactive nonstress test is shown in Figure 8-4.

ULTRASONIC ASSESSMENT

The next step in prenatal assessment is to determine the adequacy of amniotic fluid volume by real-time ultrasonography. Reduced fluid (oligohydramnios) suggests fetal compromise. Oligohydramnios can be defined as an amniotic fluid index (AFI) of less than 5. **The AFI represents the total of the linear measurements (in centimeters) of the largest amniotic fluid pockets noted on ultrasonic inspection of each of the four quadrants of the gestational sac.** When amniotic fluid is reduced, the fetus is more likely to become compromised as a result

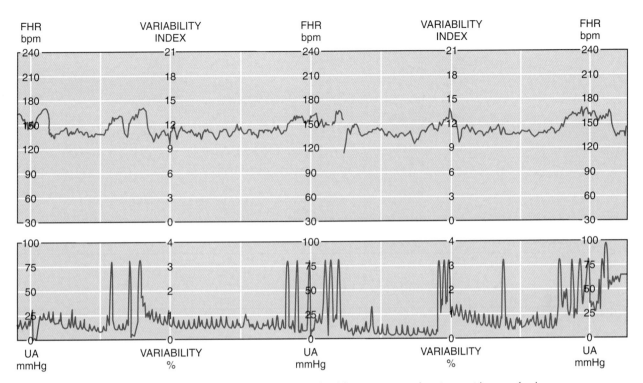

Figure 8-3. Reactive nonstress test. Note the fetal heart rate accelerations with most fetal movements, denoted by spikes above 75 mm Hg in lower panel.

of umbilical cord compression. Excessive amniotic fluid (polyhydramnios; AFI > 23) can be a sign of poor control in a diabetic pregnancy or an indication that the fetus may have an anomaly. **Fetal breathing (chest wall movements) and fetal movements (stretching and rotational movements) are also used to assess the fetus.** A fetus who has at least 30 breathing movements in 10 minutes or 3 body movements in 10 minutes is considered healthy. A combination of a **reactive nonstress test, adequate amniotic fluid, adequate fetal breathing, adequate fetal movements, and adequate tone** is frequently referred to as a **normal biophysical profile.** Each parameter is given a score of 2. A normal profile equals 10. Table 8-6 lists the recommended frequency for biophysical profile testing based on the high-risk condition.

CONTRACTION STRESS TEST

The contraction stress test is a test for uteroplacental dysfunction, a condition that may occur in a high-risk pregnancy. **A dilute infusion of oxytocin is given to establish at least 3 uterine contractions in 10 minutes. If late decelerations are observed with each contraction, the test is positive (abnormal).** If only one deceleration is observed, the test is suspicious. When the test is positive, the baby should usually be delivered.

PREVENTIVE HEALTH CARE

Management prior to and during pregnancy presents an opportunity for patient education and the practice of preventive medicine. **Childbirth preparation classes for both the patient and her husband are very educational, particularly during the first pregnancy.** The presence and encouragement of the baby's father can be most helpful during labor and delivery. These classes provide an important opportunity for both parents to enhance bonding to the infant before birth.

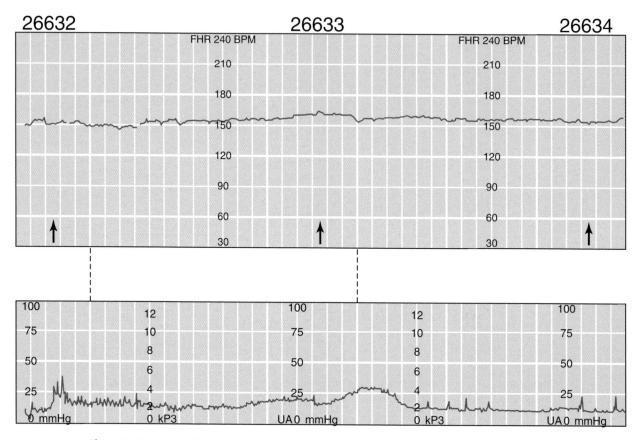

Figure 8-4. Nonreactive nonstress test. Note the lack of beat-to-beat variability and the lack of acceleration of the fetal heart rate with fetal movements *(arrows)*.

Although preconception, prenatal, and obstetric information is of primary importance, other topics that may have lifelong relevance can be introduced and emphasized during antepartum care. The pregnancy itself is frequently a strong motivator for women to eliminate potentially harmful habits or dietary patterns and to become more aware of their general health. Therefore, a systematic approach to the dissemination of preventive health care information is generally well received by the pregnant woman.

Table 8-6. Recommended frequency for biophysical profile testing	
High-Risk Condition	Frequency
IUGR	
Mild	Weekly
Moderate*	Twice weekly
Diabetes mellitus	
Class A	Weekly, 37 to 40 wk Twice weekly, beyond 40 wk
Class B and worse	Twice weekly, beginning at 34 wk
Post-term pregnancy	Twice weekly, beginning at 42 wk
Decreased fetal movements	Weekly
Other high-risk conditions	Weekly
Maternal or physician concern	Weekly

IUGR, Intrauterine growth restriction.
*For severe IUGR, delivery is usually indicated.

Suggested Reading

American College of Medical Genetics Policy Statement: Fragile X syndrome: Diagnostic and carrier testing. Am J Med Genet 53:380–381, 1994.

American College of Obstetricians and Gynecologists: Teratology, Bulletin No. 236. Washington, DC, ACOG, 1997.

American College of Obstetricians and Gynecologists Committee Opinion: Genetic Evaluation of Stillbirths and Neonatal Death, Bulletin No. 178. Washington, DC, ACOG, 1997.

American College of Obstetricians and Gynecologists: Preconceptional Care, ACOG Technical Bulletin 205. Washington, DC, ACOG, 1995.

American Academy of Pediatrics and the American College of Obstetricians and Gynecologists: Guidelines for Perinatal Care, 4th ed. Elk Grove Village, Ill, American Academy of Pediatrics, 1997.

Enkin M, Keirse MJNC, Renfrew M, Neilson J: A Guide to Effective Care in Pregnancy and Childbirth, 2nd ed. Oxford, Oxford University Press, 1999.

Korenbrot CC, Moss NE: Preconception, prenatal, perinatal and postnatal influences on health. *In* Smedley BD, Syme SL, (eds): Promoting Health: Intervention Strategies from Social and Behavioral Research. Washington, DC, National Academy Press, 2000.

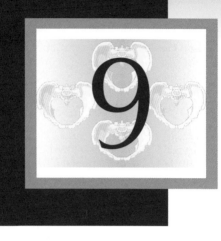

9

Normal Labor, Delivery, and Postpartum Care: Anatomic Considerations, Obstetric Analgesia and Anesthesia, and Resuscitation of the Newborn

Calvin J. Hobel and Anita Backus Chang

Labor is a physiologic process that permits a series of extensive physiologic changes in the mother to allow for the delivery of her fetus through the birth canal. **It is defined as progressive cervical effacement and dilatation resulting from regular uterine contractions that occur at least every 5 minutes and last 30 to 60 seconds.**

The role of the obstetrician is to anticipate and manage abnormalities that may occur to either the maternal or the fetal process. When a decision is made to intervene, it must be considered carefully, because each intervention carries not only potential benefits, but also potential risks. In the vast majority of cases, the best management may be close observation and, when necessary, cautious intervention.

ANATOMIC CHARACTERISTICS OF THE FETAL HEAD AND MATERNAL PELVIS

Vaginal delivery necessitates the accommodation of the fetal head to the bony pelvis. Therefore, it is necessary to know the key pelvic landmarks and diameters of the fetal skull and to be able to identify the important sutures and fontanelles.

FETAL HEAD

The head is the largest and least compressible part of the fetus. Thus, from an obstetric viewpoint, it is the most important part, whether the presentation is cephalic or breech.

The fetal skull consists of a base and a vault (cranium). The base of the skull has large, ossified, firmly united, and noncompressible bones. This serves to protect the vital structures contained within the brain stem.

The cranium consists of the occipital bone posteriorly, two parietal bones bilaterally, and two frontal and temporal bones anteriorly. The cranial bones at birth are thin, weakly ossified, easily compressible, and interconnected only by membranes. These features allow them to overlap under pressure and to change shape to conform to the maternal pelvis, a process known as "molding."

Sutures

The membrane-occupied spaces between the cranial bones are known as sutures. The **sagittal suture** lies between the parietal bones and extends in an anteroposterior direction between the fontanelles, dividing the head into right and left sides (Figure 9-1). The **lambdoid suture** extends from the posterior fontanelle laterally and serves to separate the occipital from the parietal bones. The **coronal suture** extends from the anterior fontanelle laterally and serves to separate the parietal and frontal bones. The frontal suture lies between the frontal bones and extends from the anterior fontanelle to the glabella (the prominence between the eyebrows).

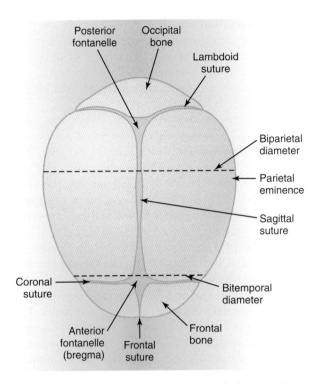

Figure 9-1. Superior view of the fetal skull showing the sutures, fontanelles, and transverse diameters.

Fontanelles

The membrane-filled spaces located at the point where the sutures intersect are known as fontanelles, the most important of which are the anterior and posterior fontanelles. Clinically, they are even more useful in diagnosing the fetal head position than the sutures.

The **posterior fontanelle** closes at 6 to 8 weeks of life, whereas the **anterior fontanelle** does not become ossified until approximately 18 months. This allows the skull to accommodate the tremendous growth of the infant's brain after birth.

The anterior fontanelle (bregma) is found at the intersection of the sagittal, frontal, and coronal sutures. It is diamond shaped and measures approximately 2 × 3 cm, and it is much larger than the posterior fontanelle. The posterior fontanelle is Y- or T-shaped and is found at the junction of the sagittal and lambdoid sutures.

Landmarks

The fetal skull is characterized by a number of landmarks. Moving from front to back, they include the following (Figure 9-2):

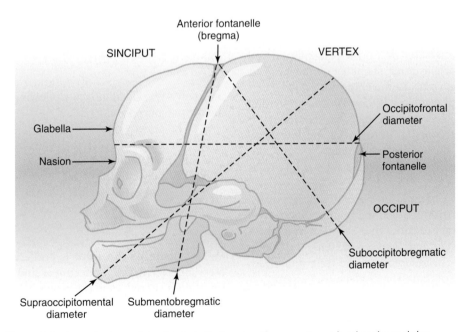

Figure 9-2. Lateral view of the fetal skull showing the prominent landmarks and the anteroposterior diameters.

1. **Nasion** (the root of the nose)
2. **Glabella** (the elevated area between the orbital ridges)
3. **Sinciput (brow)** (the area between the anterior fontanelle and the glabella)
4. **Anterior fontanelle (bregma)**—diamond shaped
5. **Vertex** (the area between the fontanelles and bounded laterally by the parietal eminences)
6. **Posterior fontanelle (lambda)**—Y- or T-shaped
7. **Occiput** (the area behind and inferior to the posterior fontanelle and lambdoid sutures)

Diameters

Several diameters of the fetal skull are important (see Figures 9-1 and 9-2). The anteroposterior diameter presenting to the maternal pelvis depends on the degree of flexion or extension of the head and is important because the various diameters differ in length. The following measurements are considered average for a term fetus:

1. **Suboccipitobregmatic (9.5 cm),** the presenting anteroposterior diameter when the head is well flexed, as in an occipitotransverse or occipitoanterior position. It extends from the undersurface of the occipital bone at the junction with the neck to the center of the anterior fontanelle.
2. **Occipitofrontal (11 cm),** the presenting anteroposterior diameter when the head is deflexed, as in an occipitoposterior presentation; it extends from the external occipital protuberance to the glabella.
3. **Supraoccipitomental (13.5 cm),** the presenting anteroposterior diameter in a brow presentation and the longest anteroposterior diameter of the head; it extends from the vertex to the chin.
4. **Submentobregmatic (9.5 cm),** the presenting anteroposterior diameter in face presentations; it extends from the junction of the neck and lower jaw to the center of the anterior fontanelle.

The transverse diameters of the fetal skull are as follows:

1. **Biparietal (9.5 cm),** the largest transverse diameter; it extends between the temporal bones.
2. **Bitemporal (8 cm),** the shortest transverse diameter; it extends between the temporal bones.

The average circumference of the term fetal head, measured in the occipitofrontal plane, is 34.5 cm.

PELVIC ANATOMY
Bony Pelvis

The bony pelvis is made up of four bones: the sacrum, coccyx, and two innominates (composed of the ilium, ischium, and pubis). These are held together by the sacroiliac joints, the symphysis pubis, and the sacrococcygeal joint. The union of the pelvis and the vertebral column stabilizes the pelvis and allows weight to be transmitted to the lower extremities.

The sacrum consists of five fused vertebrae. The anterior superior edge of the first sacral vertebra is called the **promontory,** which protrudes slightly into the cavity of the pelvis. The anterior surface of the sacrum is usually concave. It articulates with the ilium at its upper segment, with the coccyx at its lower segment, and with the sacrospinous and sacrotuberous ligaments laterally.

The coccyx is composed of three to five rudimentary vertebrae. It articulates with the sacrum forming a joint, and occasionally the bones are fused.

The pelvis is divided into the false pelvis above and the true pelvis below the linea terminalis. The false pelvis is bordered by the lumbar vertebrae posteriorly, an iliac fossa bilaterally, and the abdominal wall anteriorly. Its only obstetric function is to support the pregnant uterus.

The true pelvis is a bony canal and is formed by the sacrum and coccyx posteriorly and by the ischium and pubis laterally and anteriorly. Its internal borders are solid and relatively immobile. The posterior wall is twice the length of the anterior wall. The true pelvis is the area of concern to the obstetrician because its dimensions are sometimes not adequate to permit passage of the fetus.

Pelvic Planes

The pelvis is divided into the following four planes for descriptive purposes:

1. The pelvic inlet
2. The plane of greatest diameter
3. The plane of least diameter
4. The pelvic outlet

These planes are imaginary, flat surfaces that extend across the pelvis at different levels. Except for the plane of greatest diameter, each plane is clinically significant.

The **plane of the inlet** is bordered by the pubic crest anteriorly, the iliopectineal line of the innominate bones laterally, and the promontory of the sacrum posteriorly. The fetal head enters the pelvis through this plane in the transverse position.

The **plane of greatest diameter** is the largest part of the pelvic cavity. It is bordered by the posterior midpoint of the pubis anteriorly, the upper part of the obturator foramina laterally, and the junction of the 2nd and 3rd sacral vertebrae posteriorly. The fetal head rotates to the anterior position in this plane.

The **plane of least diameter** is the most important from a clinical standpoint, because most instances of arrest of descent occur at this level. It is bordered by the lower edge of the pubis anteriorly, the ischial spines and sacrospinous ligaments laterally, and the lower sacrum posteriorly. Low transverse arrests generally occur in this plane.

The **plane of the pelvic outlet** is formed by two triangular planes with a common base at the level of the ischial tuberosities. The anterior triangle is bordered by the subpubic angle at the apex, the pubic rami on the sides, and the bituberous diameter at the base. The posterior triangle is bordered by the sacrococcygeal joint at its apex, the sacrotuberous ligaments on the sides, and the bituberous diameter at the base. This plane is the site of a low pelvic arrest.

Pelvic Diameters

The diameters of the pelvic planes represent the amount of space available at each level. The key measurements for assessing the capacity of the maternal pelvis include the following:

1. The obstetric conjugate of the inlet
2. The bispinous diameter
3. The bituberous diameter
4. The posterior sagittal diameter at all levels
5. The curve and length of the sacrum
6. The subpubic angle

Table 9-1. Average length of pelvic plane diameters

Pelvic Plane	Diameter	Average Length (cm)
Inlet	True conjugate	11.5
	Obstetric conjugate	11
	Transverse	13.5
	Oblique	12.5
	Posterior sagittal	4.5
Greatest diameter	Anteroposterior	12.75
	Transverse	12.5
Midplane	Anteroposterior	12
	Bispinous	10.5
	Posterior sagittal	4.5–5
Outlet	Anatomic anteroposterior	9.5
	Obstetric anteroposterior	11.5
	Bituberous	11
	Posterior sagittal	7.5

The average lengths of the diameters of each pelvic plane are listed in Table 9-1.

Pelvic Inlet

The pelvic inlet has five important diameters (Figure 9-3). The anteroposterior diameter is described by one

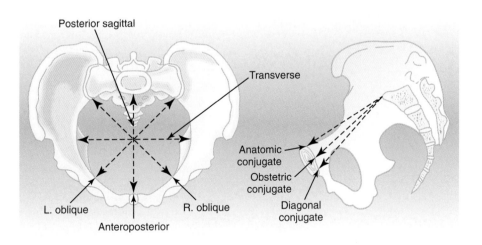

Figure 9-3. Pelvic inlet and its diameters.

of two measurements. The **true conjugate (anatomic conjugate)** is the anatomic diameter and extends from the middle of the sacral promontory to the superior surface of the pubic symphysis. The **obstetric conjugate** represents the actual space available to the fetus and extends from the middle of the sacral promontory to the closest point on the convex posterior surface of the symphysis pubis.

The **transverse diameter** is the widest distance between the iliopectineal lines. Each **oblique diameter** extends from the sacroiliac joint to the opposite iliopectineal eminence.

The **posterior sagittal diameter** extends from the anteroposterior and transverse intersection to the middle of the sacral promontory.

Plane of Greatest Diameter

The plane of greatest diameter has two noteworthy diameters. The **anteroposterior diameter** extends from the midpoint of the posterior surface of the pubis to the junction of the 2nd and 3rd sacral vertebrae.

Plane of Least Diameter (Midplane)

The plane of least diameter has three important diameters. The **anteroposterior diameter** extends from the lower border of the pubis to the junction of the fourth and fifth sacral vertebrae. The **transverse (bispinous) diameter** extends between the ischial spines. The **posterior sagittal diameter** extends from the midpoint of the bispinous diameter to the junction of the fourth and fifth sacral vertebrae.

Pelvic Outlet

The pelvic outlet has four important diameters (Figure 9-4). The **anatomic anteroposterior diameter** extends from the inferior margin of the pubis to the tip of the coccyx, whereas the **obstetric anteroposterior diameter** extends from the inferior margin of the pubis to the sacrococcygeal joint. The **transverse (bituberous) diameter** extends between the inner surfaces of the ischial tuberosities, and the **posterior sagittal diameter** extends from the middle of the transverse diameter to the sacrococcygeal joint.

PELVIC SHAPES

Based on the general bony architecture, the pelvis may be classified into four basic types (Fig. 9-5).

Gynecoid

The gynecoid pelvis is the classic female type of pelvis and is found in approximately 50% of women. It has the following characteristics:
1. Round at the inlet, with the widest transverse diameter only slightly greater than the anteroposterior diameter
2. Side walls straight

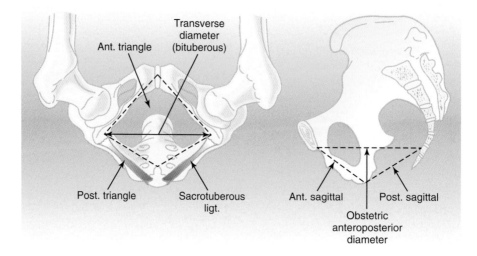

Figure 9-4. Pelvic outlet and its diameters.

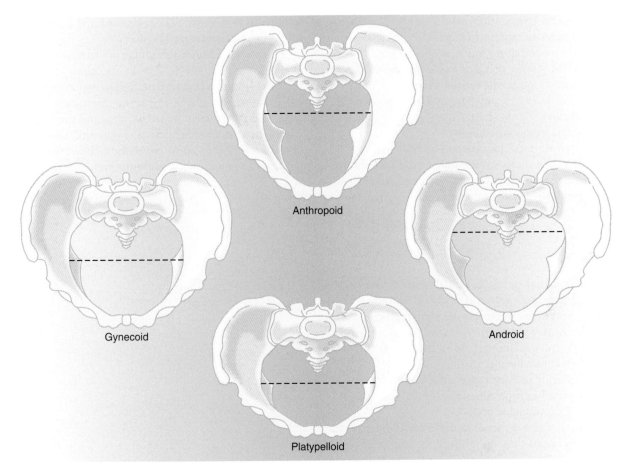

Figure 9-5. The four basic pelvic types. The *dotted line* indicates the transverse diameter of the inlet. Note that the widest diameter of the inlet is posteriorly situated in an android or anthropoid pelvis.

3. Ischial spines of average prominence
4. Well-rounded sacrosciatic notch
5. Well-curved sacrum
6. Spacious subpubic arch, with an angle of approximately 90 degrees

These features create a cylindrical shape that is spacious throughout. The fetal head generally rotates into the occipitoanterior position in this type of pelvis.

Android

The android pelvis is the typical male type of pelvis, and it is found in less than 30% of women and has the following characteristics:

1. Triangular inlet with a flat posterior segment and the widest transverse diameter closer to the sacrum than in the gynecoid type

2. Convergent side walls with prominent spines
3. Shallow sacral curve
4. Long and narrow sacrosciatic notch
5. Narrow subpubic arch

This type of pelvis has limited space at the inlet and progressively less space as one moves down the pelvis, owing to the funneling effect of the side walls, sacrum, and pubic rami. Thus, the amount of space is restricted at all levels. The fetal head is forced to be in the occipitoposterior position to conform to the narrow anterior pelvis. Arrest of descent is common at the midpelvis.

Anthropoid

The anthropoid pelvis resembles that of the anthropoid ape. It is found in approximately 20% of women and has the following characteristics:

1. A much larger anteroposterior than transverse diameter, creating a long narrow oval at the inlet
2. Side walls that do not converge
3. Ischial spines that are not prominent but are close, owing to the overall shape
4. Variable, but usually posterior, inclination of the sacrum
5. Large sacrosciatic notch
6. Narrow, outwardly shaped subpubic arch

The fetal head can engage only in the anteroposterior diameter and usually does so in the occipitoposterior position, because there is more space in the posterior pelvis.

Platypelloid

The platypelloid pelvis is best described as being a flattened gynecoid pelvis. It is found in only 3% of women, and it has the following characteristics:

1. A short anteroposterior and wide transverse diameter creating an oval-shaped inlet
2. Straight or divergent side walls
3. Posterior inclination of a flat sacrum
4. A wide bispinous diameter
5. A wide subpubic arch

The overall shape is that of a gentle curve throughout. The fetal head has to engage in the transverse diameter.

ENGAGEMENT

Engagement occurs when the widest diameter of the fetal presenting part has passed through the pelvic inlet. In cephalic presentations, the widest diameter is biparietal; in breech presentations, it is intertrochanteric.

The station of the presenting part in the pelvic canal is defined as its level above or below the plane of the ischial spines. The level of the ischial spines is assigned as "zero" station, and each centimeter above or below this level is given a minus or plus designation, respectively.

In the majority of women, the bony presenting part is at the level of the ischial spines when the head has become engaged. The fetal head usually engages with its sagittal suture in the transverse diameter of the pelvis. The head position is considered to be **synclitic** when the biparietal diameter is parallel to the pelvic plane and the sagittal suture is midway between the anterior and posterior planes of the pelvis.

When this relationship is not present, the head is considered to be **asynclitic** (Figure 9-6).

There is a distinct advantage to having the head engage in asynclitism in certain situations. In a synclitic presentation, the biparietal diameter entering the pelvis measures 9.5 cm; but when the parietal bones enter the pelvis in an asynclitic manner, the presenting diameter measures 8.75 cm. Therefore, asynclitism permits a larger head to enter the pelvis than would be possible in a synclitic presentation.

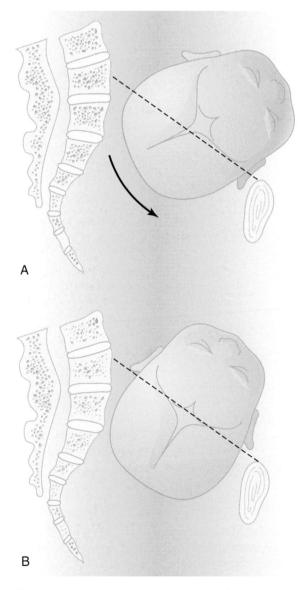

A

B

Figure 9-6. Anterior asynclitism entering the pelvis (A), and synclitism in the pelvis (B).

CLINICAL PELVIMETRY

It is not possible to assess all of the pelvic dimensions by clinical measurement. The diameters that can be clinically evaluated can be assessed at the time of the first prenatal visit to screen for obvious pelvic contractions, although some obstetricians believe that it is better to wait until later in pregnancy when the soft tissues are more distensible and the examination is less uncomfortable and possibly more accurate.

The clinical evaluation is started by assessing the pelvic inlet. The pelvic inlet can be evaluated clinically for its anteroposterior diameter. The obstetric conjugate can be estimated from the diagonal conjugate, which is obtained on clinical examination.

The diagonal conjugate is approximated by measuring from the lower border of the pubis to the sacral promontory using the tip of the second finger and the point where the index finger meets the pubis (Figure 9-7). The **obstetric conjugate** is then estimated by subtracting 1.5 to 2 cm, depending on the height and inclination of the pubis. Often the middle finger of the examining hand cannot reach the sacral promontory; thus, the obstetric conjugate is considered adequate. If the diagonal conjugate is greater than or equal to 11.5 cm, the anteroposterior diameter of the inlet is considered to be adequate.

The anterior surface of the sacrum is then palpated to assess its curvature. The usual shape is concave. A flat or convex shape may indicate anteroposterior constriction throughout the pelvis.

The midpelvis cannot accurately be measured clinically in either the anteroposterior or transverse diameter. A reasonable estimate of the size of the midpelvis, however, can be obtained as follows. **The pelvic side walls can be assessed to determine if they are convergent rather than having the normal, almost parallel, configuration.** The ischial spines are palpated carefully to assess their prominence, and several passes are made between the spines to approximate the bispinous diameter. The length of the sacrospinous ligament is assessed by placing one

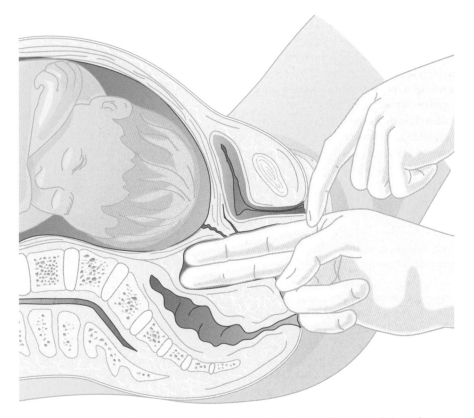

Figure 9-7. Clinical estimation of the diagonal conjugate diameter of the pelvis.

finger on the ischial spine and one finger on the sacrum in the midline. The average length is three fingerbreadths. If the sacrosciatic notch that is located lateral to the ligament can accommodate two-and-a-half fingers, the posterior midpelvis is most likely of adequate dimensions. A short ligament suggests a forward inclination of the sacrum and a narrowed sacrosciatic notch.

Finally, the pelvic outlet is assessed. This is done by first placing a fist between the ischial tuberosities. An 8.5 cm distance is considered to indicate an adequate transverse diameter. The posterior sagittal measurement should also be greater than 8 cm. The infrapubic angle is assessed by placing a thumb next to each inferior pubic ramus and then estimating the angle at which they meet. An angle of less than 90 degrees is associated with a contracted transverse diameter in the midplane and outlet.

Radiologic Assessment of the Pelvis

X-ray pelvimetry is rarely used today. When an accurate measurement of the pelvis is indicated, nuclear magnetic resonance imaging (MRI) may be used. The advantage of MRI over x-ray or computerized tomography (CT) for pelvic assessment is the lack of ionizing radiation exposure.

Indications
   1. Clinical evidence or obstetric history suggestive of pelvic abnormalities.
   2. A history of pelvic trauma.

It should always be questioned whether the results obtained by radiologic assessment will have sufficient influence on the patient's management to make the investigation worthwhile.

PREPARATION FOR LABOR

Before actual labor begins, a number of physiologic preparatory events usually occur.

Lightening

Two or more weeks before labor, the fetal head in most primigravid women settles into the brim of the pelvis. In multigravida, this often does not occur until early in labor. Lightening may be noted by the mother as a flattening of the upper abdomen and an increased prominence of the lower abdomen.

False Labor

During the last 4 to 8 weeks of pregnancy, the uterus undergoes irregular contractions that normally are painless. Such contractions appear unpredictably and sporadically and can be rhythmic and of mild intensity. In the last month of pregnancy, these contractions may occur more frequently, sometimes every 10 to 20 minutes, and with greater intensity. These Braxton Hicks contractions are considered false labor in that they are not associated with progressive cervical dilatation or effacement. They may serve, however, a physiologic role in preparing the uterus and cervix for true labor.

Cervical Effacement

Prior to the onset of parturition, the cervix is frequently noted to soften as a result of increased water content and collagen lysis. Simultaneous effacement, or thinning of the cervix, occurs as it is taken up into the lower uterine segment (Figure 9-8). Consequently, patients often present in early labor with a cervix that is already partially effaced. As a result of cervical effacement, the mucous plug within the cervical canal may be released. The onset of labor may thus be heralded by the passage of a small amount of blood-tinged mucus from the vagina ("bloody show").

STAGES OF LABOR

There are four stages of labor, each of which is considered separately. These stages in actuality are definitions of progress during labor, delivery, and the puerperium.

The first stage is from the onset of true labor to complete dilation of the cervix. The second stage is from complete dilation of the cervix to the birth of the baby. The third stage is from the birth of the baby to delivery of the placenta. The fourth stage is from delivery of the placenta to stabilization of the patient's condition, usually at about 6 hours postpartum.

First Stage of Labor

Phases. The first stage of labor consists of two phases: a latent phase, during which cervical effacement and early dilatation occur, and an active phase, during which more rapid cervical dilatation occurs (Figure 9-9). Although cervical

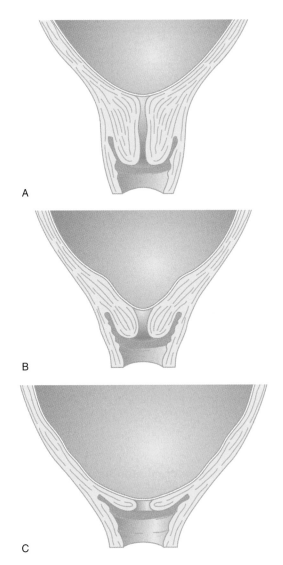

Table 9-2. **Characteristics of normal labor**		
Characteristic	Primipara	Multipara
Duration of first stage	6–18 hr	2–10 hr
Rate of cervical dilatation during active phase	1 cm/hr	1.2 cm/hr
Duration of second stage	30 min to 3 hr	5–30 min
Duration of third stage	0–30 min	0–30 min

Figure 9-8. *A,* The absence of cervical effacement prior to labor. *B,* Cervix being progressively taken up into the lower segment of the uterus (approximately 50% effaced). *C,* Cervix fully taken up (i.e., cervix is completely effaced).

softening and early effacement may occur before labor, during the first stage of labor the entire cervical length is retracted into the lower uterine segment.

Length. The length of the first stage may vary in relation to parity; primiparous patients generally experience a longer first stage than do multiparous patients (Table 9-2). Because the latent phase may overlap considerably with the preparatory phase of labor, its duration is highly variable. It may also be influenced by

other factors, such as sedation and stress. The active phase begins when the cervix is 3 to 4 cm dilated in the presence of regularly occurring uterine contractions. **The minimal dilatation during the active phase of the first stage is nearly the same for primiparous and multiparous women: 1 and 1.2 cm/hour, respectively.** If progress is slower than this, evaluation for uterine dysfunction, fetal malposition, or cephalopelvic disproportion should be undertaken.

Measurement of progress. During the first stage, the progress of labor may be measured in terms of cervical effacement, cervical dilatation, and descent of the fetal head. The clinical pattern of the uterine contractions alone is not an adequate indication of progress. After completion of cervical dilatation, the second stage commences. Thereafter, only the descent, flexion, and rotation of the presenting part are available to assess the progress of labor.

Clinical management of the first stage. Certain steps should be taken in the clinical management of the patient during the first stage of labor.

MATERNAL POSITION. The mother may ambulate during the first stage of labor provided that intermittent monitoring ensures fetal well-being and the presenting part is engaged in patients with ruptured membranes. **If she is lying in bed, the lateral recumbent position should be encouraged** to ensure perfusion of the uteroplacental unit.

ADMINISTRATION OF FLUIDS. Because of decreased gastric emptying during labor, **oral fluids are best avoided.** Placement of a 16- to 18-gauge venous catheter is advisable during the active phase of labor. This intravenous route is used to hydrate the patient with crystalloids during labor, to administer oxytocin after the delivery of the placenta, and for the treatment of any unanticipated emergencies.

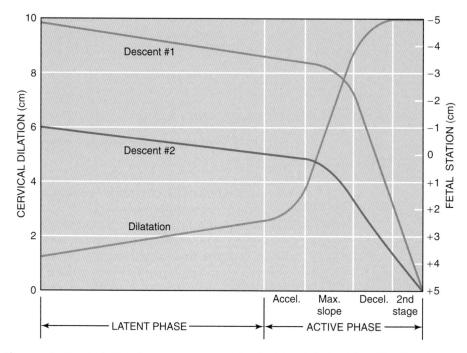

Figure 9-9. Cervical dilatation and descent of the fetal head during labor. The first descent curve represents a fetus with a floating presenting part at the onset of labor, whereas the second represents a fetus with the presenting part fixed in the pelvis prior to labor. *Modified from Friedman EA: Labor: Evaluation and Management, 2nd ed. East Norwalk, CT, Appleton-Century-Crofts, 1978, p 41.*

INVESTIGATIONS. Every woman admitted in labor should have a hematocrit or hemoglobin measurement and a blood clot held in the event that a crossmatch is needed. Blood group, rhesus (Rh) type, and an antibody screen should be done if these are not known. It is also important to know the hepatitis-B status of the mother so that a pediatrician can be notified if the mother is positive. Additionally, a voided urine specimen should be checked for the presence of protein and glucose.

MATERNAL MONITORING. Maternal pulse rate, blood pressure, respiratory rate, and temperature should be recorded every 1 to 2 hours in normal labor and more frequently if indicated. Fluid balance, particularly urine output and intake, should be monitored carefully.

ANALGESIA. Adequate analgesia is important during the first stage of labor (see later in this chapter).

FETAL MONITORING. The fetal heart rate should be evaluated by either auscultation with a DeLee stethoscope, **by external monitoring with Doppler equipment, or by internal monitoring with a fetal scalp electrode.** In uncomplicated pregnancies, continuous electronic fetal monitoring is not necessary, as several studies have demonstrated that intermittent auscultation of the fetal heart rate, when performed in conjunction with a 1:1 nurse-to-patient ratio, results in outcomes comparable to those of electronic heart rate recording. **In patients with no significant obstetric risk factors, the fetal heart rate should be auscultated or the electronic monitor tracing evaluated at least every 30 minutes in the active phase of the first stage of labor and at least every 15 minutes in the second stage of labor. In patients with obstetric risk factors, the fetal heart rate should be auscultated or the electronic monitoring tracing evaluated at least every 15 minutes during the active phase of the first stage of labor (immediately following a uterine contraction), and at least every 5 minutes during the second stage.**

UTERINE ACTIVITY. Uterine contractions should be monitored every 30 minutes by palpation for their frequency, duration, and intensity. **For high-risk pregnancies, uterine contractions should be monitored continuously along with the fetal heart rate.** This can be achieved electronically using either an external tocodynamometer or an internal pressure catheter in the amniotic cavity. The latter is particularly of value when a patient's labor is being augmented with oxytocin (Pitocin).

VAGINAL EXAMINATION. During the latent phase, particularly when the membranes are ruptured, vaginal examinations should be done sparingly to decrease the risk of an intrauterine infection. **In the active phase, the cervix should be assessed approximately every 2 hours to determine the progress of labor.** Cervical effacement and dilatation, the station and position of the presenting part, and the presence of molding or caput in vertex presentations should be recorded.

AMNIOTOMY. The artificial rupture of fetal membranes may provide information on the volume of amniotic fluid and the presence or absence of meconium. In addition, rupture of the membranes may cause an increase in uterine contractility. **Amniotomy incurs risks of chorioamnionitis if labor is prolonged and of umbilical cord compression or cord prolapse if the presenting part is not engaged.**

Second Stage of Labor

At the beginning of the second stage, the mother usually has a desire to bear down with each contraction. This abdominal pressure, together with the uterine contractile force, combines to expel the fetus. During the second stage of labor, fetal descent must be monitored carefully to evaluate the progress of labor. Descent is measured in terms of progress of the presenting part through the birth canal.

In cephalic presentations, the shape of the fetal head may be altered during labor, making the assessment of descent more difficult. **Molding** is the alteration of the relationship of the fetal cranial bones to each other as a result of the compressive forces exerted by the bony maternal pelvis. Some molding is necessary for delivery under normal circumstances. If cephalopelvic disproportion is present, the amount of molding will be more pronounced. **Caput** is a localized, edematous swelling of the scalp caused by pressure of the cervix on the presenting portion of the fetal head. The development of both molding and caput can create a false impression of fetal descent.

The second stage generally takes from 30 minutes to 3 hours in primigravid women and from 5 to 30 minutes in multigravid women.

Mechanism of labor. Six movements of the baby enable it to adapt to the maternal pelvis: descent, flexion, internal rotation, extension, external rotation, and expulsion (Figure 9-10). These movements are discussed here for both an occipitoanterior and occipitoposterior position at engagement. The mechanism of labor for other presentations is discussed in Chapter 14.

DESCENT. Descent is brought about by the force of the uterine contractions, maternal bearing-down (Valsalva) efforts, and, if the patient is upright, gravity.

FLEXION. Partial flexion exists before labor as a result of the natural muscle tone of the fetus. During descent, resistance from the cervix, walls of the pelvis, and pelvic floor cause further flexion of the cervical spine, with the baby's chin approaching its chest. **In the occipitoanterior position, the effect of flexion is to change the presenting diameter from the occipitofrontal to the smaller suboccipitobregmatic** (see Figure 9-2). In the occipitoposterior position, complete flexion may not occur, resulting in a larger presenting diameter, which may contribute to a longer labor.

INTERNAL ROTATION. In the occipitoanterior positions, the fetal head, which enters the pelvis in a transverse or oblique diameter, rotates so that the occiput turns anteriorly toward the symphysis pubis. Internal rotation probably occurs as the fetal head meets the muscular sling of the pelvic floor. It is often not accomplished until the presenting part has reached the level of the ischial spines (zero station) and therefore is engaged. In the occipitoposterior positions, the fetal head may rotate posteriorly so the occiput turns toward the hollow of the sacrum. Alternatively, the fetal head may rotate more than 90 degrees, positioning the occiput under the pubic symphysis and thus converting to an occipitoanterior position.

EXTENSION. The flexed head in an occipitoanterior position continues to descend within the pelvis. Because the vaginal outlet is directed upward and forward, extension must occur before the head can pass through it. As the head continues its descent,

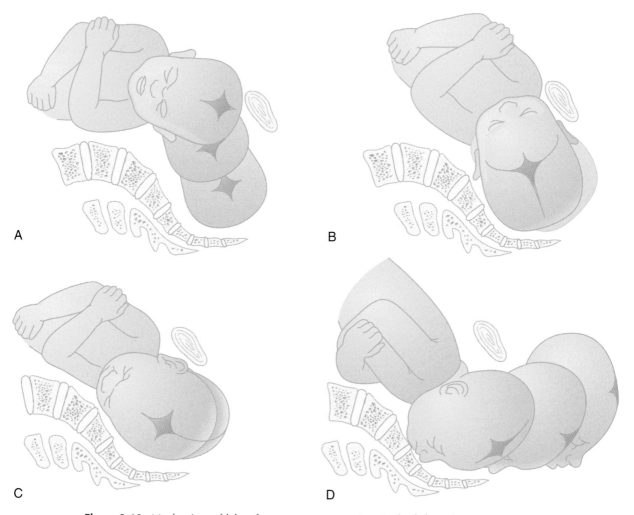

Figure 9-10. Mechanism of labor for a vertex presentation in the left occipitotransverse position. *A,* Flexion and descent. *B* and *C,* Continued descent and commencement of internal rotation. *D,* Completion of internal rotation to the occipitoanterior position followed by delivery of the head by extension.

there is bulging of the perineum followed by crowning. **Crowning** occurs when the largest diameter of the fetal head is encircled by the vulvar ring. At this time, the vertex has reached station +5. When necessary, an incision in the perineum **(episiotomy)** may aid in reducing perineal resistance, although current management is to allow the fetus to deliver without an episiotomy. The head is born by rapid extension as the occiput, sinciput, nose, mouth, and chin pass over the perineum.

In the occipitoposterior position, the head is born by a combination of flexion and extension. At the time of crowning, the posterior bony pelvis and the muscular sling encourage further flexion. The forehead, sinciput, and occiput are born as the fetal chin approaches the chest. Subsequently, the occiput falls back as the head extends, and the nose, mouth, and chin are born.

EXTERNAL ROTATION. In both the occipitoanterior and occipitoposterior positions, the delivered head now returns to its original position at the time of engagement to align itself with the fetal back and shoulders. Further head rotation may occur as the shoulders undergo an internal rotation to align themselves anteroposteriorly within the pelvis.

EXPULSION. Following external rotation of the head, the anterior shoulder delivers under the symphysis pubis, followed by the posterior shoulder over the perineal body and the body of the child.

Clinical management of the second stage. As in the first stage, certain steps should be taken in the clinical management of the second stage of labor.

MATERNAL POSITION. With the exception of avoiding the supine position, the mother may assume any comfortable position for effective bearing down.

BEARING DOWN. With each contraction, the mother should be encouraged to hold her breath and bear down with expulsive efforts. This is particularly important for patients with regional anesthesia because their reflex sensations may be impaired.

FETAL MONITORING. During the second stage, the fetal heart rate should be monitored continuously or evaluated every 5 minutes in patients with obstetric risk factors. Fetal heart rate decelerations (head compression or cord compression) with recovery following the uterine contraction may occur normally during this stage.

VAGINAL EXAMINATION. Progress should be recorded approximately every 30 minutes during the second stage. Particular attention should be paid to the descent and flexion of the presenting part, the extent of internal rotation, and the development of molding or caput. During the second stage of labor, the retracted cervix is no longer palpable.

DELIVERY OF THE FETUS. When delivery is imminent, the patient is usually placed in the lithotomy position, and the skin over the lower abdomen, vulva, anus, and upper thighs is cleansed with an antiseptic solution. Uncomplicated deliveries, particularly in multiparous women, may be carried out in the supine position with the thighs flexed. The left lateral position may be used to deliver patients with hip or knee joint deformities that prevent adequate flexion, or for patients with a superficial or deep venous thrombosis in one of the lower extremities.

As the perineum becomes flattened by the crowning head, an episiotomy may be performed to prevent perineal lacerations. **Recent studies indicate that the performance of episiotomies may result in a higher proportion of lacerations that involve the anal sphincter (third degree) or anal mucosa (fourth degree). Although these more extensive lacerations may be surgically repaired, there is an increasing awareness of the occasional complication of anal incontinence of gas or feces following vaginal delivery.**

To facilitate delivery of the fetal head, a Ritgen maneuver is performed (Figure 9-11). The right hand, draped with a towel, exerts upward pressure through the distended perineal body, first to the supraorbital ridges and then to the chin. This upward pressure, which increases extension of the head and prevents it from slipping back between contractions, is counteracted by downward pressure on the occiput with the left hand. The downward pressure prevents rapid extension of the head and allows a controlled delivery.

Once the head is delivered, the airway is cleared of blood and amniotic fluid using a bulb suction device. The oral cavity is cleared initially and then the nares are cleared. Suction of the nares is not performed if fetal distress or meconium-stained liquor is present because it may result in gasping and aspiration of pharyngeal contents. A second towel is used to wipe secretions from the face and head.

After the airway has been cleared, an index finger is used to check whether the umbilical cord encircles the neck. If so, the cord can usually be slipped over the infant's head. If the cord is too tight, it can be cut between two clamps.

Following delivery of the head, the shoulders descend and rotate into the anteroposterior diameter of the pelvis and are delivered (Figure 9-12). **Delivery of the anterior shoulder is aided by gentle downward traction on the externally rotated head. The brachial plexus may be injured if excessive force is used.** The posterior shoulder is delivered by elevating the head. Finally, the body is slowly extracted by traction on the shoulders.

After delivery, blood will be infused from the placenta into the newborn if the baby is held below the mother's introitus. Usually, the cord is clamped and cut within 15 to 20 seconds. Delayed cord clamping can result in neonatal hyperbilirubinemia as additional blood is transferred to the newborn infant. The newborn is then placed under an infant warmer.

Third Stage of Labor

Immediately after the baby's delivery, the cervix and vagina should be thoroughly inspected for lacerations and surgical repair performed if necessary. The cervix,

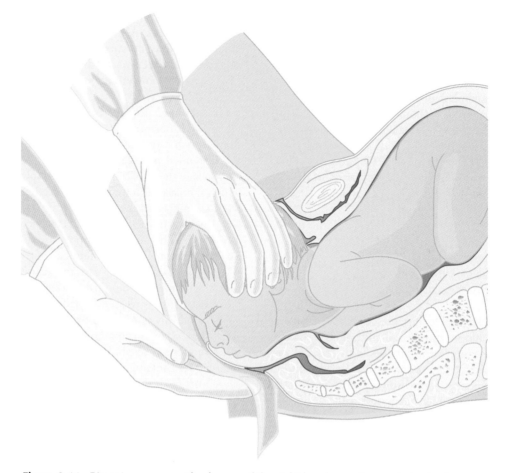

Figure 9-11. Ritgen's maneuver. The fingers of the right hand, pressing posterior to the rectum, are used to extend the head while counterpressure is applied to the occiput by the left hand to allow a controlled delivery of the fetal head.

vagina, and perineum may be more readily examined before the separation of the placenta, as no uterine bleeding should be present to obscure visualization at this time.

Delivery of the placenta. Separation of the placenta generally occurs within 2 to 10 minutes of the end of the second stage of labor. Squeezing of the fundus to hasten placental separation is not recommended because it may increase the likelihood of passage of fetal cells into the maternal circulation.

Signs of placental separation are as follows: (1) a fresh show of blood from the vagina, (2) the umbilical cord lengthens outside the vagina, (3) the fundus of the uterus rises up, and (4) the uterus becomes firm and globular. Only when these signs have appeared should the assistant attempt traction on the cord. With gentle traction and counterpressure between the symphysis and fundus to prevent descent of the uterus into the pelvis, the placenta is delivered.

Following delivery of the placenta, attention should be paid to any uterine bleeding that may originate from the placental implantation site. Uterine contractions, which reduce this bleeding, may be hastened by uterine massage and the use of oxytocin. It is routine to add 20 U of oxytocin to the intravenous infusion after the baby has been delivered. The placenta should be examined to ensure its complete removal and to detect placental abnormalities. If the patient is at risk of postpartum hemorrhage (e.g., because of anemia, prolonged oxytocic augmentation of labor, multiple gestation, or hydramnios), manual removal of the placenta, manual exploration of the uterus, or both may be necessary.

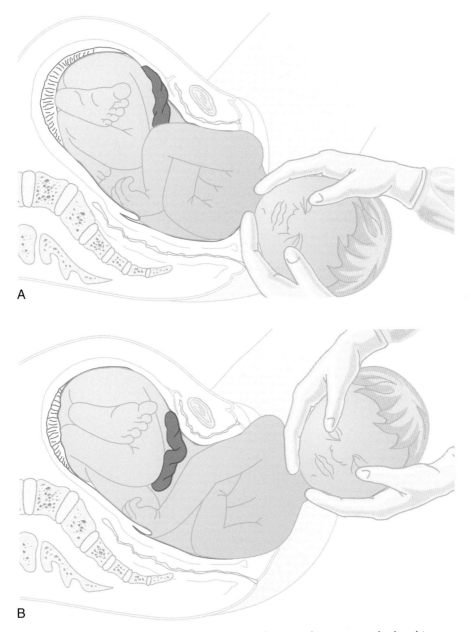

A

B

Figure 9-12. Delivery of the shoulders. *A,* Gentle downward traction on the head is applied to deliver the anterior shoulder. *B,* Gentle upward traction is used to deliver the posterior shoulder.

Perineal lacerations. Perineal lacerations, with or without episiotomy, may be classified as follows:

First degree: A laceration involving the vaginal epithelium or perineal skin

Second degree: A laceration extending into the subepithelial tissues of the vagina or perineum with or without involvement of the muscles of the perineal body

Third degree: A laceration involving the anal sphincter

Fourth degree: A laceration involving the rectal mucosa

If an episiotomy has been performed (Figure 9-13), it should be repaired as illustrated in Figure 9-14. Absorbable sutures (00) should be used, and a rectal examination should ensure that the sutures have not inadvertently transected the rectal mucosa. A third-degree tear (Figure 9-15) should be repaired as shown in Figure 9-16.

Fourth Stage of Labor

The hour immediately following delivery requires close observation of the patient. Blood pressure, pulse rate, and uterine blood loss must be monitored closely. It is during this time that postpartum hemorrhage commonly occurs, usually because of uterine relaxation, retained placental fragments, or unrepaired lacerations. Occult bleeding (e.g., vaginal hematoma formation) may manifest as pelvic pain. An increase in pulse rate, often out of proportion to any decrease in blood pressure, may indicate hypovolemia.

INDUCTION AND AUGMENTATION OF LABOR

Induction of labor is the process whereby labor is initiated by artificial means; **augmentation** is the artificial stimulation of labor that has begun spontaneously.

The natural onset of labor at term involves complex interactions between the fetus and mother, which are discussed in Chapter 6. In the absence of the natural onset of labor, pharmacologic methods may be used to initiate labor. However, labor should be induced only after appropriate assessment of the mother and fetus and an explanation to the patient of the indications for induction. In the absence of a medical indication for

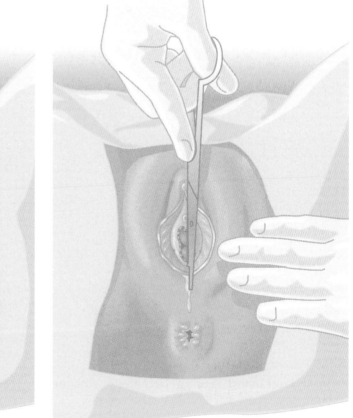

A

B

Figure 9-13. *A,* Mediolateral episiotomy. *B,* Midline episiotomy.

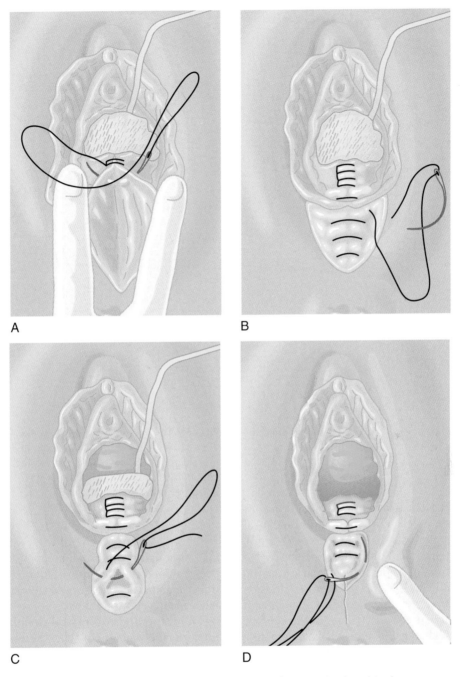

A

B

C

D

Figure 9-14. *A,* Repair of a midline episiotomy. A taped sponge is placed in the upper vagina and a continuous locked 00 or 000 absorbable suture closes the vaginal epithelium from the apex to the hymeneal ring. *B,* Three interrupted sutures are used to close the deep perineal fascia (of Colles) and underlying levator ani muscles. The vaginal epithelial suture is brought below the skin into the subcutaneous tissue. *C,* The same continuous suture is used to close the superficial fascia down to the anal edge of the episiotomy. *D,* The same suture is used as a subcuticular stitch coming back to the hymeneal ring, where it is doubly tied. The sponge is then removed (this is very important).

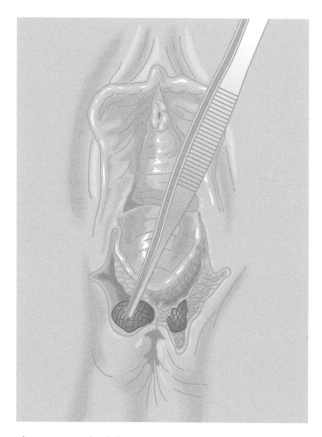

Figure 9-15. Third-degree perineal tear extending into the rectum and avulsing the circular rectal sphincter.

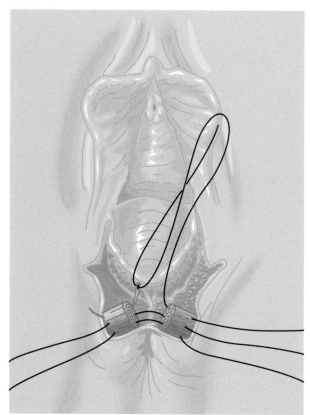

Figure 9-16. Repair of a third-degree tear involves approximating the fascia surrounding the rectal sphincter muscle and reapproximating the vaginal tears with locked continuous sutures. The process is then completed as with a midline episiotomy repair.

labor induction, fetal maturity should be confirmed by either appropriate pregnancy dating, ultrasonic measurements, or amniotic fluid analysis (e.g., L/S ratio).

Cervical effacement and softening (ripening) occur prior to the onset of spontaneous labor. Cervical ripening frequently does not occur prior to a decision for labor induction, yet the success of induction is dependent on these necessary changes in the cervix. **Several mechanical and pharmacologic approaches promote cervical ripening prior to the actual induction of uterine contractions. Local application of prostaglandins may be used.** Currently approved pharmacologic treatments include intravaginal application of prostaglandin E$_2$ using a vaginal insert called **cervidil** (on a string), which can be removed quickly if the medication causes hyperstimulation. Recently **cytotec**, a synthetic prostaglandin E$_1$ analogue, has been approved for cervical ripening. One 25 µg tablet placed intravaginally has been shown to effectively initiate cervical ripen-

ing. Although prostaglandin administration has been demonstrated to shorten the duration of labor induction, the impact on cesarean section rates due to failed induction has been minimal.

Other methods of cervical ripening may include intrauterine placement of catheters or the use of osmotic dilators (see Figure 27-5). Manual separation of the chorioamnion from the lower uterine segment does not necessarily speed the onset of labor. Although controversial, artificial rupture of the membranes may be utilized to increase uterine activity, and perhaps to speed cervical change, when performed in conjunction with administration of oxytocin.

In addition to cervical ripening, induction of labor requires the initiation of effective uterine contractions. Oxytocin is identical to the natural pituitary peptide, and it is the only drug approved for induction and augmentation of labor. Pitocin is the synthetic preparation. The physician must be fully aware of the indications and the contraindications for the use of oxytocin (Table 9-3). **In general, induction of labor before term is indicated only when the continuation of pregnancy represents a significant risk to the fetus or mother. In some situations, induction may be indicated at term, as in the case of premature rupture of the membranes.** Induction at term for convenience is not appropriate unless the patient has a history of previous precipitous delivery (less than 3 hours) or lives an unusually long distance from the hospital.

In general, any condition that makes normal labor dangerous for the mother or fetus is a contraindication to induction or augmentation of labor. The most common contraindication has been prior uterine surgery in which there has been complete transection of the uterine wall. However, **a previous lower transverse incision is no longer considered a contraindication to a trial of labor.** This is referred to as vaginal birth after cesarean, or VBAC.

Induction of labor prior to term for maternal or fetal indications must not be undertaken without the assessment of fetal pulmonary maturity, provided that a delay will not jeopardize the mother or fetus. Fetal lung maturity can most often be accelerated within 24 to 48 hours by the use of glucocorticoids.

TECHNIQUE FOR INDUCTION AND AUGMENTATION

A hospital obstetric service must establish guidelines for the proper use of oxytocin for induction and augmentation of labor. In general, an assessment and plan of management must be outlined in the patient's medical record. Indications for induction of labor should be clearly stated. It is helpful to assess the likelihood of success by a careful pelvic examination to determine the **Bishop score,** which evaluates the status of the cervix and the station of the fetal head (Table 9-4). A high score (9 to 13) is associated with a high likelihood of a vaginal delivery, whereas a low score (<5) is associated with a decreased likelihood of success (65% to 80%). Before induction is begun, the

Table 9-3. Indications and contraindications for induction and augmentation of labor

Induction	Augmentation
INDICATIONS	
MATERNAL	
Preeclampsia	Abnormal labor (in the
Diabetes mellitus	presence of
Heart disease	inadequate uterine
	activity)
	Prolonged latent phase
	Prolonged active phase
FETOPLACENTAL	
Prolonged pregnancy	
Intrauterine growth	
restriction (IUG-R)	
Abnormal fetal testing	
Rh incompatibility	
Fetal abnormality	
Premature rupture of	
membranes (PROM)	
Chorioamnionitis	
CONTRAINDICATIONS	
MATERNAL	
ABSOLUTE	Same contraindications
	as for maternal and
	fetoplacental
Contracted pelvis	
RELATIVE	
Prior uterine surgery	
Classic cesarean section	
Complete transection of	
uterus (myomectomy,	
reconstruction)	
Overdistended uterus	
FETOPLACENTAL	
Preterm fetus without lung	
maturity	
Acute fetal distress	
Abnormal presentation	

Table 9-4. Bishop score to assess likelihood of successful induction of labor

Physical Findings	RATING			
	0	1	2	3
CERVIX				
Position	Posterior	Mid	Anterior	—
Consistency	Firm	Medium	Soft	—
Effacement (%)	0–30	40–50	60–70	≥80
Dilatation (cm)	0	1–2	3–4	≥5
FETAL HEAD				
Station	−3	−2	−1	+1

patient's blood must be typed and screened for antibodies. A blood specimen should be held in the laboratory in case crossmatching becomes necessary. **Continuous electronic monitoring of the fetal heart rate and uterine activity is required during induction.** An internal uterine catheter for monitoring uterine pressure is suggested if intensity cannot be adequately assessed.

Oxytocin Infusion

Several principles should be followed when oxytocin is used to induce or augment labor:

1. **Oxytocin must be given intravenously** to allow it to be discontinued quickly if a complication such as uterine hypertonus or fetal distress develops. Because oxytocin has a half-life of 3 to 5 minutes, its physiologic effect will diminish quickly (within 15 to 30 minutes) after discontinuation.

2. **A dilute infusion must be used and "piggybacked" into the main intravenous line** so that it can be stopped quickly if necessary, without interrupting the main intravenous route.

3. **The drug is best infused with a calibrated infusion pump** that can be easily adjusted to effect the required infusion rate accurately.

4. **The induction of labor for a specific indication generally should not exceed 72 hours.** In patients with a low Bishop score, it is not unusual for an induction to progress slowly. If the cervix effaces and dilates, it is recommended that the membranes be ruptured on the third day. If adequate progress is not made within 12 hours of rupturing the membranes, a cesarean section may be performed.

5. **If adequate labor is established, the infusion rate and the concentration may be reduced,** especially during the 2nd stage of labor. This principle avoids the risks of hyperstimulation and fetal distress, which frequently occur once labor has been established.

Substantial variation exists regarding the initial dose, incremental dose, and time interval between dose increments when oxytocin is used for labor induction and augmentation. Well-performed clinical studies have supported both low-dose (1 to 30 mU/min) and high-dose (4 to 40 mU/min) protocols as seen in Table 9-5. It is not surprising that many protocols utilize "moderate" doses of oxytocin. Generally,

Table 9-5. Method of oxytocin infusion for induction/augmentation

Solution
10 units of oxytocin in 1000 mL of 5% dextrose or balanced salt solution (10 mU/mL)

Administration
Piggyback into main IV line; administer solution by infusion pump

	Low-Dose Protocol	High-Dose Protocol
Starting dose	1 mU/min	4 mU/min
Increment	1 mU/min	4 mU/min
Interval	20 min	20 min
Limited by	5 contractions in 10 min	7 contractions in 15 min
Maximal dose	20–30 mU/min	40 mU/min

intervals between dose increments should be no less than 20 minutes to permit time for steady-state plasma levels of oxytocin to be achieved and to prevent an increased risk of uterine hyperstimulation.

Complications. The use of oxytocin for the induction and augmentation of labor can cause three major complications. Firstly, an excessive infusion rate can cause **hyperstimulation** and thereby cause fetal distress from ischemia. In rare situations, a tetanic contraction can occur and lead to **rupture of the uterus.** Secondly, since oxytocin has a similar structure to antidiuretic hormone, it has an intrinsic **antidiuretic effect** and will increase water reabsorption from the glomerular filtrate. Severe water intoxication with convulsions and coma can occur rarely when oxytocin is infused continuously for more than 24 hours. Thirdly, prolonged infusion of oxytocin can result in **uterine muscle fatigue** (nonresponsiveness) and **postdelivery uterine atony** (hypotonus), which can increase the risk of postpartum hemorrhage.

PUERPERIUM

The puerperium consists of the period following delivery of the baby and placenta to approximately 6 weeks postpartum. During the puerperium, the reproductive organs and maternal physiology return toward the prepregnancy state, although menses may not return for much longer.

ANATOMIC AND PHYSIOLOGIC CHANGES
Involution of the Uterus

Through a process of tissue catabolism, the uterus rapidly decreases in weight from about 1000 g at delivery to 100 to 200 g at approximately 3 weeks postpartum. The cervix similarly loses its elasticity and regains its prepregnancy firmness. For the first few days after delivery, the uterine discharge (lochia) appears red **(lochia rubra)** owing to the presence of erythrocytes. After 3 to 4 days, the lochia becomes paler **(lochia serosa),** and by the tenth day, it assumes a white or yellow-white color **(lochia alba).** Foul-smelling lochia suggests endometritis.

Vagina

Although the vagina may never return to its prepregnancy state, the supportive tissues of the pelvic floor gradually regain their former tone. Women who deliver vaginally should be taught and encouraged to perform Kegel exercises (intermittent tightening of the perineal muscles) to maintain and improve the supportive tissues of the pelvic floor.

Cardiovascular System

Immediately following delivery, there is a marked increase in peripheral vascular resistance due to the removal of the low-pressure uteroplacental circulatory shunt. The cardiac output and plasma volume gradually return to normal during the first 2 weeks of the puerperium. As a result of the loss of plasma volume and the diuresis of extracellular fluid, a marked weight loss occurs in the first week.

Psychosocial Changes

It is fairly common for women to exhibit a mild degree of depression a few days following delivery. The **"postpartum blues"** are probably due to both emotional and hormonal factors. With understanding and reassurance from both family and physician, this usually resolves without consequence. **Any prolonged episodes of depression during or after pregnancy should receive urgent attention.**

Return of Menstruation and Ovulation

In women who do not nurse, menstrual flow usually returns by 6 to 8 weeks, although this is highly variable. Although ovulation may not occur for several months, particularly in nursing mothers, contraceptive counseling and use should be emphasized during the puerperium to avoid an undesired pregnancy.

BREASTFEEDING

There are many advantages to breastfeeding. First, **breast milk is the ideal food for the newborn, is inexpensive, and is usually in good supply.** Second, **nursing accelerates the involution of the uterus** because suckling stimulates the release of oxytocin, thereby causing increased uterine contractions. Third, and probably most important, **there are immunologic advantages for the baby from breastfeeding.** Various types of maternal antibodies are present in breast milk. The predominant immunoglobulin is secretory IgA, which provides protection in the infant's gut by preventing attachment of harmful bacteria (e.g., *Escherichia coli*) to cells on the mucosal surface. This prevents the bacteria from penetrating the bowel wall. It is also thought that maternal lymphocytes pass through the infant's gut wall and initiate immunologic processes that are not yet well understood. Breastfeeding thereby provides the newborn with passive immunity against certain infectious diseases until its own immune mechanisms become fully functional by 3 to 4 months.

LACTATION

Various hormones, such as estrogen, progesterone, human chorionic gonadotropin, cortisol, insulin, prolactin, and placental lactogen, play an important role in preparing the breasts for lactation. **At delivery, two events are instrumental in initiating lactation. Firstly, the drop in placental hormones, particularly estrogen.** Prior to delivery, these hormones interfere with the lactogenic action of prolactin. **Secondly, suckling stimulates the release of prolactin and oxytocin.** The latter causes contraction of the myoepithelial cells in the alveoli and milk ducts. The suckling stimulus is thought to be important for milk production, as well as for the ejection of colostrum and milk.

On approximately the second day after delivery, colostrum is secreted. Its content is composed mostly of protein, fat, and minerals. It is the colostrum that contains secretory IgA. **After about 3 to 6 days, the colostrum is replaced by mature milk.** The content of milk varies considerably depending on the nutritional status of the mother and the gestational age at the time of delivery. In general, the major components of breast milk are proteins, lactose, water, and fat. The major proteins synthesized in the human breast, which are unique and are not found in cows' milk, are casein, lactalbumin, and β-lactoglobulin. Essential amino acids are delivered from the mother's blood, and some of the nonessential amino acids can be synthesized in the breast. In addition, breast milk is a source of omega-3 fatty acids, which are important for early brain development.

LACTATION SUPPRESSION

When the mother chooses not to breastfeed, lactation suppression is indicated. **The simplest, and probably safest, method to accomplish this is to use a tight-fitting bra.** If breast distention does occur, pumping only makes the situation worse. Ice packs should be applied and the discomfort managed with analgesics

COMPLICATIONS OF BREASTFEEDING
Cracked Nipples

If the nipples of the breast become fissured, nursing may become difficult. Since fissures are also a portal of entry for bacteria, they should be managed aggressively with a nipple shield and an appropriate cream, such as lanolin or Masse breast cream. Further breastfeeding should be temporarily stopped. Milk can be expressed manually until the nipples heal, at which time breast-feeding can be resumed.

Mastitis

This is an uncommon complication of breastfeeding and usually develops after 2 to 4 weeks. The first symptoms are usually slight fever and chills. These are followed by redness of a segment of the breast, which becomes indurated and painful. **The etiologic agent is usually *Staphylococcus aureus*, which originates from the infant's oral pharynx.** Milk should be obtained from the breast for culture and sensitivity, and the mother should be started on a regimen of antibiotics immediately. **Because the majority of staphylococcal organisms are penicillinase-producing, a penicillinase-resistant antibiotic, such as dicloxacillin, should be used.** Breastfeeding may be discontinued but is not contraindicated. An appropriate antibiotic should be continued for 7 to 10 days. If a breast abscess ensues, it should be surgically drained. A breast pump can used to maintain lactation until the infection has cleared if nursing is discontinued.

Drug Passage to the Newborn

Because an infant may ingest up to 500 mL of breast milk per day, maternally administered drugs that pass into breast milk may have a significant effect on the infant. The amount of drug found in breast milk depends on the maternal dose, the rate of maternal clearance, the physicochemical properties of the drug, and the composition of the breast milk with respect to fat and protein. The gestational age of the infant may also be a determinant of the ultimate drug effect. Table 9-6 lists selected drugs with their reported newborn effects.

INTERCONCEPTION CARE

Women who have poor pregnancy outcomes, such as preterm births and perinatal deaths, are at greater risk for having the same problem(s) with subsequent pregnancies. Programs are now offering comprehensive interconception care to address conditions that have been shown to cause poor outcomes with interventions that could mitigate or eliminate any recurrence. The rationale for this approach is to provide continuous obstetric care rather than episodic care triggered by another pregnancy. Studies are underway to determine the value of these programs.

OBSTETRIC ANALGESIA AND ANESTHESIA

The goal of obstetric analgesia and anesthesia is to provide effective pain relief for the mother during the course of labor and delivery that is safe for her and her baby and that has minimal or no adverse effects on the progress and outcome of labor. Anesthetic practices have evolved to include an increased reliance on highly effective and safe regional anesthetic techniques, utilizing low concentration combinations of narcotics and local anesthetics in order to minimize the adverse effects of each. Maternal anesthetic risk has also declined due to the increased awareness of the safety benefits of regional over general anesthesia for cesarean section.

UTERINE BLOOD FLOW

Adequate uterine blood flow is critical to supply oxygen and essential nutrients to the fetus. Uterine

Table 9-6.	Effects of maternal drug ingestion on breastfeeding infants
Drug	**Reported Infant Effects**
Sedative-hypnotics	
Diazepam	Sedation
Antipsychotics	
Chlorpromazine	No adverse effects reported
Haloperidol	No adverse effects reported
Nonnarcotic analgesics	
Acetaminophen	No adverse effects reported
Salicylates	Theoretical risk of platelet dysfunction
Anticonvulsants	
Phenobarbital	Sedation
Phenytoin	Sedation, decreased sucking
Narcotics	
Heroin	May cause addiction
Methadone	Infant death reported
Meperidine	No adverse effects reported
Antibiotics	
Penicillin	May modify bowel flora, cause allergy, or interfere with sepsis work-up
Ampicillin	Same as for penicillin
Erythromycin	Same as for penicillin
Nitrofurantoin	Theoretical risk of hemolytic anemia in infants with G6PD deficiency
Tetracycline	Same as for penicillin; theoretical risk of discoloration of teeth and inhibition of bone growth
Digoxin	No adverse effects reported
Thyroid drugs	
Thyroxine	May interfere with screening for hypothyroidism
Propylthiouracil	Nodular goiter
Antihypertensives	
Methyldopa	No adverse effects reported
Propranolol	No adverse effects reported
Theophylline	One case of infant irritability following maternal administration of a rapidly absorbed oral preparation

G6PD, Glucose-6-phosphate dehydrogenase.

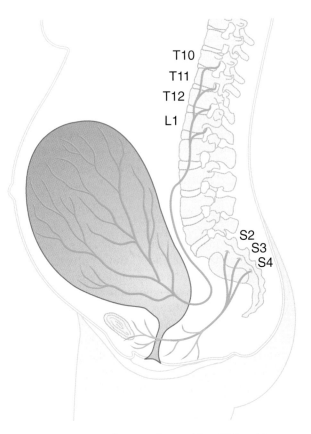

Figure 9-17. Pain pathways of parturition. T10 to L1 supply innervation to the uterus, L1 to S4 supply pain pathways to the vagina and deep pelvic structures, S2 to S4 supply nerve fibers to the pudendal nerve.

PAIN PATHWAYS

The pain pathways of parturition are shown in Figure 9-17.

ADVERSE EFFECTS OF LABOR PAIN

In addition to the mother's subjective sensation of discomfort, labor pain can have measurable adverse physiologic effects on the mother and fetus. Maternal hyperventilation during contractions causes respiratory alkalosis that results in (1) a shift of the oxyhemoglobin dissociation curve to the left, (2) increased affinity of maternal hemoglobin for oxygen, and (3) decreased oxygen offloading to the fetus. The cyclical nature of contraction pain may cause a hyperventilation/hypoventilation syndrome whereby the mother blows off so much carbon dioxide during a contraction that she hypoventilates between contractions and may

blood flow at term accounts for 700 to 900 cc/min (about 12% of maternal cardiac output) and is not autoregulated. Regional analgesia/anesthesia may increase uterine blood flow, especially in preeclamptic patients, by relieving pain and stress and reducing circulating catecholamines. Regional analgesia/anesthesia may also decrease uterine blood flow if hypotension occurs and is not properly and promptly treated.

even become mildly hypoxemic between contractions. This syndrome is exacerbated by systemic narcotics, since they do not adequately relieve the pain of the contraction, but add to the respiratory depression between contractions. Hypoxemia between contractions may be attenuated by providing supplemental oxygen. Finally, labor pain results in increased levels of circulating catecholamines. The α-adrenergic effects of the catacholamines may reduce uterine blood flow, while the beta-2 adrenergic effects may impair uterine contractility.

OPTIONS FOR LABOR PAIN RELIEF

Labor pain may be treated by many methods both nonpharmacologic and pharmacologic. **Nonpharmacologic methods** include psychoprophylaxis (Lamaze method), emotional support, massage, hydrotherapy, biofeedback, transcutaneous electrical nerve stimulation (TENS), acupuncture, and hypnosis. Scientific assessment of these methods has yielded inconsistent results, and there is no definitive evidence that any of these techniques effectively relieves labor pain or improves labor outcome. These techniques tend to work best early in the first stage of labor when the pain is least intense.

Pharmacologic treatment options for labor pain relief include: parenteral narcotics, regional analgesia (epidural, spinal, combined spinal-epidural, paracervical, caudal, and pudendal nerve block) and inhalational analgesia.

Parenteral narcotics have very limited efficacy for the relief of labor pain. They work best in the early first stage when the pain is primarily visceral and less intense. All opioids readily cross the placental barrier and may cause neonatal respiratory depression depending on the dose and timing relative to delivery. They may also cause decreased fetal heart rate variability (not reflective of fetal acidosis) and impair neonatal breastfeeding. Fentanyl and nalbuphine have the shortest neonatal half-lives of the commonly used parenteral narcotics.

Neuraxial analgesia (medication injected into the spinal column) is undoubtedly the most effective form of labor pain relief. **Lumbar epidural analgesia is the most common form of neuraxial analgesia used to treat labor pain,** and its use has been steadily increasing. It may be used to provide pain relief for the first and second stages of labor and, by injecting a higher concentration of local anesthetic, the block may be intensified and extended to provide surgical anesthe-

sia for cesarean delivery or postpartum tubal ligation. There is no degree of cervical dilation at which it is too early or too late to provide epidural analgesia as long as the patient is having regular, painful contractions associated with cervical change. The timing of placement should be made on an individualized basis taking into account such factors as the patient's and the fetus' medical status and the patient's degree of pain and response to alternative methods. Modern epidural management includes an initial bolus of local anesthetic (bupivacaine, ropivacaine, or levo-bupivacaine) and narcotic (fentanyl) to achieve a T10 sensory level, followed by an infusion of a dilute solution of the same agents until delivery. **The goal is to avoid motor block** so as to minimize any adverse effects on maternal expulsive efforts in the second stage.

A pudendal nerve block anesthetizes somatic afferent nerve fibers entering the spinal cord at sacral segments S2-S4. It **is usually effective at relieving the perineal pain of the second stage of labor,** along with the pain of episiotomy and episiotomy repair. It does not affect the ongoing pain of uterine contractions.

ANESTHESIA FOR CESAREAN DELIVERY

The type of anesthesia selected for cesarean delivery is determined by the urgency of the surgery, the presence or absence of a preexisting epidural catheter for labor, and the patient's medical condition, including the presence of any contraindications to regional anesthesia. Absolute and relative contraindications to regional anesthesia are listed in Table 9-7. All patients

Table 9-7. Contraindications to regional anesthesia	
Absolute Contraindications	Relative Contraindications (selected)
Patient refusal	Prior back surgery (including Harrington rod placement)
Coagulopathy	Certain cardiac lesions, especially stenotic valvular lesions (e.g., aortic stenosis)
Sepsis or infection at needle insertion site	Increased intracranial pressure
Uncorrected hypovolemia (e.g., ongoing hemorrhage)	

requiring anesthesia for surgery must have an airway examination regardless of how urgent the surgery is. A brief history must also be elicited. **If the history or the physical examination suggests that the intubation will be difficult, then the patient must have a regional anesthetic or an awake intubation, or the operation must be started under local anesthesia.** All patients are premedicated with a nonparticulate antacid. Routine monitors are placed including noninvasive blood pressure monitors, electrocardiograph, and pulse oximeter, and adequate left uterine displacement is assured. Supplemental oxygen is provided. A crystalloid preload of 10 to 15 cc/kg is given prior to regional anesthesia.

For elective or urgent cesarean delivery (nonemergency) regional anesthesia is preferred because the airway is maintained. Complications involving loss of the airway are the leading causes of anesthetic-related maternal mortality and are usually associated with general anesthesia. (Table 9-8) Parturients have a higher risk of airway complications than nonpregnant patients because they have (1) an eight-times higher chance of failed intubation, (2) a 60% increased oxygen consumption, (3) a decreased functional residual capacity (FRC) resulting in a lower store of oxygen, and (4) an increased risk of aspiration. If a labor epidural is already in place and functioning well, the block is extended and intensified using a concentrated solution of local anesthetic (2% lidocaine, 3% 2-chloroprocaine, 0.5% ropivacaine, or 0.5% bupivacaine). **If no epidural is in place, a spinal block is frequently utilized unless the patient would benefit from one of the advantages of an epidural** (e.g., flexible duration for repeat or more complex surgery, slower onset of sympathectomy in patients with certain cardiac lesions or pulmonary hypertension). A comparison of the characteristics of spinal and epidural anesthesia is shown in Table 9-9.

Occasionally combined spinal and epidural (CSE) anesthesia is used for cesarean delivery. This is particularly indicated when a rapid onset of anesthesia with a flexible duration is required, i.e., an urgent surgery that may be prolonged. The main disadvantage of this technique is that there is no assurance that the epidural catheter will function satisfactorily if needed, since the beginning of surgery will be performed under spinal block. If the epidural fails to provide satisfactory surgical anesthesia when activated intraoperatively, the patient may require general anesthesia.

General anesthesia is employed for cesarean delivery in three situations: (1) there is extreme urgency without a preexisting, functional epidural

Table 9-8. Causes of anesthetic-related maternal deaths in the United States, 1979–1990	
Causes	Anesthesia Deaths (%)
Airway problems	
Aspiration	23
Induction/intubation problems	12
Inadequate ventilation	12
Respiratory failure	2
Local anesthetic toxicity	13
High spinal/epidural	9
Cardiac arrest	23
Overdosage	1
Anaphylaxis	1

Table 9-9. Comparison of spinal and epidural anesthesia	
Spinal	Epidural
ADVANTAGES	**ADVANTAGES**
Faster	Can tailor duration to need
Technically easier	Lower chance of postdural puncture headache
More reliable	Slower onset
• Defined endpoint	• Beneficial in patients with cardiac and hypertensive disorders
• Minimal chance of patchy block	
Denser block	
Lower drug exposure for mother and fetus	
No chance of systemic toxicity	
DISADVANTAGES	**DISADVANTAGES**
Defined (limited) duration	Slower onset
Higher chance of postdural puncture headache (limited by use of small-bore, pencil point needles)	Higher risk of systemic toxicity due to accidental IV injection
	Risk of high spinal due to inadvertant intrathecal or subdural injection
	Risk of "patchy block" due to inadequate or asymmetrical dermatomal spread

catheter, (2) there is a contraindication to regional anesthesia, or (3) regional anesthesia has failed. When a relative contraindication to regional anesthesia is present, the benefits of regional anesthesia frequently outweigh the risks in the pregnant patient.

The protocol for general anesthesia for cesarean section includes routine monitoring and left uterine displacement, preoxygenation for at least four vital capacity breaths, and rapid sequence induction of anesthesia with cricoid pressure followed by intubation to prevent regurgitation and pulmonary aspiration of gastric contents. Once the correct position of the endotracheal tube has been confirmed by end-tidal CO_2 and ascultation of the lungs, surgery may begin.

Induction agents for general anesthesia include thiopental (most commonly), propofol, etomidate (when cardiovascular stability is particularly desired), and ketamine (indicated for hypovolemic or asthmatic patients). The muscle relaxant used to facilitate intubation is succinylcholine (unless contraindicated) due to its rapid onset and brief duration. If contraindicated, vecuronium or rocuronium may be used. **Oxygen delivery is maintained at 100% until delivery if the baby is stressed.** After delivery, nitrous oxide may be added. After induction, a potent inhalational agent is administered and then the concentration is reduced after delivery to minimize its uterine relaxing effects. Narcotics may be administered after delivery to reduce the need for inhalational anesthesia and provide post-operative pain relief. **The patient must be extubated only when fully awake in order to minimize the risk of aspiration.**

PATIENTS WHO BENEFIT FROM EARLY ANESTHESIA CONSULTATION

General anesthesia presents an increased risk for most parturients compared with regional anesthesia if surgery is necessary. General anesthesia can usually be avoided if an epidural catheter is already in place. Therefore it is helpful to identify those patients who are at increased risk of requiring surgery and those patients who have a normal chance of needing surgery but would pose an especially high anesthetic risk if they did. Patients in the former group include patients with a past history of cesarean section and patients with possible fetal indications for surgery (e.g., breech presentation, multiple gestation, prematurity, macrosomia, poor fetal heart rate tracing). These fetuses may also benefit from the controlled or possibly instrumented delivery that epidural analgesia allows.

Mothers who are at particularly high anesthetic risk should they require emergency surgery include patients with a difficult airway, significant respiratory, cardiac, or neurologic disease, severe preeclampsia, and suspected or known susceptibility to malignant hyperthermia.

Indicators of a difficult airway include: (1) a history of intubation problems, (2) craniofacial deformity (congenital or acquired), (3) limited mouth opening or small mouth, (4) facial or oropharyngeal swelling, (5) limited neck mobility, (6) protruding incisors, (buck teeth), (7) small mandible, (8) morbid obesity, and (9) neck tumor. The patients described above benefit from early outpatient or inpatient anesthesia consultation.

Unintended Consequences of Regional Anesthesia/Analgesia

Patients who receive epidural analgesia for labor pain have a similar duration of the first stage of labor, but the second stage is prolonged by 15 minutes on average. Theoretically, a prolongation of the second stage could arise from effects on the release of oxytocin, prostaglandin $F_{2\alpha}$, and other hormones responsible for the propagation of labor. Prolongation of the second stage could also be due to impaired ability to push (unlikely as long as motor block is avoided by appropriate adjustment of the epidural infusion), or decreased maternal urge to push due to sensory blockade. The latter can usually be overcome by appropriate coaching and decreasing or halting the epidural infusion.

Other side effects and complications of regional anesthesia/analgesia include fever, headache, and backache. The association with maternal fever may be due to (1) an alteration in the thermoregulatory set-point, (2) interference with peripheral thermoreceptor input to the CNS, or (3) an imbalance between maternal heat production and loss (decreased hyperventilation, decreased lower body sweating, increased shivering).

The risk of headache is about 1% to 3% with spinal anesthesia using a small-bore (24 gauge or less), pencil-point needle. The risk of headache is lower with an epidural (less than 1%) and occurs when there is an unintended dural puncture ("wet tap"). **Postdural puncture headaches are self-limited, usually resolving within 5–7 days.** They may be palliated with intravenous or oral caffeine or treated with an epidural blood patch.

There appears to be no association between newonset, long-term back pain and labor epidural analgesia. The risk of new, chronic back pain in parturients is high whether or not they have had an epidural.

RESUSCITATION OF THE NEWBORN

Improved surveillance using antenatal and intra-partum fetal heart rate monitoring, real-time ultrasonography, amniocentesis, and umbilical artery Doppler assessments has allowed the clinician to recognize the fetus at risk who may need special care at birth. The goals of an organized approach to neonatal resuscitation are to reverse any intrauterine hypoxia and to prevent postnatal asphyxia, which may result in acute major organ damage and lifelong handicaps.

PREPARATION FOR EXTRAUTERINE LIFE

Prematurity is the leading cause of poor neonatal outcome because the fetus has not yet progressed through complete stages of anatomic development and biochemical maturation. Even the fetus delivered at term undergoes changes prior to and with the onset of labor.

During pregnancy, fetal thyroxine (T_4) is converted to reverse triiodothyronine (rT_3), which is metabolically inactive. **Several days before the onset of term labor, cortisol levels increase in the fetus and induce a change in thyroid hormone dynamics. Cortisol induces the enzyme system, allowing the conversion of T_4 to triiodothyronine (T_3), which is metabolically more active and necessary for neonatal thermogenesis.** At birth, there is a surge of thyroid stimulating hormone (TSH), and at no time during life does this hormone reach such high levels as it does 30 minutes after birth. This is followed by a hyperthyroid neonatal state for several days, which is necessary for the newborn to maintain its body temperature.

A second change that occurs with the onset of labor is a change in fetal breathing activity. Fetal breathing, as observed by real-time ultrasonography, is rarely observed once labor is established. This is thought to be associated with a decrease in pulmonary fluid dynamics that may be important for the onset of respiration after delivery and the retention of surfactant in the lungs.

Finally, labor is a stress to the fetus that stimulates the release of catecholamines. This may be responsible for the mobilization of glucose, lung fluid absorption, alterations in the perfusion of organ systems, and, possibly, the onset of respiration. Only at times of severe stress later in life are catecholamine levels as high as those at birth.

ETIOLOGY OF NEONATAL CARDIORESPIRATORY DEPRESSION

At term, 0.5% of infants will require vigorous resuscitation (positive pressure ventilation for more than 1 minute). At earlier stages of gestation, almost all infants require some type of supportive care.

FACILITATING NEONATAL ADAPTATION

The physician performing the delivery should delegate the responsibility for neonatal resuscitation. All nurses working in the delivery room should be trained in techniques of neonatal assessment and resuscitation. If risk factors increase the likelihood of delivering a depressed infant, a pediatrician trained in neonatal resuscitation should be summoned.

Following delivery of a normal newborn, the following important steps should occur:

CLEAR THE AIRWAY

Descent through the birth canal causes compression of the chest wall, resulting in the discharge of fluid from the mouth and nose. When the head emerges from the vagina, the physician should use a towel or gauze pad to remove secretions from the face. In addition, a bulb suction may be used to aspirate secretions from the oropharynx. **Initially, the bulb suction should not be used to suction the nose because nasal stimulation may initiate a gasp and cause bradycardia.** Also, nasal stimulation may cause aspiration of meconium if it is present. If a moderate amount of meconium is present, placing a nasal tracheal catheter into the oral pharynx and applying suction prior to delivering the body is thought to decrease the risk of meconium aspiration.

DRY THE NEWBORN

An important part of neonatal adaptation is the initiation of thermogenesis. Excessive cooling from exposure of the wet skin is detrimental to all pre-term infants and to depressed full-term infants. The physician should dry off the infant with a towel before cutting the cord. This also serves to stimulate the onset of respiration.

CLAMP THE CORD

The umbilical arteries usually close spontaneously within 45 to 60 seconds of birth, whereas the umbilical vein remains patent for 3 to 5 minutes or longer. Delayed cord clamping significantly increases the neonatal blood volume, which increases the likelihood of neonatal jaundice and tachypnea. **The ideal time for clamping the cord is 20 to 30 seconds after birth.**

ENSURE ONSET OF RESPIRATION

The onset of respiration is normally within a few seconds of birth but may be delayed for up to 30 seconds. In the absence of clinical data to suggest a biochemical abnormality (hypoxia-acidosis), it is usually best to adopt an expectant policy of standing back and giving the infant a chance to breathe spontaneously, because overstimulation can cause apnea.

CORRECT SURFACTANT DEFICIENCY

For the premature infant, surfactant deficiency is the basic defect responsible for the development of the respiratory distress syndrome. Exogenous surfactant replacement varies from synthetic surfactant to modified or unmodified extracts of natural surfactant. These substances can be given by tracheal injection at birth to prevent the respiratory distress syndrome, or they can be given after the syndrome has developed to reduce its severity and prevent mortality.

APGAR SCORE

The Apgar score is an excellent tool for assessing the overall status of the newborn soon after birth (1 minute) and after a 5 minute period of observation (Table 9-10). A normal Apgar score is 7 or greater at 1 minute and 9 or 10 at 5 minutes.

RESUSCITATION OF THE ASPHYXIATED INFANT

The delivery of an asphyxiated infant should be systematic, based on a careful clinical assessment of those factors associated with biochemical abnormalities. **During the past 10 years, increasing emphasis has been placed on transferring the mother with a high-risk pregnancy to a tertiary care regional center before labor,** rather than transferring the sick neonate after delivery.

Ideally, at the time of delivery, a segment of cord should be doubly clamped to allow blood gas determinations on cord arterial and venous blood. These serve as a baseline to assess the severity of the neonatal hypoxia and acidosis.

A stepwise sequence of procedures is necessary to enable a smooth transition to a normal metabolic state. This sequence is referred to as the ABCs of resuscitation and is summarized in Figure 9-18.

ESTABLISH AN AIRWAY

In any infant with a high likelihood of asphyxia, suctioning of the airway should be initiated after the delivery of the head. The asphyxiated neonate usually has meconium present in the upper airway, which must be cleared with an oral suction catheter (DeLee trap) before delivery of the shoulders. Immediately following the delivery of the infant, an endotracheal tube should be inserted to remove thick mucus or meconium from the trachea and upper airway.

INITIATE BREATHING

With an established airway, either bag-mask ventilation or ventilation via an endotracheal tube should be initiated to deliver 100% oxygen to the lungs at a rate of 40 to 60 breaths per minute. Usually, the heart rate increases rapidly after the apnea is corrected, and intermittent bag-mask ventilation with supplemental oxygen can be given until spontaneous respiration commences.

Table 9-10. **The apgar score for determining the condition of a newborn infant**			
	SCORE		
Sign	0	1	2
1. Heart rate	Absent	<100 beats/min	>100 beats/min
2. Respiratory effort	Absent	Slow, weak cry	Good, strong cry
3. Muscle tone	Limp	Some flexion of extremities	Active motion
4. Reflex irritability (response to stimulation of sole of foot)	None	Grimace	Strong cry
5. Color	Pale, blue	Body, pink; extremities, blue	Completely pink

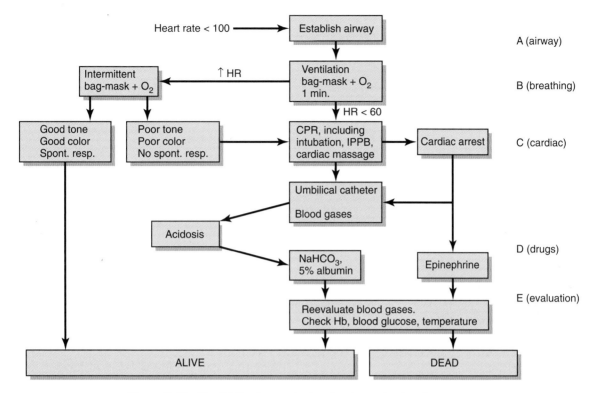

Figure 9-18. The ABCs of resuscitation for the asphyxiated neonate.

ENSURE CARDIAC PERFORMANCE

If cardiac performance is poor (heart rate less than 60 beats/minute during ventilation with 100% oxygen), external cardiac massage should be initiated. **The best technique for cardiac massage in the newborn is to compress the middle third of the sternum with two fingers at a rate of 2 compressions/second with a 1 to 2 second pause after every third compression for ventilation.** The middle finger and either the index or ring finger should be used (Figure 9-19). The sternum should be depressed to a depth of approximately 2 cm. Placement of the other hand beneath the infant's back can facilitate compression of the heart between the sternum and spine. Cardiac arrest is rare. **If cardiac massage and artificial ventilation are not successful in reestablishing cardiac function, an endotracheal or intravenous injection of a dilute solution of epinephrine may be given.** When the heart rate is above 80 beats/minute, sternal compression may be discontinued while ventilation is continued.

CORRECT BIOCHEMICAL ABNORMALITIES

Acidosis

In the case of a very sick newborn, an umbilical arterial catheter is placed and blood gas analyses are obtained to monitor the severity of the acidosis and the effectiveness of the resuscitation. Severe acidosis can be corrected by the infusion of sodium bicarbonate.

Anemia

On rare occasions, the newborn may have abnormal perfusion secondary to blood loss (e.g., from vasa previa, abruptio placentae, or a feto-maternal transfusion), which can be corrected only by immediate transfusion with blood from the mother, a blood bank, or a safe walk-in donor. A solution of 5% albumin can be used to temporarily maintain an adequate vascular volume.

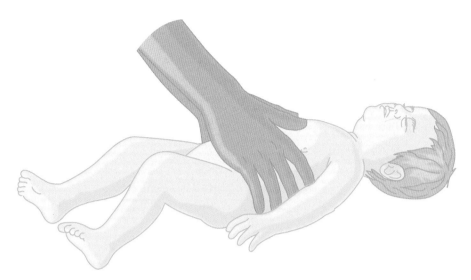

Figure 9-19. Technique for cardiac massage in the neonate. Note that both thumbs are used to depress the lower one-third of the sternum, while the remaining fingers support the infant's back.

Narcotic Depression

Respiratory depression secondary to medication is unusual with the increased use of conduction anesthesia. If neonatal respiratory depression from excessive use of narcotics is suspected, naloxone (Narcan) is an effective antidote. It is just as effective and more easily administered intramuscularly than intravenously.

Toxicity to neonatal naloxone is low, so dosage is less critical than for most drugs. Table 9-11 lists the drugs that are commonly used in resuscitation and their dosages.

Hypoglycemia

Hypoglycemia can also contribute to unsuccessful resuscitation, especially in infants with intrauterine

Table 9-11.	**Drugs used to resuscitate the neonate**			
Medication	Concentration to Administer	Preparation	Dosage/Route	Rate/Precautions
Epinephrine	1:10,000	1 mL	0.01–0.03 mg/kg 0.1–0.3 mL/kg IV or ET	Give rapidly May dilute with normal saline to 1–2 mL if giving ET
Volume expanders	Whole blood 5% Albumin-saline Normal saline Ringer's lactate	40 mL	10 mL/kg IV	Give over 5–10 min Give by syringe or IV drip
Sodium bicarbonate	0.5 mEq/mL (4.2% solution)	20 mL or 2 10-mL prefilled syringes	2 mEq/kg IV only (4 mL/kg)	Give slowly, over at least 2 minutes Give only if infant is being effectively ventilated
Naloxone hydrochloride	0.4 mg/mL	1 mL	0.1 mg/kg (0.25 mL/kg) IV, ET, IM, SQ	Give rapidly
	1.0 mg/mL	1 mL	0.1 mg/kg (0.1 mL/kg) IV, ET, IM, SQ	IV, ET preferred; IM, SQ acceptable

IV, intravenous; ET, endotracheal; IM, intramuscular; SQ, subcutaneous.

growth retardation or those with diabetic mothers. Glucose administration should be considered after the other issues have been addressed. **The use of high concentrations of glucose (e.g., 25% to 50%) is contraindicated in asphyxiated newborns because the glucose is converted to lactic acid in the absence of oxygen, which may increase the likelihood of brain damage.**

Evaluate Other Factors

Following a systematic resuscitative effort, other contributing factors must be identified if cardiorespiratory depression persists. **Hypothermia** is one of the most critical aggravating factors, and temperature control must be continuously supported. A **pneumothorax** is not uncommon following a difficult resuscitation (especially with intubation). It must be recognized promptly and decompressed with a chest tube. Also, a **diaphragmatic hernia** can result in the displacement of the stomach, bowel, or both, into the thoracic cavity, thus limiting the expansion of the left lung. Decreased breath sounds and failure to improve pulmonary function should alert the team to this possibility.

Neonatal Respiratory Failure

Neonates in imminent danger of death from a narrow range of conditions causing hypoxemia and respiratory distress not responsive to conventional forms of therapy are now candidates for **extracorporeal membrane oxygenation** (ECMO). Infants with a congenital diaphragmatic hernia, severe meconium aspiration, or other forms of persistent pulmonary hypertension have been saved using this procedure performed in selected regional centers. Data concerning long-term outcome of infants treated with extracorporeal membrane oxygenation are limited. **Carotid artery and/or jugular vein ligation, prolonged anti-coagulation, and long-term circulatory bypass are necessary with this procedure, and concerns exist about their long-term consequences.**

LONG-TERM OUTCOME

Low birth weight (<2500 g), whether a result of prematurity or intrauterine growth restriction, is an independent risk factor for cerebral palsy. By contrast, for infants weighing more than 2500 g, Apgar scores less than or equal to 3 at 5 minutes are generally not associated with an increased risk of cerebral palsy, provided that there is no associated obstetric complication. If both a low Apgar score and an obstetric complication are present, there is an increased risk of cerebral palsy.

Suggested Reading

Lopez-Zeno JA, Peaceman AM, Adashek JA, et al: A controlled trial of a program for the active management of labor. N Engl J Med 326:450, 1992.

ACOG Practice Bulletin #10: Induction of Labor, November, 1999.

ACOG Practice Bulletin #36: Obstetric anesthesia and analgesia, Obstet Gynecol 100(1):177–191, 2002.

Niermeyer S, Van Reempts P, Kattwinisel J, et al: Resuscitation of newborns. Ann Emerg Med 37:5110–5125, 2001.

Fujiwara T, Konishi M, Chida S, et al: Surfactant replacement therapy with a single postventilatory dose of a reconstituted bovine surfactant in preterm neonates with respiratory distress syndrome: Final analysis of a multicenter, double blind, randomized trial and comparison with similar trials. Pediatrics 86:753, 1990.

Practice Guidelines for Obstetrical Anesthesia: A Report by the American Society of Anesthesiologists Task Force on Obstetrical Anesthesia. Anesthesiology 90(2):600–611, 1999.

Leuthner SR, Jansen RD, Hageman JR: Cardiopulmonary resuscitation of the newborn: An update. Pediatr Clin North Am 41:893, 1994.

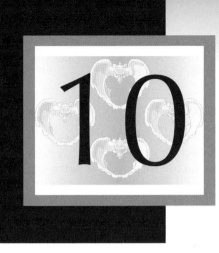

Fetal Surveillance During Labor

Richard A. Bashore and Klaus J. Staisch

Fetal surveillance during labor is an essential element of good obstetric care because of the fact that intrapartum hypoxia and acidosis may develop in any pregnancy. Unfortunately, currently available risk assessment profiles do not predict all instances of intrapartum fetal distress. **On the basis of antepartum maternal history, physical examination, and laboratory data, 20% to 30% of pregnancies may be designated high risk, and 50% of perinatal morbidity and mortality occurs in this group.** However, the remaining 50% occurs in pregnancies that are considered to be normal at the onset of labor.

METHODS OF MONITORING FETAL HEART RATE
AUSCULTATION OF FETAL HEART RATE

The time-honored technique of evaluating the fetus during labor has been auscultation of the fetal heart. Optimally, ausculatation of the fetal heart is performed every 15 minutes after a uterine contraction during the first stage of labor, and at least every 5 minutes in the second stage of labor. Some studies have suggested that intermittent auscultation of the fetal heart is comparable to continuous electronic monitoring in terms of neonatal outcome, if performed at the intervals stated above with a 1:1 patient-to-nurse ratio.

CONTINUOUS ELECTRONIC FETAL MONITORING

Electronic fetal monitoring (EFM) during labor was developed to detect fetal heart rate (FHR) patterns that were frequently associated with delivery of infants in a depressed condition. It was reasoned that early recognition of changes in heart rate patterns that may be associated with such fetal conditions as hypoxia and umbilical cord compression would serve as a warning and enable the physician to intervene to prevent fetal death in utero or irreversible brain injury.

Electronic fetal monitoring allows continuous reporting of the FHR and uterine contractions (FHR-UC) by means of a monitor that prints results on a two-channel strip chart recorder. **Uterine contractions represent a stress for the fetus, and the alteration in FHR correlates with fetal oxygenation.**

The FHR-UC record can be obtained using external transducers that are placed on the maternal abdomen. This technique is used in early labor. **Internal monitoring** is carried out by placing a spiral electrode onto the fetal scalp to monitor heart rate and placing a plastic catheter transcervically into the amniotic cavity to monitor uterine contractions (Figure 10-1). To carry out this technique, the fetal membranes must be ruptured, and the cervix must be dilated to at least 2 cm.

Internal monitoring gives better FHR tracings because the rate is computed from the sharply defined R-wave peaks of the fetal electrocardiogram, whereas with the external technique, the rate is computed from the less precisely defined first heart sound obtained with an ultrasonic transducer. The internal uterine catheter allows precise measurement of the intensity of the contractions in millimeters of mercury, whereas the external tocotransducer measures only frequency and duration, not intensity.

In the clinical setting, internal and external techniques are often combined by using a scalp electrode for precise heart rate recording and the external tocotransducer for contractions. This approach minimizes possible side effects from invasive internal monitoring.

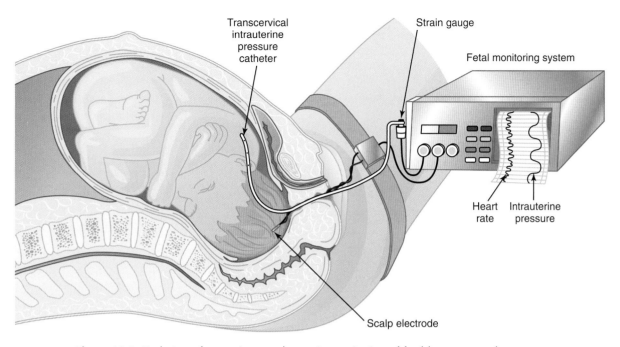

Figure 10-1. Technique for continuous electronic monitoring of fetal heart rate and pressure of uterine contractions.

ETIOLOGY OF HYPOXIA, ACIDOSIS, AND FETAL HEART RATE CHANGES

The developing fetus presents a paradox. Its arterial blood oxygen tension is only 25 ± 5 mm Hg compared with adult values of about 100 mm Hg. The rate of oxygen consumption, however, is twice that of the adult per unit weight, and its oxygen reserve is only enough to meet its metabolic needs for 1 to 2 minutes. Blood flow from the maternal circulation, which supplies the fetus with oxygen through placental exchange of respiratory gases, is momentarily interrupted during a contraction. **A normal fetus can withstand the stress of labor without suffering from hypoxia because sufficient oxygen exchange occurs during the interval between contractions.**

Under normal circumstances, the FHR is determined by the atrial pacemaker. Modulation of the rate occurs physiologically through innervation of the heart by the vagus (decelerator) and sympathetic (accelerator) nerves. A fetus whose oxygen supply is marginal cannot tolerate the stress of contractions and will become hypoxic. Under hypoxic conditions, baroreceptors and chemoreceptors in the central circulation of the fetus influence the FHR by giving rise to contraction-related or "periodic" FHR changes. The hypoxia will also result in anaerobic metabolism.

Pyruvate and lactic acid accumulate, causing fetal acidosis. **The degree of fetal acidosis can be measured by sampling blood from the presenting part. The pH of fetal scalp blood normally varies between 7.25 and 7.30. Values below 7.20 are considered to be abnormal but not necessarily indicative of fetal compromise.** Clinical and experimental data indicate that fetal death occurs when 50% or more of the transplacental oxygen exchange is interrupted.

Fetal oxygenation can be impaired at different anatomic locations within the uteroplacental-fetal circulatory loop. For example, impairment of oxygen transportation to the intervillous space may occur as a result of maternal hypertension or anemia; oxygen diffusion may be impaired in the placenta because of infarction or abruption; or the oxygen content in the fetal blood may be impaired because of hemolytic anemia in Rh-isoimmunization. Figure 10-2 summarizes the clinical conditions that may be associated with fetal distress during labor.

FETAL HEART RATE PATTERNS

The assessment of the FHR depends on an evaluation of the baseline pattern and the periodic changes related to uterine contractions.

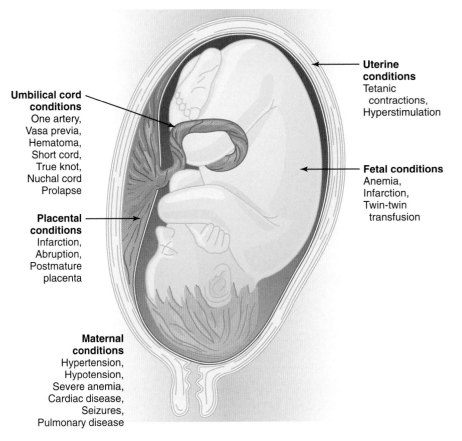

Umbilical cord conditions
One artery,
Vasa previa,
Hematoma,
Short cord,
True knot,
Nuchal cord
Prolapse

Placental conditions
Infarction,
Abruption,
Postmature
placenta

Maternal conditions
Hypertension,
Hypotension,
Severe anemia,
Cardiac disease,
Seizures,
Pulmonary disease

Uterine conditions
Tetanic
contractions,
Hyperstimulation

Fetal conditions
Anemia,
Infarction,
Twin-twin
transfusion

Figure 10-2. Clinical conditions associated with fetal distress in labor.

Baseline Assessment

This requires determination of the rate (in beats per minute) and the variability. Normal and abnormal rates are listed in Table 10-1. Baseline variability can be divided into short- and long-term intervals. These are described as follows:

1. **Short-term or beat-to-beat variability.** This reflects the interval between either successive fetal electrocardiogram signals or mechanical events of the cardiac cycle. **Normal short-term variability fluctuates between 5 and 25 beats/minute.** Variability below 5 beats/minute is considered to be potentially abnormal. When associated with decelerations, a variability of less than 5 beats/minute usually indicates severe fetal distress.

2. **Long-term variability.** These fluctuations may be described in terms of the frequency and amplitude of change in the baseline rate. **The normal long-term variability is 3 to 10 cycles per minute.** Variability is physiologically decreased during the state of quiet sleep of the fetus, which usually lasts for about 25 minutes until transition occurs to another state.

Periodic Fetal Heart Rate Changes

These are changes in baseline FHR related to uterine contractions. The responses to uterine contractions may be categorized as follows:

Table 10-1. Baseline fetal heart rates	
Rate	Beats/Min
Normal	120–160
Abnormal	
Tachycardia	>160
Bradycardia	<120

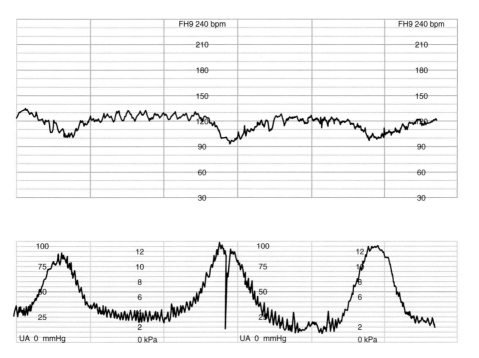

Figure 10-3. Early deceleration. Note that the deceleration starts and ends with the uterine contraction. Good beat-to-beat variability is demonstrated.

1. **No change.** The FHR maintains the same characteristics as in the preceding baseline FHR.
2. **Acceleration.** The FHR increases in response to uterine contractions. This is a normal response.
3. **Deceleration.** The FHR decreases in response to uterine contractions. Decelerations may be *early, late, variable,* or *mixed.* All except early decelerations are abnormal.

Types of Patterns

Early deceleration (head compression). This pattern usually has an onset, maximum fall, and recovery that is coincident with the onset, peak, and end of the uterine contraction (Figure 10-3). The nadir of the FHR coincides with the peak of the contraction. This pattern is seen when engagement of the fetal head has occurred. **Early decelerations are not thought to be associated with fetal distress.** The pressure on the fetal head leads to increased intracranial pressure that elicits a vagal response similar to the Valsalva maneuver in the adult. The vagal reflex can be abolished by the administration of atropine, but this approach is not used clinically.

Late deceleration (uteroplacental insufficiency). This pattern has an onset, maximal decrease, and recovery that is shifted to the right in relation to the contraction (Figure 10-4). The severity of late decelerations is graded by the magnitude of the decrease in FHR at the nadir of the deceleration (Table 10-2).

Table 10-2. Principles of grading late and variable decelerations

	GRADING CRITERIA		
	Mild	Moderate	Severe
Late deceleration: amplitude of drop in FHR	<15 beats/min	15–45 beats/min	>45 beats/min
Variable deceleration: duration of deceleration	<30 sec	30–60 sec	>60 sec

Data from Kubli FW, Hon EH, Khazin AF, et al: Observations on heart rate and pH in the human fetus during labor. Am J Obstet Gynecol 104:1190, 1969.

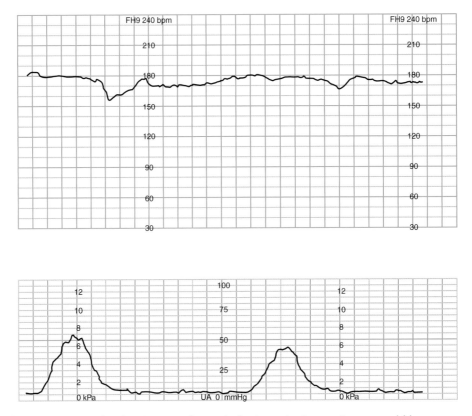

Figure 10-4. Late decelerations on electronic fetal monitoring tracing as would be recorded with a severely distressed fetus. Note the fetal tachycardia, lack of beat-to-beat heart rate variability, and the late decelerations (*upper panel*). Uterine contractions are recorded in the lower panel.

Fetal hypoxia and acidosis are usually more pronounced with severe decelerations. **Late decelerations are generally associated with low scalp blood pH values and high base deficits,** indicating metabolic acidosis from anaerobic metabolism. The partial pressure of carbon dioxide (PCO_2) in the fetal blood is usually in the normal range, and the fetal blood oxygen partial pressure (PO_2) is only slightly below normal because of the Bohr effect—the shift to the left of the oxygen dissociation curve caused by the acidosis.

Variable deceleration (cord compression). This pattern has a variable time of onset and a variable form and may be nonrepetitive. Variable decelerations are caused by umbilical cord compression. Partial or complete compression of the cord causes a sudden increase in blood pressure in the central circulation of the fetus. The bradycardia is mediated via baroreceptors. This reflex can be abolished or ameliorated by atropine (e.g., chemical vagotomy), although this approach is not used clinically. Fetal blood gases indicate respiratory acidosis with a low pH and high CO_2. When cord compression has been prolonged, hypoxia is also present, showing a picture of combined respiratory and metabolic acidosis in fetal blood gases.

The severity of variable decelerations is graded by their duration (see Table 10-2). When the FHR falls below 80 beats/minute during the nadir of the deceleration, there is usually a loss of the P-wave in the fetal electrocardiogram, indicating a nodal rhythm or a second-degree heart block.

Combined or mixed patterns. These patterns may be difficult to define and may exhibit characteristics of any of the aforementioned patterns.

Decreased beat-to-beat variability. A flat baseline can be the result of several conditions: fetal acidosis, quiet sleep state, or maternal sedation with drugs.

STRATEGIES FOR INTERVENTION

A normal FHR pattern on the electronic monitor indicates a greater than 95% probability of fetal well-being. Abnormal patterns may occur, however, in the absence of fetal distress. The false-positive rate (i.e., good Apgar scores and normal fetal acid-base status in the presence of abnormal FHR patterns) is as high as 80%. Therefore, **electronic fetal monitoring is a screening rather than a diagnostic technique.** Failure to appreciate this limitation may lead to inappropriate intervention and contribute to a high rate of cesarean deliveries.

Strategies for intervention always depend on the clinical circumstances. When abnormal FHR patterns are seen, the first step should be a search for the underlying cause. When the cause is identified, such as maternal hypotension, steps should be taken to correct the problem. **In general, a term-sized fetus tolerates ominous fetal heart patterns better than a preterm fetus.** A fetus with additional risk factors, such as intrauterine infection from chorioamnionitis, may deteriorate sooner than a fetus in a normal parturient. Other considerations in the management of fetal distress include the maternal condition and the stage of labor.

VARIABLE DECELERATIONS

The most frequently encountered abnormal FHR pattern is that of variable decelerations. A change in maternal position to the right or left side generally relieves fetal pressure on the cord and abolishes the decelerations. One hundred percent **oxygen** should be given by face mask to the mother. If the pattern is persistent, placing the mother in the Trendelenburg position or elevating the presenting part by vaginal examination may be tried. If an oxytocic infusion is running, it should be discontinued. A tocolytic agent such as **Terbutaline** may also be used to diminish uterine activity.

Variable decelerations of severe degree are most frequently seen during the second stage of labor, with the patient pushing during uterine contractions. **Amnioinfusion, which is the replacement of amniotic fluid with normal saline infused through a transcervical intrauterine pressure catheter, has been reported to decrease both the frequency and severity of variable decelerations.** Amnioinfusion results in reduced cesarean deliveries for fetal distress and fewer low Apgar scores at birth without apparent maternal or fetal distress. The use of a double-lumen uterine catheter is recommended because it allows a continuous infusion while simultaneously measuring uterine tone to guard against overdistention from excessive fluid accumulation.

The safest intervention to deliver the fetus with cord compression is often low or outlet forceps. When progressive acidosis occurs, as determined by serial scalp blood pH determinations, cesarean section should be performed if vaginal delivery is not imminent. Another circumstance requiring immediate intervention is a prolonged deceleration. This condition occurs when the FHR falls to 60 to 90 beats/minute for more than 2 minutes.

NONREACTIVE FETAL HEART RATE TRACING

A nonreactive tracing with loss of FHR-accelerations and lack of beat-to-beat variability needs further evaluation because it may be associated with fetal acidosis. By placing an artificial larynx with 120 dB of sound on the maternal abdomen in the vicinity of the vertex, **acoustic stimulation can be used to try to induce FHR-accelerations.** A response of greater than 15 beats/minute lasting at least 15 seconds always ensures the absence of fetal acidosis. Conversely, the chance of acidosis occurring in the fetus who fails to respond to such stimulation is about 50%.

LATE DECELERATIONS

Late decelerations of the FHR are most commonly seen in pregnancies associated with uteroplacental insufficiency. The following steps are taken in rapid succession to alleviate fetal distress and to determine the underlying cause:

1. **Change the maternal position from supine to left or right lateral.** The supine hypotension syndrome is caused by compression of the vena cava and aorta by the heavy uterus, leading to lowering of maternal cardiac output and underperfusion of the placenta. In addition, the weight of the term uterus can compress the internal and external iliac vessels, resulting in poor perfusion of the uterus and fetal bradycardia. When this occurs, the femoral pulse cannot be palpated on the affected side. This is called the Poseiro effect.
2. **Give oxygen by face mask.** This can increase fetal PO_2 by 5 mm Hg.

3. **Stop any oxytocic infusion** to exclude uterine hyperstimulation.
4. **Inject intravenously a bolus of a tocolytic drug** (e.g., magnesium sulfate, 2.0 g, or terbutaline, 0.25 mg) to relieve uterine tetany.
5. **Monitor maternal blood pressure** to exclude hypotensive episodes that can occur as a consequence of epidural analgesia.

When late decelerations persist for greater than 30 minutes despite the aforementioned maneuvers, fetal scalp blood pH measurements are indicated. To interpret pH values properly, notation should be made by means of an event marker on the fetal monitor indicating the timing of the scalp blood sample.

Operative delivery should be considered for fetal distress when fetal acidosis is present (pH less than 7.2) **or when late decelerations are persistent in early labor and the cervix is insufficiently dilated** to allow blood sampling from the presenting part.

FETAL TACHYCARDIA

As a baseline change, tachycardia is not a very reliable sign of fetal distress. In general, fetal tachycardia occurs to improve placental circulation when the fetus is stressed. Brief periods of tachycardia (15 to 30 minutes) are usually associated with excessive oxytocic augmentation of labor, after which the heart rate returns to baseline when the augmentation is discontinued. **Prolonged periods of tachycardia are usually associated with elevated maternal temperature or an intrauterine infection,** which should be ruled out. The acid-base status is usually normal.

MECONIUM

The presence of meconium in the amniotic fluid may be a sign of fetal distress. Classification of meconium into early and late passage facilitates a clearer understanding of its importance.

Early passage occurs any time prior to rupture of the membranes and is classified as light or heavy, based on its color and viscosity. Light meconium is lightly stained yellow or greenish amniotic fluid. Heavy meconium is dark green or black and is usually thick and tenacious. Light passage is not associated with poor outcome. Heavy passage is associated with lower 1- and 5-minute Apgar scores and is associated with the risk of meconium aspiration.

Late passage usually occurs during the second stage of labor, after clear amniotic fluid has been noted earlier. Late passage, which is most often heavy, is usually associated with some event (e.g., umbilical cord compression or uterine hypertonus) late in labor that causes fetal distress.

A decrease in meconium-related respiratory complications in the infants of patients who receive amnioinfusion has been reported, presumably as a result of the dilutional effect of the infused fluid. A common technique is to infuse a bolus of up to 800 mL of normal saline at a rate of 10 to 15 mL/minute over a period of 50 to 80 minutes. This is followed by a maintenance dose of 3 mL/minute until delivery. Overdistention of the uterine cavity can be avoided by maintaining the baseline uterine tone in the normal range and at less than 20 mm Hg.

FETAL BLOOD SAMPLING

Fetal scalp blood sampling for pH determination is indicated when fetal distress is suggested by clinical parameters, such as heavy meconium, or by moderate to severely abnormal FHR patterns. Blood is obtained from the fetus by placing an amnioscope transvaginally against the fetal skull (Figure 10-5). Cervical mucus is removed with cotton swabs. Silicone grease is applied to the skull for blood bead formation. A 2×2-mm lancet is used for a stab incision, and a drop of blood is aspirated into a long heparinized glass capillary tube.

Fetal blood pH correctly predicts neonatal outcome 82% of the time, as measured by the Apgar score. The false-positive rate is about 8%, and the false-negative rate about 10%. Determinations of PO_2, PCO_2, and base deficit from scalp blood are possible, but they are not particularly useful clinically. A pH value can be obtained from a 7-cm column of blood in a collecting glass capillary tube (0.015 mL). For PO_2 and PCO_2 determinations, a 25-cm blood column is necessary. This requires a longer sampling time and often leads to clotting within the tube during collection. Clotted blood cannot be aspirated into the gas analyzer. Furthermore, **PO_2 and PCO_2 do not correlate as well with the Apgar score as does pH.** Determination of base deficit can be helpful in differentiating between respiratory and metabolic acidosis.

UMBILICAL CORD BLOOD SAMPLING

The Apgar scoring system has been classically used to assess the newborn condition. Over time, however, the

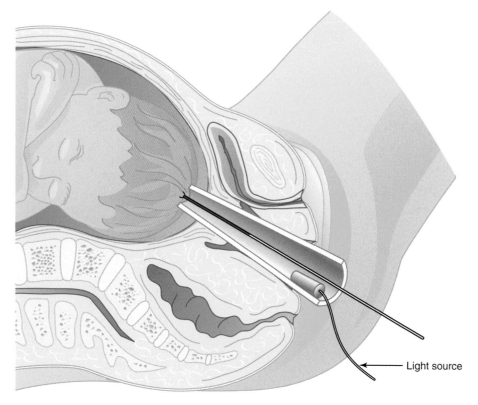

Light source

Figure 10-5. Technique of fetal scalp blood sampling via an amnioscope. After making a small stab incision in the fetal scalp, the blood is drawn off through a long capillary tube.

Apgar score has come to be used inappropriately to define asphyxia, which is a misapplication, because many other conditions (e.g., prematurity, maternal drug administration) can result in low scores that are not reflective of asphyxia. **Asphyxia implies hypoxia of sufficient degree to cause metabolic acidosis. Thus, the Apgar score alone cannot be used to define asphyxia.** A more appropriate tool for defining this condition is assessment of the fetal and neonatal acid-base status. Normal ranges for these indices are given in Table 10-3. One reasonable protocol for umbilical cord blood pH and blood gas analysis is as follows:

1. Doubly clamp a segment of umbilical cord immediately after birth in all deliveries.

Blood	pH	P_{CO_2} (mm Hg)	P_{O_2} (mm Hg)	Base Deficit (mEq/L)
SCALP BLOOD				
Early labor	7.34–7.38	43–57	20–24	(–0.2)–(0.4)
Active phase	7.34–7.40	36–54	20–24	(–2.0)–(0.0)
Complete cervical dilatation	7.26–7.42	36–60	20–24	(–3.3)–(–0.3)
CORD BLOOD				
Artery	7.22–7.34	32–64	14–22	(–7.8)–(–2.2)
Vein	7.29–7.41	25–53	23–35	(–6.2)–(–1.8)

Table 10-3. Normal ranges for fetal scalp and cord blood indices

Data from Hobel CJ: Intrapartum clinical assessment of fetal distress. Am J Obstet Gynecol 110:336, 1971.

2. If there have been problems during the delivery or concern with the infant's condition, obtain an umbilical artery blood specimen for pH and acid-base determination in a syringe flushed with heparin.

3. If a specimen cannot be obtained from the umbilical artery, obtain a specimen from an artery on the chorionic surface of the placenta.

4. If the 5-minute Apgar score is satisfactory and the newborn appears stable and vigorous, the segment of the umbilical cord can be discarded.

Fetal pulse oximetry employs a device which can be used to continually monitor fetal oxygen saturation in cases in which a nonreassuring heart pattern is present. The technique is applicable after membrane rupture in a singleton vertex presentation when cervical dilatation has reached at least 2 cm. The device is placed against the cheek of the fetus and is held in place by pressure exerted by the uterine wall. Fetal oxygen saturation normally varies between 30% and 70% during labor. Values below 30% persisting for more than 2 minutes have been associated with fetal compromise. The overall value of this new technology is currently being studied.

Ultrasonic Doppler velocimetry, for blood flow measurements in umbilical and fetal blood vessels, and **percutaneous umbilical blood sampling** (PUBS) have been used antepartum but are generally not feasible methods for labor management.

Newborn cerebral dysfunction, manifested as seizures and attributable to true birth asphyxia, does not seem to occur unless the Apgar score at 5 minutes is 3 or less, the umbilical artery blood pH is less than 7, and resuscitation is necessary at birth. The later onset of cerebral palsy can occur without these abnormalities and may be attributed to untoward events occurring earlier in the pregnancy. The impact of lesser degrees of asphyxia, as measured by the Apgar score and acid-base status at birth, requires further study. Figure 10-6 is an algorithm for the management of abnormal heart rate tracings during fetal monitoring.

COMPLICATIONS OF FETAL MONITORING

The introduction of a catheter into the uterine cavity and application of a scalp electrode may cause a slight increase in the incidence of maternal infection, but length of labor, rupture of the membranes, and the number of vaginal examinations are of much greater importance in this regard. **The incidence of fetal scalp abscesses and soft tissue injuries from**

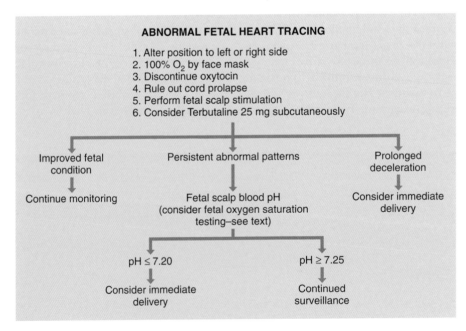

Figure 10-6. Algorithm for the management of an abnormal heart tracing during fetal monitoring.

electrode applications is less than 5%. Scalp abscesses are managed by opening the intradermal vesicle to allow drainage. These small abscesses heal without the need for antibiotic therapy. Spread of the infection into adjacent tissues is rare.

The incidence of scalp abscesses from microblood sampling is less frequent than infection from electrode application. After fetal scalp blood sampling, a cotton swab should always be applied throughout the next uterine contraction and the puncture site inspected for hemostasis during the second contraction. If these precautions are followed, hemorrhage does not occur with scalp blood sampling.

CONTROVERSIES ABOUT FETAL MONITORING IN THE DIAGNOSIS AND TREATMENT OF FETAL DISTRESS

After more than 30 years of routine use of electronic monitoring for assessing FHR in labor, there is still no conclusive evidence of its advantage in long-term fetal outcome. **In 12 prospective, randomized, controlled trials involving more than 55,000 infants worldwide, EFM appears to have little documented benefit over intermittent auscultation with respect to perinatal mortality and long-term neurologic outcome.** The increase in the rate of cesarean deliveries in the United States and elsewhere during recent decades has not been reflected in a decrease in the incidence of cerebral palsy.

The prevalence of intrapartum fetal asphyxia is on the order of 2%. Most of these children have no evidence of brain damage.

When the decision has been made to monitor the FHR, the particular method used can be left to the woman and her obstetrician. Both intermittent and continuous monitoring of the heart rate are regarded as acceptable by the American College of Obstetricians and Gynecologists. Either method will have a similar outcome in terms of the overall incidence of long-term neurologic damage, including cerebral palsy. Intrapartum events appear to play only a small part in the overall incidence of this disorder, and newer methods must be introduced to determine the actual prenatal event that leads to cerebral palsy.

Despite the "intensive obstetrics" of the past 25 years, with increasing attention directed to prenatal care, reduction of birth trauma, and greater use **of cesarean section for high-risk deliveries, the frequency of cerebral palsy remains unchanged at about 2 cases per 1000 term infants.** There is a pressing need to inform the public, as well as the medical profession, that cerebral palsy is not often caused by events during labor, and that the cause in most cases remains unknown.

The current technical approaches to fetal assessment are likely to remain. There are many common conditions in obstetrics in which evaluation of uterine contractility is of primary interest to the physician, with FHR being of secondary significance. Among the indications for contraction measurements are arrest disorders of labor (see Chapter 9). In patients who undergo induction of labor for maternal or fetal reasons, the response to oxytocic stimulation in terms of contraction response can be quantified in Montevideo units, which many physicians prefer to palpation of the uterus to assess strength of labor. Recently, equipment for pulse oximetry to measure oxygen saturation in maternal blood and Doppler blood pressure recorders have been incorporated into the housing of the fetal monitor.

Until new concepts for monitoring are validated, the type of fetal monitoring needs to take into consideration the wishes of the informed patient, the capabilities of the nursing service to carry out monitoring, and the requirements of the physician managing the labor.

Suggested Reading

American College of Obstetricians and Gynecologists: Fetal Heart Rate Patterns: Monitoring, Interpretation and Management, Technical bulletin No. 207. Washington, DC, ACOG, July 1995.

Garite TJ, Dildy GA, NcNamara H, et al: A multicenter controlled trial of fetal pulse oximetry in the intrapartum management of nonreassuring fetal heart rate patterns. Am J Obstet Gynecol 183: 1049, 2000.

Katz VL, Bowes Wa: Meconium aspiration syndrome: Reflections on a murky subject, Am J Obstet Gynecol 166: 171, 1992.

Parer JT, King T: Fetal heart rate monitoring: Is it salvageable? Am J Obstet Gynecol 182: 982, 2000.

Thacker SB, Stroup DF, Peterson HB: Efficacy and safety of intrpartum electronic monitoring: An update, Obstet Gynecol 86: 613, 1995.

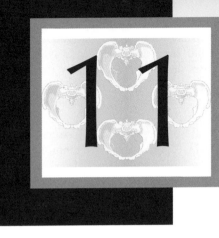

Obstetric Hemorrhage and Puerperal Sepsis

Robert H. Hayashi and Joseph C. Gambone

The three most common causes of maternal death are hemorrhage, infection, and hypertensive disease. In this chapter, the problems of third-trimester bleeding, postpartum hemorrhage, and infection are discussed. These problems are associated not only with maternal and fetal mortality but also with significant morbidity and prolonged hospitalization.

ANTEPARTUM HEMORRHAGE

Vaginal bleeding in the third trimester complicates 4% of all pregnancies. It is considered an obstetric emergency because hemorrhage remains the most frequent cause of maternal death in the United States and often leads to fetal death. It is critical for the well-being of both the mother and fetus that the patient who presents with third-trimester bleeding be managed expediently. The differential diagnosis of third-trimester bleeding is outlined in Box 11-1.

INITIAL EVALUATION

If a patient is bleeding profusely, a team approach to the assessment and management should be instituted to maintain hemodynamic stability. This team should include an obstetrician, an anesthesiologist, and nurses who are knowledgeable about the management of the critically ill patient. At least one large-bore intravenous line should be placed. A central venous pressure line, or preferably a Swan-Ganz catheter, is helpful in the management of hypovolemic shock.

Medical history should be checked for known bleeding disorders or liver disease. The vital signs and amount of bleeding should be checked immediately, as should the patient's mental status. **A pelvic examination should not be performed until placenta previa has been excluded by ultrasonography.** Once placenta previa has been excluded, a sterile speculum examination can be safely done to rule out genital tears or lesions (e.g., cervical cancer) that may be responsible for the bleeding. If none are identified, a digital examination may be performed to determine whether cervical dilatation is present.

A complete blood count should be obtained and compared with previous evaluations to help assess the amount of blood loss. An assessment of the patient's coagulation profile should be done by obtaining a platelet count, serum fibrinogen level, prothrombin time, and partial thromboplastin time. The patient should be typed and crossmatched for at least 4 units of blood (packed cells).

The most accurate means of determining the cause of third-trimester bleeding is with ultrasonography. The ultrasonographic evaluation should include not only the location and character of the placenta but also an assessment of gestational age, an estimate of fetal weight, a determination of the fetal presentation, and a screening for fetal anomalies. Uterine activity and the fetal heart rate should be assessed with a monitored strip to rule out labor and establish fetal well-being.

PLACENTA PREVIA

The incidence of placenta previa is 0.5%. Bleeding from a placenta previa accounts for approximately 20% of all cases of antepartum hemorrhage. Seventy percent of patients with placenta previa present with painless vaginal bleeding in

Box 11-1. Causes of antepartum bleeding

COMMON
Placenta previa
Abruptio placentae

UNCOMMON
Uterine rupture
Fetal (chorionic) vessel rupture
Cervical or vaginal lacerations
Cervical or vaginal lesions including cancer
Congenital bleeding disorder
Unknown

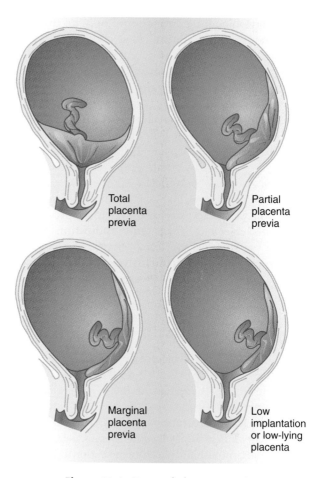

Figure 11-1. Types of placenta previa.

the third trimester, 20% have contractions associated with bleeding, and 10% have the diagnosis made incidentally by ultrasonography or at term.

PREDISPOSING FACTORS

Factors that have been associated with a higher incidence of placenta previa include (1) multiparity, (2) increasing maternal age, (3) prior placenta previa, and (4) multiple gestation. Patients with a placenta previa have a 4% to 8% risk of having placenta previa in a subsequent pregnancy.

CLASSIFICATION

Placenta previa is classified according to the relationship of the placenta to the internal cervical os (Figure 11-1). **Complete placenta previa** implies that the placenta totally covers the cervical os. A complete placenta previa may be central, anterior, or posterior, depending on where the center of the placenta is located relative to the os. **Partial placenta previa** implies that the placenta partially covers the internal cervical os. **A marginal placenta previa** is one in which the edge of the placenta extends to the margin of the internal cervical os.

DIAGNOSIS

The classic presentation of placenta previa is painless vaginal bleeding in a previously normal pregnancy. The mean gestational age at onset of bleeding is 30 weeks, with one-third presenting before 30 weeks. Placenta previa is almost exclusively diagnosed today by ultrasonography. Between 4% and 6% of

patients have some degree of placenta previa on ultrasonic examination before 20 weeks' gestation. With the development of the lower uterine segment, a relative upward placental migration occurs, with 90% of these resolving by the third trimester. Complete placenta previa is the least likely to resolve, with only 10% of cases resolving by the third trimester. **When placenta previa is diagnosed in the second trimester, a repeat sonogram is indicated at 30 to 32 weeks for follow-up evaluation.**

Transabdominal ultrasonography has an accuracy of 95% for placenta previa detection. If the placenta is implanted posteriorly and the fetal vertex is low, the lower margin of the placenta may be obscured and the diagnosis of placenta previa missed. **Transvaginal ultrasonography can accurately diagnose placenta previa in virtually 100% of cases. Theoretically, transvaginal ultrasonography could**

precipitate bleeding, so it should only be done in a hospital setting with informed consent.

Clinically, the diagnosis of placenta previa can be made by palpating the placenta through the cervical os during a procedure called a **double set-up examination.** Although the double set-up was used frequently in the past, the introduction of high-resolution ultrasonography has left little indication for it today. The double set-up procedure dictates that the patient be in the operating room prepared for cesarean delivery. A complete surgical team must be ready to operate should the vaginal examination (performed to determine whether a placenta previa exists) precipitate substantial bleeding. **The only indication for a double set-up in modern obstetrics is when ultrasonography is inconclusive and the patient is in labor with non-life-threatening vaginal bleeding.**

MANAGEMENT

Once the diagnosis of placenta previa is established, management decisions depend on the gestational age of the fetus and the extent of the vaginal bleeding. **With a preterm pregnancy, the goal is to attempt to obtain fetal maturation without compromising the mother's health.** If bleeding is excessive, delivery must be accomplished by cesarean section regardless of gestational age. When the bleeding episode is not profuse or repetitive, the patient is managed expectantly in the hospital on bed rest. With expectant management, 70% of patients will have recurrent vaginal bleeding prior to completion of 36 weeks' gestation and will require delivery. **If the patient reaches 36 weeks, fetal lung maturity should be determined by amniocentesis and the patient delivered by cesarean section if the fetal lungs are mature.** Elective delivery is preferable, as spontaneous labor places the mother at greater risk for hemorrhage and the fetus at risk for hypovolemia and anemia.

LOW-LYING PLACENTA

A patient with a low-lying placenta may present in the same way as a patient with placenta previa. It may be difficult to distinguish a low-lying placenta from a marginal placenta previa, and a double set-up examination may be done if the diagnosis is uncertain. **A vaginal delivery is usually accomplished, although it should be done in a well-controlled manner and setting.**

MATERNAL-FETAL RISKS

The maternal mortality from placenta previa has dropped precipitously over the past 60 years from 30% to less than 1%. This has primarily been the result of the liberal use of cesarean section and careful expectant management. **The rare maternal death is generally associated with complications of cesarean section or uncontrolled hemorrhage from the placental site (usually posterior).** Disseminated intravascular coagulopathy (DIC) may result if a massive hemorrhage or an associated abruption occurs.

The risk of antepartum or intrapartum hemorrhage, or both, is a constant threat to the patient with placenta previa. Bleeding may be caused by an associated placenta accreta, uterine atony, or the placenta previa itself. **Placenta accreta implies an abnormal attachment of the placenta through the uterine myometrium as a result of defective decidual formation (absent Nitabuch's layer).** This abnormal attachment may be superficial **(accreta),** or the placental villi may invade partially through the myometrium **(increta)** or extend to the uterine serosa **(percreta). Two-thirds of patients with this complication require hysterectomy.** Patients with a history of uterine surgery are at greatest risk of developing an accreta. In fact, **those with a prior cesarean section carry a 25% risk.**

Preterm delivery poses the greatest risk to the fetus. Fortunately, primarily as a result of advances in obstetric and neonatal care, the perinatal mortality rate (PMR) has declined over the past decade. The PMR is, however, significantly higher than in the general population and is presently quoted as 40 to 80 deaths per 1000 births. **Twenty percent of pregnancies will be complicated by intrauterine growth restriction (IUGR), and there is a twofold higher incidence of congenital abnormalities. The incidence of malpresentation is 30%. In addition, there is a higher incidence of preterm premature rupture of the membranes in pregnancies complicated by placenta previa.**

ABRUPTIO PLACENTAE

Abruptio placentae, or premature separation of the normally implanted placenta, complicates 0.5% to 1.5% of all pregnancies (1 in 120 births). Abruption severe enough to result in fetal death occurs in 1 per 500 deliveries.

PREDISPOSING FACTORS

Factors associated with an increased incidence of abruption are noted in Box 11-2. The most common of these risk factors is maternal hypertension, either chronic or as a result of preeclampsia. The risk of recurrent abruption is high: 10% after one abruption and 25% after two.

PATHOPHYSIOLOGY

Placental separation is initiated by hemorrhage into the decidua basalis with formation of a decidual hematoma. The resulting separation of the decidua from the basal plate predisposes to further separation and bleeding, as well as compression and destruction of placental tissue. The inciting cause of placental separation is unknown. It has been postulated that it may be due to an inherent weakness or anomaly in the spiral arterioles. Blood may either dissect upward toward the fundus, resulting in a **concealed hemorrhage,** or extend downward toward the cervix, resulting in an external or **revealed hemorrhage.**

DIAGNOSIS AND MANAGEMENT

Clinically, the diagnosis of a placental abruption is entertained if a patient presents with painful vaginal bleeding in association with uterine tenderness, hyperactivity, and increased tone. The signs and symptoms of placental abruption are, however, variable. The most common finding is vaginal bleeding, seen in 80% of cases. **Abdominal pain and uterine tenderness are seen in 66% of cases, fetal distress in 60%, uterine hyperactivity and increased uterine tone in 34%, and fetal demise in 15%.**

The diagnosis of placental abruption is primarily a clinical one. **Ultrasonography may detect only 2%**

Box 11-2. Risk factors for abruptio placentae

Maternal hypertension
Placental abruption in a prior pregnancy
Trauma
Polyhydramnios with rapid decompression
Premature rupture of membranes
Short umbilical cord
Tobacco use
Folate deficiency

---

of abruptions. Because placental abruption may coexist with a placenta previa, the reason for doing an initial ultrasonic examination is to exclude the latter diagnosis.

Management of the patient with an abruption includes careful maternal hemodynamic monitoring, fetal monitoring, serial evaluation of the hematocrit and coagulation profile, and delivery. Intensive monitoring of both the mother and the fetus is essential because rapid deterioration of either one's condition can occur. Blood products for replacement should always be available, and a large-bore (16- to 18-gauge) intravenous line must be secured. Red blood cells should be given liberally if indicated.

MATERNAL-FETAL RISKS

Abruption places the fetus at significant risk of hypoxia and, ultimately, death. **The perinatal mortality rate due to placental abruption is presently 35%,** and the condition accounts for 15% of third-trimester stillbirths. Fifteen percent of live-born infants have significant neurologic impairment.

Placental abruption is the most common cause of DIC in pregnancy. This results from release of thromboplastin from the disrupted placenta and the subplacental decidua into the maternal circulation, causing a consumptive coagulopathy. Clinically significant DIC complicates 20% of cases and is most commonly seen when the abruption is massive or fetal death has occurred. **Hypovolemic shock and acute renal failure due to massive hemorrhage may be seen with a severe abruption if hypovolemia is left uncorrected. Sheehan's syndrome** (amenorrhea as a result of postpartum pituitary necrosis) may be a delayed complication resulting from coagulation within the portal system of the pituitary stalk.

UTERINE RUPTURE

Uterine rupture implies complete separation of the uterine musculature through all of its layers, ultimately with all or a part of the fetus being extruded from the uterine cavity. The overall incidence is 0.5%.

Uterine rupture may be spontaneous, traumatic, or associated with a prior uterine scar, and it may occur during or before labor or at the time of delivery. **A prior uterine scar is associated with 40% of cases.** With a prior lower-segment transverse incision, the risk for rupture is <1%, whereas the **risk with a**

vertical (classical) scar is 4–7%. Sixty percent of uterine ruptures occur in previously unscarred uteri.

DIAGNOSIS AND MANAGEMENT

The signs and symptoms of uterine rupture are highly variable. **Classically, rupture is characterized by the sudden onset of intense abdominal pain and some vaginal bleeding.** Impending rupture may be heralded by hyperventilation, restlessness, agitation, and tachycardia. After the rupture has occurred, the patient may be free of pain momentarily and then complain of diffuse pain thereafter. The most consistent clinical finding is an abnormal fetal heart rate pattern. The patient may or may not have vaginal bleeding, and if it occurs it can range from spotting to severe hemorrhage. **The presenting part may be found to have retracted on pelvic examination, and fetal parts may be more easily palpable abdominally.** Abnormal contouring of the abdomen may also be seen. Fetal distress develops commonly, and fetal death or long-term neurologic sequelae may occur in 10% of cases.

A high index of suspicion is required. Immediate laparotomy is essential. **In most cases, total abdominal hysterectomy is the treatment of choice,** although debridement of the rupture site and primary closure may be considered in women of low parity who desire more children.

MATERNAL-FETAL RISK

Delay in management places both mother and child at significant risk. The major risk to the mother is hemorrhage and shock. Although **the associated maternal mortality rate is now less than 1%,** if the mother is left untreated she will almost certainly die. For the fetus, rapid intervention will minimize morbidity and mortality. **The associated fetal mortality rate today is still about 30%.**

FETAL BLEEDING

Rupture of a fetal vessel complicates 0.1% to 0.8% of pregnancies. **This often results when the cord insertion is velamentous,** implying that the vessels of the cord insert between the amnion and chorion away from the placenta. The incidence of velamentous cord insertion varies from 1% in singleton pregnancies to 10% in twins and 50% in triplets. If the

unprotected vessels pass over the cervical os, this is termed a **vasa previa.** The incidence of vasa previa is 1 per 5000 pregnancies. Velamentously inserted vessels need not pass over the os to rupture, although the risk of rupture is greatest with a vasa previa. Rupture of a fetal vessel necessitates immediate abdominal delivery. **Vasa previa alone carries a perinatal mortality rate of 50%, which increases to 75% if the membranes rupture.**

BLEEDING OF UNKNOWN ETIOLOGY

In many cases of antepartum hemorrhage, no definite cause is ever found. The bleeding is usually minimal in amount. This diagnosis can be made only after exclusion of all other causes.

POSTPARTUM HEMORRHAGE

Postpartum hemorrhage is defined as blood loss in excess of 500 mL at the time of vaginal delivery. There is normally a greater blood loss **following delivery by cesarean section;** therefore, **blood loss in excess of 1000 mL** is considered a postpartum hemorrhage in such patients. The excessive blood loss usually occurs in the immediate postpartum period but can occur slowly over the first 24 hours. **Delayed postpartum hemorrhage can occasionally occur, with the excessive bleeding commencing more than 24 hours after delivery.** This is usually a result of subinvolution of the uterus and disruption of the placental site "scab" several weeks postpartum or of the retention of placental fragments that separate several days after delivery. **Postpartum hemorrhage occurs in about 4% of deliveries.**

Etiology

Most of the blood loss occurs from the myometrial spiral arterioles and decidual veins that previously supplied and drained the intervillous spaces of the placenta. As the contractions of the partially empty uterus cause placental separation, bleeding occurs and continues until the uterine musculature contracts around the blood vessels and acts as a physiologic-anatomic ligature. Failure of the uterus to contract after placental separation (uterine atony) leads to excessive placental site bleeding. Other causes of postpartum hemorrhage are listed in Box 11-3.

Box 11-3. Causes of postpartum hemorrhage

Uterine atony
Genital tract trauma
Retained placental tissue
Low placental implantation
Uterine inversion
Coagulation disorders
    Abruptio placentae
    Amniotic fluid embolism
    Retained dead fetus
    Inherited coagulopathy

UTERINE ATONY

The majority of postpartum hemorrhages (75% to 80%) are due to uterine atony. The factors predisposing to postpartum uterine atony are shown in Box 11-4.

GENITAL TRACT TRAUMA

Trauma during delivery is the second most common cause of postpartum hemorrhage. During vaginal delivery, lacerations of the cervix and vagina may occur spontaneously, but they are more common following the use of forceps or a vacuum extractor. The vascular beds in the genital tract are engorged during pregnancy, and bleeding can be profuse. Lacerations are particularly prone to occur over the perineal body, in the periurethral area, and over the ischial

Box 11-4. Factors predisposing to postpartum uterine atony

Overdistention of the uterus
Multiple gestations
Polyhydramnios
Fetal macrosomia
Prolonged labor
Oxytocic augmentation of labor
Grand multiparity (a parity of 5 or more)
Precipitous labor (one lasting <3 hr)
Magnesium sulfate treatment of preeclampsia
Chorioamnionitis
Halogenated anesthetics
Uterine leiomyomata

spines along the posterolateral aspects of the vagina. The cervix may lacerate at the two lateral angles while rapidly dilating in the first stage of labor. Uterine rupture may occasionally occur. At the time of delivery by low transverse cesarean section, an inadvertent lateral extension of the incision can damage the ascending branches of the uterine arteries; an extension inferiorly can damage the cervical branches of the uterine artery.

RETAINED PLACENTAL TISSUE

Normally, a layer of fibrinoid material, called **Nitabuch's layer,** is found at the base of the placenta. When the partially empty uterus contracts, the placenta cleanly separates through this layer. If the placental anchoring villi grow down into the myometrium and disrupt this fibrinoid layer, placental separation will be incomplete or may not occur at all. Extensive growth of placental tissue into the myometrium without an intervening fibrinoid layer is called **placenta accreta.** A complete placenta accreta will not cause bleeding because the placenta remains attached, but the partial type may cause profuse bleeding, as the normal part of the placenta separates and the myometrium cannot contract sufficiently to occlude the placental site vessels. **In about half of the patients with delayed postpartum hemorrhage, placental fragments are present when uterine curettage is performed with a large curette.**

LOW PLACENTAL IMPLANTATION

Low implantation of the placenta can predispose to postpartum hemorrhage because the relative content of musculature in the uterine wall decreases in the lower uterine segment, which may result in insufficient control of placental site bleeding.

COAGULATION DISORDERS

Peripartum coagulation disorders are high-risk factors for postpartum hemorrhage but fortunately are quite rare. Patients with coagulation problems, such as occur with thrombotic thrombocytopenic purpura, amniotic fluid embolism, abruptio placentae, idiopathic thrombocytopenic purpura, or von Willebrand's disease, may develop postpartum hemorrhage because of their inability to form a stable blood clot in the placental site.

Patients with **thrombotic thrombocytopenia** have a rare syndrome of unknown etiology characterized by thrombocytopenic purpura, microangiopathic hemolytic anemia, transient and fluctuating neurologic signs, renal dysfunction, and a febrile course. In pregnancy, the disease is usually fatal. An **amniotic fluid embolus** is also fairly rare and is associated with an approximately 80% mortality. This syndrome is characterized by a fulminating consumption coagulopathy, intense bronchospasm, and vasomotor collapse. It is triggered by an intravascular infusion of a significant amount of amniotic fluid during a tumultuous or rapid labor in the presence of ruptured membranes. During the process of **placental abruption,** a small amount of amniotic fluid may leak into the vascular system, and the thromboplastin in the amniotic fluid may trigger a consumption coagulopathy without the other elements of a large amniotic fluid embolus. Patients with **idiopathic thrombocytopenic purpura** have platelets with abnormal function or a shortened life span. This causes thrombocytopenia and a bleeding tendency. Circulating antiplatelet antibodies of the IgG type may occasionally cross the placenta and result in fetal and neonatal thrombocytopenia as well. **Von Willebrand's disease** is an inherited coagulopathy characterized by a prolonged bleeding time due to factor VIII deficiency. During pregnancy, these patients are likely to have a decreased bleeding diathesis, because pregnancy elevates factor VIII levels. In the postpartum period, they are susceptible to delayed bleeding as factor VIII levels fall.

UTERINE INVERSION

Uterine inversion is the "turning inside out" of the uterus in the third stage of labor. It is quite rare, occurring in only about 1 in 20,000 pregnancies. Just after the second stage, the uterus is somewhat atonic, the cervix open, and the placenta attached. **Improper management of the third stage of labor can cause an iatrogenic uterine inversion.** If the inexperienced physician exerts fundal pressure while pulling on the umbilical cord before complete placental separation (particularly with a fundal implantation of the placenta), uterine inversion may occur. As the fundus of the uterus moves through the vagina, the inversion exerts traction on peritoneal structures, which can elicit a profound vasovagal response. The resulting vasodilatation increases bleeding and the risk of hypovolemic shock. **If the placenta is completely or partially separated, the uterine atony may cause profuse bleeding, which compounds the vasovagal shock.**

OBSTETRIC SHOCK

Hypotension without significant external bleeding may occasionally develop in an obstetric patient. This condition is called obstetric shock. **The causes of obstetric shock include concealed hemorrhage, uterine inversion, and amniotic fluid embolism.**

An improperly sutured episiotomy can lead to a concealed postpartum hemorrhage. If the first suture at the vaginal apex of the episiotomy incision does not incorporate the cut and retracted arterioles, they can continue to bleed, creating a hematoma that can dissect cephalad into the retroperitoneal space. This may cause shock without external evidence of blood loss. **A soft tissue hematoma, usually of the vulva, may occur following delivery in the absence of any laceration or episiotomy and may also contribute to occult blood loss.**

Spontaneous uterine rupture during labor is rare (1 in 1900 deliveries), but it usually results in significant intraperitoneal bleeding. Uterine rupture can also occur secondary to blunt abdominal trauma at the time of an automobile accident.

DIFFERENTIAL DIAGNOSIS

Identification of the cause of postpartum hemorrhage or obstetric shock requires a systematic approach. The fundus of the uterus should be palpated through the abdominal wall to determine the presence or absence of **uterine atony.** Next, a quick but thorough inspection of the vagina and cervix should be performed to ascertain whether any **lacerations** may be compounding the bleeding problem. Any uterine inversion or **pelvic hematoma** should be excluded during the pelvic examination. If the cause of bleeding has not been identified, **manual exploration of the uterine cavity** should be performed, under general anesthesia if necessary. With fingertips together, a gloved hand is slipped through the open cervix, and the endometrial surface is palpated carefully to identify any retained products of conception, uterine wall lacerations, or partial uterine inversion. If no cause for the bleeding is found, a **coagulopathy** must be sought.

MANAGEMENT OF POSTPARTUM HEMORRHAGE AND OBSTETRIC SHOCK

The first steps toward good management are the identification of patients at risk for postpartum hemorrhage and the institution of prophylactic measures during labor to minimize the possibility of maternal mortality. Patients with any predisposing factors for postpartum hemorrhage, including a history of postpartum hemorrhage, should be screened for anemia and atypical antibodies to ensure that an adequate supply of type-specific blood is on hand in the blood bank. An intravenous infusion via a large-bore needle or catheter should be commenced prior to delivery, and blood should be held in the laboratory for possible crossmatching.

During the diagnostic workup of an established hemorrhage, the patient's vital signs must be monitored closely. Four units of packed red blood cells must be typed and cross-matched, and intravenous crystalloids (such as normal saline or lactated Ringer's solution) infused to restore intravascular volume. **Resuscitation with normal saline usually requires a volume of three times the estimated blood loss.**

UTERINE ATONY

If uterine atony is determined to be the cause of the postpartum hemorrhage, a rapid continuous intravenous infusion of dilute oxytocin (40 to 80 U in 1 L of normal saline) should be given to increase uterine tone. If the uterus remains atonic and the placental site bleeding continues during the oxytocic infusion, **ergonovine maleate or methylergonovine,** 0.2 mg, may be given intramuscularly. The ergot drugs are contraindicated in patients with hypertension, because the pressor effect of the drug may increase blood pressure to dangerous levels.

Analogues of prostaglandin $F_{2\alpha}$ given intramuscularly are quite effective in controlling postpartum hemorrhage caused by uterine atony. The 15-methyl analogue (Hemabate) has a more potent uterotonic effect and longer duration of action than the parent compound. The expected time of onset of the uterotonic effect when the 15-methyl analogue (0.25 mg) is given intramuscularly is 20 minutes, whereas when injected into the myometrium it may take up to 4 minutes.

Failing these pharmacologic treatments, **a bimanual compression and massage of the uterine corpus may control the bleeding and cause the uterus to contract. Although packing the uterine cavity is not widely practiced,** it may occasionally control postpartum hemorrhage and obviate the need for surgical intervention. The vital signs, hematocrit, and fundal height should be monitored frequently while the packing is in place, because continued bleeding will not be initially evident through the packing. The packing may be removed in 1 to 24 hours. Usually, the bleeding will be controlled.

If uterine bleeding persists in an otherwise stable patient, she could be transported to the angiocatheterization laboratory, where radiologists can **place an angiocatheter into the uterine arteries for injection of thrombogenic materials to control blood flow and hemorrhaging.**

Operative intervention is a last resort. If the patient has completed her childbearing, a **supracervical or total abdominal hysterectomy** is definitive therapy for intractable postpartum hemorrhage caused by uterine atony. If reproductive potential is important to the patient, **ligation of the uterine arteries** adjacent to the uterus will lower the pulse pressure distal to the ligatures. This procedure is more successful in controlling uterine placental site hemorrhage and is easier to perform than bilateral hypogastric artery ligation.

GENITAL TRACT TRAUMA

When postpartum hemorrhage is related to genital tract trauma, surgical intervention is necessary. Repair of genital tract lacerations requires the implementation of an important principle: **The first suture must be placed well above the apex of the laceration to incorporate any retracted bleeding arterioles into the ligature.** Repair of vaginal lacerations requires good light and good exposure, and the tissues should be approximated without dead space. A running lock suture technique provides the best hemostasis. **Cervical lacerations need not be sutured unless they are actively bleeding (Figure 11-2).** Large, expanding hematomas of the genital tract require surgical evacuation of clots and a search for bleeding vessels that can be ligated, then packed for hemostasis. Stable hematomas can be observed and treated conservatively. A retroperitoneal hematoma generally begins in the pelvis. If the bleeding cannot be controlled from a vaginal approach, a laparotomy and bilateral hypogastric artery ligation may be necessary.

The intraoperative laceration of the ascending branch of the uterine artery during delivery through a

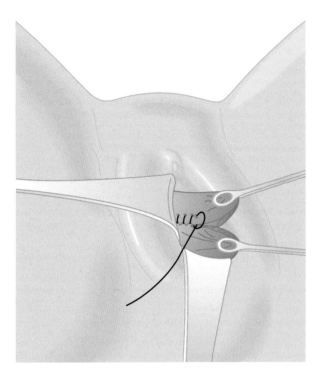

Figure 11-2. Suturing a cervical laceration. The first suture must be placed above the apex of the laceration.

low transverse cesarean section can be easily controlled by the placement of a large suture ligature through the myometrium and broad ligament below the level of the laceration. A uterine rupture usually necessitates subtotal or total abdominal hysterectomy, although small defects may be repaired.

RETAINED PRODUCTS OF CONCEPTION

When the placenta cannot be delivered in the usual manner, manual removal of the placenta is necessary (Figure 11-3). This should be performed urgently if bleeding is profuse. Otherwise, it is reasonable to delay 30 minutes to await spontaneous separation. General anesthesia may be required. Following manual removal of the placenta or placental remnants, the uterus should be scraped with a large curette.

UTERINE INVERSION

The management of a uterine inversion requires quick thinking. The patient rapidly goes into shock, and **immediate intravascular volume expansion with intravenous crystalloids is required.** An anesthesi-

ologist should be summoned. When the patient's condition is stable, the partially separated placenta should be completely removed and an attempt made to replace the uterus by placing a cupped hand around the fundus and elevating it in the long axis of the vagina. If this is unsuccessful, a further attempt should be made using IV nitroglycerin (100 µg) to relax the uterine muscle. Once replaced, a dilute oxytocin infusion should be started to cause the uterus to contract before removing the intrauterine hand. **Rarely, the uterus cannot be replaced from below, and a surgical procedure may be required.** At laparotomy, a vertical incision should be made through the posterior portion of the cervix to incise the constriction ring and allow the fundus to be replaced into the peritoneal cavity. Suturing of the cervical incision will complete this procedure.

AMNIOTIC FLUID EMBOLUS

The principal objectives of treatment for amniotic fluid embolism are to support the respiratory system, correct the shock, and replace the coagulation factors. These necessitate immediate cardiopulmonary resuscitation, usually with mechanical ventilation; rapid volume expansion with an electrolyte solution; positive inotropic cardiac support; placement of a bladder catheter to monitor urine output; correction of the red cell deficit by transfusion with packed red blood cells; and reversal of the coagulopathy with the use of platelets, fibrinogen, and other blood components.

COAGULOPATHY

When postpartum hemorrhage is associated with coagulopathy, the specific defect should be corrected by the infusion of blood products, as outlined in Box 11-5 and Table 11-1. **Patients with thrombocytopenia require platelet concentrate infusions; those with von Willebrand's disease require factor VIII concentrate or cryoprecipitate.**

A packed red cell infusion is given to a patient who has bled enough to drop the circulating red cell population sufficiently to compromise the delivery of oxygen to the tissues. Therefore, institution of blood transfusion is best judged by symptoms of oxygen deprivation rather than by some empirical hemoglobin level. No important physiologic impairment has been noted at hemoglobin levels as low as 6 to 8 g/dL (hematocrit, 18% to 24%). **In general, a 1 U**

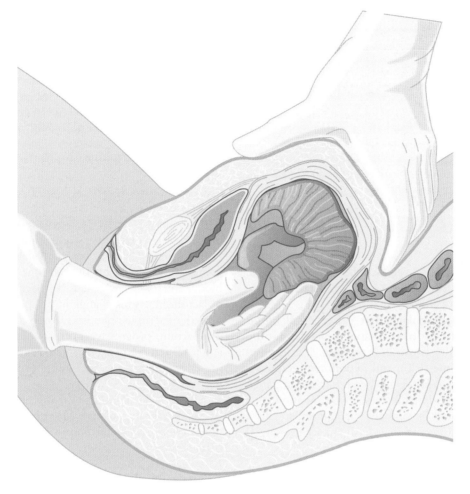

Figure 11-3. Manual removal of the placenta. The abdominal hand provides counterpressure on the uterine fundus against the shearing force of the fingers in the uterus.

Table 11-1. Blood products used to correct coagulation defects

Blood Product	Volume (mL) in 1 U*	Effect of Transfusion
Platelet concentrate	30–40	Increases platelet count by about 20,000 to 25,000
Cryoprecipitate	15–25	Supplies fibrinogen, factor VIII, and factor XIII (3–10 times more concentrated than the equivalent volume of fresh plasma)
Fresh-frozen plasma	200	Supplies all factors except platelets (1 g of fibrinogen)
Packed red blood cells	200	Raises hematocrit 3%–4%

*1 U, Quantity obtained from 1 U (500 mL) of fresh whole blood.

Box 11-5. Laboratory evaluation of disseminated intravascular coagulation

- **Platelet count** (normal range = $150-450 \times 10^9$/L): 1 unit of platelets will raise the platelet count by 5–10 $\times 10^9$/L
- **Plasma fibrinogen** (normal range = 175–600 mg/dL): Fresh frozen plasma (FFP): 1 unit = 1 g of fibrinogen; 4 units of FFP will raise the plasma fibrinogen by 5–10 mg/dL
- **Cryoprecipitate:** 1 bag = 0.25 g of fibrinogen; 16 bags raises the plasma fibrinogen by 5–10 mg/dL
- **Fibrin split products**
  Normal range = <0.05 µg/mL (D-dimer method)

---

transfusion of packed red blood cells will increase the hemoglobin level by 1 g/dL (and the hematocrit by 3% to 4%).

Massive blood replacement (when total blood volume is replaced in a 24-hour period) may be associated with thrombocytopenia, prolonged prothrombin time (PT), and hypofibrinogenemia. Thrombocytopenia is the most common abnormality, so platelet transfusion following determination of a low platelet count is not an uncommon scenario. Fresh-frozen plasma may be transfused for prolonged PT or hypofibrinogenemia.

PUERPERAL SEPSIS

Puerperal sepsis still accounts for significant postpartum maternal morbidity and mortality. **Patients with a puerperal genital tract infection are susceptible to the development of septic shock, pelvic thrombophlebitis, and pelvic abscess.**

Following a vaginal delivery, approximately 6% or 7% of women demonstrate febrile morbidity, defined as a temperature of 100.4°F (38°C) or higher that occurs for more than 2 consecutive days (exclusive of the first postpartum day) during the first 10 postpartum days. **Following primary cesarean section, the incidence of febrile morbidity is about twice that following vaginal delivery. The majority of these fevers are caused by endometritis.**

ETIOLOGY

The pathophysiology of puerperal sepsis is closely related to the various microbial inhabitants of the vagina and cervix. The vaginal flora during gestation resembles that in the nonpregnant state, although there is a trend toward isolating more *Mycoplasma genitalis* and anaerobic streptococci in the last trimester. **Potentially pathogenic organisms can be cultured from the vagina in approximately 80% of pregnant women. These organisms include enterococci, hemolytic and nonhemolytic streptococci, anaerobic streptococci, enteric bacilli, pseudodiphtheria bacteria, and *Neisseria* species other than *N. gonorrhoeae*.** Excessive overgrowth of these organisms during pregnancy is inhibited by the acidity of the vagina (pH 4 to 5), primarily as a result of the production of lactic acid by the lactobacilli.

The uterine cavity is normally free of bacteria during pregnancy. After parturition, the pH of the vagina changes from acidic to alkaline because of the neutralizing effect of the alkaline amniotic fluid, blood, and lochia, as well as the decreased population of lactobacilli. This change in pH favors an increased growth of aerobic organisms. Approximately 48 hours postpartum, progressive necrosis of the endometrial and placental remnants produces a favorable intrauterine environment for the multiplication of anaerobic bacteria.

About 70% of puerperal infections are caused by anaerobic organisms. Most of these are anaerobic cocci (*Peptostreptococcus*, *Peptococcus*, and *Streptococcus*), although mixed infections with *Bacteroides fragilis* are encountered in up to one-third of cases. **Of the aerobic organisms, *Escherichia coli* is the most common pathogen,** followed by enterococci. Puerperal infection from clostridia is rare.

Intrauterine staphylococcal infection is rare. This organism is frequently responsible for infection of perineal wounds and abdominal incisions. *Trichomonas vaginalis* and *Candida albicans* are frequent inhabitants of the vagina, but no connection with puerperal sepsis has been established. ***Mycoplasma* organisms have been shown to contribute to puerperal endometritis.**

PREDISPOSING FACTORS

Predisposing factors to the development of a puerperal genital tract infection are shown in Box 11-6.

After delivery, the placental site vessels are clotted off, and there is an exudation of lymph-like fluid along with massive numbers of neutrophils and other white cells to form the lochia. Vaginal microorganisms readily enter the uterine cavity and may become path-

> **Box 11-6. Factors predisposing to the development of puerperal genital tract infection**
>
> Poor nutrition and hygiene
> Anemia
> Premature rupture of the membranes (PROM)
> Prolonged rupture of the membranes
> Prolonged labor
> Frequent vaginal examinations during labor
> Cesarean delivery
> Forceps or vacuum delivery
> Cervical/vaginal lacerations
> Manual removal of the placenta
> Retained placental fragments or fetal membranes

ogenic at the placental site, depending on such variables as the size of the inoculum, the local pH, and the presence or absence of devitalized tissue. The latter may include tissue incorporated in the suture line of a cesarean section.

The normal body defense mechanisms usually prevent any progressive infection, but a breakdown of these defenses allows the bacteria to invade the myometrium. Further invasion into the lymphatics of the parametrium can cause lymphangitis, pelvic cellulitis, and the possibility of widespread infection from septic emboli.

Endomyoparametritis is a potentially life-threatening condition. It commonly begins with retention of secundines (placental and amnio-chorionic membrane fragments) that block the normal lochial flow, allowing accumulation of intrauterine lochia, which in turn changes the local pH and acts as a culture medium for bacterial growth. Unless normal lochial flow is established, bacterial invasion progresses.

CLINICAL FEATURES

Puerperal infection manifests as rising fever and increasing uterine tenderness on postpartum day 2 or 3. With the development of parametritis (pelvic cellulitis), the temperature elevation will be sustained, and signs of pelvic peritonitis may develop. Erratic temperature fluctuations and severe chills suggest bacteremia and dissemination of septic emboli, with the particular likelihood of spread to the lungs.

When the usual relative pelvic venous stasis is combined with a large inoculum of pathogenic anaerobic bacteria, a pelvic vein thrombophlebitis is likely to develop, usually on the right side of the pelvis. **The clinical picture of pelvic thrombophlebitis is characterized by a persistent spiking fever for 7 to 10 days after delivery, despite antibiotic therapy.**

DIAGNOSIS

Evaluation of a febrile postpartum patient should include a careful history and physical examination. Extrapelvic causes of fever, such as breast engorgement, mastitis, aspiration pneumonia, atelectasis, pyelonephritis, thrombophlebitis, or wound infection, should be excluded.

Although a pelvic examination is generally not helpful in diagnosing pelvic thrombophlebitis, it may allow the palpation of tender, thrombosed, and edematous ovarian, parauterine, or iliac veins. An abdominal pelvic computed tomographic scan or ultrasonographic scan may be helpful. This diagnosis is usually made by exclusion, however, and by the prompt regression of fever following commencement of heparin anticoagulant therapy.

Before the institution of antibiotic therapy for puerperal endometritis, aerobic and anaerobic cultures should be obtained from the blood, endocervix, and uterine cavity, and a catheterized urine specimen should be obtained for culture. The antibiotic sensitivities from these cultures may be used to determine appropriate second-line drug therapy in the event of failure of the first-line drugs. Antibiotics should commence following diagnosis, because receiving culture results for anaerobic organisms may take several days.

MANAGEMENT

A febrile puerperal patient with cessation of lochial flow should undergo a pelvic examination and removal of any secundines that may be occluding the cervical os.

The antibiotic treatment of puerperal infection usually follows two major principles. **First, early antibiotic treatment should be instituted** to confine then eliminate the infectious process. **Second, the antibiotics should provide anaerobic coverage** because these organisms are involved in 70% of puerperal infections. Antibiotics should be continued for at least 48 hours after the patient becomes afebrile. Anaerobic organisms especially require prolonged chemotherapy for elimination.

Broad-spectrum antibiotics, such as ampicillin and the cephalosporins, are effective first-line

drugs for mild and moderate cases of puerperal infection. When the infection is moderate to severe, a penicillin-aminoglycoside combination has traditionally been used as first-line therapy. The major pelvic pathogen resistant to this combination, however, is *Bacteroides fragilis*, which is usually sensitive to either clindamycin or chloramphenicol. Therefore, **the use of clindamycin with either an aminoglycoside or Ampicillin should provide better first-line coverage.**

When pelvic thrombophlebitis or thromboembolism is suspected or clinically diagnosed, unfractionated heparin therapy should be instituted to increase the clotting time (Lee-White method) or activated prothrombin time to two to three times normal. Only 2 to 3 weeks of anticoagulant therapy are needed for uncomplicated pelvic thrombophlebitis. Patients with femoral thrombophlebitis require 4 to 6 weeks of heparin therapy followed by the administration of oral anticoagulants for a few months.

If the patient does not respond to heparin therapy and the clinical course is one of unrelenting fever and pelvic tenderness, a diagnosis of **pelvic abscess** must be entertained. Diagnosis is made by pelvic examination and confirmed by pelvic ultrasonography or computed tomographic scan. The finding of a tender, pelvic parametrial mass suggests an abscess. Ultrasonography will confirm that the mass is fluid-filled rather than solid. **The presence of a pelvic abscess demands surgical drainage.**

Suggested Reading

Preventing postpartum hemorrhage: Managing the third stage of labor. Maternal Neonatal Health 19(3): 2001.

Crane S, Chun B, Acker D: Treatment of obstetrical hemorrhagic emergencies. Curr Opin Obstet Gynecol 5:675, 1993.

Lavery JP: Placenta previa. Clin Obstet Gynecol 33:414, 1990.

Lucas WF: Postpartum hemorrhage. Clin Obstet Gynecol 23:637, 1980.

Sweet RL, Ledger WJ: Puerperal infectious morbidity: A two-year review. Am J Obstet Gynecol 117:1093, 1973.

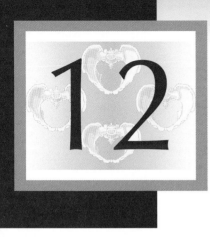

12 Uterine Contractility and Dystocia

Richard A. Bashore and Robert H. Hayashi

Although the definition of **dystocia** is **"difficult childbirth,"** the term is used interchangeably with **dysfunctional labor** and characterizes labor that does not progress normally. **The problem may be caused by (1) ineffective uterine expulsive forces; (2) an abnormal lie, presentation, position, or fetal structure;** or **(3) disproportion** between the size of the fetus and pelvis, resulting in mechanical interference with the passage of the fetus through the birth canal. The cause or causes of abnormal labor should be determined as accurately as possible so that an effective and safe management plan can be developed.

PHYSIOLOGIC CHANGES OF LABOR

The pregnant uterus is a large smooth-muscle organ consisting of billions of smooth-muscle cells. Each smooth-muscle cell becomes a contractile element when the intracellular ionic calcium concentration increases to trigger an enzymatic process that results in the formation of the actin-myosin element. Also, stimulation of oxytocin and/or prostaglandin receptors on the plasma membrane further activates the formation of the actin-myosin element.

Contractions occur in localized areas of the uterus during gestation, but during parturition the entire uterus contracts in an organized way to empty itself. These coordinated smooth-muscle contractions occur as a result of the involvement and action of special gap junction structures. **Gap junctions are protein structures that form along the interface of two smooth-muscle cell membranes** and that act by promoting the movement of action potentials throughout the myometrium.

The pregnant cervix must also be structurally altered from a firm, intact sphincter to a soft, pliable, dilatable structure through which the products of conception can pass at the appropriate time. **These structural changes are the result of collagenolysis and increased water content,** which probably occur in response to an increase in the estrogen-progesterone ratio, prostaglandin E_2, and enzymatic remodeling of cervical tissue.

NORMAL LABOR

The early part, or **latent phase,** of labor is involved with softening and effacement of the cervix with minimal dilatation. This is followed by a more rapid rate of cervical dilatation, known as the **active phase of labor,** which is **further divided into the acceleration (maximum slope) and deceleration phases.** The descent of the fetal presenting part usually begins during the active phase of labor, then progresses at a more rapid rate toward the end of the active phase, and continues after the cervix is completely dilated. A useful method for assessing the progress of labor and detecting abnormalities in a timely manner is to plot the rate of cervical dilatation and descent of the fetal presenting part (Figure 12-1).

Normal cervical dilatation and descent of the fetus take place in a progressive manner and occur within a well-defined time period. Dysfunctional labor occurs when rates of dilatation and descent exceed these time limits. The phase of labor during which the abnormality occurs and the configuration of the abnormal labor curve may indicate the potential causes for the abnormal labor.

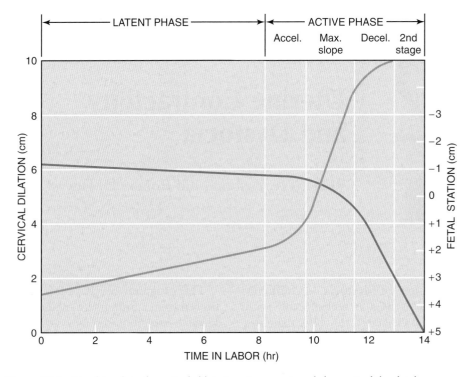

Figure 12-1. Graphic plot of cervical dilatation (in green) and descent of the fetal presenting part (in red) during labor. *From Cohen WR, Friedman EA (eds): Management of Labor. Gaithersburg, MD, Aspen Publishers, 1983, p 13.*

ABNORMALITIES OF THE LATENT PHASE OF LABOR

The normal limits of the latent phase of labor extend up to 20 hours for nulliparous patients and up to 14 hours for multiparous patients. A latent phase that exceeds these limits is considered prolonged and may be caused by hypertonic uterine contractions, premature or excessive use of sedatives or analgesics, or less commonly, hypotonic uterine contractions. **Hypertonic contractions are ineffective and painful** and are associated with increased uterine tone, whereas **hypotonic contractions are usually less painful** and are characterized by an easily indentable uterus during the contraction. Hypotonic contractions occur more frequently during the active phase of labor. A long, closed, firm cervix requires more time to efface and to undergo early dilatation than does a soft, partially effaced cervix, but it is doubtful that a cervical factor alone causes a prolonged latent phase. **Some patients who appear to be developing a prolonged latent phase are shown eventually to be in false labor, with no progressive dilatation of the cervix.**

The identification of the cause or causes of a prolonged latent phase is usually not difficult. Palpation or recording of uterine contractions and observation of the patient over a period of time usually suggests whether uterine activity is hypotonic or hypertonic or whether the patient is in false labor. The outcome of a prolonged latent phase is generally favorable for both the mother and the fetus, provided that no other abnormalities of labor subsequently occur.

MANAGEMENT

The management of a prolonged latent phase depends on its cause. **A prolonged latent phase caused by premature or excessive use of sedation or analgesia usually resolves spontaneously after the effects of the medication have disappeared. Hypertonic activity** responds erratically to oxytocin but **usually responds to a therapeutic rest with morphine sulfate or an equivalent drug.**

Hypocontractile dysfunction usually responds well to an intravenous infusion of oxytocin. One technique that has been recommended for stimulation of labor involves the addition of 10 U of oxytocin to 1000 mL of intravenous solution for a final concentration of 10 mU of oxytocin to each 1 mL of solution. An infusion of this solution is begun at a rate of between 0.5 to 1.0 mU/min and is increased by approximately 50% increments every 20 to 45 minutes until uterine contractions of the desired frequency and intensity are obtained.

For many years, artificial rupture of the membranes has been regarded as an effective method for management of a prolonged latent phase, but this approach continues to be controversial. When undertaken during the latent phase of labor, this procedure carries the added risk of intrauterine infection, particularly if it does not expedite delivery.

ABNORMALITIES OF THE ACTIVE PHASE OF LABOR

When the cervix dilates to approximately 3 to 4 cm, the rate of dilatation progresses more rapidly. Cervical dilatation of less than 1.2 cm/hour in nulliparous women and 1.5 cm in multiparous women constitute a **protraction disorder of the active phase of labor.**

During the latter part of the active phase, the fetal presenting part also descends more rapidly through the pelvis and continues to descend through the second stage of labor. A rate of descent of the presenting part of less than 1.0 cm/hour in nulliparous women and 2.0 cm/hour in multiparous women is considered to be a **protraction disorder of descent** (Figure 12-2). If a period of 2 hours or more elapses during the active phase of labor without progress in cervical dilatation, an **arrest of dilatation** has occurred; a period of more than 1 hour without a change in station of the fetal presenting part is defined as an **arrest of descent** (Figure 12-3).

In the absence of cephalopelvic disproportion or fetal malposition, protraction or arrest disorders are usually caused by hypotonic uterine contractions, conduction anesthesia, or excessive sedation. The maternal pelvis should be evaluated, and the presenting fetal part should also be evaluated under these conditions.

MANAGEMENT

Protraction disorders do *not* respond to oxytocic stimulation, therapeutic rest, or artificial rupture

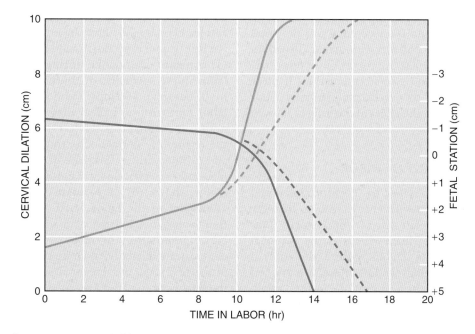

Figure 12-2. Normal dilatation (in green) and descent (in red) curves of normal labor ——— and curves depicting protracted dilatation and descent abnormalities of labor - - - - - *Modified from Friedman EA: Labor: Clinical Evaluation and Management. 2nd ed. New York, Appleton-Century-Crofts, 1978, p 65.*

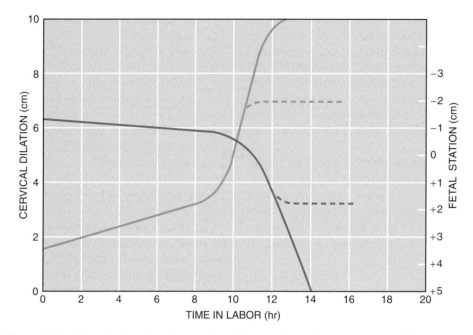

Figure 12-3. Normal dilatation (in green) and descent (in red) curves of normal labor ——— and curves depicting arrest disorders of dilatation and descent - - - - -. *Modified from Friedman EA: Labor: Clinical Evaluation and Management, 2nd ed. New York, Appleton-Century-Crofts, 1978, p 66.*

of the membranes. Patients with this disorder should be treated expectantly as long as the fetal heart rate remains satisfactory and labor continues to progress. A large percentage of patients with **arrest disorders** unrelated to cephalopelvic disproportion or fetal malposition *do* respond to oxytocic stimulation. If these disorders are related to oversedation, normal labor patterns will resume if the effect of the drug is allowed to wear off.

ACTIVE MANAGEMENT OF LABOR

Active management of labor has been proposed and utilized in the nulliparous patient as a strategy to lower the incidence of cesarean delivery for dystocia. This approach was initiated in the 1960s at the National Maternity Hospital in Dublin, where the rate of cesarean births is relatively low. Recent published studies of this approach in institutions in the United States and Canada have been controversial with respect to the lowering of cesarean birth rates, but all studies have reported lower rates of intervention in general when active management of labor is employed.

The criteria and components of this program are as follows: **(1) nulliparous pregnant patient with spontaneous onset of labor and a singleton fetus in a cephalic presentation; (2) prenatal education classes** and intrapartum reassurances to set realistic patient expectations and lower patient anxiety; **(3) constant attendance during labor, usually by a labor nurse specialist or midwife; (4) peer review of all cesarean sections; (5) nonadmittance to the labor unit without a clear diagnosis of labor** (based not on the amount of cervical dilation but rather on the quality of contractions, which should be regular and painful with at least one of the following: complete cervical effacement, rupture of membranes, or bloody show); **(6) performance of amniotomy on admission to the labor ward** and regular examination for progress in cervical dilatation; and **(7) oxytocic augmentation of labor** if the patient fails to demonstrate dilatation at a rate of 1 cm/hour or more in the first stage of labor or if there is no descent of the fetal head for 1 hour in the second stage.

Most active management protocols use an initial infusion rate and increments of 4 to 6 mU/min of oxytocin with only 15 minutes between increments. **An abnormal fetal heart rate pattern may lead to further fetal evaluation** before operative delivery is initiated. With a nonreassuring fetal heart pattern, a fetal scalp stimulation might be done, looking for fetal heart rate acceleration as a reassuring response. If this procedure fails to elicit a fetal heart acceleration, fetal evaluation may involve **determining the pH of blood from the fetal scalp.**

Many active management of labor programs have reported no compromise of perinatal outcomes and no cases of uterine rupture.

DYSTOCIA CAUSED BY ABNORMAL PRESENTATION AND POSITION

Presentations other than vertex and positions other than occipitoanterior are considered to be abnormal in the laboring patient. Disorders of the dilatation and descent phases of labor occur with increased frequency in cases of abnormal presentation or position because of the altered relationship between the presenting part of the fetus and the maternal pelvis. Fetal malpresentations are discussed further in Chapter 14.

Persistent Occipitotransverse Position

The fetal head normally enters and engages in the maternal pelvis in an occipitotransverse (OT) position. It subsequently rotates to an occipitoanterior position or, in a small percentage of cases, to an occipitoposterior position. This rotation occurs because the head flexes as the leading part of the vertex encounters the pelvic floor and then rotates to adjust to the shape of the gynecoid pelvis. In a small number of cases, the head fails to flex and rotate and persists in an occipitotransverse position. This position may be caused by cephalopelvic disproportion; altered pelvic architecture, such as in a patient with a platypelloid or android pelvis; or a relaxed pelvic floor, brought about by epidural anesthesia or multiparity. The diagnosis of a persistent OT position may be difficult at times, owing to the obscuring of suture lines and fontanelles by the excessive molding and caput formation that often accompany this abnormal position.

A persistent OT position with arrest of descent for a period of 1 hour or more is known as transverse arrest. Arrest occurs because of the deflexion that accompanies the persistent OT position, resulting in the larger occipitofrontal diameter (11 cm) becoming the presenting diameter. Until the head undergoes flexion and rotation, further descent cannot take place. Transverse arrest commonly occurs with the vertex at a +2 to +3 station.

The management of transverse arrest at a +2 to +3 station is complex, in part, because at these stations the widest part of the fetal head is at or above the level of the ischial spines. If the midpelvis is compromised, cesarean delivery is indicated. If the pelvis is judged to be of normal size and the fetus is not macrosomic, oxytocic stimulation of labor may be appropriate if uterine contractions are inadequate.

Manual rotation using the fingers of the examiner's hand or forceps rotation using Kielland forceps may be indicated if the pelvis is of normal size and shape. **Forceps delivery of a persistent OT position at a +2 to +3 station has been referred to as a midpelvic or midforceps delivery.** When the pelvis is of a platypelloid or android type (see Figure 9-5), rotation may not be feasible.

Because of the marked degree of molding and caput formation that usually occurs in this position, the bony part of the vertex of the fetal head may be at a +1 station or higher, although the scalp may be visible at the introitus. Thus, what appears to be an uncomplicated low forceps operation may actually be a midforceps procedure. One method for avoiding this mistake involves a clinical evaluation of the relationship between the fetal head and the sacrum. If the fetal head fills the hollow of the sacrum, the biparietal diameter is usually at or below the spines, and an attempt at forceps delivery can be considered.

Persistent Occipitoposterior Position

The head generally rotates from OT to occipitoanterior (OP) during the descent through the maternal pelvis. Even if the head initially rotates to an occipitoposterior position, most fetuses will eventually rotate spontaneously during labor to occipitoanterior, leaving only a small percentage (5% to 10%) of fetuses with a persistent OP position.

The course of labor in the presence of a persistent OP position is usually normal except for a tendency for the second stage to be prolonged (>2 hours). It is also associated with considerably more discomfort. As with the persistent OT position, the fetal head may become markedly molded with extensive caput formation, which may cause difficulty in diagnosing its correct station and position. Observation of a prolonged second stage of labor is appropriate, provided that labor continues to be progressive and the fetal heart rate is normal.

Delivery of the head may occur spontaneously in the OP position, but if the perineum provides undue resistance to delivery, a low forceps-assisted delivery may be required (e.g., using Simpson's forceps). In the past a Kielland forceps rotation was usually performed, but because of a lack of experience and training, fetuses in the OP position are usually now delivered without rotation. **Use of a vacuum extractor with a cup designed for a safe and secure posterior application may be performed.** Sometimes the head will rotate, but it will usually deliver in the OP position. A wide mediolateral episiotomy should be performed to lessen the resistance of the outlet to the delivery of the fetal head.

DYSTOCIA CAUSED BY ABNORMALITIES OF FETAL STRUCTURE
Macrosomia and Shoulder Dystocia

A fetus weighing 4500 g or more in a nondiabetic mother is above the 90th percentile of fetal weight for a term pregnancy and is considered to be excessively large. Macrosomia may result from genetic determinants, maternal diabetes, multiparity, or postterm gestation. **In general, the larger the fetus, the longer the labor and the greater the incidence of midforceps operations and of shoulder dystocia.** Also, the greater the amount by which the fetus exceeds 4500 g, the higher the rate of perinatal mortality and morbidity resulting from birth trauma, especially shoulder dystocia.

An accurate estimate of fetal weight is elusive, even with the aid of sonographic techniques for the evaluation of fetal head and body size. **Errors in the estimation of fetal weight can be 15% to 20% or more.** Additionally, when the fetus is excessively large, the occurrence of shoulder dystocia depends on the size of the maternal pelvis in relation to the size of the fetus, a clinical correlation that is difficult to make. Although the mean duration of labor is prolonged for excessively large fetuses, **it is not unusual to encounter unexpected shoulder dystocia after a labor that has been entirely normal up to the moment of delivery.**

Shoulder dystocia is not overcome by traction on the fetal head but, instead, by one or more maneuvers designed to displace the anterior shoulder from behind the symphysis pubis. The **first maneuver** involves downward or lateral pressure with the hand over the maternal suprapubic region in an effort to guide the anterior shoulder under or away from the symphysis pubis. Next, the **McRoberts maneuver** may be employed. The maternal thighs are sharply flexed against the maternal abdomen to reduce the angle between the sacrum and spine, thus freeing the impacted shoulder. If this is not successful, **pressure is applied with the operator's fingers against the scapula of the posterior shoulder in an attempt to rotate (screw) the posterior shoulder upward until it becomes the anterior shoulder.** If this maneuver does not correct the problem, **a hand is inserted into the vagina and the posterior arm is grasped and pulled across the chest, resulting in delivery of the posterior shoulder and displacement of the anterior shoulder from behind the symphysis pubis.** Fracture of the humerus may result from this maneuver, but the bone heals quickly in the neonate. **If none of these maneuvers is successful, one or both clavicles are fractured,** preferably by pressure on the clavicle directed away from the pleural cavity to prevent traumatic puncture of the lungs. **Excessive traction on the head may result in damage to the brachial plexus, with the possibility of a permanent Erb's palsy.** The maneuvers described here to overcome shoulder dystocia (especially by downward pressure of the anterior shoulder toward the floor) may also result in brachial plexus damage.

A maneuver has been described, attributed to Zavanelli, to manage shoulder dystocia that is not corrected successfully by the methods already described. In this last-resort procedure, the fetal head is manually returned to its prerestitution position and then slowly replaced into the vagina by steady upward pressure against the head. Delivery is subsequently accomplished by cesarean section. A uterine relaxant may be required to carry out this procedure.

Developmental Abnormalities

Localized abnormalities of fetal anatomy may lead to dystocia. **Internal hydrocephalus** may cause enlargement of the fetal head to the extent that vaginal delivery is not possible. The diagnosis is usually made by ultrasonography performed because of the clinical suspicion, or it may appear as an unexpected finding on ultrasonography performed for other indications.

Several options are available for the delivery of the fetus with hydrocephalus. Excessive cerebrospinal fluid may be removed by inserting a needle directly into the ventricular space through the dilated cervix during labor, or fluid may be removed transabdominally with the aid of ultrasonic visualization of the fetal head before or during labor. Alternatively, the fetus may be delivered by cesarean section to avoid the risk of infection, which can result from transvaginal or trans-abdominal drainage.

Intrauterine shunting of the fetal ventricular system into the amniotic fluid compartment is an experimental procedure, and it is unclear at this time whether the long-term results justify the procedure.

The accumulation of **ascites** in the fetal abdomen or **enlargement of fetal organs, such as the bladder or liver, may result in unexpected dystocia after the fetal head is delivered. Rhesus disease and nonimmune hydrops are potential causes of these abnormalities.** If they are present, careful ultrasonic evaluation before or during labor should be carried out to identify excessive enlargement of the fetal abdomen. Ascitic fluid or urine from a massively enlarged bladder may be removed by transabdominal drainage with a needle before vaginal delivery. Cesarean delivery may be indicated if the fetal abdomen cannot be sufficiently decompressed.

A defect in the fetal lumbosacral vertebrae may result in the protrusion of a meningeal sac (**meningocele**) or a sac containing spinal cord (**meningomyelocele**). These defects are usually detected as a result of abnormal serum or amniotic fluid α-fetoprotein values or by ultrasonography. If the sac is large, abdominal delivery is advisable to avoid dystocia or rupture of the sac and potential infection. If the sac is small and is covered by fetal skin, as reflected by a normal α-fetoprotein value, vaginal delivery may be appropriate.

DYSTOCIA CAUSED BY MATERNAL PELVIC ABNORMALITIES

Cephalopelvic disproportion (CPD) exists if the maternal bony pelvis is not of sufficient size and of appropriate shape to allow the passage of the fetal head. This problem may occur as a result of contraction of one of the planes of the pelvis. Relative CPD may exist with a normal pelvis, if the fetal head is excessively large or if it is in an abnormal position. Contraction of the maternal pelvis may occur at the level of the inlet or midpelvis, but **contraction of the outlet is extremely unusual** unless it is found in association with a midpelvic contraction.

Cephalopelvic disproportion at the level of the pelvic inlet causes a failure of descent and engagement of the head. The finding of an unengaged head in a nulliparous patient at the start of labor indicates an increased likelihood of CPD at the pelvic inlet, but an unengaged fetal head in a multiparous patient in labor is not an unusual occurrence. Relative CPD can occur in the multiparous patient (the "multip trap"), however, and should be kept in mind.

The management of a nulliparous patient with an unengaged fetal head in labor should begin with a careful clinical evaluation of the maternal pelvis. If the capacity of the inlet is normal, expectant management with observation of the labor pattern is appropriate. If uterine contractions are ineffective, oxytocic stimulation of labor may be considered.

The occurrence of CPD at the level of the midpelvis occurs more frequently than inlet dystocia because the capacity of the midpelvis is smaller than that of the inlet and also because deflection or positional abnormalities of the fetal head are more likely to occur at that level. The occurrence of bony dystocia at the level of the midpelvis is usually indicated by an arrest of descent of the head at a +2 to +3 station. With CPD and arrest of descent, application of the head to the cervix is poor, resulting in the loss of part of the force needed for cervical dilatation. Thus CPD may be associated with a protracted or expected rate of cervical dilatation before an arrest of descent is apparent.

DYSTOCIA CAUSED BY CONDUCTION ANESTHESIA

The use of epidural anesthesia for pain control during the first stage of labor has gained wide acceptance. Refinement of the epidural technique has allowed a segmental block and titratable continuous infusion of narcotics and local anesthetics to better tailor pain control, with less interference with the process of labor (see Chapter 9).

The incidence of epidural anesthesia interfering with the progress of labor is variable, and the issue is controversial.

Suggested Reading

American College of Obstetricians and Gynecologists: Operative vaginal delivery, Technical bulletin No. 196. Washington, DC, ACOG, 1994.

Frigoletto FD, Lieberman E, Lang JM, et al: A clinical trial of active management of labor. N Engl J Med 333:745, 1995.

Garfield RE, Sims J, Daniel EE: Gap junctions: Their presence and necessity in myometrium during gestation. Science 198:958, 1977.

Gonik B: An alternative maneuver for management of shoulder dystocia. Am J Obstet Gynecol 145:882, 1983.

Hannah ME, Hannah WJ, Hewson SA, et al: Planned cesarean section versus planned vaginal birth for breech presentation at term: A randomized multicentre trial. Lancet 356:1375–1383, 2000.

13

Obstetric Complications: Preterm Labor, PROM, IUGR, Postterm Pregnancy, and IUFD

Calvin J. Hobel

PRETERM LABOR

Preterm labor and delivery are major causes of perinatal morbidity and mortality. **Although fewer than 10% of all infants born in the United States are preterm infants, their contribution to neonatal morbidity and mortality ranges from 50% to 70%.** To decrease the medical and economic impact of preterm delivery, a major goal of obstetric care is not only to reduce the incidence of the condition, but also to increase the gestational age of infants whose preterm births are unavoidable.

DEFINITION AND INCIDENCE

Preterm birth is defined as that occurring after 20 weeks and before 37 completed weeks of gestation. Labor that occurs between these gestational ages is defined as preterm labor.

Preterm births in the United States have increased from 9.8% in 1981 to 11.8% in 2000. Between 1988 and 1999, the mortality rate for white infants declined by 49% to 7.1 infant deaths per 1000 live births and the mortality rate for black infants declined 45% to 13.8. Because prematurity is the leading cause of infant mortality, the prevention of prematurity has become a high priority.

ETIOLOGY AND RISK FACTORS

There are three etiologic subtypes of preterm birth as outlined in Table 13-1. These subtypes are **spontaneous preterm birth** (idiopathic), **preterm premature rupture of the membranes,** and **induction of labor for medical indications.** Private patients have a much higher proportion of idiopathic preterm labor, whereas black patients in public institutions have a higher proportion of deliveries due to premature rupture of the membranes. Attempts have been made to define further the idiopathic subgroup, which some experts now believe includes undiagnosed conditions and/or problems of placental origin, silent infection, immunologic etiology, or uterine and/or cervical origin. The "true" idiopathic subgroup would only represent a small percentage as these other conditions are identified. Recently, genetic thrombophilias have been shown to account for a significant proportion of the uteroplacental problems leading to intrauterine growth restriction and preeclampsia, the two major reasons for the early induction of labor to avoid fetal death. A variety of socioeconomic, psychosocial, and medical conditions have been found to carry an increased risk of preterm delivery.

Socioeconomic Factors

In the United States, the incidence of preterm deliveries in the black population is twice as high as that in the white population. This factor cannot be viewed as a single entity but probably encompasses other characteristics of the population, such as poor access to and procurement of antenatal care, high stress levels, and poor nutritional status.

Medical and Obstetric Factors

When one preterm birth has occurred, the relative risk of preterm delivery in the next pregnancy is 3.9, and the risk increases to 6.5 with two previous preterm deliveries.

Table 13-1. Etiology of preterm labor and delivery

Patients	Idiopathic (Intact Membranes)	Preterm Premature Rupture of the Membranes (PPROM)	Medical Indications for Induction of Labor
Private institution	54%	27%	19%
Public institution			
White	44%	36%	20%
Black	28%	51%	21%

Data from Meis PJ, Ernest JM, Moore ML, et al: Causes of low birth weight births in public and private patients. Am J Obstet Gynecol 156:1165, 1987; and Lettieri L, Vintzileos AM, Rodis JF, et al: Does "idiopathic" preterm labor resulting in preterm birth exist? Am J Obstet Gynecol 168:1480, 1993.

Second-trimester abortions seem to carry an increased risk for subsequent preterm delivery, especially if a previous preterm birth has also occurred. The risk associated with induced 1st-trimester abortions is controversial. **Repeated spontaneous 1st-trimester abortions,** however, do **increase the risk.**

Other medical and obstetric factors associated with an increased risk of delivering preterm include bleeding in the 1st trimester, urinary tract infections, multiple gestation, uterine anomalies, polyhydramnios, and incompetent cervix.

Recently, attention has been directed toward maternal employment, physical activity, nutritional status, genital tract infections, stress, and anxiety as major risk factors for preterm birth.

PREVENTION

Current strategies for prevention are based on at least three potential causal pathways. Beginning in 1980, the focus was on patient education to identify early signs and symptoms, so that patients could be admitted early for tocolytic therapy. Multiple studies in the United States have failed to support this approach. In France, programs were more successful because the focus was directed not only to education about early signs and symptoms, but also about the risk factors causing symptoms. In addition, they included work leave, rest, and home care.

Thus, **the current strategy is to first identify the patient at risk.** Several scoring systems have been developed to identify the highest risk group, which represents about 30% of the population. However, because almost half of preterm deliveries occur in low-risk patients, this group cannot be overlooked. Therefore, a prevention strategy must be applied to all patients. Three potential pathways leading to preterm delivery have been identified:

1. Infection-cervical
2. Placental-vascular
3. Stress-strain

These pathways provide direction for the identification of patients at risk and the application of potential interventions.

Infection-Cervical Pathway

Bacterial vaginosis has been shown to be associated with preterm delivery, independent of other recognized risk factors. **Treatment of bacterial vaginosis has reduced the incidence of preterm delivery.** In addition, treating women in preterm labor with antibiotics significantly prolongs the time from the onset of treatment to delivery, compared to that in patients who do not receive antibiotics. Thus, addressing the issue of these relatively asymptomatic infections is an important strategy for preventing preterm birth.

There is a link between vaginal-cervical infections and progressive changes in the cervical length, as measured by vaginal ultrasonography. The relative risk of preterm birth increases significantly from 2.4 for a cervical length of 3.5 cm (50th percentile) to 6.2 for a length of 2.5 cm (10th percentile). Short cervices appear to be more common in women who have had prior preterm births and pregnancy terminations.

The most recent test to be developed is cervical and vaginal fetal fibronectin. This substance is a basement membrane protein produced by the fetal membranes. When the fetal membranes are disrupted, as with repetitive uterine activity, shortening of the cervix, and/or in the presence of infection, fibronectin is secreted into the vagina and can be tested. **A positive fetal fibronectin test at 22 to 24 weeks**

predicts more than half of the spontaneous preterm births that occur before 28 weeks. A positive test for fetal fibronectin is significantly associated with a short cervix, vaginal infections, and uterine activity. A negative test is the best predictor of a low risk of preterm delivery.

Placental-Vascular Pathway (PVP-1)

The placental-vascular pathway (PVP-1) begins early in pregnancy at the time of implantation, when there are important changes taking place at the placental/decidual/myometrial interface. First, there are important immunologic changes, with a switch from a Th-1 type of immunity, which may be embryotoxic, to Th-2 antibody profile, in which blocking antibody production is thought to prevent rejection. At the same time, the trophoblasts are invading the spiral arteries of the decidua and myometrium, thus assuring that a low resistance vascular connection is established. Alterations in both of these early changes are currently thought to play an important role in the pathophysiology of poor fetal growth, an important component of preterm birth, fetal growth restriction, and preeclampsia.

Stress-Strain Pathway

Both mental (cognitive) and work-related stress and strain are postulated to initiate a stress response that increases release of cortisol and catecholamines. Cortisol from the adrenal gland initiates placental corticotrophin-releasing hormone (CRH), which is known to initiate labor at term. Catecholamines released during the stress response not only affect blood flow to the uteroplacental unit but also cause uterine contractions. Poor nutrition in the form of reduced calories and/or abnormal patterns of intake (fasting) are known stressors and have been associated with a significantly increased risk of preterm birth. **In support of the stress pathway are the studies that have shown that the level of CRH, a mediator of the stress response, increases significantly in the weeks prior to the onset of preterm labor.** Stress reduction and improved nutrition are the only current interventions that can be applied to this pathway.

DIAGNOSIS

The diagnosis of preterm labor occurring between 20 and 37 weeks is based on the following criteria in patients with ruptured or intact membranes: (1) **documented uterine contractions** (4 per 20 minutes or 8 per 60 minutes) and (2) **documented cervical change** (cervical effacement of 80% or cervical dilatation of 2 cm or more).

MANAGEMENT

Provided that membranes are not ruptured and there is no contraindication to a vaginal examination (e.g., placenta previa), **an initial assessment must be done to ascertain cervical length and dilatation and the station and nature of the presenting part.** The patient should also be evaluated for the presence of any underlying correctable problem, such as a urinary tract or vaginal infection. She should be placed in the lateral decubitus position, monitored for the presence and frequency of uterine activity, and reexamined for evidence of cervical change after an appropriate interval, unless she already meets the preceding criteria for preterm labor. During the period of observation, either oral or parenteral hydration should be initiated.

With adequate hydration and bed rest, uterine contractions cease in approximately 20% of patients. These patients, however, remain at high risk for recurrent preterm labor.

Because of the role of cervical colonization and vaginal infection in the etiology of preterm labor and premature rupture of membranes, **cultures should be taken for group B Streptococcus.** Other organisms that may be important are Ureaplasma, Mycoplasma, and *Gardnerella vaginalis.* The latter is associated with bacterial vaginosis, a diagnosis that can be made by the presence of three of four clinical signs (vaginal pH >4.5, amine odor after addition of 10% potassium hydroxide (KOH), and presence of clue cells and/or milky discharge).

Because randomized trials suggest treatment efficacy, **it is acceptable to administer antibiotics to patients who are in preterm labor.** For patients who are not allergic to penicillin, a 7-day course of ampicillin and/or erythromycin can be given. Those allergic to penicillin can be given clindamycin or vacomycin.

Once the diagnosis of preterm labor has been made, the following laboratory tests should be obtained: complete blood cell count, random blood glucose level, serum electrolytes level, urinalysis, and urine culture and sensitivity. An ultrasonic examination of the fetus should be performed to assess fetal weight, document presentation, assess cervical length, and rule out the presence of any accompanying congenital malformation. The test may also detect an underlying etiologic factor, such as twins or a uterine anomaly.

If the patient does not respond to bed rest and hydration, tocolytic therapy is instituted, provided that there are no contraindications. Measures implemented at 28 weeks should be more aggressive than those initiated at 35 weeks. Similarly, a patient with advanced cervical dilatation on admission requires more aggressive management than one whose cervix is closed and minimally effaced.

UTERINE TOCOLYTIC THERAPY

It is assumed that physiologic events leading to the initiation of labor also occur in preterm labor. The pharmacologic agents presently being used all seem to inhibit the availability of calcium ions, but they may also exert a number of other effects. The agents currently available and used and their dosages are presented in Box 13-1.

Box 13-1. Uterine tocolytic agents

MAGNESIUM SULFATE
Solution: Initial solution contains 6 g (12 mL of 50% MgSO$_4$) in 100 mL of 5% dextrose. Maintenance solution contains 10 g (20 mL of 50% MgSO$_4$) in 500 mL of 5% dextrose
Initial dose: 6 g over 15–20 min, parenterally
Titrating dose: 2 g/hr until contractions cease; follow serum levels (5–7 mg/dL); maximal dose, 4 g/hr
Maintenance dose: Maintain dose for 12 hr, then 1 g/hr for 24–48 hr; may switch to oral β-agonist therapy before discontinuing*

NIFEDIPINE
Preparation: Oral gelatin capsules of 10 or 20 mg
Loading dose: 30 mg; if contractions persist after 90 min, give an additional 20 mg (second dose); if labor is suppressed, a maintenance dose of 20 mg is given orally every 6 hr for 24 hr and then every 8 hr for another 24 hr
Failure: If contractions persist 60 min after the second dose, treatment should be considered a failure

PROSTAGLANDIN SYNTHETASE INHIBITORS
Short-term use only

---

* Oral Terbutaline 2.5–5.0 mg every 4–6 hr; titrate frequently to pulse rate; begin ½ hr prior to discontinuing parenteral therapy.

Magnesium Sulfate

Magnesium sulfate has become the drug of choice for initiating tocolytic therapy. In addition, it is the drug of choice for patients with diabetes mellitus or heart disease. **Magnesium acts at the cellular level by competing with calcium for entry into the cell at the time of depolarization.** Successful competition results in an effective decrease of intracellular calcium ions, resulting in myometrial relaxation.

Although magnesium levels required for tocolysis have not been critically evaluated, it appears that the levels needed may be higher than those required for prevention of eclampsia. Levels from 5.5 to 7.0 mg/dL appear to be appropriate. These can be achieved using the dosage regimen outlined in Box 13-1. After the loading dose is given, a continuous infusion is maintained, and plasma levels should be determined until therapeutic levels are reached. The drug should be continued at therapeutic levels until contractions cease. Because magnesium is excreted by the kidneys, adjustments must be made in patients with underlying renal disease and an abnormal creatinine clearance. Once successful tocolysis has been achieved, the infusion is continued for at least 12 hours, and then the infusion rate is weaned over 2 to 4 hours and then discontinued. In very high risk patients (advanced cervical dilation or continued labor in very low birth weight cases), the infusion can be continued until the fetus has been exposed to glucocorticoids to enhance lung maturity.

A common minor side effect of magnesium therapy is a feeling of warmth and flushing on first administration. Respiratory depression is seen at magnesium levels of 12 to 15 mg/dL, and cardiac conduction defects and arrest are seen at higher levels.

In the fetus, plasma magnesium levels approach those of the mother, and a low plasma calcium level may also be demonstrated. The neonate may show some loss of muscle tone and drowsiness, resulting in a lower Apgar score. These effects are prolonged in the preterm neonate because of the decrease in renal clearance.

Long-term parenteral magnesium therapy has been used for control of preterm labor in selected patients. Although it has not been well studied, an important side effect seems to be loss of calcium, which in one reported case led to osteoporosis and a vertebral fracture. The effect of fetal calcium metabolism has not been well studied, especially in terms of bone growth and calcification. It may be important in such patients to institute calcium therapy on a prophylactic basis.

Nifedipine

Nifedipine, a calcium-entry blocker, has been shown to be an effective uterine relaxant by inhibiting the slow, inward current of calcium ions during the second phase of the action potential of uterine smooth-muscle cells. **Nifedipine as an oral agent is very effective in suppressing preterm labor with minimal maternal and fetal side effects. Nifedipine may gradually replace intravenous magnesium sulfate.** The only side effects are headache, cutaneous flushing, hypotension, and tachycardia. The latter two side effects can be partially avoided by making certain the patient is well hydrated and by the use of support stockings, such as TED hose.

Prostaglandin Synthetase Inhibitors

Prostaglandins induce myometrial contractions at all stages of gestation, both in vivo and in vitro. Because prostaglandins are locally synthesized and possess a relatively short half-life, prevention of their synthesis within the uterus could abort labor. **These agents are used on a short-term basis** in special circumstances where prostaglandin production may be the inciting factor in preterm labor, such as with the presence of uterine fibroids. **Indomethacin is the most commonly used prostaglandin inhibitor; it can be administered both orally and rectally, with some slight delay in absorption from rectal administration as compared with the oral route.** Peak serum levels of indomethacin occur 1.5 to 2 hours after oral administration. Excretion of the intact drug occurs in maternal urine. It can result in oligohydramnios and premature closure of the fetal ductus arteriosus, which in turn may lead to neonatal pulmonary hypertension and cardiac failure. In addition, **indomethacin decreases fetal renal function, and indomethacin-exposed infants have a greater risk of necrotizing enterocolitis, intracranial hemorrhage, and patent ductus arteriosus.** Short-term use may be acceptable, but if patients are given indomethacin, the fetus should be evaluated with ultrasonography for ductus arteriosus flow.

Efficacy of Tocolytic Therapy

Although the advent of tocolytic agents has failed to decrease preterm births in large population studies, their use has shifted the distribution of births by gestational age to more prolonged gestations. There has also been an improvement in neonatal survival, a decreased incidence of respiratory distress syndrome (RDS), and an increase in the birth weight of infants treated with these agents. Benefits do not accrue to infants older than 34 weeks' gestational age.

Antibiotic Therapy

A number of studies have advocated the use of antibiotic prophylaxis in patients with preterm labor. Such patients may have a higher incidence of subclinical chorioamnionitis than previously thought.

Diagnostic amniocentesis in patients with idiopathic preterm labor has identified about 15% of these patients whose amniotic cavity is colonized with pathogens. If bacteria find their way into the amniotic cavity in this 15%, it is reasonable to assume that a proportion of the remaining cases will have bacteria in the decidual cell space between the chorion and the myometrium. Thus **it is reasonable to use prophylactic antibiotics in women with preterm labor in an attempt to prevent the progression of a silent infection to clinical amnionitis and the risk of fetal infection.**

Contraindications to Tocolytic Therapy

Contraindications include severe preeclampsia, severe bleeding from placenta previa or abruptio placentae, chorioamnionitis, intrauterine growth restriction, fetal anomalies incompatible with life, and fetal demise. Because of the low success rate, advanced cervical dilatation may also preclude tocolytic therapy, although therapy may delay delivery sufficiently for glucocorticoid administration to accelerate fetal lung maturity. Management of patients should be individualized, and even if the patient's cervix is dilated 6 cm and she is having infrequent contractions, it is advisable to employ tocolysis and administer glucocorticoid therapy.

USE OF GLUCOCORTICOIDS FOR FETAL PULMONARY MATURATION

Antenatal corticosteroid therapy for fetal pulmonary maturation reduces mortality and the incidence of RDS and intraventricular hemorrhage (IVH) in preterm infants. These benefits extend to a broad range of gestational ages (24 to 34 weeks) and are not limited by gender or race. **Treatment consists of 2 doses of 12 mg of**

betamethasone, given intramuscularly 24 hours apart or 4 doses of 6 mg of dexamethasone given intramuscularly 12 hours apart. Optimal benefit begins 24 hours after initiation of therapy and lasts 7 days. Because treatment with corticosteroids for less than 24 hours is still associated with significant reductions in neonatal mortality, RDS, and IVH, antenatal corticosteroids should be given unless immediate delivery is anticipated.

LABOR AND DELIVERY OF THE PRETERM INFANT

A certain number of patients will not respond to tocolytic therapy. The goal in these patients is to conduct both labor and delivery in an optimal manner so as not to contribute to the morbidity or mortality of the preterm infant. All parameters for assessing gestational age and fetal weight must be considered. With modern neonatal care, the lower limit of potential viability is 24 weeks or 500 g, although these limits vary with the expertise of the neonatal intensive care unit.

Fetal heart rate patterns that are relatively innocuous in the term fetus may indicate a more ominous outcome for the preterm fetus. Continuous fetal heart monitoring and prompt attention to abnormal fetal heart rate patterns are extremely important. Acidosis at birth adversely affects respiratory function by destroying surfactant and delaying its release.

With a vertex presentation, vaginal delivery is preferred, independent of gestational age, provided that fetal acidosis and delivery trauma are avoided. Use of outlet forceps and an episiotomy to shorten the second stage are advocated. Some reports recommend cesarean section for delivery of the very low birth weight baby.

Approximately 23% of infants present as a breech at 28 weeks, compared with about 4% at term. This presentation carries an increased risk of cord prolapse or compression. In addition, cervical entrapment of the aftercoming fetal head may occur at delivery because, prior to term, the head is proportionally larger than the buttocks. For the breech fetus estimated at less than 1500 g, neonatal outcome is improved by cesarean section.

PREMATURE RUPTURE OF THE MEMBRANES
DEFINITION AND INCIDENCE

Premature rupture of the membranes (PROM) is defined as amniorrhexis (spontaneous rupture of membranes as opposed to amniotomy) prior to the onset of labor at any stage of gestation. It has been suggested that the term preterm PROM (PPROM) should be used to define those patients who are preterm with ruptured membranes, whether or not they have contractions.

ETIOLOGY AND RISK FACTORS

The etiology of PROM remains unclear, but a variety of factors are purported to contribute to its occurrence, including vaginal and cervical infections, abnormal membrane physiology, incompetent cervix, and nutritional deficiencies.

DIAGNOSIS

Diagnosis of PROM is based on the history of vaginal loss of fluid and confirmation of amniotic fluid in the vagina. Episodic urinary incontinence, leukorrhea, or loss of the mucus plug must be ruled out. Management of the patient presenting with this history depends on the gestational age. Because of the risk of introducing infection and the usually long latency period from the time of examination until delivery, the examiner's hands should not be inserted into the vagina of a patient who is not in labor, whether preterm or term. A sterile vaginal speculum examination should be performed to confirm the diagnosis, to assess cervical dilatation and length, and if the patient is preterm, to obtain cervical cultures and amniotic fluid samples for pulmonary maturation tests.

On examination, pooling of amniotic fluid in the posterior vaginal fornix can usually be seen. A Valsalva maneuver or slight fundal pressure may expel fluid from the cervical os, which is diagnostic of PROM. Confirmation of the diagnosis can be made by (1) testing the fluid with nitrazine paper, which will turn blue in the presence of the alkaline amniotic fluid, and (2) placing a sample on a microscopic slide, air drying, and examining for ferning. False-positive nitrazine test results occur in the presence of alkaline urine, blood, or cervical mucus. In the presence of blood, which is usually seen in patients who are also in early labor, the pattern may appear to be skeletonized, and a distinct ferning may not be seen. As in the case of preterm labor with intact membranes, a complete ultrasonic examination should be carried out to rule out fetal anomalies and to assess gestational age and amniotic fluid volume.

MANAGEMENT
General Considerations

An intact amniotic sac serves as a mechanical barrier to infection, but in addition, amniotic fluid has some bacteriostatic properties that may play a role in preventing chorioamnionitis and fetal infections. Intact membranes are not an absolute barrier to infection because bacterial colonization occurs in 10% of patients in term labor with intact membranes and in up to 25% of patients in preterm labor.

For preterm fetuses with PPROM, the risks associated with preterm delivery must be balanced against the risks of infection and sepsis that may make in utero existence even more problematic. For the mother, the risks include not only the development of chorioamnionitis but also the possibility of failed induction in the presence of an unfavorable cervix, resulting in subsequent cesarean section.

Management is dictated to a large extent by the gestational age at the time of membrane rupture, although **the quantity of amniotic fluid remaining after PPROM may be as important as gestational age in determining pregnancy outcome.**

Ultrasonic definition of oligohydramnios has been standardized. Objective criteria include measurement of the vertical axis of amniotic fluid present in four quadrants, the total being called the **amniotic fluid index (AFI).** A value of less than 5 cm is considered abnormal.

Oligohydramnios associated with PROM in the fetus at less than 24 weeks' gestation may lead to the development of pulmonary hypoplasia. Factors that may be responsible include fetal crowding with thoracic compression, restriction of fetal breathing, and disturbances of pulmonary fluid production and flow. The duration of membrane rupture is an important consideration. Constraints placed on fetal movements in utero can also result in a variety of positional skeletal abnormalities, such as talipes equinovarus.

If PROM occurs at 36 weeks or later and the condition of the cervix is favorable, labor should be induced after 6 to 12 hours if no spontaneous contractions occur. In the presence of an unfavorable cervical condition with no evidence of infection, it is reasonable to wait 24 hours prior to induction of labor to decrease the risk of failed induction and maternal febrile morbidity. The following discussion applies when premature membrane rupture occurs prior to 36 weeks' gestational age.

Laboratory Tests

In addition to the laboratory tests obtained for the patient in preterm labor, sufficient amniotic fluid can usually be obtained from the vaginal pool for pulmonary maturation studies. Because of the higher incidence of chorioamnionitis in association with PROM, amniotic fluid should also be examined with Gram stain and culture.

Conservative Expectant Management

Conservative management applies to the care of patients with PPROM who are observed with the expectation of prolonging gestation. **Because the risk of infection appears to increase with the duration of membrane rupture, the goal of expectant management is to continue the pregnancy until the lung profile is mature.** Careful surveillance must be maintained to diagnose chorioamnionitis at an early enough stage to minimize fetal and maternal risks. In its fulminant state, chorioamnionitis is associated with a high maternal temperature and a tender, sometimes irritable, uterus.

In cases of subclinical infection, diagnosis and treatment may be delayed. A combination of factors should alert the clinician to the possibility of chorioamnionitis, including maternal temperature greater than 100.4°F (38°C) in the absence of any other site of infection, fetal tachycardia, a tender uterus, and uterine irritability on nonstress testing.

The presence of bacteria by Gram stain or culture of amniotic fluid obtained at amniocentesis correlates with subsequent maternal infection in about 50% of cases and with neonatal sepsis in about 25%. The presence of white blood cells alone in amniotic fluid is less predictive of infection. The decision to perform amniocentesis is based on the gestational age, the presence of early signs of infection, and the AFI as measured by real-time ultrasonography. Recently investigators have described elevation of inflammatory cytokines in the amniotic fluid and fetal circulation in preterm infants who subsequently developed chronic lung disease during the neonatal period. A similar response may be associated with a greater risk of damage to the preterm baby's brain, thus increasing the risk of cerebral palsy. Thus the management of patients with PROM is critical for the prevention of neonatal morbidity.

Ampicillin or erythromycin significantly prolongs the interval to delivery in patients with PPROM. The neonates delivered from patients receiving prophylaxis also have less morbidity.

Management of Chorioamnionitis

Once chorioamnionitis is diagnosed, antibiotic therapy should be delayed only until appropriate cultures have been taken. Ampicillin and tobramycin in combination are the drugs of choice. In the penicillin-sensitive patient, cephalosporins may be indicated, noting the 12% incidence of crossover sensitivity. Once antibiotics have been started, labor should be induced. **If the condition of the cervix is unfavorable, and there is evidence of fetal involvement, it may be necessary to perform a cesarean section.**

The presence of active genital herpes is an important concern in the presence of ruptured membranes. Herpes infection at a site remote from the cervix and vagina is probably not associated with an increased risk of fetal infection, so the site of infection should be taken into consideration before recommending immediate cesarean section.

Tocolytic Therapy

The use of tocolytics to control preterm labor in patients with PROM is controversial. The arguments against their use are that they may mask evidence of maternal infection (e.g., tachycardia) and that contractions associated with the membrane rupture may be indicative of uterine infection. Arguments for their use are that PROM is sometimes initially associated with evidence of uterine contractions, and time is gained for pulmonary maturation. In the presence of infection, tocolysis is usually unsuccessful.

Use of Corticosteroids

There appears to be a decreased incidence of RDS in infants who are born after 16 to 72 hours of membrane rupture compared with infants of similar gestational age born without PPROM. However, the current recommendation is to give steroids with PPROM prior to 34 weeks.

Outpatient Management

After inpatient observation for 2 to 3 days without any evidence of infection, outpatient management can be considered. To be eligible for such management, the patient should be reliable, fully informed regarding the risks involved, and prepared to participate in her own care. The fetus should be presenting as a vertex, and the cervix should be closed to minimize the chance of cord prolapse. At home, restricted physical activity is advised, no coital activity should occur, and the patient must monitor her temperature at least four times per day. Instructions should be given to return immediately if the temperature exceeds 100°F (37.8°C).

The patient should be seen weekly, at which time her temperature is taken, nonstress testing is done after 28 weeks, and the baseline fetal heart rate and AFI are evaluated. Ultrasonic evaluation of fetal growth should also be carried out every 2 weeks. **Any patient with oligohydramnios is not a candidate for outpatient management.**

Labor and Delivery

The same considerations discussed under preterm labor apply to patients with PROM. The decrease in amniotic fluid that is sometimes seen can result in early cord compression and the presence of variable fetal heart decelerations. This is true of both vertex and breech presentations; therefore, there is a necessity for abdominal delivery in a large number of cases unless fluid replacement can be instituted by amnioinfusion.

TESTS OF PULMONARY MATURITY

By far, the major determinant of successful extrauterine existence is the ability of the neonate to maintain successful oxygenation. Pulmonary maturation involves changes in pulmonary anatomy in addition to alterations of physiologic and biochemical parameters. Beginning at about 24 weeks, the terminal bronchioles divide into three or four respiratory bronchioles. Type II pneumocytes, which are important in surfactant synthesis, begin to proliferate during this phase.

Surfactant is required for successful lung function in the fetus and is a complex mixture of phospholipids, neutral lipids, proteins, carbohydrates, and salts. It is important in decreasing alveolar surface tension, maintaining alveoli in an open position at a low internal alveolar diameter, and decreasing intraalveolar lung fluid. **Synthesis takes place in the type II pneumocytes by incorporation of choline, and significant recycling seems to occur by resorption and secretion.**

Initially, the important phospholipid was thought to be phosphatidylcholine (lecithin), but it is apparent that other components, such as phosphatidylinositol (PI) and phosphatidylglycerol (PG), are also important. These substances are produced and secreted in increasing amounts as gestation advances, and the continued egress of tracheal fluid into the amniotic fluid results in their increasing presence near term.

Measurement of these substances in the amniotic fluid obtained by amniocentesis allows prediction of the risk of development of RDS in the neonate. Lecithin (L) levels increase rapidly after 35 weeks' gestation, whereas sphingomyelin (S) levels remain relatively constant after this gestational age. The lecithin and sphingomyelin concentrations are measured by thin-layer chromatography and are expressed as the L/S ratio. The presence of blood or meconium in the amniotic fluid will affect the L/S ratio; meconium will decrease it and blood will normalize it to a value of 1.4.

LUNG PROFILE

Using two-dimensional thin-layer chromatography, both PG and PI can be measured. Along with the L/S ratio, these make up the lung profile. RDS is rare when the L/S ratio is greater than 2 and PG is present, whereas when the L/S ratio is less than 2 and no PG is present, more than 90% of infants develop RDS. **If the L/S ratio indicates pulmonary immaturity (L/S <2) but PG is present, fewer than 5% of infants develop RDS.** The lung profile offers a more reliable predictor of pulmonary maturity, especially in infants of diabetic mothers. Other advantages of using PG are that contamination with vaginal secretions or blood, as occurs in cases of ruptured membranes and vaginal pool sampling, does not interfere with the detection of PG.

RAPID TESTS FOR FETAL LUNG MATURITY

There has been a search for a rapid test to assess fetal lung maturity, which could then be followed up with the more standard tests. Recent interest has focused on the assessment of **lamellar body number density (LBND)**, which is assessed using an electronic cell counter (Coulter). This test can be completed within 2 hours by any hospital clinical laboratory. Normal ranges have been developed and depend on the individual laboratory (maturity $\geq$46,000 μL LBND), and the sensitivity and predictive value are as good if not better than the standard L/S ratio. This test may become more popular as laboratories and clinicians gain experience with its use.

SURFACTANT THERAPY

RDS in preterm infants is caused by a lack of surfactant. Production of surfactant by type II pneumocytes may be induced by corticosteroids and thyroid-releasing hormone, but many premature infants still develop RDS. Several ovine studies using instillation of surfactant into the pulmonary tree immediately postpartum have shown dramatic improvements in lung mechanics and survival of the preterm lamb. These studies have been confirmed in human trials, with all studies reporting a decrease in the incidence and severity of RDS as well as the incidence of chronic neonatal lung disease. A wide variety of surfactant preparations are now available, including synthetic surfactants and surfactants derived from animal sources.

INTRAUTERINE GROWTH RESTRICTION

Intrauterine growth restriction (IUGR) by definition occurs when the birth weight of a newborn infant is below the 10th percentile for a given gestational age. The terms, small for gestational age (SGA) and IUGR, should not be used synonymously. SGA merely indicates that a fetus or neonate is below a defined reference range of weight for a gestational age, whereas IUGR refers to a small group of fetuses or neonates whose growth potential has been limited by pathologic processes in utero, with resultant increased perinatal morbidity and mortality. **Growth-restricted fetuses are particularly prone to problems such as meconium aspiration, asphyxia, polycythemia, hypoglycemia, and mental retardation.**

ETIOLOGY

The causes of IUGR can be grouped into three main categories: maternal, placental, and fetal. Combinations of these are frequently found in pregnancies with IUGR.

Maternal

Maternal causes include poor nutritional intake, cigarette smoking, drug abuse, alcoholism, cyanotic heart disease, and pulmonary insufficiency. In recent years, the **antiphospholipid syndrome** (autoantibody production) has been identified as a cause of IUGR in some women, both with and without hypertension. Antiphospholipid antibodies such as lupus-like anticoagulant and anticardiolipin antibodies are autoimmune (acquired) conditions, which contribute to the formation of vascular lesions in both the uterine and the placental vasculature that may result in impaired fetal growth and demise. Recently, several hereditary thrombophilias have been identified, which have been associated with a greater risk for IUGR, abruption, and preeclampsia. These conditions result in vascular lesions within the spinal arteries supplying the placenta. Identification and treatment with low-dose heparin and low-dose aspirin have been shown to reduce the risk of IUGR.

Placental

This category is representative of circumstances in which there is inadequate substrate transfer because of placental insufficiency. **Conditions that lead to this state include essential hypertension, chronic renal disease, and pregnancy-induced hypertension.** If the latter occurs late in pregnancy and is not accompanied by chronic vascular or renal disease, significant IUGR is unlikely to occur. A small fraction of IUGR cases may be attributed to placental or cord abnormalities (e.g., velamentous cord insertion).

Fetal

In this case, inadequate or altered substrate is present. Examples of fetal causes include **intrauterine infection** (listeriosis and TORCH [*t*oxoplasmosis, *o*ther infections, *r*ubella, *c*ytomegalovirus infection, and *h*erpes simplex] agents) and **congenital anomalies.**

CLINICAL MANIFESTATIONS

Two types of fetal growth restriction have been described: symmetric and asymmetric. In fetuses with symmetric growth restriction, growth of both

the head and the body is inadequate. The head-to-abdominal circumference ratio may be normal, but the absolute growth rate is decreased. Symmetric growth restriction is most commonly seen in association with intrauterine infections or congenital fetal anomalies. **When asymmetric growth restriction occurs, usually late in pregnancy, the brain is preferentially spared at the expense of "nonvital" abdominal viscera.** As a result, the head size is proportionally larger than the abdominal size.

DIAGNOSIS

Growth restriction may go undiagnosed unless the obstetrician establishes the correct gestational age of the fetus (Box 13-2), identifies high-risk factors from the obstetric data base, and serially assesses fetal growth by fundal height or ultrasonography.

Fetal or neonatal IUGR is usually defined as weight at or below the 10th percentile for gestational age. **The 10th percentile is most commonly used as a defining point.**

Serial uterine fundal height measurements should serve as the primary screening tool for IUGR. A more thorough sonographic assessment should be undertaken when (1) the fundal height lags more than 3 cm behind a well-established gestational age or (2) the mother has high-risk conditions such as preexisting hypertension; chronic renal disease; advanced diabetes with vascular involvement; preeclampsia; viral disease; addiction to nicotine, alcohol, or hard drugs; or the presence of serum lupus anticoagulant or antiphospholipid antibodies.

Box 13-2. Factors to be evaluated in dating a pregnancy
Accuracy of the date of the last normal menstrual period.
Evaluation of uterine size on pelvic examination in the 1st trimester.
Evaluation of uterine size in relation to gestational age during subsequent antenatal visits (concordance or size-for-dates discrepancy).
Gestational age when fetal heart tones were first heard using a Doppler ultrasonic device (usually at 12–14 wk).
Date of quickening (usually 18–20 wk in a primigravida and 16–18 wk in a multigravida).
Sonographic measurement of fetal length (crown-rump) in 1st trimester is most accurate.

Recently, interest has focused on the prediction of patients at risk for IUGR at midpregnancy. Patients with abnormal triple screens (AFP, hCG, and EU₃) who do not have abnormal fetuses by ultrasound and amniocentesis may be at risk for IUGR. In addition, elevations of umbilical artery and uterine artery Doppler assessments (increased resistance) as early as midpregnancy are associated with a greater risk of IUGR as pregnancy progresses.

At present, a number of sonographic parameters are used to diagnose IUGR: (1) **biparietal diameter** (BPD), (2) **head circumference,** (3) **abdominal circumference** (Figure 13-1), (4) **head-to-abdominal circumference ratio,** (5) **femoral**

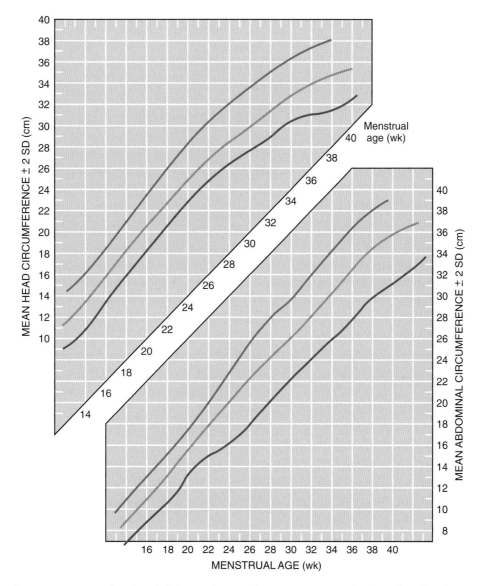

Figure 13-1. Mean head and abdominal circumferences (green) with 5th (red) and 95th (blue) percentile confidence limits between 16 and 40 weeks' menstrual age. *Adapted from Campbell S, Griffin D, Roberts A, et al: Early prenatal diagnosis of abnormalities of the fetal head, spine, limbs, and abdominal organs. In Orlandi C, Polani PE, Bovicelli L (eds): Recent Advances in Prenatal Diagnosis: Proceedings of the First International Symposium on Recent Advances in Prenatal Diagnosis, Bologna, September 15–16, 1980, New York, John Wiley & Sons, 1980.*

length, (6) **femoral-length-to-abdominal-circumference ratio,** (7) **amniotic fluid volume,** (8) **calculated fetal weight,** and (9) **umbilical and uterine artery Doppler.** Of these, **the abdominal circumference is the single most effective parameter for predicting fetal weight because it is reduced in both symmetric and asymmetric IUGR.** Most formulas for estimating fetal weight incorporate two or more parameters to reduce the variance of measurements.

During advancing gestation, the head circumference remains greater than the abdominal circumference until approximately 34 weeks, at which point the ratio approaches 1 (Figure 13-2). **Following 34 weeks, the normal pregnancy is associated with an abdominal circumference that is greater than the head circumference.** When asymmetric growth restriction occurs, usually in the 3rd trimester, the BPD is essentially normal, whereas the ratio of head to abdominal circumference is abnormal. With symmetric growth restriction, the head-to-abdominal circumference ratio may be normal, but the absolute growth rate is decreased, and estimated fetal weight is reduced.

From 50% to 90% of infants with manifestations of IUGR at birth can be identified with serial prenatal ultrasonography. The accuracy depends on the quality of the assessments, the criteria used for diagnosis, and the effect of interventions applied when this diagnosis is made. For example, it is not unusual to observe an improvement in fetal growth after interventions such as work stoppage, bed rest, dietary modification, and curtailment of the use of tobacco, hard drugs, and alcohol.

It is worthwhile to plot out each serial measurement on a standard growth curve. For example, a fetus measuring near the 10th percentile in midgestation may continue to grow along that curve (SGA) or, conversely, may fall well below the 10th percentile (IUGR) later in pregnancy.

MANAGEMENT
Prepregnancy

An important part of preventive medicine is to anticipate risks that can be modified before a woman becomes pregnant. Improving nutrition and stopping smoking are two approaches that should improve fetal growth in women who are underweight, who smoke, or both. **For women with antiphospholipid antibodies associated with the delivery of a prior IUGR infant, low-dose aspirin (81 mg/day) in early pregnancy may reduce the likelihood of recurrent IUGR.** For patients with one of the hereditary

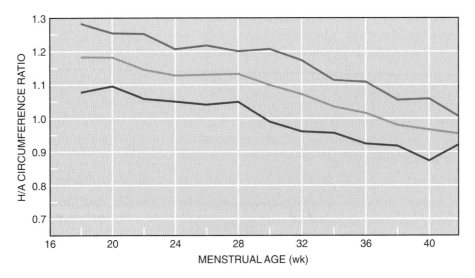

Figure 13-2. Graphic representation of the mean head-to-abdominal circumference ratios (green) with 5th (red) and 95th (blue) percentile confidence limits from 17 to 42 weeks' menstrual age. *From Campbell S, Thomas A: Ultrasound measurement of the fetal head to abdominal circumference ratio in the assessment of growth retardation. Br J Obstet Gynaecol 84:165, 1977.*

thrombophilias, low-dose heparin (5000 U twice daily) with or without low-dose aspirin has also been shown to reduce the risk of recurrent IUGR.

Antepartum

Once a fetus has been identified as having decreased growth, the obstetrician should direct his or her efforts toward modifying any associated factors that can be changed. Because **poor nutrition and smoking** exert their main effects on birth weight in the latter half of pregnancy, cessation of smoking and improved nutrition can have a positive impact. The working woman who becomes fatigued is more likely to have a low-birth-weight infant. Work leave or, in some cases of maternal disease, hospitalization will increase uterine blood flow and may improve the nutrition of the fetus at risk.

The most important clinical decisions revolve around the timing and mode of delivery. **The objective is to expedite delivery before the occurrence of fetal compromise but after fetal lung maturation.** This requires regular fetal monitoring with a twice-weekly nonstress test (NST) and biophysical profile. Most institutions use a modified biophysical profile that includes an NST and AFI. The oxytocin challenge test (OCT) is rarely used because its false-positive rate approaches 50%.

Fetuses clinically suspected of IUGR could be approached as follows:

1. For cases in which results of fetal monitoring are normal and ultrasonic findings strongly suggest normal growth, no clinical intervention is warranted.

2. **For cases in which ultrasonic findings strongly suggest IUGR, with or without abnormal fetal surveillance, delivery is indicated at gestational ages of 34 weeks or later, or at any reasonable gestational age if pulmonary maturity is documented.** In the presence of severe oligohydramnios, amniocentesis may not be safe or feasible. Delivery should be strongly considered without assessing lung maturity because these fetuses are at great risk of asphyxia, and the stress associated with IUGR usually accelerates fetal pulmonary maturity.

3. For those cases in which ultrasonic findings are equivocal for IUGR, bed rest, fetal surveillance, and serial ultrasonic measurements at three weekly intervals are indicated.

A simple technique is available whereby a pregnant woman can help in the assessment of fetal well-being. She assesses **fetal movement** (kick count) each evening while resting comfortably on her left side. If she does not perceive 10 movements in 1 hour, she is instructed to call her health care provider to schedule a biophysical assessment. Some providers instruct their patients, irrespective of their risk, to begin a fetal kick count chart at 28 weeks' gestation.

Recently, a series of studies have indicated that Doppler-derived umbilical artery systolic-to-diastolic ratios are abnormal in IUGR fetuses. Fetuses with growth restriction tend to have increased resistance to flow and to demonstrate low, absent, or reversed diastolic flow. This noninvasive technique can be used to evaluate high-risk patients, and may help in the timing of delivery when used in conjunction with the modified biophysical profile.

LABOR AND DELIVERY

IUGR per se is not a contraindication for induction of labor, but there should be a low threshold to perform a cesarean section because of the poor capacity of the IUGR fetus to tolerate asphyxia. As a result, **during labor, these high-risk patients must be electronically monitored to detect the earliest evidence of fetal distress.**

A combined obstetric-neonatal team approach to delivery is mandatory because of the likelihood of neonatal asphyxia.

After birth, the infant should be carefully examined to rule out the possibility of congenital anomalies and infections. **The monitoring of blood glucose levels is important, because the fetuses do not have adequate hepatic glycogen stores, and hypoglycemia is a common finding.** Furthermore, hypothermia is not uncommon in these infants. **Respiratory distress syndrome is more common in the presence of fetal distress,** because fetal acidosis reduces surfactant synthesis and release.

PROGNOSIS

The long-term prognosis for infants with IUGR must be assessed according to the varied etiologies of the growth restriction. If infants with chromosomal abnormalities, autoimmune disease, congenital anomalies, and infection are excluded, the outlook for these newborns is generally good.

POSTTERM PREGNANCY

The prolonged or postterm pregnancy is one that persists beyond 42 weeks (294 days) from the onset of the last normal menstrual period. **Estimates of the incidence of postterm pregnancy range from 6% to 12% of all pregnancies.**

Perinatal mortality is two to three times higher in these prolonged gestations. Much of the increased risk to the fetus and neonate can be attributed to development of the **fetal postmaturity (dysmaturity) syndrome.** Occurring in 20% to 30% of postterm pregnancies, **this syndrome is related to the aging and infarction of the placenta,** resulting in placental insufficiency with impaired oxygen diffusion and decreased transfer of nutrients to the fetus. Some of these fetuses meet the criteria for having IUGR and should not have been allowed to advance to term. If evidence of intrauterine hypoxia is present (such as meconium staining of the umbilical cord, fetal membranes, skin, and nails), perinatal mortality is even further increased.

The fetus with postmaturity syndrome typically has loss of subcutaneous fat, long fingernails, dry, peeling skin, and abundant hair. The 70% to 80% of postdate fetuses not affected by placental insufficiency continue to grow in utero, many to the point of **macrosomia (birth weight greater than 4000 g). This macrosomia often results in abnormal labor, shoulder dystocia, birth trauma, and an increased incidence of cesarean birth.**

ETIOLOGY

The cause of postdate pregnancy is unknown in most instances. Prolonged gestation is common in association with an anencephalic fetus and is probably linked to the lack of a fetal labor-initiating factor from the fetal adrenals, which are hypoplastic in anencephalic fetuses. **Prolonged gestation may also be associated rarely with placental sulfatase deficiency and extrauterine pregnancy.** Paternal genes, as expressed by the fetus, play a role in the timing of birth and the risk of repeating a prolonged pregnancy.

DIAGNOSIS

The diagnosis of postterm pregnancy is often difficult. The key to appropriate classification and subsequent successful perinatal management is the accurate dating of gestation. It is estimated that uncertain dates are present in 20% to 30% of all pregnancies; hence, the importance of early and accurate assessment of gestational age cannot be overemphasized.

MANAGEMENT
Antepartum

The appropriate management of prolonged pregnancy revolves around **identification of the low percentage of fetuses with postmaturity syndrome** who are truly at risk of intrauterine hypoxia and fetal demise. When biophysical tests of fetal well-being are available, the time of delivery for each patient should be individualized. **However, if the gestational age is firmly established at 42 weeks, the fetal head is well fixed in the pelvis, and the condition of the cervix is favorable, labor usually should be induced.**

The two clinical problems that remain are (1) patients with good dates at 42 weeks' gestation with an unripe cervix and (2) patients with uncertain gestational age seen for the first time with a possible or probable diagnosis of prolonged pregnancy.

In the first group of patients, a twice-weekly NST and biophysical profile should be performed. The AFI is an important ultrasonic measurement that should also be used in the management of these patients. The AFI is the sum of the vertical dimensions (in centimeters) of amniotic fluid pockets in each of the four quadrants of the gestational sac. **Delivery is indicated if there is any indication of oligohydramnios (AFI ≤5) or if spontaneous fetal heart rate decelerations are found on the NST.** So long as these parameters of fetal well-being are reassuring, labor need not be induced unless the cervical condition becomes favorable, the fetus is judged to be macrosomic, or there are other obstetric indications for delivery.

Some institutions begin weekly testing at 41 weeks to avoid missing the few fetuses who are stressed prior to 42 weeks. **At 42 weeks' gestation with firm dates, delivery is initiated by the appropriate route, regardless of other factors,** in view of the increasing potential for perinatal morbidity and mortality.

When the patient presents very late in gestation for initial assessment of prolonged pregnancy, but the gestational age is in question and fetal assessment is normal, an expectant approach is often acceptable. The risk of intervention with the delivery of a preterm infant must be considered. The woman herself can participate in the fetal assessment by doing fetal kick counts during the postterm period.

INTRAPARTUM

Continuous electronic fetal monitoring must be employed during the induction of labor. The patient should be encouraged to lie on her left side. **The fetal membranes should be ruptured as early as is feasible in the intrapartum period so that internal electrodes can be applied and the color of the amniotic fluid assessed.** Cesarean section is indicated for fetal distress. It should not be delayed because of the decreased capacity of the postterm fetus to tolerate asphyxia and the increased risk of meconium aspiration. If meconium is present, neonatal asphyxia should be anticipated, and a neonatal resuscitative team should be present at delivery.

INTRAUTERINE FETAL DEMISE

Intrauterine fetal demise (IUFD) is fetal death after 20 weeks' gestation but before the onset of labor. It complicates about 1% of pregnancies. With the development of newer diagnostic and therapeutic modalities over the past 2 decades, the management of IUFD has shifted from watchful expectancy to more active intervention.

ETIOLOGY

In more than 50% of cases, the etiology of antepartum fetal death is not known or cannot be determined. Associated causes include hypertensive diseases of pregnancy, diabetes mellitus, erythroblastosis fetalis, umbilical cord accidents, fetal congenital anomalies, fetal or maternal infections, fetomaternal hemorrhage, antiphospholipid antibodies and hereditary thrombophilias.

DIAGNOSIS

Clinically, fetal death should be suspected when the patient reports the absence of fetal movements, particularly if the uterus is small for dates or if the fetal heart tones are not detected using a Doppler device. Because the placenta may continue to produce hCG, a positive pregnancy test does not exclude an IUFD.

Diagnostic confirmation has been greatly facilitated since the advent of ultrasonography. **Real-time ultrasonography confirms the lack of fetal movement and absence of fetal cardiac activity.**

MANAGEMENT

Fetal demise between 13 and 28 weeks allows for two different approaches: watchful expectancy and induction of labor.

Watchful Expectancy

About 80% of patients experience the spontaneous onset of labor within 2 to 3 weeks of fetal demise. The patient's feeling of personal loss and guilt may create such anxiety, however, that this conservative approach may prove unacceptable. Thus, in general, the management of women who fail to go into labor spontaneously is active intervention by induction of labor or dilation and evacuation (D&E).

Induction of Labor

Justifications for such intervention include the emotional burden on the patient associated with carrying a dead fetus, the slight possibility of chorioamnionitis, and the 10% risk of disseminated intravascular coagulation when a dead fetus is retained for more than 5 weeks in the 2nd or 3rd trimester.

Vaginal suppositories of prostaglandin E_2 (dinoprostone [Prostin E2]) have received the approval of the Food and Drug Administration (FDA) for use from the 12th to the 28th week of gestation. Dinoprostone is an effective drug with an overall success rate approaching 97%. Although at least 50% of patients receiving dinoprostone experience nausea and vomiting or diarrhea with temperature elevations, these side effects are transient and can be minimized with premedication (i.e., prochlorperazine [Compazine]). There have been reported cases of uterine rupture and cervical lacerations, but with properly selected patients, the drug is safe. The maximum recommended dose is a 20-mg suppository every 3 hours until delivery. Dinoprostone usage in this range is contraindicated in patients with prior uterine incisions (e.g., cesarean, myomectomy) because of the unacceptable risk of uterine rupture. Furthermore, prostaglandins are contraindicated in patients with a history of bronchial asthma or active pulmonary disease, although the E series act primarily as bronchodilators. Recently, **misoprostol (Cytotec, a synthetic prostaglandin E_1 analogue)** vaginal tablets have been found to be quite effective with little or no gastrointestinal side effects, and they are less expensive than dinoprostone.

After 28 weeks' gestation, if the condition of the cervix is favorable for induction and there are no contraindications, Cytotec followed by oxytocin are the drugs of choice.

Monitoring of Coagulopathy

Regardless of the mode of therapy chosen, **weekly fibrinogen levels should be monitored during the period of expectant management, along with a hematocrit and platelet count.** If the fibrinogen level is decreasing, even a "normal" fibrinogen level of 300 mg/dL may be an early sign of consumptive coagulopathy in cases of fetal demise. An elevated prothrombin and partial thromboplastin time, the presence of fibrinogen-fibrin degradation products, and a decreased platelet count may clarify the diagnosis.

If laboratory evidence of mild disseminated intravascular coagulation is noted in the absence of bleeding, delivery by the most appropriate means is recommended. If the clotting defect is more severe or if there is evidence of bleeding, blood volume support or use of component therapy (fresh-frozen plasma) should be given prior to intervention.

FOLLOW-UP

Physician responsibilities do not end with delivery of the fetus. In addition to emotional support of the parents, a search should be undertaken to determine the cause of the intrauterine death. **TORCH and parvovirus studies and cultures for *Listeria* are indicated.** In addition, **all women with a fetal demise should be tested for the presence of anticardiolipin antibodies. Testing for the hereditary thrombophilias should also be considered. If** congenital abnormalities are detected, fetal chromosomal studies and total body radiographs should be done, in addition to a complete autopsy. The autopsy report, when available, must be discussed in detail with both parents. In a stillborn fetus, the best tissue for a chromosomal analysis is the fascia lata, obtained from the lateral aspect of the thigh. The tissue can be stored in saline or Hanks' solution. **A significant number of cases of IUFD are the result of fetomaternal hemorrhage,** which can be detected by identifying fetal erythrocytes in maternal blood **(Kleihauer-Betke test).** Subsequent pregnancies occurring in a woman with a history of IUFD must be managed as high-risk cases.

Suggested Reading

Bugalho A, Bique C, Machungo F, et al: Induction of labor with intravaginal misoprostol in intrauterine fetal death. Am J Obstet Gynecol 71:538–541, 1994.

Campbell S: Ultrasound measurement of the fetal head to abdominal circumference ratio in assessment of growth retardation. Br J Obstet Gynaecol 84:165, 1977.

Gomez R, Romero R, Ghezzi F, et al: The fetal inflammatory response syndrome. Am J Obstet Gynecol 179:194–202, 1998.

Hannah ME, Hannah WJ, Hellman J, et al: Induction of labor as compared with serial antenatal monitoring in post-term pregnancy: A randomized controlled trial. The Canadian Multicenter Post-term Pregnancy Trial Group. N Engl J Med 326:1587, 1992.

Iams JD: Prediction and early detection of preterm labor. Obstet Gynecol 101:402–412, 2003.

Kupferminc MJ, Eldor A, Seinman N, et al: Increased frequency of genetic thrombophilia in women with complications of pregnancy. N Engl J Med 340:9–13, 1999.

14 Multifetal Gestation and Malpresentation

Thomas R. Moore

MULTIPLE GESTATION

Multiple gestation may be defined as any pregnancy in which two or more embryos or fetuses exist simultaneously. It is of utmost importance to recognize multiple gestation as a complication of pregnancy. **Because the mean gestational age of delivery of twins is approximately 36 weeks, the perinatal mortality and morbidity in multiple gestation exceeds that of singleton gestations disproportionately.** Because of the additional physiologic stresses associated with two fetuses and placentas and a rapidly enlarging uterus, maternal morbidity is also increased.

ETIOLOGY AND CLASSIFICATION OF TWINNING

Multiple gestation occurs either as the result of the splitting of an embryo (i.e., **identical or monozygotic twinning**) or the fertilization of two or more eggs produced in a single menstrual cycle (i.e., **fraternal or dizygotic twinning**). Because **dizygotic twins** arise from separate eggs, they are structurally distinct pregnancies coexisting in a single uterus, each with its own amnion, chorion, and placenta. **Monozygotic twins** arise from cleavage of a single fertilized egg at various stages during embryogenesis, and thus the arrangement of the fetal membranes and placentas will depend on the time at which the embryo divides (Table 14-1). The earlier the embryo splits, the more separate the membranes and placentas will be. If division occurs within the first 72 hours of fertilization, the membranes will be **diamniotic, dichorionic** with a thick, four-layered intervening membrane. If division occurs after 4 to 8 days of development, when the chorion has already formed, **monochorionic, diamniotic** twins

will evolve with a thin, two-layer septum. If splitting occurs after 8 days, when both amnion and chorion have already formed, the result will be **monochorionic, monoamniotic, twins** residing in a single sac with no septum. Of all monozygotic twins, 30% are dichorionic, diamniotic, and 69% are monochorionic, diamniotic. Only 1% of twins are monoamnionic. Because twins share a sac in this type, without an intervening membrane, the risk of umbilical cord entanglement is high, resulting in a net mortality in these twins of almost 50% (Figure 14-1).

INCIDENCE AND EPIDEMIOLOGY

Twins account for approximately 1% of all US births. The frequency of **monozygotic** twinning, which depends on a very infrequent biologic event (embryo splitting), is constant in all populations studied at about 1 in 250 births. However, **the frequency of dizygotic twins, which arises from multiple ovulations in the mother, is strongly influenced by family history, ethnicity, and maternal age.** A family history of dizygotic but not monozygotic twins in the

Table 14-1. The relationship between the timing of cleavage and the nature of the membranes in twin gestations	
Time of Cleavage*	Nature of Membranes
0–72 hr	Diamniotic, dichorionic
4–8 days	Diamniotic, monochorionic
9–12 days	Monoamniotic, monochorionic

*Time interval between ovulation and cleavage of the egg.

MONOCHORIONIC TWIN PLACENTATION   DICHORIONIC TWIN PLACENTATION

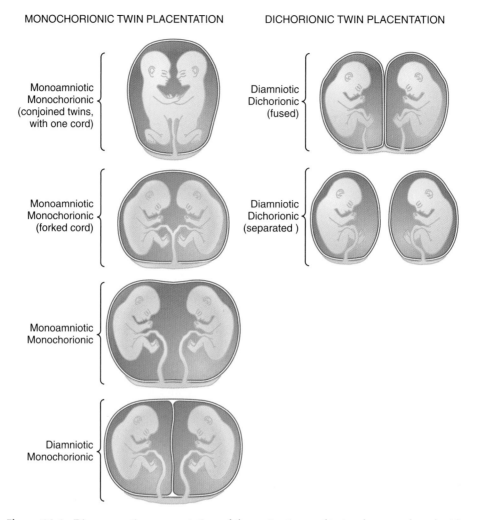

Monoamniotic
Monochorionic
(conjoined twins,
with one cord)

Monoamniotic
Monochorionic
(forked cord)

Monoamniotic
Monochorionic

Diamniotic
Monochorionic

Diamniotic
Dichorionic
(fused)

Diamniotic
Dichorionic
(separated)

Figure 14-1. Diagrammatic representation of the major types of twin placentas found with monozygotic twins. *Redrawn from Benirschke K, Driscoll SG: Pathology of the Human Placenta. New York, Springer-Verlag, 1974, p 263.*

maternal pedigree increases the likelihood of dizygotic twinning in subsequent generations. In western Nigeria, twinning occurs in 1 in 22 gestations, whereas in the Native American and Inuit populations, twinning is less than one-fifth of that rate. Twins are twice as common in women over 35 years of age as in women at 25 years of age. Given these statistics, approximately **two-thirds of spontaneously conceived twins are fraternal** and one-third are identical (monozygotic). However, in recent years, the incidence of multizygotic multifetal gestation has increased markedly, with the more widespread use of ovulation induction agents. The incidence of multiple

gestation with the use of clomiphene is about 6% to 8% and about 20% to 30% following gonadotropin therapy.

DETERMINATION OF ZYGOSITY

The prognosis and expected morbidity with twins is strongly dependent on zygosity: monozygotic twins are more likely to involve congenital anomalies, twin-twin transfusion syndrome, and premature delivery. Thus **determination of zygosity is the most important next step after multifetal pregnancy has been first diagnosed.**

Ultrasonic evaluation of the pregnancy is frequently very helpful in determining zygosity. Imaging of discordant fetal gender confirms a dizygotic gestation. Visualization of a thick amnion-chorion septum is suggestive of dizygotic twins, as is the presence of a "peak" or inverted "V" at the base of the membrane septum. Because an early embryonic split can infrequently result in dichorionic, diamniotic membranes with separate placentas, these findings are not definitive. **Confident diagnosis of zygosity may require detailed examination after delivery.** Thirty percent of twins will be of different sex and are, therefore, dizygotic. Twenty-three percent will have monochorionic placentas and are, therefore, monozygotic. Twenty-seven percent will have the same sex, dichorionic placentas, but different blood groupings, and must be, therefore, dizygotic. **Twenty percent will have the same sex, dichorionic placentas, and identical blood groupings. For the latter group, further studies, such as human leukocyte antigen (HLA) typing or DNA analysis, allow determination of zygosity.**

ABNORMALITIES OF THE TWINNING PROCESS

Among monozygotic multiple gestations, abnormalities in the twinning process are relatively common and include conjoined twins, interplacental vascular anastomoses, twin-twin transfusion syndrome, fetal malformations, and umbilical cord abnormalities.

Conjoined Twins

If division of the embryo occurs very late (after 13 days, when the embryonic disc has completely formed), cleavage of the embryo will be incomplete, resulting in **conjoined twins.** Fortunately, this is a very rare event, occurring **once in 70,000 deliveries.** Conjoined twins are classified according to the anatomic location of the incomplete splitting: **thoracopagus** (anterior), **pygopagus** (posterior), **craniopagus** (cephalic), **or ischiopagus** (caudal). The majority of such twins are thoracopagus. Delivery of conjoined twins frequently requires cesarean delivery, but postnatally these gestations have a surprisingly optimistic prognosis in many cases. More advanced contemporary imaging has allowed detailed mapping of the shared organs and more successful surgical separation procedures.

Interplacental Vascular Anastomoses

Interplacental vascular anastomoses occur almost exclusively in monochorionic twins at a rate of 90% or more. The most common type is arterial-arterial, followed by arterial-venous and then venous-venous. Vascular communications between the two fetuses via the placenta may give rise to a number of problems, including abortion, hydramnios, twin-twin transfusion syndrome, and fetal malformations. Overall, the incidence of both minor and major congenital malformations in twins is twice that in singletons, with the greater incidence of malformations occurring in monochorionic twins.

Twin-Twin Transfusion Syndrome

The presence of unbalanced anastomoses in the placenta (typically arterial-venous connections) leads to a syndrome in which one twin's circulation perfuses the other (i.e., the twin-twin transfusion syndrome) in approximately **10% of monozygotic twins.** In this syndrome, arterial blood from the "donor twin" enters the placenta (via the umbilical artery) and is taken up by the umbilical venous system belonging to the "recipient twin," which results in a net transfer of blood from the "donor" to the recipient twin. **Fetal complications include hypovolemia, hypotension, anemia, oligohydramnios, and growth restriction in the donor twin, and hypervolemia, hydramnios, hyperviscosity, thrombosis, hypertension, cardiomegaly, polycythemia, edema, and congestive heart failure in the recipient twin.** Both twins are at risk of demise from the circulatory derangement, and the pregnancy is predisposed further for preterm delivery due to uterine overdistention with hydramnios.

Fetal Malformations

Arterial-arterial placental anastomoses can result in a number of fetal structural malformations. In this situation, the arterial blood from the donor twin enters the arterial circulation of the recipient twin, and the reversed blood flow may cause thrombosis within critical organs or atresias due to trophoblastic embolization. The recipient twin, being perfused in a reverse direction with relatively poorly oxygenated blood, fails to develop normally.

Umbilical Cord Abnormalities

Abnormalities of the umbilical cord occur with a higher frequency in twins and are primarily associated with monochorionic twins. Absence of one umbilical artery occurs in about 3% to 4% of twins, as opposed to 0.5% to 1% of singletons. **The absence of one umbilical artery is significant because in 30% of such cases, it is associated with other congenital anomalies (e.g., renal agenesis).** Marginal and velamentous umbilical cord insertions also occur more frequently in twins.

Retained Dead Fetus Syndrome

It is not unusual for one twin to die in utero remote from term, whereas the remaining twin and the pregnancy continue to be viable. Over time (after 3 weeks or more in pregnancies that have progressed beyond 20 weeks), the **retained dead fetus syndrome can develop, which involves disseminated intravascular coagulopathy in the mother** as a result of transfer of nonviable fetal material with thromboplastin-like activity into her circulation. In such cases, the maternal platelet count and fibrinogen level should be checked once a week to identify possible coagulation abnormalities. The dead fetus is reabsorbed if the demise occurs prior to 12 weeks' gestation. Beyond this time, the fetus shrinks and becomes dehydrated and flattened **(fetus papyraceus).**

ALTERED MATERNAL PHYSIOLOGIC ADAPTATION WITH MULTIPLE FETUSES

A number of normal maternal physiologic responses to pregnancy are exaggerated with multiple gestation. Whereas in normal pregnancy, maternal blood volume is augmented by 40% (2 L) over nonpregnant baseline, in twins this increase may be 3 L or more. **The increased blood volume and demand for iron and folate increase the risk of anemia in the mother** and makes the patient less able to tolerate the stresses of infection, labor, and premature labor therapy. **Preeclampsia and gestational hypertension are almost doubled in multifetal gestation.** The increased uterine size associated with multiple fetuses can cause **maternal respiratory embarrassment, orthostatic hypotension due to compression of the vena cava, and compromise of renal function due to compression of the ureters.**

DIAGNOSIS

Historical factors such as a maternal family history of dizygotic twinning, the use of fertility drugs, a maternal sensation of feeling larger than with previous pregnancies, or a sensation of excessive fetal movements should raise the suspicion of twins. Physical signs, including excessive weight gain, excessive uterine fundal growth, and auscultation of fetal heart rates in separate quadrants of the uterus are suggestive but not diagnostic. **The diagnosis of multiple gestation requires a sonographic examination demonstrating two separate fetuses and heart activities.** An obstetric ultrasound should be performed when multiple gestation is suspected. This diagnosis can be made as early as 6 weeks of gestation.

ANTEPARTUM MANAGEMENT

Because of the high risk of preterm birth, intensive antepartum management schemes are directed at prolonging gestation and increasing birth weight in order to decrease perinatal morbidity and mortality. The complications of multiple gestation are shown in Box 14-1.

Box 14-1. Complications of multiple gestations

MATERNAL
Anemia
Hydramnios
Hypertension
Premature labor
Postpartum uterine atony
Postpartum hemorrhage
Preeclampsia
Cesarean delivery

FETAL
Malpresentation
Placenta previa
Abruptio placentae
Premature rupture of the membranes (PROM)
Prematurity
Umbilical cord prolapse
Intrauterine growth restriction (IUGR)
Congenital anomalies
Increased perinatal morbidity
Increased perinatal mortality

First and Second Trimesters

In the late 1st and early 2nd trimester, the patient is seen every 2 weeks for cervical assessment because **incompetent cervix is more common with multiple gestations.** A suture (cerclage) can be placed in the cervix if marked shortening is noted in the absence of contractions. Adequacy of maternal diet is assessed due to the increased need for overall calories, iron, vitamins, and folate. The Institute of Medicine (IOM) recommends women with twins gain a total of 16.0 to 20.5 kg (35 to 45 lb) during the pregnancy.

Third Trimester

In the 3rd trimester, **prevention of prematurity is of utmost importance.** The cervix is monitored closely with ultrasonographic measurements for early effacement and dilation that may precede frank premature labor. A cervical length <25 mm at 24 to 28 weeks is associated with doubling of the risk of premature birth. Interventions to prolong the length of twin pregnancy, such as bed rest, serial uterine activity monitoring, hospitalization, and prophylactic tocolytic therapy, have been carried out but have not been consistently shown to prolong gestation. Nevertheless, most experts utilize a combination of these therapies, individualized for the patient's circumstances.

Discordant fetal growth, which is signified by one fetus flattening its growth, is a cause of morbidity and mortality. Fetal growth is monitored by ultrasound every 4 to 6 weeks beginning at 24 weeks, with additional fetal surveillance (e.g., biophysical testing, nonstress fetal heart rate assessment) when fetal growth falls below the normal curve. **The patient is monitored closely for signs of preeclampsia,** including the development of nondependent edema, urinary protein, and rising arterial blood pressure.

Because twins experience higher rates of stillbirth and growth restriction than singletons, **fetal well-being should be confirmed at least weekly by non-stress testing (NST) or biophysical profile (BPP) from 36 weeks onward,** and earlier in the presence of complications such as intrauterine growth restriction (IUGR), discordant growth, hypertension, or polyhydramnios. The use of the contraction stress test (CST) is particularly useful in cases with IUGR or a nonreactive NST, but because these pregnancies are already predisposed to result in preterm labor, a CST should be used judiciously.

INTRAPARTUM MANAGEMENT
TREATMENT OF PRETERM LABOR

The treatment of preterm labor is discussed elsewhere, but multiple gestations present special challenges. **Relative contraindications to tocolysis in these pregnancies include a gestational age of 34 weeks or more, growth failure of one or more fetuses, and preeclampsia.** Aggressive tocolysis typically involves use of agents with adverse cardiovascular effects in the mother, such as beta-mimetics and magnesium sulfate. These agents, particularly when combined with antenatal corticosteroid therapy, have been associated with maternal volume overload and congestive heart failure. Box 14-2 provides a list of necessary prerequisites for the management of labor in pregnancies complicated by multiple gestation.

VERTEX-VERTEX PRESENTATIONS

To choose the safest route of delivery for mother and babies, the presentations of the fetuses must be accurately known. By convention, the presenting twin is designated as twin A and the second twin as twin B. **Vertex (twin A)-vertex (twin B) occurs most**

Box 14-2. Prerequisites for the intrapartum management of multiple gestation

A secondary or tertiary care center.
A delivery room equipped for immediate cesarean section, if necessary.
A well-functioning large-bore intravenous line (e.g., 16-gauge) for rapid administration of fluids and blood.
Blood available for transfusion.
The capability to continuously monitor the fetal heart rates simultaneously.
An anesthesiologist who is immediately available to administer general anesthesia should intrauterine manipulation or cesarean section be necessary for delivery of the second twin.
Two obstetricians scrubbed and gowned for the delivery, one of whom is skilled in intrauterine manipulation and delivery of the second twin.
Imaging techniques (i.e., sonography) for determining the precise presentations of the twins.
Two pediatricians, one of whom is skilled in the immediate resuscitation of the newborn.
An appropriate number of nurses to assist in the delivery and care of the newborn infants.

frequently (50% of the time), followed by vertex-breech, breech-vertex, and breech-breech.

Vertex-vertex twins are managed similarly to a singleton vertex presentation. Both fetal heart rates should be monitored continuously during labor. Oxytocin (Pitocin) can be used to manage hypotonic contractions. After delivery of the first twin, the cord is clamped (identified as twin A) and cut, but cord blood samples are not obtained until the second fetus has been delivered to prevent potential hemorrhage from the undelivered fetus through placental vascular anastomoses. A vaginal examination is then performed to assess the presentation and station of the second twin. If the second twin is still in a vertex presentation, spontaneous delivery is expected. If necessary, forceps or vacuum can be used to assist delivery of a vertex second twin.

After delivery of the second fetus, the cord blood samples are obtained and the placenta is delivered. Care should be taken to not disrupt the fetal membranes, as these will often reveal the zygosity of the twins. Following delivery of the placenta, uterine tone should be closely monitored, as the incidence of postpartum atony and hemorrhage is increased in multiple gestation.

MANAGEMENT OF OTHER PRESENTATIONS

Increased risk of fetal injury exists with delivery of a breech fetus. For this reason, breech-breech and breech-vertex twins are usually delivered by cesarean section. When delivery of vertex-breech or vertex-transverse twins is contemplated, informed consent by the mother and skill of the obstetrician are determining factors in choosing between cesarean and vaginal delivery. **Although there is presently no scientific evidence that cesarean delivery is superior for the vertex-breech presentation, difficulty in extracting the breech second twin can result in umbilical cord prolapse, head entrapment, neck injury, and asphyxia.** Unless the obstetrician is comfortable with managing these problems, planned cesarean is the only reasonable choice.

PERINATAL OUTCOME

The high perinatal mortality rate in twin gestations (30 to 50 per 1000 births), which is approximately five times that in singleton gestations, is largely attributable to prematurity and congenital anomalies (Box 14-3). Birth asphyxia is also a significant factor, and

---

Box 14-3. Causes of perinatal morbidity and mortality in twins
Respiratory distress syndrome
Birth trauma
Cerebral hemorrhage
Birth asphyxia
Birth anoxia
Congenital anomalies
Stillbirths
Prematurity

---

thus it is not surprising that second twins have twice the perinatal mortality of first-born twins. **Compared to singletons, death from complications of birth trauma is four times more frequent with second-born twins and twice as frequent in first-born twins.** Congenital anomalies and stillbirths account for about a third of the perinatal mortality rate. **Stillbirths occur twice as frequently in twins as in singletons.** Cerebral hemorrhage, asphyxia, and anoxia account for one-tenth of the overall perinatal mortality rate.

Twin gestations experience a fourfold increase in cerebral palsy. The increased morbidity in multiple gestations is related to placental, anatomic, and delivery abnormalities. **Low birth weight** (mean birth weight in twins is 2395 g vs. 3377 g for singletons), **prematurity, and IUGR may predispose to permanent brain injury.** The increased frequency of congenital anomalies and injuries during delivery (with both cesarean and vaginal routes) contributes to the increase in suboptimal outcome in newborns from multiple gestations. Postnatally, twins on average are shorter and lighter than singletons of similar birth weight until 4 years of age.

MULTIPLE GESTATION WITH MORE THAN TWO FETUSES

Although higher order multiple gestations (triplets and higher) can result from embryo splitting and polyovulation, today the most frequent cause is iatrogenic from the use of ovulation induction agents. The incidence of spontaneous triplets is 1 in 8000 and that of spontaneous quadruplets 1 in 700,000 births. However, because of the widespread use of assisted reproductive technologies, current estimates of the incidence of triplets is 1 in 3000 births. This rate has tripled in the last two decades.

Prematurity increases as the number of fetuses increases. The average length of gestation is 33 weeks for triplets but only 29 weeks for quadruplets, with mean birth weights 1818 g and 1395 g, respectively. Theoretically, delivery of higher order multiples can follow the principles outlined above for twins. However, in contemporary practice, almost all high order multiples are delivered by cesarean to decrease the risk of morbidity in these very premature pregnancies. **The perinatal mortality rate for triplets and quadruplets is 50 to 100 per 1000 births, a rate that is twice that of twins.**

FETAL MALPRESENTATION

The term *malpresentation* encompasses any fetal presentation other than vertex, including breech, face, brow, shoulder, and compound presentations. Both fetal and maternal factors contribute to the occurrence of malpresentation. The most common malpresentation is breech.

BREECH PRESENTATION

Breech presentation occurs when the fetal buttocks or lower extremities present into the maternal pelvis.

The incidence of breech presentation is 4% of all deliveries. Prior to 28 weeks, approximately 25% of fetuses are in a breech presentation position. As the fetus grows and occupies more of the uterus, it tends to assume a vertex presentation to accommodate best to the confines and shape of the uterus. By 34 weeks' gestation, most fetuses have assumed the vertex presentation position.

Etiology

The major factor predisposing to breech presentation is prematurity. Approximately 20% to 30% of all singleton breeches are of low birth weight (<2500 g). However, fetal structural anomalies (e.g., hydrocephalus) may restrict the ability of the fetus to present as a vertex. In breech presentations, the incidence of structural anomalies is greater than 6%, or two to three times that of a vertex. Other etiologic factors include uterine anomalies (e.g., bicornuate uterus), multiple gestation, placenta previa, hydramnios, contracted maternal pelvis, and pelvic tumors that obstruct the birth canal.

Classification

There are three types of breech presentation: **frank, complete, and incomplete or footling** (Figure 14-2). **Frank breech** occurs when both fetal thighs are

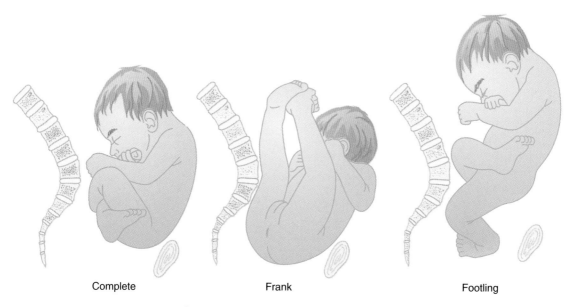

Complete   Frank   Footling

Figure 14-2. Types of breech presentation.

flexed and both lower extremities are extended at the knees. **A complete breech** has both thighs flexed and one or both knees flexed (sitting in a "squat" position). **An incomplete (or footling) breech** has one or both thighs extended and one or both knees or feet lying below the buttocks. At term, 65% of breech fetuses are frank, 25% are complete, and 10% are incomplete.

Diagnosis

The diagnosis of breech presentation can often be made by the Leopold examination (see Chapter 8), in which the firm fetal head is palpated in the fundal region and the softer, smaller breech occupies the lower uterine segment above the symphysis pubis. In a frank breech in labor, the fetal buttocks, anus, sacrum, and ischial tuberosities can be palpated on vaginal examination. With a complete breech, the feet, ankles, and often the buttocks are palpable through the dilated cervix. Vaginal examination of an incomplete breech reveals one or both fetal feet but may require ultrasound for definitive diagnosis.

Pregnancy Management

Exclude fetal and uterine anomalies. If breech presentation is suspected after 34 weeks, the prenatal records and any prior ultrasonic examinations should be reviewed for the presence of uterine myomata, müllerian anomaly or fetal structural abnormality. If suspicious, a thorough ultrasonic examination should be ordered.

External cephalic version. External cephalic version (ECV) is a procedure in which the obstetrician manually converts the breech fetus to a vertex presentation via external uterine manipulation under ultrasonic guidance. ECV may be considered in a breech presentation at term before the onset of labor. Version is not carried out prior to 36 to 37 weeks' gestation because of the tendency for the premature fetus to revert spontaneously to a breech presentation. The procedure must be carried out in a hospital that is equipped to perform an emergency cesarean section because of the small risk of placental abruption or cord compression. The patient should have nothing by mouth for 8 hours prior to the version attempt in case emergency delivery is necessary. **Evidence of utero-placental insufficiency, hypertension, intrauterine** **growth restriction, oligohydramnios, or a history of previous uterine surgery is a contraindication to external cephalic version.** The success rate of external version is about 60% regardless of whether systemic tocolytics or regional anesthesia is used. Only 2% of successful term versions revert to breech.

Labor Management

Vaginal Delivery. Until the publication of recent randomized trials demonstrating that vaginal breech delivery is associated with increased perinatal morbidity when compared to planned cesarean, vaginal breech deliveries were performed in selected centers in patients who met strict criteria. These criteria are summarized in Box 14-4. **The standard of care now in most practices is to deliver all breeches by cesarean section** to avoid the potential morbidities of umbilical cord prolapse, head entrapment, birth asphyxia, and birth trauma.

Assisted Breech Delivery. Because the breech presentation can present in a setting in which cesarean section is impossible or unsafe, vaginal delivery of the breech continues to be an important practitioner skill. Once the fetus has delivered spontaneously to the

---

Box 14-4. Criteria for vaginal delivery of a breech presentation

Fetus must be in a frank or complete breech presentation.
Gestational age should be at least 36 weeks.
Estimated fetal weight should be between 2500 and 3800 g.
Fetal head must be flexed.
Maternal pelvis must be adequately large, as assessed by x-ray pelvimetry* or tested by prior delivery of a reasonably large baby.
There must be no other maternal or fetal indication for cesarean section.
Anesthesiologist must be in attendance.
Obstetrician must be experienced.
Assistant must be scrubbed and prepared to guide the fetal head into the pelvis.

---

*Inlet: Anteroposterior (AP) diameter, ≥11.0 cm; transverse diameter, ≥12.0 cm. Midpelvis: AP diameter ≥11.5 cm; transverse diameter, ≥10.0 cm.

umbilicus (Figure 14-3), gentle downward traction is exerted until the scapulae appear at the introitus. After delivery of the scapulae, the shoulders are delivered by sweeping each arm in turn across the fetal chest until only the fetal head remains undelivered. Once the shoulders have been delivered, the head is delivered by manual flexion of the fetal head with the operator's fingers applied to the fetal maxilla or with Piper forceps. Some obstetricians use Piper forceps routinely because this method has been shown to result in delivery of the head with the least amount of trauma to the fetus.

Cesarean Delivery

During the process of breech vaginal delivery, successively larger parts of the fetus deliver, with the largest part, the fetal head, delivering last. In the very premature infant whose abdomen is much smaller than the head, the lower extremities, abdomen, and trunk may deliver through an incompletely dilated cervix, leaving the fetal head trapped and leading to fetal asphyxia and birth trauma. **Premature breech fetuses are thus preferentially delivered by cesarean section because of the head-abdomen size disparity.** Cesarean delivery is currently preferred for both preterm and term breech infants, although significant trauma can still occur if care is not taken with delivery of the arms and head.

Complications and Outcome

Even with optimal management, the perinatal mortality of breech fetuses is approximately 25 per 1000 live

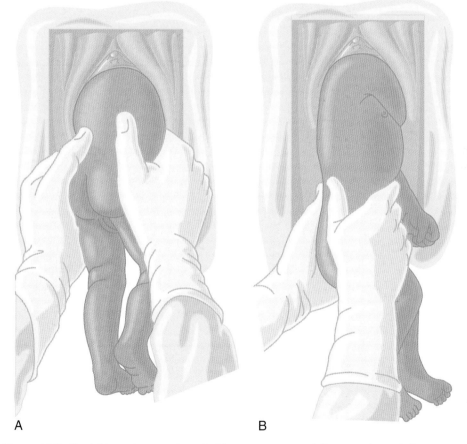

A   B

Figure 14-3. Partial breech extraction. *A,* After spontaneous delivery to the umbilicus, traction is applied to the infant's pelvis. When the scapulae are visible, rotation of the trunk allows delivery of the anterior shoulder. *B,* Delivery of the anterior shoulder by downward traction. *Continued*

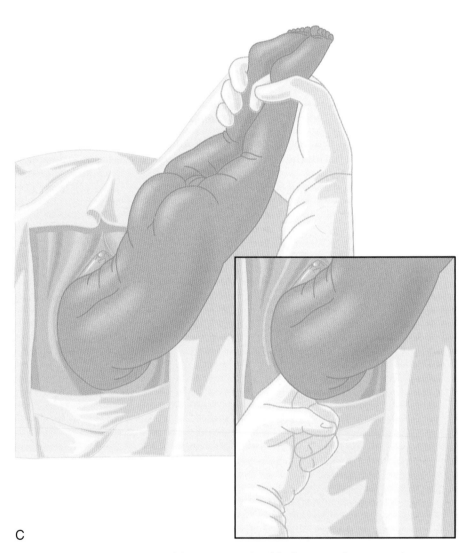

C

Figure 14-3, cont'd *C,* Delivery of the posterior shoulder by upward traction. The posterior arm is freed digitally by splinting the fetal humerus (inset).   *Continued*

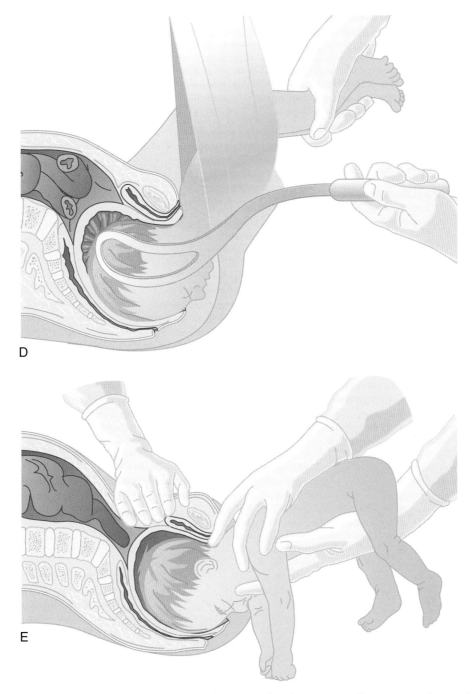

D

E

Figure 14-3, cont'd *D,* Delivery of the aftercoming head using Piper forceps. *E,* Delivery of the aftercoming head using the Mauriceau-Smellie-Veit maneuver. Abdominal pressure is applied to maintain flexion of the fetal head.

births, vs. 12 to 16 per 1000 for nonbreech fetuses. When prematurity and multiple gestations are excluded, the perinatal mortality for breech fetuses is still significantly higher than for vertex fetuses. **Factors that contribute to increased perinatal morbidity and mortality include lethal congenital anomalies, prematurity, birth trauma, and asphyxia.** Asphyxia typically results from umbilical cord prolapse during labor or entrapment of the after-coming head. Birth trauma can occur whenever force-ful traction is exerted on the fetus and can involve the brachial plexus **(Erb's palsy),** pharynx, and liver.

FACE PRESENTATION

Face presentation occurs when the fetal head is hyper-extended such that the fetal face, between the chin and orbits, is the presenting part. **The incidence is about 1 in 500 deliveries.**

Etiology

The etiology of face presentation is somewhat enig-matic. During normal vertex delivery, the fetal head is markedly flexed, with the fetal occiput as the leading part. Factors that permit the fetus to enter the pelvis with a markedly extended head include extreme pre-maturity, high maternal parity, and congenital anom-alies such as fetal goiter. In the majority, however, no etiologic factor is evident.

Diagnosis

The diagnosis of face presentation is usually made at the time of vaginal examination during labor, when the soft tissues of the fetal mouth and nose are noted adjacent to the malar bones and orbital ridges. Face presentation is then confirmed by sonography or by radiography. Because anencephalic fetuses uniformly present face first, **anencephaly should be ruled out when face presentation is suspected.**

Mechanism of Labor

The position of the presenting face is classified accord-ing to the location of the fetal chin (mentum). Approx-imately 60% of face presentations are mentum anterior at the time of diagnosis, whereas 15% are mentum transverse and 25% mentum posterior. The mechanism of labor with a face presentation is similar to the vertex presentation in that the longest diameter (mentum to brow) enters the pelvis transversely. As labor proceeds and the face descends to the midplane, internal rotation occurs into the vertical axis. If the mentum rotates anteriorly under the symphysis pubis, vaginal delivery should be expected. Forceps, but not vacuum, can be applied to assist if prerequisites are met. However, **if the mentum rotates posteriorly, the fetal head will be unable to extend farther to complete the expulsive process.** Thus mentum pos-terior cases and those with persistent mentum trans-verse must be delivered by cesarean section. However, since final rotation from mentum transverse may occur only after a significant period of maternal pushing, patience is necessary. Approximately half of the mentoposterior and mentotransverse presentations spontaneously rotate to a mentoanterior position. When delivered by spontaneous vaginal delivery (Figure 14-4) or low forceps (Figure 14-5), perinatal morbidity and mortality for face presentations are similar to those for vertex presentations.

OTHER PRESENTATIONS

Brow presentation occurs when the presenting part of the fetus is between the facial orbits and anterior fontanelle (Figure 14-6). This type of presentation arises as the result of extension of the fetal head such that it is midway between flexion (vertex presentation) and hyperextension (face presentation). **The inci-dence is about 1 in 1400 deliveries. With a brow presentation, the presenting diameter is the supra-occipitomental diameter,** which is much longer than the presenting diameter for a face or a vertex presentation.

The intrapartum management is expectant, because the brow presentation is an unstable one. Fifty percent to 75% will convert to either a face presentation, through extension, or a vertex presentation, through flexion, and will subsequently deliver vaginally. **With a persistent brow presentation, the large present-ing diameter makes vaginal delivery impossible, unless the fetus is very small or the maternal pelvis is very large, and delivery must be accomplished by cesarean section.** There is an increased incidence of both prolonged labor (30% to 50%) and dysfunc-tional labor (30%). As with face presentations, mid-pelvic delivery and methods to convert the brow presentation to a vertex presentation are contraindi-cated. Perinatal morbidity and mortality are similar to those for vertex presentations.

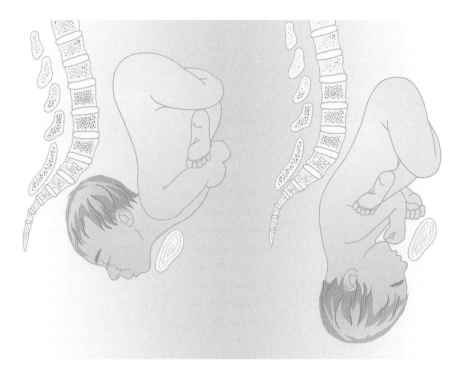

Figure 14-4. Spontaneous delivery of a mentum anterior face presentation. Note the flexion of the head under the symphysis pubis. The chin appears first, followed by the nose, brow, vertex, and occiput.

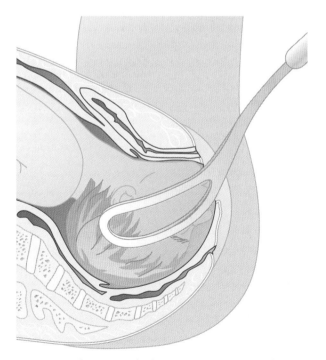

Figure 14-5. Simpson forceps applied to a mentum anterior face presentation.

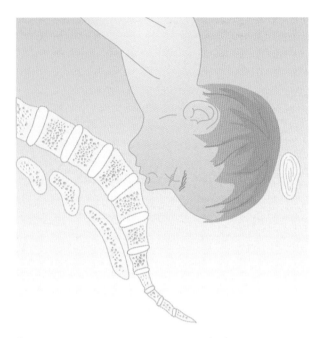

Figure 14-6. Brow presentation. Note the large presenting diameter (occipitomental).

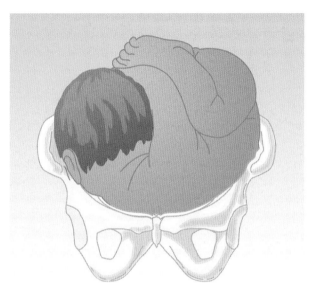

Figure 14-7. Shoulder presentation. Note the transverse lie of the fetus with the back down, which cannot be delivered vaginally.

A **compound presentation** occurs when a fetal extremity (usually the hand) prolapses alongside the presenting part (the head) and both parts enter the maternal pelvis at the same time. This presentation occurs more frequently with premature gestations. The incidence of a hand or arm prolapsing alongside the presenting fetal head is 1 in 700 deliveries and management is expectant. Usually, the prolapsed part of the fetus does not interfere with labor. If the arm prolapses, it is best to wait to see if it moves out of the way as the head descends. If it does not, the arm may be gently pushed upward while the head is simultaneously pushed downward by fundal pressure. If the complete extremity prolapses and the fetus then converts to a **shoulder presentation** (Figure 14-7), delivery must be accomplished by cesarean section.

Suggested Reading

American College of Obstetricians and Gynecologists: Committee Opinion Number 265: Mode of term single breech delivery. Obstet Gynecol 98(6):1189–1190, 2001.

Bell D, Johansson D, McLean FH, et al: Birth asphyxia, trauma and mortality in twins: Has cesarean section improved outcome? Am J Obstet Gynecol 154:235, 1986.

Benirschke K: The biology of the twinning process: How placentation influences outcome. Semin Perinatol 19:342, 1995.

Hannah ME, Hannal WJ, Hewson SA, et al: Planned caesarean section versus planned vaginal birth for breech presentation at term: A randomised multicentre trial. Term Breech Trial Collaborative Group. Lancet 21:356(9239):1375–1383, 2000.

Planned caesarean section for term breech delivery. Cochrane Database Syst Rev (1):CD000166, 2001.

15 Hypertensive Disorders of Pregnancy

Lony C. Castro

The hypertensive disorders of pregnancy are major contributors to maternal and perinatal morbidity and mortality. **In the mother, they can cause placental abruption, disseminated intravascular coagulation (DIC), renal failure, hepatic failure, central nervous system (CNS) hemorrhage, and stroke. Fetal and neonatal complications include growth restriction, prematurity, and perinatal death.** The Centers for Disease Control (CDC) have recently reported that preeclampsia/eclampsia is the third leading cause of maternal mortality in the United States, primarily due to CNS hemorrhage. The combined incidence of hypertensive disorders in pregnancy varies depending on the population being studied and on the criteria used but is reported to range from 12% to 22%, whereas the preeclampsia/eclampsia syndrome occurs in approximately 5% to 8% of pregnancies.

CLASSIFICATION AND DEFINITIONS

The general classification of hypertensive disorders recommended by the Working Group Report on High Blood Pressure in Pregnancy (2000) and adopted by the American College of Obstetricians and Gynecologists (ACOG) in 2002 (Box 15-1). **Toxemia** should not be used, as it represents the entire spectrum of hypertensive disorders of pregnancy and may also refer to isolated proteinuria.

Blood pressure readings vary depending on maternal position and the gestational age of the pregnancy. Maternal blood pressure tends to be lower in the left lateral decubitus position and higher in the sitting position. In the supine position, some pregnant women will have elevated pressures, whereas others will have supine hypotension due to compression of the vena cava by the uterus. In addition to positional variations, arterial blood pressure normally declines during the 1st and 2nd trimesters of pregnancy and rises to prepregnant levels in the 3rd trimester.

The diagnosis of hypertension should be reserved for patients with a systolic blood pressure of greater than or equal to 140 mm Hg or a diastolic of greater than or equal to 90 mm Hg. Blood pressure measurements should be taken in the sitting position after the woman has rested at least 10 minutes. Arterial pressures may also be taken in the lateral decubitus position, but the measurements should be corrected to the level of the right atrium. In the hospitalized patient, either sitting or lateral decubitus measurements may be used, but consistency is advised. The length of the blood pressure cuff should be at least 1.5 times the circumference of the upper arm and the fifth Korotkoff sound (disappearance) should be used for determining diastolic pressure.

PREECLAMPSIA/ECLAMPSIA

Preeclampsia is a syndrome unique to pregnancy characterized by the new onset of hypertension and proteinuria in the latter half of gestation. Preeclampsia is classically considered to be a disease affecting the first pregnancy, but it also occurs in multiparas, especially if there are predisposing risk factors such as twins, diabetes mellitus, and chronic hypertension. **When it arises in the early second trimester (14 to 20 weeks), a hydatidiform mole or choriocarcinoma should be considered.**

The following two criteria are essential for the diagnosis of preeclampsia: (1) the development of

> **Box 15-1. General classification of hypertensive disorders of pregnancy**
>
> - Preeclampsia/eclampsia (hypertension and proteinuria unique to pregnancy)
> - Chronic hypertension
> - Chronic hypertension with superimposed preeclampsia
> - Gestational or transient hypertension

Based on the National Institutes of Health Working Group Report on High Blood Pressure in Pregnancy, 2000.

hypertension (systolic blood pressures ≥140 mm Hg or diastolic blood pressures ≥90 mm Hg), **in a woman whose blood pressures were previously normal, after the 20th week of pregnancy; (2) proteinuria, which is defined as ≥0.3 g protein in a timed 24-hour urine collection.** This usually correlates with a 1+ dipstick reading or greater on a clean catch urine sample.

In the past, a 30-mm Hg rise in systolic blood pressure or a 15-mm Hg rise in diastolic pressure was considered to be a sign of preeclampsia. Because of the previously described physiologic rise in blood pressure during the 3rd trimester and the frequent lack of accurate prepregnant blood pressures for use as a baseline, this rise is no longer considered diagnostic if the blood pressure remains under 140/90 mm Hg. Despite this, **rising blood pressures should be of concern** because they may precede the development of the full preeclampsia syndrome. Similarly, **preeclampsia is often preceded by, or associated with, the development of generalized edema.** Dependent edema (edema of the lower extremities) is very common in normal pregnancies. Hand and facial edema are more likely to be associated with preeclampsia, but if unaccompanied by hypertension and proteinuria, they are not diagnostic of the preeclampsia syndrome.

Preeclampsia is divided into mild and severe forms, depending on the severity of the hypertension, the amount of proteinuria, and the degree to which other organ systems are affected. Box 15-2 lists specific criteria for the diagnosis of severe preeclampsia. If any of the signs or symptoms listed in Box 15-2 is present in a woman with preeclampsia, it is very likely that she has severe disease, which is associated with much greater maternal and perinatal morbidity.

A variant of severe preeclampsia with particularly high morbidity is the HELLP syndrome. This syndrome occurs in preeclamptic women with evidence of *h*emolysis, *e*levated *l*iver enzymes and *l*ow *p*latelets (thrombocytopenia). In contrast to more typical presentations of preeclampsia, the patient with HELLP syndrome is more likely to be multiparous, older than 25 years, and at less than 36 weeks' gestation. Hypertension may be initially absent in 20% of the patients, whereas 30% will have mild elevations in blood pressure, and 50% will have severe elevations.

ECLAMPSIA

Eclampsia is the presence of tonic-clonic seizures in a woman that cannot be attributed to other causes. Patients with severe preeclampsia are at the greatest risk of developing seizures, but the seizures can occur in so-called mild preeclamptics. Eclamptic seizures can also occur prior to classic signs of preeclampsia. **In general, 25% of patients with eclampsia develop the seizures before labor, 50% during labor, and 25% after delivery** (usually within the first 24 to 48 hours' postpartum). It is especially important to consider other causes of seizures, especially in atypical cases of eclampsia (i.e., more than 48 hours' postpartum or previous evidence of only mild disease).

CHRONIC HYPERTENSION

The diagnosis of chronic hypertension requires at least one of the following: known hypertension prior to pregnancy, the development of hypertension prior to 20 weeks' gestation, or, in cases where hypertension is first noted during pregnancy, persistence of elevated blood pressures greater than 12 weeks' postpartum.

Most pregnant women with chronic hypertension will have essential hypertension, but a small percentage will have secondary hypertension due to renal, vascular, or endocrinologic causes. Depending on the associated signs and symptoms and response to medication, a workup to determine the etiology of the hypertension may be indicated. In fact, it is not uncommon for the physiologic stress of pregnancy to bring to clinical attention for the first time a previously inapparent or subclinical vascular or renal disease. In these situations, it may be very difficult to differentiate between preeclampsia and an aggravated chronic hypertensive condition. Sometimes only careful follow-up postpartum will indicate the correct diagnosis.

CHRONIC HYPERTENSION WITH SUPERIMPOSED PREECLAMPSIA

Preeclampsia may become superimposed on chronic hypertensive disease. Often, an underlying hypertensive disorder of renal or other origin is present, and the process is aggravated by pregnancy. Superimposed preeclampsia can be very difficult to distinguish from poorly controlled chronic hypertension, especially if the woman is not seen until after the 20th week of gestation, but the two conditions are managed differently, and superimposed preeclampsia carries a worse prognosis than does either chronic hypertension or preeclampsia alone.

Superimposed preeclampsia should be reserved for those women with chronic hypertension who develop new-onset proteinuria ($\geq$0.3 g in a 24-hour collection) after the 20th week of gestation. In pregnant women with preexisting hypertension and proteinuria, the diagnosis of superimposed preeclampsia should be considered if they experience sudden significant increases in blood pressure or proteinuria or any of the other signs and symptoms consistent with severe preeclampsia listed in Box 15-2, including thrombocytopenia or abnormally elevated liver enzymes.

GESTATIONAL HYPERTENSION

The diagnosis of gestational hypertension is made if hypertension without proteinuria first appears after 20 weeks' gestation or within 48 to 72 hours after delivery and resolves by 12 weeks' post-partum. It is extremely difficult to differentiate this condition from the early stages of preeclampsia. A significant percentage of women with apparent gestational hypertension will go on to develop proteinuria and the full preeclampsia syndrome at a later stage in pregnancy. Others will have previously unrecognized chronic hypertension. **The diagnosis of gestational hypertension can only be made in retrospect, if the pregnancy has been completed without the development of proteinuria and if the blood pressure has returned to normal prior to the 12th week postpartum.**

PREECLAMPSIA/ECLAMPSIA
ETIOLOGY

Genetic, immunologic, endocrinologic, nutritional, and even infectious agents have been proposed as causes of preeclampsia, thus the disease is called a "disease of theories." Despite extensive research, no definite cause has been identified. **Because of the prompt resolution of the disease after delivery, most attention has been focused on the placenta and its membranes and the fetus.**

Uteroplacental ischemia may be central to the development of the disease, which has been attributed to failure of the normal physiologic changes in the spiral and radial arteries of the uterus. Ischemia could also be due to underlying vascular disease such as what occurs in chronic hypertension or to immunologically mediated placental vascular damage. Alternatively, ischemia could be caused by increased intramural resistance in the myometrial vessels, which could be related to a heightened myometrial tension produced by a large fetus in a primiparous woman, by twins, or by hydramnios.

It is postulated that uteroplacental ischemia results in the production and release of toxins that enter the circulation and cause widespread endothelial dysfunction. The nature of these toxins has not yet been identified but may involve oxygen free radicals and lipid peroxides. Endothelial dysfunction leads to an imbalance between different classes of locally produced vasoconstrictors and vasodilators. Preeclampsia is associated with a disturbance in prostaglandin production, with a decrease in the ratio of the vasodilators prostaglandin E_2 (PGE_2) and prostacyclin to the vasoconstrictor PGF series and thromboxanes.

In normal pregnancy, prostacyclin (PGI_2) synthesis increases fourfold to fivefold, whereas thromboxane A_2

Box 15-2. **Criteria for severe preeclampsia**

- Severe hypertension (systolic BP $\geq$160 or diastolic BP $\geq$110 mm Hg) at rest, on two occasions at least 6 hr apart
- Heavy proteinuria (at least 5 g in a 24-hr collection or a qualitative value of 3+ in urine samples collected 4 hr apart
- Oliguria (<500 mL in 24 hr)
- Cerebral or visual disturbances
- Pulmonary edema or cyanosis
- Epigastric or right upper quadrant pain
- Impaired liver function (elevated liver enzymes)
- Thrombocytopenia
- Fetal growth restriction

Data from American College of Obstetricians and Gynecologists: Practice Bulletin No. 33, Washington, DC, ACOG, 2002.

production remains relatively unchanged or increases slightly. PGI$_2$ is associated with decreased vascular resistance and decreased platelet aggregation. **In hypertensive pregnancies, PGI$_2$ production does not increase to the same degree as in normal pregnancy, and thromboxane A$_2$ is reported to be unchanged.** The result is a relatively reduced PGI$_2$-to-thromboxane A$_2$ ratio compared with that in a normotensive pregnant woman, leading to increased peripheral vascular resistance and platelet activation.

Endothelial changes also appear to involve a relative deficiency in the production of nitric oxide, a vasodilator and inhibitor of platelet aggregation, along with increased production of endothelin-I. Endothelin-I is an extremely potent vasoconstrictor and activator of platelets. This shift in the production of locally acting vasoactive substances could enhance vasoconstriction in response to circulating pressor hormones. The net effect would be to cause widespread arteriolar constriction leading to hypoxic/ischemic damage in different vascular beds, systemic hypertension, and worsening placental ischemia. The relative severity of the signs and symptoms of preeclampsia in any given individual afflicted with the disease would vary on the basis of which specific organ systems were most affected.

PATHOPHYSIOLOGY

Although the cause of preeclampsia is unknown, the underlying pathophysiologic abnormality is generalized vasospasm. A rise in blood pressure could be elicited by an increase in cardiac output or systemic vascular resistance. Cardiac output in untreated pregnant patients with preeclampsia and eclampsia is not significantly different from that of normal pregnant subjects in the last trimester of pregnancy; matched for gestational age, however, the systemic vascular resistance is significantly elevated.

Renal blood flow and glomerular filtration rate (GFR) in patients with preeclampsia and eclampsia are significantly lower than in those patients with a normal pregnancy of a comparable gestational period. The decrease in renal blood flow results from constriction of the afferent arteriolar system. **This afferent vasoconstriction may eventually lead to damage to the glomerular membranes, thereby**

increasing their permeability to proteins and leading to proteinuria. The renal vasoconstriction and decrease in GFR also account for oliguria.

The cerebral vascular resistance is always high in patients with preeclampsia and eclampsia. In hypertensive patients without convulsions, cerebral blood flow may remain within normal limits as a result of autoregulatory phenomena. In patients with convulsions, however, cerebral blood flow and oxygen consumption are significantly less than in normal pregnant subjects. Likewise, there is decreased blood flow and increased vascular resistance in the uteroplacental circulation in preeclamptic patients. Color-flow Doppler studies of the uteroplacental circulation suggest changes that are consistent with the development of increased vascular resistance in patients with preeclampsia.

PATHOLOGY

Three major pathologic lesions are classically associated with preeclampsia and eclampsia: (1) lack of decidualization of the myometrial segments of the spiral arteries; (2) glomerular capillary endotheliosis; and (3) hemorrhage and necrosis in many organs, presumably secondary to arteriolar constriction. The uteroplacental pathology in preeclampsia/eclampsia is characterized by a lack of "decidualization" of the myometrial segments of the spiral arteries.

Under normal circumstances, the invasion of trophoblast results in the replacement of the muscular and elastic layers of the spiral arteries by fibrinoid and fibrous tissue, resulting in large, tortuous, low-resistance channels that extend through the myometrium. In preeclampsia, this change is mostly limited to the decidual segments of the vessels and may result in a 60% reduction in the diameter of the myometrial segment of a spiral artery. The extent of placental infarction is increased in almost all preeclamptic pregnancies.

The typical renal lesion of preeclampsia/eclampsia is "glomerular capillary endotheliosis," which is best seen by electron microscopy. This disorder is manifested by marked swelling of the glomerular capillary endothelium and deposits of fibrinoid material in and beneath the endothelial cells. On light microscopy, the glomerular diameter is increased, with protrusion of the glomerular tufts into the neck of the proximal tubules and variable degrees of endothelial and mesangial cellular swelling.

Arteriolar vasospasm of relatively short duration (1 hour) can cause hypoxia and necrosis of sensitive parenchymal cells. Vasospasm of longer duration (3 hours) can lead to infarction of vital organs, such as the liver, placenta, and brain. In the liver, periportal necrosis and hemorrhage may occur, with subcapsular hematoma being a rare complication. In the brain, focal areas of hemorrhage and necrosis may occur. In the retina, the clinical window to the arterial vasculature, vasospasm may be visualized on ophthalmoscopic examination. **Retinal hemorrhage is considered to be an extremely ominous sign** because it may signal similar phenomena in other vital organs.

CLINICAL AND LABORATORY MANIFESTATIONS

Many of the clinical and laboratory manifestations of preeclampsia and eclampsia can be explained on the basis of endothelial dysfunction and vasospasm.

ANGIOTENSIN SENSITIVITY

One of the earliest signs of developing preeclampsia is a lowering of the effective pressor dose of infused angiotensin II. In normal pregnancy, the amount of angiotensin necessary to increase the diastolic pressure 20 mm Hg is increased, whereas in patients destined to develop preeclampsia, the effective pressor dose is lower.

WEIGHT GAIN AND EDEMA

Abnormal weight gain and edema occur early and reflect an expansion of the extravascular fluid compartment. This expansion is related to the increased capillary permeability that allows fluid to diffuse from the intravascular to the extravascular space. Thus, many preeclamptics have an increase in total body fluid volume but are intravascularly volume depleted. **The hematocrit may also increase, reflecting the relative hypovolemia and hemoconcentration.**

ELEVATION OF BLOOD PRESSURE

The next sign usually detected is an elevation of blood pressure, particularly the diastolic pressure, which more closely mirrors changes in peripheral vascular resistance. In the antepartum period, the blood pressure changes may occur days to weeks after the onset of pathologic fluid retention.

PROTEINURIA

In the antepartum period, proteinuria may occur days or weeks after the onset of hypertension. If the disease first manifests during labor or in the immediate postpartum period, this progression of events is compressed into hours and sometimes minutes. The proteinuria of preeclampsia/eclampsia is likely due to afferent arteriolar constriction with increased glomerular permeability to proteins.

RENAL FUNCTION

The earliest change may be an increase in serum uric acid concentration. Creatinine clearance may decrease, and serum creatinine and blood urea nitrogen levels may rise. Renal involvement may progress to significant oliguria and frank renal failure.

THE COAGULATION SYSTEM

Thrombocytopenia is the most common abnormality. Although platelet counts tend to decline even in normal pregnancies, a value <100,000 cells/mm^3 is clearly pathologic and, if accompanied by other signs of preeclampsia, is evidence of severe disease. **DIC may occur** especially if there is a placental abruption. **The specific combination of hemolysis, elevated liver function tests, and low platelet levels (the HELLP syndrome)** can occur without clinical manifestations of DIC and **is a sign of severe preeclampsia** even if blood pressures are normal or only minimally elevated.

LIVER FUNCTION

In the liver, vasospasm may result in focal hemorrhages and infarctions leading to right upper quadrant or epigastric pain and elevated serum enzyme levels (alanine aminotransferase and aspartate aminotransferase). Hepatic rupture is a rare, ominous complication of preeclampsia that is usually associated with the HELLP syndrome. If significant hemolysis is present, bilirubin levels will often be elevated.

PLACENTAL FUNCTION

Vasospasm in the uteroplacental vascular bed results in placental infarction and decreased uteroplacental perfusion. This ultimately leads to fetal compromise in the form of intrauterine growth restriction (IUGR), oligohydramnios, or fetal heart rate abnormalities. **Extensive placental infarctions can result in retroplacental hemorrhage or abruption,** which is an important cause of perinatal morbidity and mortality.

CENTRAL NERVOUS SYSTEM EFFECTS

Visual disturbances, such as blurred vision, spots, and scotomata, represent degrees of retinal vasospasm. **Increased reflex irritability or hyperreflexia are extremely worrisome signs** of CNS involvement and may connote imminent seizures.

EVALUATION AND MANAGEMENT OF PREECLAMPSIA

There are three important questions the clinician must ask when managing a woman with preeclampsia. First, is the disease process mild or severe? Second, is there evidence of fetal compromise (i.e., growth restriction, oligohydramnios, or heart rate abnormalities)? Third, is the fetus mature enough for a reasonably uncomplicated course after delivery?

Delivery is the only definitive cure for preeclampsia so it is always beneficial for the mother but may result in the delivery of a very preterm neonate. The goal of management is to decrease or prevent the maternal complications of severe preeclampsia, while minimizing the neonatal complications arising from prematurity. A woman with mild preeclampsia, without evidence of fetal compromise, will generally not be delivered unless the gestational age is 34 weeks or older, whereas **a woman with severe preeclampsia or eclampsia should be delivered after a period of stabilization, regardless of the gestational age of the fetus.**

The initial maternal assessment involves a complete medical history, physical examination, and laboratory evaluation. The history should focus on whether there is any past history of elevated blood pressures or renal disease either prior to pregnancy or during previous pregnancies. The patient should be carefully questioned regarding symptoms of severe preeclampsia or its complications, including headache, visual changes, nausea, vomiting, abdominal or epigastric pain, and vaginal bleeding. The chart should be reviewed to determine when in the current pregnancy blood pressures started to rise and when proteinuria developed.

The physical examination should focus on the assessment of blood pressure, weight gain, edema, fundal height, and reflexes and a qualitative assessment of urinary protein excretion with a dipstick. In addition, findings consistent with severe preeclampsia such as epigastric or right upper quadrant tenderness, uterine tenderness, petechiae due to low platelets, and signs of pulmonary edema should be sought. If there is severe headache or visual symptoms, an ophthalmic examination may be indicated. The initial laboratory studies recommended are outlined in Box 15-3.

A careful fetal evaluation is also indicated. This should begin with an accurate determination of fetal gestational age based on clinical and sonographic data, if available. A fetal ultrasound should be performed to evaluate fetal growth and amniotic fluid volume. **A nonstress test (NST) or biophysical profile should also be done** to determine if there is evidence of acute fetal compromise.

It is generally advisable to hospitalize patients with a presumed diagnosis of preeclampsia to determine the disease's severity and maternal and fetal stability. After the initial evaluation, **if the mother's disease is mild and if there is no evidence of fetal compromise, management consists of rest and observation.** There is no evidence that chronic antihypertensive therapy or diuretic therapy prevents the progression of mild preeclampsia to severe preeclampsia or improves maternal or fetal outcomes. Depending on the special circumstances surrounding each case, management can be carried out in the hospital or in some cases as an outpatient. The mother will require frequent reassessment of symptoms, blood pressure, and qualitative urine protein excretion along with weekly laboratory tests. The fetus needs to be followed with monitoring of fetal activity, heart rate reactivity, and amniotic fluid volume. **The patient should be delivered by the time she reaches 38 weeks, develops signs or symptoms of worsening disease, or if there is evidence of fetal compromise.**

If the initial evaluation is consistent with the diagnosis of severe preeclampsia the patient should remain hospitalized for the remainder of the pregnancy. After 32 to 34 weeks' gestation, stabilization and delivery are appropriate for most patients. For those patients less than 32 weeks with severe preeclampsia, the decision regarding delivery needs to be individualized after carefully weighing the risks to the neonate of prematurity vs. the potential maternal and fetal risks of continuing the pregnancy. Both the mother and fetus require very close monitoring with maternal laboratory parameters and fetal assessment testing repeated daily if necessary. **In some instances, stabilization of the patient with bed rest, along with medical control of severe hypertension and corticosteroids for fetal lung maturity will moderate the disease process and allow delivery to be delayed in the hopes of advancing gestational age.** Deterioration in clinical status (e.g., uncontrollable hypertension, oliguria, pulmonary edema, evidence of HELLP or coagulopathy, CNS symptoms, abruption, or abnormal fetal testing) requires delivery.

INTRAPARTUM MANAGEMENT OF PREECLAMPSIA

Labor should be induced (or spontaneous labor allowed to continue) in the absence of obstetric indications for cesarean delivery such as failure to progress in labor, nonreassuring fetal status, or nonvertex presentation. The mother and fetus must be carefully monitored during labor and delivery. **Two of the most important maternal issues to be dealt with are seizure prophylaxis and control of hypertension.** Other potential maternal problems that may develop are oliguria, pulmonary edema, and thrombocytopenia or the HELLP syndrome.

If the fetus is growth restricted or if placental abruption occurs, the fetal heart rate tracing may show evidence of late decelerations, bradycardia, or other signs of fetal compromise necessitating cesarean delivery. In most instances, epidural anesthesia is the anesthetic of choice for operative delivery or pain relief during labor unless there is evidence of coagulopathy.

SEIZURE PROPHYLAXIS

Because of the risk of seizures and their attendant morbidity and even mortality, a great deal of attention must be given to the level of CNS irritability. Peripheral reflexes, particularly of the patella and ankle, are most extensively used as determinants of heightened instability. **In patients with preeclampsia, severe headaches, sustained clonus, or a positive Chvostek's sign can be prodromal symptoms or signs of eclampsia.**

Table 15-1. Anticonvulsive magnesium sulfate therapy

Type of Treatment	IV	IM
Prophylactic loading	4 g over 15–20 min in 100 mL fluid	5 g in each buttock
Maintenance	2 g/hr controlled IV infusion	5 g/4 hr

IV, intravenous; IM, intramuscular.

Seizure prophylaxis should be instituted in most patients with preeclampsia during the intrapartum period and continued for about 24 hours after delivery. In addition, patients with severe preeclampsia should have seizure prophylaxis instituted on admission and continued during the initial period of stabilization. **Randomized controlled trials have confirmed that magnesium sulfate is the agent of choice for the prevention and treatment of eclamptic seizures because it is efficacious and is associated with low neonatal morbidity.** Both intramuscular (IM) and intravenous (IV) routes are effective for prophylaxis, but the IM injections can be very painful.

Table 15-1 outlines the protocols for magnesium administration, and Table 15-2 reviews the relationship between serum magnesium concentrations, clinical response, and signs of toxicity. Therapeutic levels are generally accepted to be in the range of 4.8 to 9.6 mg/dL, but levels should not be allowed to rise above 8 mg/dL to avoid toxicity. **The magnesium ion is excreted exclusively through the kidneys, so careful monitoring of urine output is essential.** A

Table 15-2. Clinical correlates of serum magnesium sulfate levels (therapeutic range: 4.8–9.6)

Clinical Response	Serum Levels (mg/dL)
Loss of patellar reflex	8–12
Warmth and flushing	9–12
Somnolence	10–12
Slurred speech	10–12
Paralysis and respiratory difficulty	15–17
Cardiac arrest	30–35

magnesium overdose can have severe, even fatal, consequences. Magnesium should be given by a controlled infusion pump with a fail-safe mechanism to prevent errors in administration (i.e., inadvertent bolus infusion). **Serial assessments of urine output, deep tendon reflexes, and respirations are important for detecting signs of magnesium toxicity.** These clinical assessments can be supplemented with serial measurements of serum magnesium levels or arterial O_2 saturation via pulse oximetry. Magnesium toxicity can occur even in a patient with apparently normal renal function. Magnesium toxicity is treated by stopping infusion of the drug and administering calcium gluconate, 10 mL of a 10% solution, intravenously, and initiating resuscitative measures if necessary.

ANTIHYPERTENSIVE THERAPY

Arterial blood pressure exceeding a level of 160 mm Hg systolic or 105 to 110 mm Hg diastolic must be treated promptly. In the setting of severe preeclampsia, blood pressures reaching these levels are considered to represent a hypertensive crisis. The goal of antihypertensive therapy in severe preeclampsia is to lower blood pressure carefully to prevent CNS hemorrhage. In general one should not lower the blood pressure to "normal levels" or less than 140/90 mm Hg. **Caution must always be exercised to not lower the arterial pressure too much or too rapidly, for either may result in a decreased utero-placental blood flow and fetal distress.**

The safest, most efficacious drugs for the acute control of severe hypertension complicating preeclampsia are **hydralazine and labetalol.** The clinician should be very familiar with the parenteral use of these drugs in this setting and their potential complications. Of the two, **hydralazine is the most widely used** and has theoretical advantages over labetalol in that it is a direct vasodilator, does not induce brochospasm, and is not contraindicated in the presence of heart failure. Table 15-3 details the dosage, duration of action, and potential complications of these two drugs. Oral nifedipine has been used successfully, starting at a dose of 10 mg orally and repeated in 30 minutes if necessary. **Nifedipine should be used cautiously to avoid hypotension**, particularly when used in conjunction with magnesium sulfate. **Intravenous sodium nitroprusside has the advantage of providing minute-to-minute control of blood pressure** but may cause fetal cyanide toxicity with prolonged administration, so the use of this medication is generally limited to the postpartum period.

MANAGEMENT OF FLUID BALANCE

Accurately recorded intake and output data must be kept to calculate fluid requirements. **These patients**

Table 15-3. Emergency parenteral therapy for severe hypertension during pregnancy*				
Agent	Action	Dose	Side Effects	Comment
Hydralazine	Direct vasodilator	5 mg IV over 1–2 min, then 5–10 mg IV every 10–20 min until BPs are 140–150/90–100 mmHg. If no response after 20 mg switch to another drug.	Headache, palpitations, flushing, lupus-like syndrome	Increases cardiac output and probably uterine and renal blood flow; has been drug of choice for short-term control.
Labetalol hydrochloride	Nonselective β_1- and α_1-blocker	Start with 20 mg IV bolus. If inadequate response after 10 min, give 40 mg IV followed by 80 mg IV every 10 min × two more doses if needed to lower BPs to 140–150/90–100 mmHg. Total dose not to exceed 220 mg.	Nausea, vomiting, heart block, burning sensation in throat, dizziness	Increasing experience and efficacy reported; is becoming drug of choice in many centers. Avoid if evidence of acute heart failure or asthma.

*Data from Joint National Committee: The sixth report of the Joint National Committee on Prevention, Detection, Evaluation, and Treatment of High Blood Pressure (JNC VI). Arch Intern Med 157:2413–2446, 1997.

experience vasoconstriction, have interstitial edema, and often demonstrate some degree of reduced intravascular volume, which may reduce urinary output. In addition, they may be receiving several different therapeutic infusions, such as magnesium sulfate and oxytocin, which have a direct or indirect effect on urinary output.

The most common errors that occur in the management of these patients are fluid volume overload, excessive salt restriction, and water intoxication. The conservative approach is to replace documented output plus insensible loss with an appropriate electrolyte-containing fluid. Because of the multifaceted pathophysiology of this disease, central hemodynamic monitoring using a pulmonary artery catheter may aid in the management of refractory cases of oliguria or pulmonary edema.

MANAGEMENT OF ECLAMPSIA

Eclampsia is a true obstetric emergency, and all physicians involved in the care of pregnant women should be prepared to recognize the occurrence of an eclamptic seizure and begin initial resuscitative/stabilization efforts until appropriate obstetric backup arrives. The management of these patients should be carried out by a team of physicians and well-trained nurses in an isolated labor room, with minimal noise and not too much light. As with any seizure condition, the initial requirement is to clear the airway and give oxygen by face mask to relieve airway obstruction and hypoxia. Blood pressure should be recorded every 10 minutes with the patient in the lateral position. A 16- to 18-gauge IV line should be placed for drawing blood and administering drugs and fluids. An indwelling catheter should be placed in the bladder, and laboratory tests obtained as outlined in Box 15-3.

Box 15-3. Initial laboratory evaluation on a patient with preeclampsia

- **CBC, platelet count:** If abnormal order coagulation panel, LDH, and smear
- **Renal studies:** Serum BUN and creatinine, urinalysis, 24-hr urine for protein and creatinine
- **Liver function tests:** AST, ALT, and bilirubin

LDH, lactate dehydrogenase; BUN, blood urea nitrogen; AST, serum aspartate aminotransferase; ALT, serum alanine amino transferase.

Pharmacologic stabilization consists of preventing recurrent convulsions and controlling hypertension. Randomized, controlled trials have confirmed that magnesium sulfate is the most efficacious drug for preventing recurrent eclamptic seizures and has the best safety profile for the mother and fetus. The administration of IV magnesium sulfate for the treatment of eclamptic seizures is similar to its prophylactic use as outlined in Table 15-1, except that the loading dose is generally increased from 4 to 6 g. The maintenance dose remains 2 g/hour if renal function appears normal. If diazepam (Valium) is used in addition to magnesium sulfate, personnel skilled in intubation should be readily available in case maternal respiratory depression occurs. In general, it is desirable to avoid polypharmacy.

Eclamptic seizures often induce a fetal bradycardia that usually resolves after maternal stabilization and correction of hypoxia. It is very important to stabilize the mother as previously outlined before any attempt is made to deliver the infant either vaginally or by cesarean delivery. Induction of labor or cesarean section during the acute phase may aggravate the course of the disease. Once hypoxia is corrected, convulsions controlled, and the diastolic blood pressures brought down to the 90 to 100-mm Hg range, delivery should be expedited, preferably by the vaginal route. If this is not feasible, cesarean delivery is indicated.

PROPHYLAXIS

Much more research into the genetic and molecular mechanisms of preeclampsia needs to be carried out before effective methods of prevention can be developed.

Randomized trials have failed to show any significant benefit from either low-dose aspirin or calcium for the prevention of preeclampsia. Preliminary studies suggest that antioxidants, such as vitamin C and vitamin E, or linoleic acid combined with calcium may be efficacious in decreasing the occurrence of preeclampsia in selected groups; however, much larger trials are needed.

MANAGEMENT OF CHRONIC HYPERTENSION

The major goals in the management of chronic hypertension in pregnancy are to control hypertension and to detect the development of superimposed preeclampsia in the mother and IUGR in the fetus. In the patient with uncomplicated hypertension whose blood pressures are well controlled and who does not show signs of superimposed preeclampsia or fetal growth restriction, the outcome for both the mother and fetus should be good.

When a woman with chronic hypertension is first seen during the pregnancy it is important to review previous records to determine whether she has essential hypertension or a secondary cause of high blood pressure. If no previous evaluations have been done, it may be appropriate to rule out some of the more common endocrinologic, renal, or cardiovascular causes of hypertension. Baseline laboratory tests similar to those outlined in Box 15-3, with the addition of an electrocardiogram (ECG), may be useful. The purpose of these tests is to establish a baseline should the patient later develop superimposed preeclampsia, as well as to look for evidence of end organ dysfunction.

It is important to review the antihypertensive medications being taken and to discontinue any that are potentially teratogenic. **There is little evidence that lowering blood pressures below the 140/90 to 150/100-mm Hg range benefits the pregnancy.** In fact, lowering the blood pressure too much may result in decreased uterine perfusion pressure and iatrogenic fetal growth restriction. **In many women, blood pressures will decrease to normal in the 2nd trimester and no antihypertensive medication will be needed.**

As a general rule, the safest antihypertensive medication should be used at the lowest possible dose needed to keep blood pressures about 140/90 mm Hg. Methyldopa is considered to be the safest antihypertensive medication in pregnancy, and calcium channel blockers and labetalol are also considered to be safe. **Angiotensin-converting enzyme inhibitors and angiotensin II receptor blockers should be avoided at all stages of pregnancy because of potential fetal toxicity.** Beta blockers should be used with caution because they may cause fetal growth restriction and may affect the interpretation of the NST. In addition to pharmacologic control of blood pressure, the foundations of conservative management also include reduced physical activity and bed rest.

Because these pregnancies have a high incidence of IUGR, both early and serial ultrasonic examinations are indicated. The early ultrasonogram (16 to 20 weeks) is primarily for the assessment of fetal anomalies and confirmation of pregnancy dates, whereas serial ultrasonic examinations (every 3 to 4 weeks after 24 weeks) are of great assistance in detecting growth restriction. Depending on the clinical circumstances, periodic fetal monitoring with bio-

physical profiles may start as early as 26 to 28 weeks and should be commenced by 36 weeks in all hypertensive patients.

A significant increase in hypertension or the development of proteinuria in a previously non-proteinuric patient with chronic hypertension are likely signs of superimposed preeclampsia. The incidence of superimposed preeclampsia varies from 15% to 25%. These patients should undergo repeat laboratory evaluation, as outlined in Box 15-3. Management should follow that outlined for severe preeclampsia.

The timing of delivery in the chronic hypertensive patient depends on the clinical circumstances. **For patients without evidence of fetal growth restriction in whom the blood pressure is well controlled and no signs of superimposed preeclampsia are present, a full-term gestation may be allowed, provided that fetal well-being is normal.** Any progression beyond the 40th week should be very carefully considered and probably avoided. The presence of growth restriction or blood pressure deterioration or the advent of proteinuria may dictate earlier delivery. If delivery is desirable but not imperative prior to 37 weeks, confirmation of fetal lung maturity should be obtained. **The route of delivery should be vaginal in the absence of obstetric reasons for cesarean section.**

SEQUELAE AND OUTCOME

Uncomplicated preeclampsia or eclampsia in the primigravid patient carries essentially no long-term maternal sequelae. Such patients are at no greater risk of subsequent development of hypertensive cardiovascular disease than any other individual. However they do experience a higher rate of preeclampsia in subsequent pregnancies, especially if they had a pregnancy complicated by severe preterm preeclampsia. **The female offspring of preeclamptic women experience an increased risk of preeclampsia in their own pregnancies,** providing evidence of a genetic basis to the disease.

Similarly, pregnancy does not seem to affect the subsequent course in a patient with chronic hypertension. Some of the more serious complications of preeclampsia, such as cerebrovascular accidents and renal failure, may have long-term maternal sequelae. In contrast, **women with gestational hypertension seem to have a higher incidence of developing chronic hypertension later in life.**

Overall, the mortality rate in women with hypertensive disease of pregnancy varies according to the severity of the disease, socioeconomic level, and quality of care received. Although at present there is no proven way of preventing preeclampsia, accessible, high quality prenatal care should prevent the majority of severe complications associated with the disease.

Fetal and neonatal sequelae are more difficult to determine because some of the morbidity and mortality associated with these hypertensive syndromes are related to IUGR, prematurity, and acute and chronic fetal distress. All of these may have long-term CNS effects.

Suggested Reading

American College of Obstetricians and Gynecologists: Chronic hypertension in pregnancy. ACOG Practice Bulletin No. 29. Clinical Management Guidelines for Obstetrician-Gynecologists, Washington, DC, ACOG, 2001.

American College of Obstetricians and Gynecologists: Diagnosis and management of pre-eclampsia and eclampsia. ACOG Practice Bulletin No. 33. Clinical Management Guidelines for Obstetrician-Gynecologists, Washington, DC, ACOG, 2002.

Joint National Committee: The sixth report of the Joint National Committee on Prevention, Detection, Evaluation, and Treatment of High Blood Pressure (JNC VI). Arch Intern Med 157:2413–2446, 1997.

Mackay AP, Berg CJ, Atrash HK: Pregnancy-related mortality from pre-eclampsia and eclampsia. Obstet Gynecol 533–538, 2001.

Working Group Report on High Blood Pressure in Pregnancy: National High Blood Pressure Education Program. NIH Publication No. 00-3029, 2000.

16 Rhesus Isoimmunization

Khalil Tabsh and Nancy Theroux

Rhesus (Rh) isoimmunization is an immunologic disorder that occurs in a pregnant, Rh-negative patient carrying an Rh-positive fetus. The immunologic system in the mother is stimulated to produce antibodies to the Rh antigen, which then cross the placenta and destroy fetal red blood cells.

PATHOPHYSIOLOGY

A person who lacks the specific Rh antigen on the surface of the red blood cells is called "Rh-negative," and an individual with the antigen is considered "Rh-positive." **A number of antigens make up the Rh complex, including C, D, E, c, e, and other variants, such as D^u antigen.** More than 90% of cases of Rh isoimmunization are due to D antigens. Therefore, this chapter is mainly limited to a discussion of the D antigen, although the same principles apply to any other antigen-antibody combination.

Among black Americans, about 8% are Rh-negative, whereas among white Americans, about 14% are Rh-negative. **When Rh-negative patients are exposed to Rh antigen, they may become sensitized.** Two mechanisms are proposed for this sensitization. The most likely mechanism is the occurrence of an undetected placental leak of fetal red blood cells into the maternal circulation during pregnancy. The other proposal is the "grandmother" theory. This theory suggests that an Rh-negative woman may have been sensitized from birth by receiving enough Rh-positive cells from her mother during her own delivery to produce an antibody response.

In general, two exposures to the Rh antigen are required to produce any significant sensitization, unless the first exposure is massive. The first exposure leads to primary sensitization, whereas the second causes an anamnestic response leading to the rapid production of immunoglobulins, which can cause a "transfusion reaction" or hemolytic disease of the fetus during pregnancy.

The initial response to exposure to Rh antigen is the production of IgM antibodies for a short period of time, followed by the production of IgG antibodies that are capable of crossing the placenta. If the fetus has the Rh antigen, these antibodies will coat the fetal red blood cells and cause hemolysis. If the hemolysis is mild, the fetus can compensate by increasing the rate of erythropoiesis to maintain its red cell mass. If the hemolysis is severe, it can lead to profound anemia, resulting in hydrops fetalis from congestive cardiac failure and intrauterine fetal death.

The fetal and maternal circulations are normally separated by the placental "barrier." Small hemorrhages occur in either direction across the intact placenta throughout pregnancy. With advancing gestational age, the incidence and size of these transplacental hemorrhages increase. **Most immunizations occur at the time of delivery, and antibodies appear either during the postpartum period or following exposure to the antigen in the next pregnancy.**

If a pattern of mild, moderate, or severe disease has been established with two or more previous pregnancies, the disease tends either to be of the same severity or to become progressively more severe with subsequent pregnancies. **If a woman has a history of fetal hydrops with a previous pregnancy, the risk of hydrops with a subsequent pregnancy is about 90%.** Hydrops usually develops at the same time as, or earlier than, in the previous pregnancy.

INCIDENCE

Although transplacental hemorrhage is very common, the incidence of Rh immunization within 6 months of the delivery of the first Rh-positive, ABO-compatible infant is only about 8%. In addition, the incidence of sensitization with the development of a secondary immune response prior to the next Rh-positive pregnancy is 8%. Therefore, the overall risk of immunization for the second full-term, Rh-positive, ABO-compatible pregnancy is about 1 in 6 pregnancies. The risk of Rh sensitization following an ABO-incompatible, Rh-positive pregnancy is only about 2%. The protection against immunization in ABO-incompatible pregnancies is due to the destruction of the ABO-incompatible cells in the maternal circulation and the removal of the red blood cell debris by the liver.

Transplacental hemorrhage may occur after spontaneous or induced abortions. The incidence of immunization following spontaneous abortion is 3.5%, whereas that following induced abortion is 5.5%. The risk is low in the first 8 weeks, but it rises to significant levels by 12 weeks' gestation. The risk of immunization following amniocentesis or ectopic pregnancy is less than 1%. All Rh-negative patients at 8 weeks' or more gestation should receive prophylactic Rh$_O$ D-immune globulin (Rh$_O$-GAM) following spontaneous or induced abortion, invasive gynecologic procedures, or abdominal trauma.

RECOGNITION OF THE PREGNANCY AT RISK

A blood sample from every pregnant woman should be sent at the first prenatal visit for determination of the blood group and Rh type and for antibody screening. In Rh-negative patients, the blood group and Rh status of the father of the baby should be determined. If the father is Rh-positive, his Rh genotype and ABO status should be determined. This may be done by testing the father's red blood cells with the reagents available for the antigens D, E, C, e, and c. If he is homozygous for the D antigen, every fetus he fathers will be Rh-positive and could potentially be affected. If he is heterozygous, only half of his children will be affected. Information regarding the zygosity of the father is of value in absolutely predicting the presence or absence of the Rh antigen in the fetus if the father is homozygous and in signaling the potential need for fetal antigen testing if the father is heterozygous. Approximately 56% of Rh positive whites are heterozygous for the Rh D antigen. If it is not possible to test the antigen status and zygosity of the father, it must be assumed that he is antigen positive.

The Rh-negative woman whose partner is Rh-positive and whose initial antibody screen is negative should have a repeat antibody titer at 28 weeks' gestation prior to receiving Rh$_O$-GAM prophylactically. The risk of transplacental hemorrhage increases at the time of delivery, especially with cesarean section or manual removal of the placenta. At delivery, cord blood must be sent for determination of the fetal blood group, Rh type, and for a direct Coombs' test. If a transplacental hemorrhage of greater than 30 mL of blood is suspected, a Kleihauer-Betke test is helpful in determining the volume of the hemorrhage.

MATERNAL RH-ANTIBODY TITER

Anti-D antibody titers generally provide limited information regarding the severity of fetal hemolysis in Rh disease. However, many centers continue to utilize anti-D antibody titers to help guide their decision making regarding the initiation of testing procedures (e.g., amniocentesis, percutaneous umbilical blood sampling). The American College of Obstetricians and Gynecologists (ACOG) and other independent researchers have recommended that, in an initially immunized pregnancy, the fetus is not in serious jeopardy if the titer remains below 1:16. In patients with a positive titer less than 1:16, repeat titers should be obtained every 2 to 4 weeks. If the titer rises to 1.16 or greater, invasive testing should be considered. The timing and methods of invasive testing will depend on the current clinical status of the fetus, the gestational age, and the patient's obstetric history.

AMNIOTIC FLUID SPECTROPHOTOMETRY

Analysis of amniotic fluid remains the most frequently used method of gauging the severity of fetal hemolysis. There is an excellent correlation between the amount of biliary pigment in the amniotic fluid and the fetal hematocrit, beginning at 27 weeks' gestation.

The most likely source of bilirubin in the amniotic fluid is tracheal and pulmonary efflux with some transudate from the umbilical and placental vessels. Because of the small concentrations found in the amniotic fluid, spectrophotometric analysis is the most widely used technique for estimating amniotic fluid bilirubin concentration.

The optical density deviation (ΔOD) at 450μ from a baseline drawn between the optical density values at 365 and 550μ measures the amniotic fluid unconjugated bilirubin level, which in turn correlates with the cord blood hemoglobin of the newborn at birth.

Bilirubin is oxidized to colorless pigments when it is exposed to light; therefore, the fluid should be protected from light. Heme pigments and meconium may cause falsely high spectrophotometric values.

Bilirubin is normally found in amniotic fluid in a concentration that gradually diminishes toward term. For predictive interpretation, Liley devised a spectrophotometric graph based on the correlation of cord blood hemoglobin concentrations at birth and the amniotic fluid change in optical density at 450μ. Using this method, he was able to establish predictive zones for mild, moderate, and severe disease. **The Liley chart (Figure 16-1) can be used to determine, with accuracy, the severity of the disease and the appropriate management, beginning at 27 weeks' gestation.** The Queenan curve, a modified Liley curve with four zones instead of three, is used as a predictive tool in some centers from 14 to 40 weeks gestation (Figure 16-2).

TECHNIQUE OF AMNIOCENTESIS

Ultrasonically guided amniocentesis carries very little risk to the fetus or mother and is the only appropriate method for obtaining an amniotic fluid specimen. An ultrasonic examination is performed to localize a pocket of amniotic fluid far enough away from the fetus and placenta to obtain a sample safely. A 22-gauge spinal needle is inserted and 10 mL of fluid is aspirated utilizing a sterile technique. The fluid is transferred to a dark or foil-wrapped tube to prevent deterioration owing to light exposure and is sent for assessment of the ΔOD 450. The incidence of fetal mortality from amniocentesis for hemolytic disease is reported to be less than 1:900 in experienced centers. Of potential concern is the procedure-related risk of fetomaternal hemorrhage, which may worsen the severity of the sensitization. **The incidence of fetomaternal hemorrhage is reported to be 8.4% to 11% per procedure.**

ULTRASONIC DETECTION OF RH SENSITIZATION

Serial ultrasonic examinations of a woman with a fetus at risk for hemolytic disease can be a useful adjunct to amniocentesis in confirming fetal well-being and determining the advent of fetal hydrops. The examination should include a routine fetal assessment plus a determination of placental size and thickness and hepatic size. **Both the placenta and the fetal liver are enlarged with hydrops. Fetal hydrops is easily diagnosed by the characteristic appearance of one or more of the following: ascites, pleural effusion, pericardial effusion, or skin edema.** Appearance of any of these factors during an ultrasonic examination eliminates the need for diagnostic amniocentesis and necessitates therapeutic intervention based on fetal gestational age.

Doppler assessment of peak velocity in the fetal middle cerebral artery (MCA) may prove to be the most valuable ultrasonic tool for detecting fetal anemia. A value above 1.5 multiples of the median for gestational age is considered predictive. For accurate evaluation, the Doppler gate is placed over the fetal MCA just as it bifurcates from the carotid siphon. Color Doppler is clearly advantageous for this examination. **After 35 weeks' gestation, this test may produce a higher false-positive rate (Figure 16-3).**

PERCUTANEOUS UMBILICAL BLOOD SAMPLING

Advances in fetal interventional techniques and high-resolution ultrasonography have made direct fetal blood sampling the most accurate method for the diagnosis of fetal hemolytic disease. **Percutaneous umbilical blood sampling (PUBS) can allow measurement of fetal hemoglobin, hematocrit, blood gases, pH, and bilirubin levels.** The hematologic values for normal fetuses from 15 to 30 weeks' gestation are listed in Table 16-1. The technique for fetal blood sampling is similar to that described for fetal intravenous transfusion discussed later in this chapter. One drawback to this diagnostic procedure is that it requires expertise above and beyond that required for amniocentesis. **The major risk is fetal exsanguination from tears in placental vessels,** but when performed by an experienced practitioner, the risk of this complication is only 2% or less. **However, there is a greater risk of fetomaternal hemorrhage,**

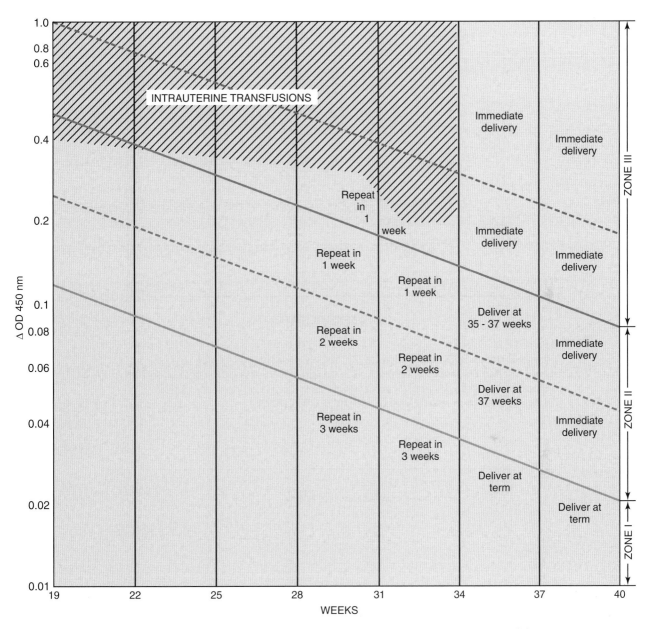

Figure 16-1. Modified Liley chart used to determine the appropriate management of the patient with isoimmunization. The ΔOD 450 nm level in the amniotic fluid at a given weeks' gestation determines whether fetal transfusion or delivery is advisable.

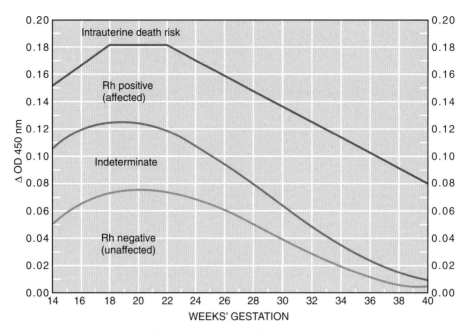

Figure 16-2. Queenan curve for ΔOD 450 values for the management of the patient with isoimmunization. OD, optical density; Rh, rhesus. *Adapted from Queenan JT, Tomai TP, Ural SH, et al: Deviations in amniotic fluid optical density at a wavelength of 450 nm in Rh-immunized pregnancies from 14 to 40 weeks' gestation: A proposal for clinical management. Am J Obstet Gynecol 168:1370–1376, 1993.*

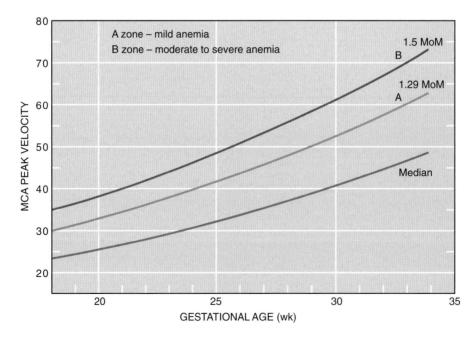

Figure 16-3. Middle cerebral artery (MCA) Doppler peak velocities based on gestational age. MoM, multiples of the median. *Data from Moise KJ, Jr: Management of Rhesus alloisoimmunization. Obstet Gynecol 100(3):600–611, 2002.*

Table 16-1. Hematologic values for normal fetuses*

Hematologic Value	GESTATIONAL AGE (WK)					
	15	16–17	18–20	21–22	23–25	26–30
Hgb, g/dL	10.9 ± 0.7	12.5 ± 0.8	11.48 ± 0.78	12.29 ± 0.89	12.4 ± 0.77	13.36 ± 1.18
RBCs, $\times 10^9$/L	2.43 ± 0.26	2.68 ± 0.21	2.66 ± 0.29	2.97 ± 0.27	3.06 ± 0.27	3.52 ± 0.32
MCV, fL (± 1)	143 ± 8	143 ± 12	133.9 ± 8.83	1.130 ± 6.17	126.2 ± 6.23	118.2 ± 5.7

Data from American College of Obstetricians and Gynecologists: Management of isoimmunization in pregnancy. Technical Bulletin No. 148. Washington, DC, ACOG, 1990.
Hgb, hemoglobin; RBCs, red blood cells; MCV, mean corpuscular volume.
*Values are for normal fetuses from 15 to 30 weeks' estimated gestational age.

reported to be as high as 40%. Percutaneous umbilical blood sampling should not be a first-line method of assessing fetal status unless clearly indicated.

DETECTING FETOMATERNAL HEMORRHAGE

The Kleihauer-Betke test is dependent on the fact that adult hemoglobin is more readily eluted through the cell membrane in the presence of acid than is fetal hemoglobin (HbF). The maternal blood is fixed on a slide with ethanol (80%) and treated with a citrate phosphate buffer to remove the adult hemoglobin. After staining with hematoxylin and eosin, the fetal cells can readily be distinguished from the empty maternal cells. All cells are then counted, and an estimate of the extent of the fetal to maternal hemorrhage (measured in milliliters) is made on the basis of the following equation:

No. of fetal cells counted/No. of maternal cells counted = Estimated fetal blood volume (mL)/Estimated maternal blood volume (mL)

NEWER TECHNIQUES FOR EVALUATING FETAL RH STATUS

In the last decade, amniocentesis has become the most commonly employed method to test fetal blood type in cases of a heterozygous paternal genotype. Most laboratories offering fetal red cell antigen typing on amniotic cells require an accompanying paternal blood sample, and with the recent discovery of an Rh D pseudogene in 21% of blacks, a maternal blood sample should also be provided. Chorionic villus sampling has been utilized to determine fetal blood type but is discouraged because of the potential for worsening fetal disease if the fetus is Rh D positive.

Flow cytometry has been successfully reported in sorting fetal cells from maternal blood. **DNA amplification** using a single fetal nucleated erythrocyte can be used to determine fetal Rh D blood type. **Free fetal DNA in maternal plasma or serum has also been utilized to detect Rh D sequences.**

CLINICAL MANAGEMENT OF THE Rh-SENSITIZED PATIENT

Because single ΔOD 450 values are helpful only if they are very high (zone III) or very low (zone I), serial sampling of amniotic fluid is generally indicated. The severity of hemolytic disease in the prior pregnancy provides an index for the timing of the first amniocentesis (Table 16-2). With serial sampling, one

Table 16-2. Guidelines for the timing of amniocentesis

Severity of Disease in Previous Pregnancies	Timing of First Amniocentesis (wk)
No disease	26–30
Mild-moderate: (delivery at 37–40 wk)	20–28
Severe without death (delivery at 34–37 wk)	20–25
Severely affected neonate with hydrops or stillbirth	20–24

of three trends will emerge. Falling ΔOD 450 values are indicative of a fetus that is either unaffected (e.g., Rh-negative) or very mildly affected. No intervention is indicated in these patients. If the ΔOD 450 is either stable or rising, frequent ΔOD 450 determinations are necessary. **If the ΔOD 450 enters zone II or III after 34 weeks' gestation, determination of fetal lung maturity and delivery is indicated. If this occurs prior to 34 weeks, however, delivery is best avoided** because of the risk of complications from prematurity. **In such cases, intrauterine transfusion is the treatment of choice** if the ΔOD 450 enters zone III. In addition to serial ΔOD 450 values, the timing of delivery should be based on the patient's obstetric history and fetal well-being assessed by nonstress testing, biophysical profiles, and fetal lung maturity testing. **The fetal lung maturity profile, including at least a lecithin-to-sphingomyelin (L:S) ratio and a phosphatidylglycerol (PG) level, will help determine the optimum time for delivery.**

INTRAUTERINE TRANSFUSION

Intrauterine transfusion, initially introduced in 1963 as an intraperitoneal transfusion, has markedly changed the prognosis for severely affected fetuses. **The goal is to transfuse fresh group O, Rh-negative packed red blood cells.** In addition to routine blood screening, the blood for transfusion is irradiated, washed, processed through a leukocyte-poor filter, and screened for cytomegalovirus. Curare is usually injected directly into the fetal thigh with a 22-gauge spinal needle prior to transfusion, regardless of method, to immobilize the fetus during the procedure. Repeat transfusions are generally scheduled at 1 to 3 week intervals. The final transfusion is typically performed at 34 to 35 weeks' gestation. In general, the fetus is delivered when the lungs are mature.

The overall survival rate following intrauterine transfusion is about 85%. In fetuses with no evidence of hydrops, the survival rate is about 90%, and for fetuses with hydrops prior to the transfusion, the survival rate is about 75%.

Fetal Intraperitoneal Transfusion

Red blood cells are absorbed via the subdiaphragmatic lymphatics and proceed via the right lymphatic duct into the fetal intravascular compartment. After transfusion, the absorption of blood may be monitored with serial transverse ultrasonic scans of the fetal abdomen.

In nonhydroptic fetuses, the blood should be absorbed within 7 to 9 days. In the presence of hydrops, absorption is variable and may necessitate removal of ascitic fluid at the time of transfusion.

Under real-time ultrasonic guidance, a 20-gauge spinal needle is inserted through the mother's abdomen into the fetal peritoneal cavity. The correct positioning of the needle is determined by injection of a small amount of normal saline and carbon dioxide, which can be easily visualized with ultrasonography. The red blood cells are slowly injected manually in 10-mL aliquots through an extension catheter attached to the spinal needle. If fetal bradycardia occurs at any time during the procedure, the transfusion is terminated.

For intraperitoneal transfusions, the volume to be infused is based on the following formula:

$$\text{Volume} = [\text{gestational age (weeks)} - 20] \times 10$$

For example, a 30-week fetus would require a 100-mL transfusion (30 weeks − 20 × 10 = 100 mL).

Intravascular Transfusion

Because many fetuses are not subjected to transfusion until ascites is present, intravenous fetal transfusion has become increasingly popular. In addition, transfusion into the peritoneal cavity can result in fetal bradycardia or a pseudosinusoidal fetal heart rate pattern following the procedure because of compression at the site of insertion of the umbilical cord.

Under ultrasonic guidance, a 22-gauge spinal needle is inserted into the umbilical vein or the hepatic part of the umbilical portal venous system. If the umbilical vein is used, the preferred sites are either at the placental cord insertion or into a loop of umbilical cord. The volume of blood to be transfused is based on the fetal body weight, as determined by ultrasonography.

OTHER MODES OF THERAPY

Maternal plasmapheresis may be helpful in severe erythroblastosis when intrauterine transfusions are not successful, but perinatal outcome with this technique has not been impressive. **Phenobarbital** has been used to induce fetal hepatic microsomal glucuronosyltransferase activity, thereby increasing uptake and excretion of bilirubin by the liver. Treatment with phenobarbital is initiated 2 to 3 weeks before delivery.

PREVENTION OF RHESUS ISOIMMUNIZATION

Because Rh isoimmunization occurs in response to exposure of an Rh-negative mother to the Rh antigen, the mainstay for prevention is the avoidance of maternal exposure to the antigen. Rh$_O$-GAM diminishes the availability of the Rh antigen to the maternal immune system, although the exact mechanism by which it prevents Rh isoimmunization is not well understood.

Rh$_O$-GAM is prepared from fractionated human plasma obtained from hyperreactive sensitized donors. The plasma is screened for hepatitis B surface antigen and anti-HIV-1, the antibody to the acquired immunodeficiency syndrome (AIDS) virus. The globulin is available in several dosages for intramuscular injection. Since the advent of its use in 1967, Rh immune globulin has dramatically reduced the incidence of Rh isoimmunization.

Because the greatest risk for fetal-to-maternal hemorrhage occurs during labor and delivery, Rh immune globulin was initially administered only during the immediate postpartum period. This resulted in a 1% to 2% failure rate, thought to be due to exposure of the mother to fetal red blood cells during the antepartum period. **The indications for the use of Rh immune globulin have therefore been broadened to include any antepartum event (such as amniocentesis) that may increase the risk of transplacental hemorrhage. The routine prophylactic administration of Rh immune globulin at 28 weeks' gestation is now the standard of care.** Despite adherence to this suggested Rh immune globulin protocol, 0.27% of primiparous Rh-negative patients still become sensitized.

INDICATIONS FOR ADMINISTRATION OF RH$_O$-GAM

The following provides a practical approach to the administration of Rh immune globulin to an Rh-negative patient with no Rh antibodies.

During a normal pregnancy, 300 μg of Rh immune globulin is administered at 28 weeks' gestation, following testing for sensitization with an indirect Coombs' test. A 300-μg dose is administered following amniocentesis at any gestational age. If a fetomaternal hemorrhage is suspected at any time during the pregnancy, a Kleihauer-Betke test should be performed. If positive, **Rh immune globulin is administered in a dose of 10 μg/mL of fetal** blood that entered the maternal circulation. Following an uncomplicated delivery, 300 μg of Rh immune globulin is given within 72 hours. If a larger than normal fetal-to-maternal hemorrhage is suspected, such as may occur in patients with abruptio placentae or those requiring cesarean section or manual removal of the placenta, a Kleihauer-Betke determination should be performed after delivery and the appropriate dose of the Rh immune globulin determined.

Establishment of fetal circulation occurs at approximately 4 weeks' gestation, and the presence of the Rh$_O$ D antigen has been demonstrated as early as 38 days following conception. Consequently, Rh isoimmunization can occur at any time during pregnancy, from the early first trimester on. Because fetal erythrocytes can be readily detected in the maternal blood following induced or spontaneous abortion, **50 μg of Rh immune globulin should be given to all Rh-negative women following any type of abortion.**

Fetal erythrocytes have been demonstrated in the maternal circulation following rupture of a tubal pregnancy. Consequently, **Rh immune globulin should be given to an Rh-negative woman with an ectopic pregnancy.** Because chorionic villi in gestational trophoblastic disease are avascular and are devoid of fetal erythrocytes, **Rh immune globulin is probably not necessary following molar pregnancy.** At least one case of sensitization following a molar pregnancy, however, has been reported.

Irregular Antibodies

Although Rh isoimmunization is the most common cause of hemolytic disease in the newborn, other blood group systems may be involved, such as Kell, Duffy, or Kidd. For example, Kell antigen may elicit a strong IgG response similar to Rh isoimmunization.

Suggested Reading

American College of Obstetricians and Gynecologists: Prevention of RhD alloimmunization in pregnancy, Practice Bulletin No. 4. Washington, DC, ACOG, 1990.

Mari G, Deti L, Oz U, et al: Accurate prediction of fetal hemoglobin by Doppler ultrasonography: Obstet Gynecol 99:589–593, 2002.

Moise KJ: Management of rhesus alloimmunization in pregnancy. Obstet Gynecol 100(3):600–611, 2002.

Common Medical and Surgical Conditions Complicating Pregnancy

Joseph C. Gambone, J. George Moore, and Brian J. Koos

The more common medical, infectious, and surgical disorders that may complicate pregnancy are covered in this chapter.

ENDOCRINE DISORDERS

Diabetes mellitus and thyroid disease are the two most common endocrine disorders complicating pregnancy.

DIABETES MELLITUS
Incidence and Classification

The incidence of diabetes mellitus in pregnancy is less than 0.5%. In addition to the uniform classification of diabetes during the nonpregnant state (Table 17-1), **White's classification of diabetes during pregnancy** is commonly used and is more descriptive (Table 17-2).

Complications

Fetal and maternal complications associated with diabetes mellitus during pregnancy are listed in Table 17-3.

Diagnosis

Screening for gestational diabetes is generally performed between 24 and 28 weeks of gestation. This timing will identify most gestational diabetics while providing several weeks of therapy to reduce potentially adverse consequences of this disorder.

If the 1-hour screening (50 g oral glucose) plasma glucose exceeds 200 mg/dL, a glucose tolerance test may not be required, particularly if the fasting plasma glucose level exceeds 95 mg/dL. However, most gravidas with abnormally high 1-hour glucose screens ($\geq$140 mg/dL) should have a 3-hour glucose tolerance test (100 g oral glucose loading), which is generally preceded by 3 days of a diet containing at least 300 g of carbohydrate (Table 17-4). The patient is considered to have A_1 gestational diabetes if at least two values are abnormal. The pregnant woman is classified as A_2 should the fasting and/or postprandial plasma glucose concentrations remain abnormally high despite appropriate dietary interventions. These gravidas will require hypoglycemic agents to maintain normal serum glucose levels.

Table 17-1. Classification of diabetes mellitus (nonpregnant)	
Type 1	Ketone prone (juvenile diabetes)
Type 2	Ketone resistant (NIDDM)*
Diabetes-Associated Condition (Impaired Glucose Tolerance)	
	Cystic fibrosis
	Cortisone-induced
	Cushing's disease

*NIDDM, Non–insulin-dependent diabetes mellitus.

Management

The diabetic team. Management of gestational diabetes requires a team approach involving patient teaching and counseling, medical-nursing assessments and interventions, strategies to achieve maternal euglycemia, and avoidance of fetal-neonatal compromise. Ideally, this team should include the patient, obstetrician, clinical nurse specialist, dietitian, psychosocial worker, and neonatologist. **The most significant change in diabetic management during pregnancy has been the inclusion of the patient as an active participant in formulating management strategies.**

Achieving euglycemia. The importance of strict metabolic control before and during pregnancy to decrease the incidence of congenital anomalies, perinatal morbidity, and perinatal mortality has been established. Diet, insulin, and exercise must be regulated to achieve euglycemia.

DIET. Caloric requirements are calculated on the basis of ideal body weight (see electronic calculator for ideal body weight in PDA): 30 kcal/kg for those patients 80% to 120% of ideal body weight; 35 to 40 kcal/kg for those <80% of ideal body weight; and 24 kcal/kg for gravidas who are 120% to 150% of ideal body weight. The diet is comprised of about 50% carbohydrate, 20% protein, and 20% fat. The diet should also contain a generous amount of fiber. The caloric intake is divided into 25% for breakfast, 30% at lunch, 30% at dinner, and 15% at a bedtime snack (for those on insulin).

THERAPY. Oral hypoglycemic agents that cross the placenta are not recommended for pregnant women because of the risks of teratogenesis and neonatal hypoglycemia. However, oral hypoglycemic agents (e.g., glyburide), which do not enter the fetal circulation in appreciable quantities, have been used successfully to treat gestational diabetes after the 1st trimester.

Insulin has been used predominantly to maintain euglycemia in pregnant women. Short-acting, intermediate-acting, or long-acting insulin may be used in a combination of dosage schedules to affect maternal euglycemia. The peak action of short-acting (regular) insulin is about 4 hours, intermediate-acting insulin about 12 hours, and long-acting insulin 14 to 20 hours. A combination of short-acting and intermediate-acting insulin is usually given as a split morning and evening dose. A method for calculating insulin dosage is shown in Box 17-1.

EXERCISE. Diabetic patients should be encouraged to exercise for about half an hour after meals. Use of a stationary bicycle or mild to moderate aerobic exercise is adequate. A hospitalized, sedentary patient who achieves euglycemia during her hospital stay may encounter frequent episodes of hypoglycemia once she is discharged and returns to her usual daily activities.

Antepartum Obstetric Management

Aside from achieving euglycemia, adequate surveillance should be maintained during pregnancy to avoid maternal complications and to ensure fetal growth and development. A detailed obstetric ultrasound study,

---

Table 17-2. White's classification of diabetes in pregnancy

Class	Description	Therapy
A_1	Gestational diabetes; glucose intolerance developing during pregnancy; fasting blood glucose normal	Diet alone
A_2	Gestational diabetes with fasting plasma glucose >105 mg/dL; or 2-hr postprandial plasma glucose >120 mg/dL	Diet and insulin
B	Overt diabetes developing after ago 20 yr and duration <10 yr	Diet and insulin
C	Overt diabetes developing before age 20 yr or duration >10 yr	Diet and insulin
D	Overt diabetes developing between the ages of 10 and 19 yr, or duration 10–19 yr, or background retinopathy	Diet and insulin
F	Overt diabetes at any age or duration with nephropathy	Diet and insulin
R	Overt diabetes at any age or duration with proliferative retinopathy	Diet and insulin
H	Overt diabetes at any age or duration with arteriosclerotic heart disease	Diet and insulin

Table 17-3. Maternal and fetal complications of diabetes mellitus

Entity	Monitoring
MATERNAL COMPLICATIONS	
Obstetric Complications	
Polyhydramnios	Close prenatal surveillance; ultrasonography
Preeclampsia	
Diabetic Emergencies	
Hypoglycemia	Blood glucose monitoring; insulin and dietary adjustment; check for infection,
Ketoacidosis	including urine culture every 6 wk
Diabetic coma	
Vascular and End-Organ Involvement or Deterioration	
Cardiac	Electrocardiogram first visit and as needed
Renal	Renal function studies, first visit and as needed
Ophthalmic	Funduscopic evaluation, first visit and as needed
Peripheral vascular	Check for ulcers, foot sores; noninvasive Doppler studies as needed
Neurologic	
Peripheral neuropathy	Neurologic and gastrointestinal consultations as needed
Gastrointestinal disturbance	
FETAL COMPLICATIONS	
Macrosomia with traumatic delivery	Repeat pelvic ultrasonography prior to delivery
Delayed Organ Maturity	
(pulmonary, hepatic, neurologic,	Amniocentesis for lung profile
pituitary-thyroid axis)	
Congenital Anomalies	
Cardiovascular	Prior to 22 wk gestation, maternal serum α-fetoprotein; HbA_{1c} monthly; pelvic
Neural tube defects	ultrasonography and fetal echocardiogram; amniocentesis and genetic
Caudal regression syndrome	counseling, if necessary
Intrauterine Growth Restriction	
Intrauterine fetal death	Repeat ultrasonography every 4 wk; NST and OCT; biophysical profile weekly
Abnormal FHR patterns	or biweekly
Small-for-dates babies	

FHR, fetal heart rate; NST, nonstress test; OCT, oxytocin challenge test.

Table 17-4. Three-hour glucose tolerance test*

Test	Whole Blood (mg/dL)	Maximal Normal Plasma Glucose (mg/dL)
Fasting	90	105
1 hr	165	195
2 hr	145	165
3 hr	125	145

*100 g of oral glucose given after an overnight fast.

fetal echocardiogram, and maternal serum α-fetoprotein level should be obtained at 16 to 20 weeks to alert the obstetrician to the presence of congenital malformations in the fetus. Maternal renal, cardiac, and ophthalmic functions are closely monitored. **The glycosylated hemoglobin levels (HbA_{1C}) should be obtained at the first prenatal visit, which is preferably scheduled early in the 1st trimester. Individuals with significantly elevated values (>8.5%) should be particularly targeted for careful ultrasonic assessment of congenital anomalies.** Regular electronic, biochemical, and ultrasonographic fetal monitoring should be performed. For diabetic classes

---

> ### Box 17-1. Method for calculation of starting dose of insulin
>
> INSULIN UNITS = BODY WEIGHT (KG)
> ×0.6 (1st trimester)
> ×0.7 (2nd trimester)
> ×0.8 (3rd trimester)
>
> DOSAGE SCHEDULE: GIVE 2/3 IN AM AND
> 1/3 IN PM
> AM: 2/3 NPH, 1/3 regular
> PM: 1/2 NPH, 1/2 regular

A, B, and C, fetal macrosomia is not uncommon and should be investigated, whereas for classes D, E, and F, fetal growth restriction occurs more commonly.

Timing of Delivery

Advances in the management of the diabetic patient, such as tight metabolic control, availability of the fetal lung profile, and fetal assessment techniques, have generally obviated the need for preterm delivery (<37 weeks gestation). **If the maternal state is stable, blood glucose is in the euglycemic range, and fetal studies indicate continued growth of a healthy baby, delivery may be delayed until term and spontaneous onset of labor.** Earlier intervention is indicated if these conditions are not met. For macrosomic babies, increased birth trauma to both mother and fetus should be kept in mind. Cesarean delivery may be elected for large fetuses (>4000 g) or for a cervix that fails to respond to normal induction methods.

Intrapartum Management

Intrapartum management of a diabetic patient requires the establishment of maternal euglycemia during labor, which may be achieved by giving a continuous infusion of regular insulin in 5% dextrose at a rate of 0.5 to 2.0 U of insulin per hour. **Plasma glucose levels are measured every hour and insulin dosage adjusted accordingly to maintain a plasma glucose level of between 80 and 120 mg/dL.** In calculating the 24-hour insulin requirements, the ratio of insulin requirements to total caloric intake per day may be used as a rough estimate. This ratio multiplied by caloric intake during labor (~600 calories) yields an estimate of anticipated total insulin requirements for the day. Provided that plasma glucose is monitored frequently and insulin administered only when plasma glucose exceeds 120 mg/dL, not all insulin-dependent patients will require exogenous insulin (in multiples of 2 U) during labor. Continuous electronic **fetal heart rate monitoring is recommended for all diabetic patients.**

Postpartum Period

After delivery of the fetus and placenta, insulin requirements drop sharply because the placenta, which is the source of many insulin antagonists, has been removed. Most insulin-dependent diabetic patients do not require exogenous insulin for the first 48 to 72 hours after delivery. **Plasma glucose levels should be obtained every 6 hours and regular insulin given when plasma glucose levels exceed 150 mg/dL.** Prior to hospital discharge, patients may be restarted on two-thirds of the prepregnancy insulin dosage, with adjustments made as necessary. Gestational diabetics (with class A_1 and A_2 disease) frequently do not need insulin therapy postpartum. A fasting blood glucose or a 75-g oral glucose tolerance test should be performed at 6 weeks postpartum.

Patients should be counseled about changes in diet. Except for gestational class A diabetics, the American Dietetic Association (ADA) diet with the same distribution of carbohydrates, proteins, and fat should be maintained. If the mother is breastfeeding, 500 calories/day should be added to the prepregnant diet.

Contraceptive counseling is an important aspect of total patient care, especially in the diabetic patient (see Chapter 27). Sterilization is recommended for consenting patients who desire permanent sterilization and those with advanced vascular involvement.

THYROID DISEASES
Normal Thyroid Physiology During Pregnancy

With the increase in glomerular filtration rate that occurs during pregnancy, the renal excretion of iodine increases and plasma inorganic iodine levels are nearly halved. Goiters due to iodine deficiency are not likely if plasma inorganic iodine levels are greater than 0.08 μg/dL. **Only patients with plasma inorganic iodine levels that are borderline before pregnancy show an increased incidence of goiter during pregnancy.** Inorganic iodine supplementation up to a total of 250 μg/day is sufficient to prevent goiter formation during pregnancy.

Thyroid function tests. The free thyroxine concentration is the only direct method of estimating thyroid function that compensates for changes in thyroxine-binding globulin (TBG) capacity. Although serum levels of bound triiodothyronine (T_3) and thyroxine (T_4) are increased during pregnancy, free thyroxine levels remain within the normal range. The uptake of triiodothyronine by resin (T_3 resin uptake), which is an indirect measure of T_4-binding capacity, tends to be in the hypothyroid range during pregnancy, an indication that more binding sites are available. Because serum T_4 level increases and the T_3 resin uptake decreases, the free T_4 index remains the same during pregnancy. Because determination of free T_4 levels is more expensive, **the free thyroxine index may be used as an indirect approximation of the free thyroxine concentration during pregnancy.** Values of thyroid function tests during pregnancy are shown in Table 17-5.

Fetal thyroid function. Prior to 10 weeks' gestation, no organic iodine is present in the fetal thyroid. By 11 to 12 weeks, the fetal thyroid is able to produce iodothyronines and T_4, and by 12 to 14 weeks it is able to concentrate iodine. **Fetal thyroid-stimulating hormone (TSH), T_4, and free thyroxine levels suggest that a mature, autonomous, thyroid-pituitary axis exists as early as 12 weeks' gestation.**

Placental transfer of thyroid hormone. Minimal transfer of T_4 and T_3 occurs across the placenta. Thyroid releasing hormone and thyroid hormone analogues, with smaller molecular weights, decreased protein binding, and increased fat solubility, cross the placental barrier much more easily and could potentially be used to affect the fetal status without producing maternal thyrotoxicosis.

Maternal Hyperthyroidism

The incidence of maternal thyrotoxicosis is about 1 per 500 pregnancies. It is accompanied by an increased incidence of prematurity, intrauterine growth restriction (IUGR), stillbirth, and neonatal morbidity and mortality. **Graves' disease, or toxic diffuse goiter, is the most common cause of hyperthyroidism associated with pregnancy.** Other causes of hyperthyroidism in pregnancy include hydatidiform mole and toxic nodular goiter. Patients with Graves' disease tend to have a remission during pregnancy and an exacerbation during the postpartum period. Evidence suggests that the increased immunologic tolerance during pregnancy may lead to a decrease in thyroid antibodies to account for any remission.

Clinical features. The clinical diagnosis of hyperthyroidism in pregnancy is difficult because many of the signs and symptoms of the hyperdynamic circulation associated with hyperthyroidism are present in a normal euthyroid pregnant individual. A resting pulse rate greater than 100 beats/minute that fails to slow with a Valsalva maneuver, eye changes, loss of weight, failure to gain weight despite normal or increased food intake, and heat intolerance are all helpful in making the clinical diagnosis.

Investigations. **The initial screening tests for a pregnant woman with possible hyperthyroidism include a serum free T_4 and TSH assays.** An elevated serum free T_4 level and a suppressed TSH level

Table 17-5. Thyroid function tests in nonpregnant women and in maternal and cord blood at term			
Test	Nonpregnant	Pregnant	Cord
Serum thyroxine (T_4) (μg/dL)	5–12	10–16	6–13
Free T_4 (ng/dL)	1.0–2.3	2.5–3.5	1.5–3.0
Serum triiodothyronine (T_3) (ng/dL)	110–230	150–250	40–60
Reverse T_3 (ng/dL)	15–30	35–65	80–360
Resin T_3 uptake (%)	20–30	10	10–15
Thyroxine-binding globulin (g/dL)	12–28	40–50	10–16
Serum thyroid-stimulating hormone (units/mL)	1.94	0–6	0–20

Modified from Burrow GN, Ferris T (eds): Medical Complications during Pregnancy. Philadelphia, WB Saunders, 1972, p 194.
Note: Absolute values for these may vary according to the method used, but the ratio between maternal and cord values should remain constant.

establish the diagnosis of hyperthyroidism. Occasionally, a free T_3 determination might be needed to diagnose T_3 thyrotoxicosis.

Therapy. Because radioactive iodine treatment is contraindicated during pregnancy, medical treatment is generally employed. The mainstay of antithyroid therapy is thioamides, which block the synthesis but not the release of thyroid hormone. It usually takes about 1 week for amelioration of symptoms and 4 to 6 weeks for full control. **Propylthiouracil and methimazole (Tapazole)** have been used interchangeably, although propylthiouracil has the added advantage of blocking conversion of T_4 to T_3.

Once a diagnosis of hyperthyroidism has been made, the patient should be started on 100 to 150 mg of propylthiouracil every 8 hours. The dose of antithyroid medication is lowered by half when free T4 levels start to decline. Antithyroid drugs are further reduced to the lowest dose that results in monthly free T4 levels within the upper range of normal (2.5 to 3.5 ng/dL) for pregnant women. In many cases, antithyroid therapy can be discontinued after 30 weeks of gestation.

Because propylthiouracil easily crosses the placenta, a major concern during maternal treatment is the development of fetal goiter and hypothyroidism. Clinical follow-up of these patients suggests that only 1% to 5% of children exposed to propylthiouracil develop goiter. The neonatal goiter associated with propylthiouracil therapy is not large and obstructive, and there is no conclusive evidence that propylthiouracil treatment can lead to cretinism. Children exposed to thioamides in utero attain full physical and intellectual development and have normal thyroid function studies. Propylthiouracil excretion in breast milk does not exceed 0.025% of the administered daily maternal dose, and no changes occur in the thyroid function tests of breast-fed neonates.

Surgical management of the hyperthyroid pregnant patient is recommended only if medical treatment fails. Today few patients undergo subtotal thyroidectomy during pregnancy. It is advisable to delay surgery until the 2nd trimester because the rate of spontaneous abortion is highest during the 1st trimester.

Thyroid Storm

The major risk for a pregnant patient with thyrotoxicosis is the development of a thyroid storm.

Precipitating factors include infection, labor, cesarean delivery, or noncompliance with medication. The maternal mortality exceeds 25% despite good medical management. The signs and symptoms associated with a thyroid storm include hyperthermia, marked tachycardia, perspiration, and severe dehydration. Specific treatment is directed at **(1) blocking β-adrenergic activity with propranolol, 20 to 80 mg every 6 hours; (2) blocking secretion of thyroid hormone with sodium iodide, 1 g intravenously; (3) blocking synthesis of thyroid hormone and conversion of T_4 to T_3 with 1200 to 1800 mg of propylthiouracil** given in divided doses; (4) further blocking the deamination of T_4 to T_3 with 8 mg of **dexamethasone** per day; (5) **replacing fluid losses** with at least 5 L of fluid; and (6) rapidly lowering the temperature with **hypothermic techniques.**

Neonatal Thyrotoxicosis

About 1% of pregnant women with a history of Graves' disease give birth to children with thyrotoxicosis. It is transient and lasts less than 2 to 3 months but is associated with a neonatal mortality rate of about 16%. Fetal thyrotoxicosis can be suspected if the baseline fetal heart rate consistently exceeds 160 beats per minute. A fetal goiter can often be identified by ultrasonography in such cases. This situation is associated with an increase in perinatal morbidity and mortality and should be treated prenatally and postnatally.

Hypothyroidism

Pregnant women on appropriate thyroid replacement can expect a normal pregnancy outcome, but untreated maternal hypothyroidism has been associated with an increased risk of spontaneous abortion, preeclampsia, premature separation of the placenta, low-birth-weight or stillborn infants, and lower intelligence levels in offspring.

The most important laboratory finding to confirm the diagnosis of hypothyroidism is an elevated TSH level. Other findings include low levels of serum T_3 and T_4 and a decreased T_3 resin uptake. Once a diagnosis of hypothyroidism has been made in a pregnant woman, thyroid replacement should be started immediately. Levothyroxine in a dose of 0.15 mg/day is usually sufficient to ameliorate the symptoms. Women in whom thyroid therapy is begun during pregnancy should have monthly measurements of TSH with appropriate adjustments in levothyrox-ine therapy to keep the TSH within the normal range. Those who have received pregestational thyroid therapy should have TSH and free T4 levels measured at the initial visit and subsequently at 16 to 20 weeks and 28 to 32 weeks of gestation.

Neonatal hypothyroidism. Thyroid hormone defi-ciency during the fetal and early neonatal periods leads to generalized developmental retardation. The sever-ity of symptoms depends on the time of onset and the severity of the deprivation. If the disease is diagnosed and treated during the early neonatal period, the damage may be greatly minimized.

The incidence of congenital hypothyroidism (cretinism) is about 1 in 4000 births. The etiologic factors include thyroid dysgenesis, inborn errors of thyroid function, and drug-induced endemic hypothy-roidism. **The most common cause of neonatal goiter is maternal ingestion of iodides present in cough syrup.** The goiters associated with maternal iodine ingestion are large and obstructive, unlike those associated with maternal propylthiouracil treatment.

HEART DISEASE

Heart disease in pregnancy can be divided into two categories: **rheumatic and congenital.** Better treat-ment of rheumatic fever and improvements in medical and surgical management of congenital heart disease has meant that in a modern tertiary referral center, about 80% of patients with cardiac disease in preg-nancy now have congenital heart disease.

RHEUMATIC HEART DISEASE

The most common lesion associated with rheumatic heart disease is mitral stenosis. Regardless of the spe-cific valvular lesion, **patients are at higher risk of developing heart failure, subacute bacterial endo-carditis, and thromboembolic disease.** They also have a higher rate of fetal wastage.

Pure mitral stenosis is found in about 90% of patients with rheumatic heart disease. During preg-nancy, the mechanical obstruction worsens as cardiac output increases. **Asymptomatic patients may de-velop symptoms of cardiac decompensation or pulmonary edema as pregnancy progresses.** Atrial fibrillation is more common in patients with severe mitral stenosis, and **nearly all women who develop atrial fibrillation during pregnancy experience congestive heart failure.** However, pulmonary con-gestion and heart failure develop in only half of women in whom atrial fibrillation predates pregnancy.

Patients with mitral insufficiency or aortic stenosis are in less danger of having cardiac decompensation in the 3rd trimester because their myocardium is able to increase its workload without decompensating.

CONGENITAL HEART DISEASE

Congenital heart disease includes atrial or ventricular septal defect, primary pulmonary hypertension (Eisen-menger's syndrome), and cyanotic heart disease. If the anatomic defect has been corrected during childhood with no residual damage, the patient will go through pregnancy without complications. Patients with per-sistent atrial or ventricular septal defects and those with tetralogy of Fallot with complete surgical cor-rection generally tolerate pregnancy well. However, **patients with primary pulmonary hypertension or cyanotic heart disease with residual pulmonary hypertension are in danger of undergoing decom-pensation during pregnancy.** Pulmonary hyperten-sion from any cause is associated with about a 30% maternal mortality during pregnancy or in the imme-diate postpartum period. In all of these patients, care should be taken to avoid overloading the circulation and precipitating pulmonary congestion, heart failure, or hypotension with reversal of the left-right shunt, all of which are conditions that may lead to hypoxia and sudden death.

CARDIAC ARRHYTHMIAS

Supraventricular tachycardia is the most common cardiac arrhythmia. It is usually benign and occurs sec-ondary to structural changes in the heart that have presumably been present since birth. Atrial fibrillation and atrial flutter are more serious and are usually asso-ciated with underlying cardiac disease.

PERIPARTUM CARDIOMYOPATHY

This entity is very rare, but it is exclusively associated with pregnancy. Patients have no underlying cardiac disease, and symptoms of cardiac decompensation appear during the last weeks of pregnancy or 1 to 6 months postpartum. **Pregnant women particularly at risk of developing cardiomyopathy are those** with a history of preeclampsia or hypertension and those who are poorly nourished. No etiologic factor has been found. Chronic hypertension, viral myocarditis, and valvular heart disease must be excluded in patients with cardiac dysfunction before the diagnosis can be made.

MANAGEMENT OF CARDIAC DISEASE DURING PREGNANCY

The New York Heart Association's functional classification of heart disease is of value in assessing the risk of pregnancy for a patient with acquired cardiac disease and in determining the optimal management during pregnancy, labor, and delivery (Table 17-6). In general, the maternal and fetal risks for patients with class I and II disease are small, whereas they are greatly increased with class III and IV disease. However, pulmonary edema leading to maternal death has been reported on rare occasions in patients with class I and II cardiac disease. This functional classification is less helpful in predicting outcome in those with congenital heart diseases, such as Eisenmenger's syndrome.

Prenatal Management

As a general principle, **all pregnant cardiac patients should be managed with the help of a cardiologist.** Frequent prenatal visits are indicated, and frequent hospital admissions may be needed, especially for patients with class III and IV cardiac disease. It is important to keep in mind principles of prenatal management for these patients.

Avoidance of excessive weight gain and edema. Cardiac patients should be placed on a low-sodium diet (2 g/day) to prevent excessive expansion of blood

Table 17-6. New York Heart Association's functional classification of heart disease

Class I	No signs or symptoms of cardiac decompensation
Class II	No symptoms at rest, but minor limitation of physical activity
Class III	No symptoms at rest, but marked limitation of physical activity
Class IV	Symptoms present at rest, discomfort increased with any kind of physical activity

and extracellular fluid volumes. They should be encouraged to rest in the left lateral decubitus position for at least 1 hour every morning, afternoon, and evening to promote diuresis, especially during the latter part of gestation. Adequate sleep should be encouraged.

Avoidance of strenuous activity. All cardiac patients should avoid strenuous activity. Individuals with significant heart disease are unable to increase their cardiac output to the same extent as healthy individuals to meet the increased metabolic demands associated with exercise. Consequently, they tend to extract more oxygen from the arterial blood, resulting in a larger arteriovenous oxygen difference. With strenuous exercise or tissue hypoxia, or both, blood is shifted from the uteroplacental circulation to other organs.

Avoidance of anemia. With anemia, the oxygen-carrying capacity of the blood decreases. Oxygen delivery to tissues is generally maintained by increased cardiac output. An increase in heart rate, especially with mitral stenosis, leads to a decrease in left ventricular filling time, so pulmonary congestion and edema may result. Another factor that might lead to cardiac decompensation is the inability of the right ventricle to efficiently pump a percentage of the venous return.

Management of Delivery and the Immediate Postpartum Period

Cardiac patients should be delivered vaginally unless obstetric indications for cesarean are present. The patient should be instructed to **avoid pushing** during the second stage of labor because the associated increase in intraabdominal pressure increases venous return and cardiac output and can lead to cardiac decompensation. The second stage of labor is assisted by performing an **outlet forceps** delivery or by the use of a **vacuum extractor.**

The immediate postpartum period presents special risks to the cardiac patient. After delivery of the placenta, the uterus contracts and about 500 mL of blood is added to the effective blood volume. **Cardiac output increases up to 80% above prelabor values in the first few hours after a vaginal delivery and up to 50% after cesarean section.** To minimize the risk of overloading the circulation, the lower extremities are kept at the level of the body by lowering the stirrups, the uterus is not routinely massaged to expedite placental separation, nor is Pitocin given after delivery of the placenta, unless bleeding is excessive.

If cardiac decompensation occurs, it should be managed as a medical emergency. Medical management should include administration of morphine sulfate, supplemental oxygen, an intravenous loop diuretic (e.g., furosemide), IV sodium nitroprusside, digitalis, and, sometimes, IV aminophylline. Phlebotomy and rotating tourniquets might be considered if the aforementioned measures are not sufficient. Continuous pulse oximetry can be very helpful in managing these patients. Monitoring with a pulmonary artery catheter can provide a good index of left ventricular function, but this is generally discouraged in those with pulmonary hypertension.

AUTOIMMUNE DISEASE IN PREGNANCY

An autoimmune disease is one in which antibodies are developed against the host's own tissues. A number of autoimmune diseases can significantly affect either the maternal or the fetal outcome in pregnancy. These include rheumatoid arthritis, systemic lupus erythematosus (SLE), idiopathic thrombocytopenic purpura (ITP), isoimmune thrombocytopenia, Graves' disease, and myasthenia gravis. A summary of the interactions of primary immunologic disorders and pregnancy is shown in Table 17-7.

IMMUNE THROMBOCYTOPENIA

Available information suggests that platelet production is normal or increased in immune thrombocy-

Table 17-7. Autoimmune disease in pregnancy

Disease	Effect of Disease on Pregnancy		Effect of Pregnancy on Disease	Antibodies That Cross Placenta
	Mother	Fetus		
Rheumatoid arthritis	No significant effect	No significant effect Teratogenic effects of medication	Improved commonly	None
Idiopathic thrombocytopenic purpura (ITP)	Antepartum, intrapartum, and postpartum hemorrhage	Fetal hemorrhage (particularly intracranial bleeding)	None	Platelet antibodies
Thrombotic thrombocytopenic purpura	No significant effect	Similar to ITP	None	Platelet antibodies
Graves' disease	No significant effect	Intrauterine growth retardation Neonatal thyrotoxicosis	Improved during pregnancy Exacerbation postpartum	Long-acting thyroid stimulator (LATS)
Myasthenia gravis	No significant effect	Transient neonatal myasthenia	Variable during pregnancy Moderate exacerbation postpartum	Anti-acetylcholinesterase
Systemic lupus erythematosus (SLE)	Increased incidence of uterine infection Increased incidence of preeclampsia	Abortion (spontaneous) Prematurity Intrauterine growth retardation Stillbirth Congenital heart block Endomyocardial fibrosis	Exacerbation of disease Deterioration of renal condition Anemia, leukopenia, and thrombocytopenia	Various tissues and membranes

topenia, but peripheral platelet destruction exceeds bone marrow production. This condition is considered to be an autoantibody disorder in which immunoglobulins attach to maternal platelets. The subsequent structural damage of these formed elements leads to platelet sequestration in the reticuloendothelial system.

Treatment

Therapy is not initiated unless platelet counts are <50,000/μL or petechial hemorrhages are present. Corticosteroids, in a dose equivalent to 1 mg/kg per day of prednisone, **are given initially,** maintained for 2 to 3 weeks, then tapered slowly. Within 2 weeks of commencing corticosteroid treatment, the platelet count increases, although it may remain below control levels.

Even in the absence of changes in the platelet count, hemostasis is improved. Fetal thrombocytopenia can accompany maternal ITP, which can increase the risk of intracranial hemorrhage. Vaginal delivery is generally carried out because there is no good evidence that the fetal outcome is improved by cesarean delivery. **Intravenous immunoglobulin can be given for corticosteroid failures** in Rh-positive women. **Splenectomy is a last resort** for patients who fail to respond to corticosteroid and immunoglobulin treatment. **Platelet transfusions are not usually recommended** except in life-threatening situations because platelets are destroyed quickly in the peripheral circulation.

ANTIPHOSPHOLIPID ANTIBODIES (LUPUS ANTICOAGULANT AND ANTICARDIOLIPIN)

Subclinical autoimmune disease and circulating antibodies to negatively charged phospholipids (lupus anticoagulant and anticardiolipin) have been implicated as a cause of recurrent abortion, early fetal loss, severe intrauterine growth restriction, early-onset severe preeclampsia, and arterial and venous thrombosis. When these conditions are present and are unexplained, it may be helpful to test for antiphospholipid antibodies, although patients with immunologic problems represent a small proportion of the total number of patients with these complications of pregnancy. Lupus anticoagulant can be screened for with an activated partial prothrombin time or the more specific dilute Russell viper venom test

(DRVVT); a sensitive and specific radioimmunoassay is available for the detection of anticardiolipin.

RENAL DISORDERS
ACUTE RENAL FAILURE

Acute renal failure during pregnancy or in the postpartum period may be due to deterioration of renal function secondary to a preexisting renal disease or to a pregnancy-induced disorder. The underlying causative factors may be prerenal, renal, or postrenal. **With prerenal causes, a history of blood or fluid loss is usually elicited** from the patient or implied from reviewing the medical history. **Renal causes are usually suspected in a patient with a history of preexisting renal disease or with a hypercoagulable state,** such as thrombotic thrombocytopenic purpura or hemolytic uremic syndrome. With prolonged hypotension, **acute cortical necrosis or acute tubular necrosis** may occur. **Postrenal causes are less common but should be suspected in situations in which urologic obstructive lesions are present** or in which there is a history of kidney stones.

Laboratory Studies

Laboratory tests are directed at assessing renal function, cardiovascular status, and the patency of the urologic tract.

Renal studies. Renal studies include urine output, blood urea nitrogen (BUN)-to-creatinine ratio, fractional excretion of sodium, and urine osmolality. **Oliguria is defined as urine output of less than 25 mL/hour,** whereas anuria is the cessation of urine output. With acute renal failure, the urine output may not decrease, although oliguria or anuria is usually present. Not infrequently, a decrease in urine output alerts the physician to an impending crisis. **During pregnancy, the serum values of BUN and creatinine decrease, but the BUN-to-creatinine ratio remains about 20:1.** A ratio greater than 20:1 suggests tubular hypoperfusion (prerenal failure).

The fractional excretion of sodium (FENa) is calculated as follows:

$$FENa = Urine\ sodium/plasma\ sodium/Urine\ creatinine/plasma\ creatinine \times 100$$

An FENa of less than 1% is suggestive of hypovolemia and tubular hypoperfusion. Alternatively, a value greater than 3% is highly indicative of tubular damage.

Urine osmolality greater than 500 mOsm/L or a urine-to-plasma osmolality ratio greater than 1.5:1 is highly suggestive of renal hypoperfusion. Urine specific gravity is of limited value, especially when the urine contains protein or hemolyzed blood.

Cardiovascular studies. Acute blood and fluid losses are usually associated with orthostatic hypotension, tachycardia, decreased skin turgor, and reduced sweating. In a pregnant hypertensive or preeclamptic patient who is in labor, many of these signs are overlooked. If indicated, a Swan-Ganz catheter allows monitoring of right and left ventricular filling pressures, cardiac output, and pulmonary capillary wedge pressure. This can help to distinguish between congestive heart failure, cardiac tamponade, and volume depletion, any of which can lead to acute renal failure.

Urologic tract studies. A Foley catheter and renal sonogram are usually sufficient to diagnose obstructive lesions. Rarely, a one-shot intravenous pyelogram is needed.

Treatment

Prerenal causes. Restoration of intravascular volume, cardiac output, and arterial pressure to normal values is sufficient to reverse oliguria. Careful attention should be given to electrolyte imbalance when large amounts of crystalloids are infused.

Renal causes. Acute tubular necrosis, acute cortical necrosis, or both, may be present. Because acute cortical necrosis is generally irreversible, treatment is directed toward preventing further damage. **A trial of diuretic therapy to increase urinary output appears to decrease the duration and severity of acute tubular necrosis and increase survival rates. Furosemide** (Lasix) 40 mg, is given initially and repeated every 4 to 6 hours for 48 hours in the presence of adequate urinary response. **If the diuretic therapy fails to increase the urine output, an oliguric fluid regimen (>500 mL/24 hr) is initiated.** Fluid intake should be limited to replacement of urine output and insensible water loss, and renal function studies should be monitored on a daily basis. For the first few days after the renal ischemic episode, renal function may worsen, but within 7 to 10 days, most patients with acute tubular necrosis show marked improvement. **If renal function deteriorates rapidly or fails to recover, hemodialysis is recommended.**

In some patients in whom acute renal failure is accompanied by oliguria, a diuretic phase coincides with the recovery period. The urine output may exceed 10 L/day, and if fluid and electrolyte losses are not replaced promptly, death ensues. **About 50% of obstetric patients who develop acute renal failure during pregnancy or the postpartum period recover enough renal function during the first year to survive without dialysis.**

Postrenal causes. In many instances, simple measures, such as turning the patient on the left side to displace the gravid uterus away from the ureters, or inserting a Foley catheter into the bladder to overcome urethral obstruction, will resolve the problem. In situations in which a ureteral or renal pelvic obstruction is present (e.g., stones), surgical intervention is indicated to relieve the obstruction.

CHRONIC RENAL FAILURE

The outcome of pregnancies complicated by chronic renal disease is less favorable. Good pregnancy outcome may be expected in nonhypertensive pregnant patients who have serum creatinine levels below 1.5 mg/dL prior to conception. **When the serum creatinine levels exceed 3 mg/dL, continuation of pregnancy to the point of fetal viability is rare. Hypertensive individuals with chronic renal disease do not fare as well as normotensive patients** with the same degree of renal impairment.

Pregnancy has no effect on the natural course of the renal disease in patients who have mild impairment of renal function and are normotensive. The deterioration in renal function, superimposition of hypertension, and substantial increase in proteinuria seen during pregnancy subside after delivery. Patients with nephrotic syndrome do well during pregnancy despite the massive urinary protein losses. In most of these individuals, proteinuria partially abates in the postpartum period.

PREGNANCY FOLLOWING RENAL TRANSPLANTATION

Pregnancy after renal transplantation should not be considered before a thorough assessment of maternal, fetal, and neonatal risk factors is undertaken. Hypertension and cesarean delivery are more common in

> ### Box 17-2. Criteria for determining suitability of pregnancy in renal transplantation patients
>
> - 2 yr posttransplant and in good health
> - Anatomic status compatible with good obstetric outcome
> - No proteinuria
> - No significant hypertension
> - No evidence of active allograft rejection
> - No evidence of pelvicaliceal distention on recent intravenous pyelogram
> - Serum creatinine <2 mg/dL
> - Prednisone dosage ≤15 mg/day and azathioprine dosage ≤2 mg/kg/day and cyclosporin dosage ≤5 mg/kg/day

Data from Davison JM, Lindheimer MD: Pregnancy in renal transplant recipients. J Reprod Med 27:613, 1982.

women with renal transplantation. **Fetal complications include steroid-induced adrenal and hepatic insufficiency, prematurity, and intrauterine growth restriction.** Decrease in thymus size, lymphopenia, and lethargy have been reported. In addition, the infant may inherit the primary disease of the mother or other family members. The mother and neonate are at increased risk of infection because of immunosuppressive therapy.

The criteria shown in Box 17-2 may be used to identify renal transplantation patients who are good candidates for pregnancy. Cyclosporin (up to 5 mg/kg/day) is usually given to pregnant women who are recipients of renal transplantation. This immunosuppressant, which may decrease glomerular filtration and raise arterial pressure, can be associated with hyperkalemia, hyperuricemia, and less frequently a hemolytic uremic syndrome.

GASTROINTESTINAL DISORDERS
NAUSEA AND VOMITING DURING PREGNANCY

About 60% to 80% of pregnant women complain of nausea and vomiting during the first 8 to 12 weeks of gestation. The symptoms are usually mild and disappear during the early part of the 2nd trimester. In a small number of patients, the severity of the symptoms necessitates hospital admission. **The underlying causes of nausea and vomiting during pregnancy are not well understood.**

Treatment is usually symptomatic. Patients are instructed to refrain from eating large and late meals, to avoid the recumbent position, especially after meals, and to use an extra pillow to elevate the head when sleeping. Patients with more severe symptoms also require solid or liquid antacids, which should be taken 1 to 3 hours after meals and at bedtime. Many patients respond to pyridoxine (vitamin B_6), while others may require antiemetics such as promethazine.

HYPEREMESIS GRAVIDARUM

This term is reserved for the intractable nausea and vomiting that occurs in about 1% of gravid women. **The overall incidence is about 1%,** but cultural, racial, and personality factors are known to influence the prevalence of this disorder. **The disorder appears more frequently with first pregnancies** but tends to recur with subsequent pregnancies. **Pregnancy outcome is usually good,** with no additional risk to the mother, fetus, or neonate, provided that appropriate therapy is given.

Clinical diagnosis is based on the history and physical findings. A history of intractable vomiting and inability to retain food and fluid is usually elicited. Physical findings of weight loss, dry and coated tongue, and decreased skin turgor are very suggestive. The initial laboratory workup includes urine tests for ketonuria and blood tests for electrolytes and acetone. Electrolyte disturbances may include hypokalemia, hyponatremia, and hypochloremic alkalosis. Treatment is symptomatic, but **if outpatient management fails, patients must be admitted for intravenous administration of fluids, electrolytes, glucose, vitamins, and antiemetics** (e.g., droperidol-diphenhydramine or metoclopramide). The few who do not respond to this therapy may require nasogastric feeding or parenteral nutrition.

REFLUX ESOPHAGITIS

Reflux esophagitis or heartburn is a common complaint in about 70% of pregnant women. The main symptoms include substernal discomfort aggravated by meals and the recumbent position and occasional hematemesis. An unusual symptom peculiar to reflux esophagitis is water brash, which is best described as the sudden filling of the mouth with clear, watery material that has a salty taste and produces a nauseous sensation.

Treatment

Treatment is usually symptomatic. Patients are instructed to refrain from eating large and late meals, to avoid the recumbent position, especially after meals, and to use an extra pillow to elevate the head when sleeping. Patients with more severe symptoms also require antacids, which should be taken 1 to 3 hours after meals and at bedtime. **H₂-blockers (cimetidine) or a proton pump blocker (omeprazole) may be indicated in severe refractory cases.**

PEPTIC ULCER

Pregnancy conveys relative protection against the development of peptic ulceration and may ameliorate an already present ulcer. Gastric acid secretion is probably not altered during pregnancy, although some studies suggest modest suppression. **The diagnosis of ulcer disease is mainly based on symptomatic improvement in response to conservative treatment.** Endoscopy is reserved for those patients who do not respond to treatment, have more severe gastrointestinal symptoms, or manifest significant gastrointestinal hemorrhage.

Treatment

Treatment involves avoiding caffeine, alcohol, tobacco, and spicy foods, all of which stimulate acid secretion. **Liquid antacids** with a low sodium content are recommended and should be continued for at least 6 weeks. These include **Maalox TC suspension, Mylanta II liquid, and Gelusil-II liquid. Antibiotic therapy is indicated for all *Helicobacter pylori*–infected ulcer patients. Cimetidine (Tagamet) or omeprazole should be reserved for complicated, recurrent, and refractory cases.** Cimetidine, an H₂-receptor antagonist, inhibits gastric acid secretion but has no effect on gastric volume, gastric emptying, or lower esophageal sphincter tone. The drug has been associated with cardiac arrhythmias, cardiac arrest, and an increased risk of gastric carcinoma. It crosses the placenta and reaches the fetus in substantial quantities.

ACID ASPIRATION SYNDROME (MENDELSON'S SYNDROME)

The pregnant patient in labor is at an increased risk of acid aspiration because of (1) delayed gastric emptying, which is made worse when associated with increased anxiety or the use of sedatives, narcotics, and anticholinergic agents; **(2) increased gastric acidity;** and **(3) increased intraabdominal and intragastric pressure,** making regurgitation more likely. Damage to the pulmonary tissue is greatest when the pH of the aspirated fluid is less than 2.5 or the volume of the aspirate is greater than 25 mL. Preventive efforts are directed at decreasing the acidity of the gastric contents or decreasing the acid secretion by the stomach. Toward this end, women in labor should be advised to eat a light meal before coming to the hospital. **Liquid magnesium and aluminum antacids given every 3 to 4 hours during labor decrease the gastric acidity** but increase the volume of the gastric acid–antacid emulsion. If the patient is to undergo any surgical procedure that requires general anesthetic, intubation should be performed.

CHRONIC INFLAMMATORY BOWEL DISEASE

The two entities described under this disorder are **Crohn disease (regional enteritis)** and **ulcerative colitis.** In about 25% of patients with inflammatory bowel disease, differentiation between these two disorders is difficult.

Patients with inflammatory bowel disease do well during pregnancy, provided that there are no acute exacerbations. It seems unlikely that the natural history of the disease changes during pregnancy. **If inflammatory bowel disease is active at the time of conception, the spontaneous abortion rate is doubled.** If surgery is required for complications of inflammatory bowel disease, fetal survival is reduced.

Treatment

Treatment of an acute exacerbation of inflammatory bowel disease is the same for pregnant and nonpregnant patients, although some of the more experimental drugs should not be used during pregnancy. **If diarrhea is the main complaint, dietary restriction of lactose, fruits, and vegetables is necessary.** If a lactose-free diet is used, calcium supplementation is needed. **Constipating agents, such as Pepto-Bismol and psyllium hydrophilic mucilloid (Metamucil), may be used daily and are quite effective.** The use of diphenoxylate-atropine (Lomotil) or loperamide (Imodium) should be restricted to patients in whom conservative management fails. **For those** patients with mild to moderate symptoms, sulfasalazine may be beneficial. The usual daily dose is 2 to 6 g.

HEPATIC DISORDERS

Liver disorders that are peculiar to pregnancy are discussed below.

INTRAHEPATIC CHOLESTASIS OF PREGNANCY

Although the pathogenesis of this syndrome is not known, some distinctive features are present: (1) **cholestasis and pruritus** without other major liver dysfunction, (2) **a tendency to recurrence** with each pregnancy, (3) **an association with oral contraceptives,** and (4) **a benign course** in that there are no maternal hepatic sequelae. The incidence is highly variable, ranging from 1 to 2 per 1000 pregnancies in low-risk cases in the United States, up to 10 to 20 per 1000 pregnancies in Scandinavia and Chile. Most probably, genetic, geographic, or environmental factors are involved. **The main symptom in a patient with cholestasis of pregnancy is itching, which may occur as early as 20 weeks of gestation.** Jaundice is rarely observed, although patients may notice darkening of the urine and passage of lighter-colored stools. Laboratory tests show elevated levels of serum bile acids. Serum levels of bilirubin and liver enzymes (e.g., aspartine and alanime transaminase) may be mildly elevated. Abdominal ultrasonography should be performed to exclude gallbladder obstruction, a hepatitis screen should be done to exclude viral hepatitis, and an autoantibody screen for primary biliary cirrhosis should also be undertaken.

Treatment

Local measures such as cold baths, bicarbonate washes, or phenol (0.5% to 1% in water-soluble creams) might be of some help. Oral glucocorticoid treatment over 7 to 10 days has been tried with excellent results. However, the pruritus is best treated with ursodeoxycliolic acid (300 mg, 2 to 3 times per day), a nontoxic bile acid that decreases the cytotoxicity of the bile acid mixture in the liver. The latter treatment usually significantly ameliorates the pruritus and reduces serum levels of bile acids, amino transferases and bilirubin. The mechanism of fetal compromise is uncertain, but maternal cholestasis causes substantial changes in fetal steroid metabolism.

This condition has been associated with sudden fetal death. **Fetal assessment and delivery by about 38 weeks of gestation are generally performed.**

ACUTE FATTY LIVER OF PREGNANCY

Fatty liver is a serious complication that is peculiar to pregnancy. The incidence is about 1 per 10,000 pregnancies. It most commonly occurs in the 3rd trimester of pregnancy or the early postpartum period. Although the cause is unknown, it may in some instances result from an inborn error of metabolism, possibly a deficiency of long-chain 3-hydroxyl coenzyme A dehydrogenase. **Presentation is variable, with abdominal pain, nausea and vomiting, jaundice, and increased irritability.** Extreme polydipsia or pseudodiabetes insipidus may be present. Hypoglycemia is infrequently present. **Hypertension and proteinuria are present in approximately 50% of patients, raising the issue of coexisting preeclampsia.**

Invariably, patients suffer hepatic coma and renal failure. Laboratory findings include an increase in prothrombin time (PT) and partial thromboplastin time (PTT), hyperbilirubinemia, hyperammonemia, hyperuricemia, and a moderate elevation of the transaminase levels. Hematemesis and spontaneous bleeding become manifest as disseminated intravascular coagulation (DIC) develops. Liver failure is indicated by elevated blood ammonia levels.

Treatment

Treatment is mainly directed at supportive measures, such as administration of intravenous fluids with 10% glucose to prevent dehydration and severe hypoglycemia. For the coagulopathy of hepatic failure, vitamin K supplementation is not effective, and fresh-frozen plasma or cryoprecipitate should be given.

Prognosis was once very poor, with about 80% of patients dying in a coma. Intrauterine fetal demise was also once the norm. With early recognition and immediate delivery, up to 72% of patients survive, and the prognosis for the fetus is also much improved.

THROMBOEMBOLIC DISORDERS

These disorders include superficial thrombophlebitis, deep venous thrombosis, and pulmonary embolism. The overall incidence of these disorders during pregnancy is about 1.4%, with about 80% occurring during the postpartum period.

Superficial Thrombophlebitis

The incidence of superficial thrombophlebitis during pregnancy is 1 in 600 during the antepartum period and 1 in 95 in the immediate postpartum period. It is more common in patients with varicose veins, obesity, and those whose physical activity is limited. **In most patients, superficial thrombophlebitis is limited to the calf area, and symptoms include swelling and tenderness of the involved extremity.** On physical examination, there is erythema, tenderness, warmth, and a palpable cord over the course of the involved superficial veins.

Superficial thrombophlebitis is not life-threatening and does not lead to pulmonary embolization. If not treated promptly and adequately, however, the inflammatory process might extend to the deep veins. Pain medications, local application of heat (thermal blanket), and elevation of the lower extremities to promote improved venous flow are often sufficient treatment. **There is no need for anticoagulants, but antiinflammatory agents may be considered.** After 5 to 7 days of bed rest and when symptoms disappear, the patient may gradually begin to ambulate. Toe-to-groin elastic stockings may replace periods of bed rest, which is controversial. Postrecovery residual effects frequently persist in the form of valvular incompetence. **Patients should be instructed to avoid standing for prolonged periods and to wear support hose** to help avoid a repeat episode.

Deep Venous Thrombosis

The incidence of deep venous thrombosis is 1 in 2000 patients antepartum and 1 in 700 patients postpartum. The risk of pulmonary embolization is high, and immediate treatment is indicated. Vascular injury, infection, and tissue trauma, coupled with the hypercoagulability and venous stasis of pregnancy, are the triggering factors for deep venous thrombosis.

Clinical features. The clinical diagnosis of deep venous thrombosis is difficult. Pain in the calf areas in association with dorsiflexion of the foot (positive Homans' sign) is a clinical sign of deep venous thrombosis in the calf veins. Acute swelling and pain in the thigh area and tenderness in the femoral triangle are suggestive of iliofemoral thrombosis.

Investigations. Noninvasive techniques, such as compression ultrasonography with Doppler flow studies and impedance plethysmography, are helpful and may be used as screening techniques, but a negative result does not necessarily exclude the diagnosis, especially in women in whom the clinical picture is highly suggestive of deep venous thrombosis. Also, magnetic resonance imaging (MRI) has been used to evaluate patients suspected of having pelvic thrombosis with a negative Doppler ultrasonic examination. Iodine 125-labeled fibrinogen and technetium 99 m scans are sensitive to calf and iliac venous thrombosis, respectively. They are infrequently used because of lack of availability or radiation hazard.

The most reliable test for deep venous (noniliac) thrombosis is a well-performed venogram, but this is not generally performed because of the 2% risk of dye-induced phlebitis and radiation exposure, the latter dosage being between 0.05 and 0.628 cGy.

Treatment. When a clinical diagnosis of deep venous thrombosis is made, anticoagulant therapy should be started and further diagnostic workup delayed several hours until adequate heparin levels have been reached. If the workup fails to identify any iliofemoral or calf thrombosis, heparin administration may be discontinued.

Treatment of proven deep venous thrombosis during pregnancy is initiated with intravenous heparin therapy. An initial dose of 10,000 U followed by a continuous infusion of intravenous heparin at a rate of about 1000 U/hour is maintained for 5 to 7 days or until symptoms disappear. **For the first 1 to 2 days, the heparin dose should be increased or decreased to keep the PTT at 2 to 2 1/2 times the normal control values.** Because anticoagulant therapy must be continued for the duration of pregnancy and up to 6 weeks' postpartum, either subcutaneous full-dose heparin or low molecular weight heparin can also be administered subcutaneously or on a per kilogram weight basis. Warfarin therapy, which crosses the placenta, carries the risks of fetal hemorrhage and teratogenesis and is less commonly used for this disorder.

Pulmonary Embolism

The incidence of pulmonary embolism during pregnancy is about 1 in 2500. **The maternal mortality is** less than 1% if treated early and greater than 80% if left untreated. In about 70% of cases, deep venous thrombosis is the instigating factor.

Clinical features. Suggestive symptoms include pleuritic chest pain, shortness of breath, air hunger, palpitations, hemoptysis, and syncopal episodes. Suggestive signs include tachypnea, tachycardia, low-grade fever, a pleural friction rub, chest splinting, pulmonary rales, an accentuated pulmonic valve second heart sound, and even signs of right ventricular failure. In most obstetric patients, the signs and symptoms of a pulmonary embolus are subtle.

Investigations. An electrocardiogram can show sinus tachycardia with or without premature heartbeats or right ventricular axis deviation. Determination, evaluation, and assessment of cardiac enzymes are not helpful. On chest film, atelectasis, pleural effusion, obliteration of arterial shadows, and elevation of the diaphragm may be present. **Arterial blood gases obtained on room air show an oxygen tension below 80 mm Hg. If there is any doubt about the diagnosis, a ^{99m}Tc ventilation-perfusion scan should be done,** which can be performed with minimal risk to the fetus. **Computed helical tomography** can also be helpful in the diagnosis. **Pulmonary angiography is rarely required,** but its main value is to diagnose a large embolus in patients for whom embolectomy is planned. Treatment of acute episodes and follow-up during pregnancy, labor, delivery, and the postpartum period are the same as for deep venous thrombosis.

Prophylactic anticoagulant therapy. In pregnant patients with a history of a pulmonary embolus or deep venous thrombosis during a previous pregnancy, prophylactic doses of heparin are given during pregnancy and the immediate postpartum period. **Minidose heparin (10,000 to 15,000 U/day)** provides sufficient prophylaxis for most patients, although some pregnant women may require full anticoagulation.

OBSTRUCTIVE LUNG DISEASE
BRONCHIAL ASTHMA

The incidence of bronchial asthma in pregnancy is approximately 1%, and about 15% of these individuals have one or more severe attacks during pregnancy. **Although the effect of pregnancy on bronchial asthma is variable, severe asthma is associated with an increased abortion rate and an increased incidence of intrauterine fetal death and fetal growth restriction, most probably as a result of intrauterine hypoxia.** Pulmonary function studies done during an acute episode show (1) increased airway resistance; (2) increased residual volume, functional residual capacity, and total lung capacity; (3) decreased inspiratory and expiratory reserve volume; (4) decreased vital capacity; and (5) decreased 1-second forced expiratory volume (FEV_1), peak expiratory flow rate, and maximum midexpiratory flow rate.

Obstetric Management

Pregnant asthmatics should be followed closely during pregnancy to ensure adequate maternal and fetal assessment. **Most asthmatics will require no drug treatment.** Adequate bed rest, the avoidance of dehydration, early and aggressive treatment of respiratory infections, and the avoidance of hyperventilation, excessive physical activity, and allergens are usually sufficient to prevent an exacerbation of symptoms. Serial measurements of peak expiratory rates can provide useful information on respiratory status. Cough medications containing iodine should be used with care because of the risk of causing a congenital goiter in the fetus.

For outpatient treatment of occasional mild asthma attacks, inhaled β-agonists are often sufficient. These agents have both a bronchodilator effect on smooth muscle cells and an inhibitory effect on release of mediators (e.g., histamine) from mast cells. Inhaled β-agonists used most frequently are the long-term selective $β_2$-agonists such as **albuterol or metaproterenol.**

The timing of delivery is dependent on the status of both the mother and the fetus. If pregnancy is progressing well, there is no need for early intervention, and it is advisable to await the spontaneous onset of labor. Early delivery can be considered for fetal growth restriction or maternal deterioration.

Management of Labor and Delivery

If the patient has been taking oral steroids during pregnancy, the intravenous administration of glucocorticoids is recommended during labor, delivery, and the postpartum period. A selective epidural block during labor benefits the patient in that it reduces pain, anxiety, hyperventilation, and respiratory work, all of which are known to aggravate the disease or precipitate an attack. **Vaginal delivery should be anticipated. Cesarean delivery is performed only for obstetric reasons.**

CYSTIC FIBROSIS

Cystic fibrosis is the most severe form of obstructive lung disease observed during pregnancy, but there is no evidence that pregnancy increases the maternal risk. However, women with pulmonary hypertension are at increased risk of heart failure and should be counseled against pregnancy. Similarly, women with malabsorption symptoms might become more emaciated during pregnancy. Preconception counseling is recommended, although prenatal diagnosis cannot exclude cystic fibrosis with complete confidence in all patients. **The fetus is at increased risk of intrauterine growth restriction and premature delivery.**

For labor and delivery, epidural analgesia is recommended. Outlet forceps or vacuum assisted delivery should also be considered. The Valsalva maneuver should be avoided because of the associated increase in maternal oxygen requirements (measured by pulse oximetry). Breastfeeding is recommended unless the maternal condition does not allow it.

SEIZURES

Seizure frequency during pregnancy may increase, decrease, or remain the same. It is difficult to relate the worsening of seizure control during pregnancy to the lower plasma levels of anticonvulsant drugs because seizure control improves in more than 50% of patients. Rarely, grand mal seizures may occur for the first time during pregnancy or in the puerperium and must be distinguished from eclampsia.

Treatment

If patients have had no seizure activity for a few years, medication may be discontinued before conception. If patients are pregnant and their seizures are well controlled, no change in therapy should be attempted unless the drugs are teratogenic. The two most commonly used drugs for seizure treatment are phenytoin (Dilantin) and phenobarbital. **Phenobarbital has fewer teratogenic effects, so it is the drug of first choice in early pregnancy.** Phenobarbital at a dose of 100 to 250 mg/day may be given in divided doses. The serum levels are monitored, and the dose is increased gradually until a therapeutic level (10 to 40 µg/mL) is reached. **Diphenylhydantoin** may be given at 300 to 500 mg/day, in single or divided doses, to achieve serum levels of 10 to 20 µg/mL (1 to 2 µg/mL free level), whereas **primidone** can be given at 750 to 1500 mg/day, in three divided doses, to achieve 5 to 15 µg/mL serum levels. Other anticonvulsant drugs, such as **clonazepam (Klonopin)** and **carbamazepine (Tegretol), should be used with care. Valproic acid (Depakene) and trimethadione pose special risks to the mother and fetus and should be used with caution.**

Maternal megaloblastic anemia and fetal congenital malformations due to folic acid deficiency occur as a rare complication of anticonvulsant therapy. Most of the reported cases have followed the administration of phenytoin. Folic acid supplementation is recommended, but careful attention should be paid to plasma levels of diphenylhydantoin because folic acid supplements are known to reduce plasma levels of phenytoin. Phenytoin is also reported to interfere with intestinal calcium absorption, leading to maternal and fetal hypocalcemia. In patients taking phenobarbital, primidone, or phenytoin, vitamin D supplements (10 mg/day) may be taken starting at about 34 weeks. Antacids and antihistamines should be avoided in patients receiving phenytoin, because they also lower plasma levels of phenytoin and may precipitate a seizure attack.

For the treatment of status epilepticus, immediate hospitalization is required. Patency of the airway should be ascertained. After blood is drawn for plasma levels of anticonvulsants, **10 mg of intravenous diazepam (Valium) should be given slowly, followed by 200 to 500 mg of diphenylhydantoin.** If seizure patterns continue, 500 mg of amobarbital sodium may be added. If these measures fail, general anesthesia may be employed. Therapeutic levels of phenytoin must be maintained during the rest of the pregnancy and postpartum period.

All patients who receive anticonvulsant therapy should have detailed ultrasonography and fetal echocardiography at about 18 weeks to specifically identify fetal congenital anomalies. Plasma anticonvulsant levels are determined monthly. **The management of labor and delivery follows obstetric indications.** During labor and in the immediate postpartum period, anticonvulsant drugs may be given intravenously. A cord blood specimen should be sent for PT because of the possibility of a coagulopathy in the neonate. Postpartum, the dose of the anticonvulsant drug may be lowered, provided that a therapeutic level is maintained. **Although anticonvulsants are excreted in breast milk in small amounts, breastfeeding is not contraindicated.**

COMPLICATIONS

Pregnant patients with epilepsy have a twofold increase in such maternal complications as preeclampsia, vaginal bleeding, hyperemesis, prolonged labor, and premature labor. A high incidence of intrauterine fetal demise, coagulopathy, and congenital anomalies is seen in the fetus. In the neonate, higher rates of coagulopathy, drug withdrawal symptoms, and neonatal morbidity and mortality are reported. **Anticonvulsants alone may not be responsible for the twofold to threefold increase in the rate of congenital anomalies.** Genetic predisposition plus other risk factors, such as frequent convulsions during early pregnancy, the increased incidence of maternal complications, and the socioeconomic status of the pregnant epileptic patient, are contributory.

HIV AND OTHER INFECTIOUS DISEASES

Infections in pregnancy are a known cause of maternal and neonatal morbidity. Acquired immunodeficiency syndrome (AIDS) in pregnancy is relatively uncommon in the United States, but it is important to recognize and treat to decrease fetal infection.

HUMAN IMMUNODEFICIENCY VIRUS

About 16.4 million women have human immunodeficiency virus (HIV) worldwide; mother-to-child transmission is the primary cause of the annual HIV infection rate of 600,000 in children. Since 1994, significant progress has been made in reducing the vertical transmission rate in developed countries.

The Virus

HIV is an RNA retrovirus. Virus-infected cells are the major source of transmission of HIV. Free virus rarely is a source of infection except if the concentration of free virus is very high. HIV replicates in certain cell types, in particular in T4 helper lymphocytes in the hematopoietic system and in cells of the central

nervous system. As with all retroviruses, HIV contains a reverse transcriptase in its core. HIV has specific surface proteins gp120 and gp41 and core proteins p18 and p24. The HIV infects a cell by first making contact with the gp120 protein. It then enters the cell, releases its core RNA, makes a DNA copy of itself with its reverse transcriptase, and inserts this DNA into the host genome. This viral gene then either enters into a latent state or begins making viral RNA and proteins with production of an infectious virus.

Laboratory Diagnosis

Serology tests commonly used for diagnosis are summarized in Box 17-3. Indirect serologic methods that detect HIV antibody include the enzyme-linked immunosorbent assay (ELISA), Western blot, and immunofluorescence assay (IFA) tests. **The sensitivity of the ELISA is 93% to 99%, and the specificity is 99%.** Although rare, false-positive ELISA results can occur, so a confirmatory test is always needed. The Western blot test, which identifies the presence of HIV core and envelope antigens, is 99% sensitive and 98.5% specific. False-positive Western blot results are extremely uncommon. Indirect serology with the capture ELISA technique can also identify HIV antigen (e.g., p24 antigen test). **The virus can also be identified by direct tissue culture or by HIV DNA polymerase chain reaction.**

Disease Course

Disease course is summarized in Box 17-4. Infection with HIV results in a chronic progressive disease. **Seroconversion typically occurs 3 to 14 weeks after exposure, but in rare instances it may take 6 months or more.** In 90% of cases, seroconversion is associated with a mononucleosis-like syndrome or aseptic meningitis. **Once the virus has been**

Box 17-3. Laboratory diagnosis of HIV infection
Enzyme-linked immunosorbent assay (ELISA)
Western blot
Immunofluorescent assay
Indirect serology with capture ELISA (p24 antigen test)
Direct tissue culture identification
HIV DNA polymerase chain reaction

Box 17-4. **Disease course after HIV infection**
Asymptomatic period (average is 10 yr) in adults
Destruction of T4 cells by HIV
Reversal of T4/T8 ratio to <1
Constitutional symptoms (malaise, anorexia, fever, weight loss, nausea)
Secondary cancers (Kaposi's sarcoma, non-Hodgkin's lymphoma)
Dementia and neuropathies
Opportunistic infections
Pneumocystis carinii pneumonia
Tuberculosis
Cryptococcal meningitis
Cytomegalovirus retinitis
Atypical mycobacterial disease
Severe herpes
Cryptosporidiosis
Cerebral toxoplasmosis

acquired, the patient enters an asymptomatic period, but lifetime infection should be assumed. Because HIV has a predilection for helper (T4) cells, a gradual destruction of the patient's cell-mediated immunity occurs, rendering the host susceptible to opportunistic infections. Eventual reversal of the T4/T8 ratio to less than 1 is seen on laboratory analysis.

Typically, the patient develops asymptomatic lymphadenopathy, followed by the onset of constitutional symptoms (anorexia, fever, weight loss, diarrhea, nausea, and vomiting). Eventually, opportunistic infections, secondary cancers (Kaposi's sarcoma, non-Hodgkin's lymphoma) or neurologic diseases (dementia, neuropathy) develop. Opportunistic infections that may be seen include the following: *Pneumocystis carinii* pneumonia (PCP), tuberculosis, cryptococcal meningitis, cytomegalovirus (CMV) retinitis, atypical mycobacterial disease, cerebral toxoplasmosis, severe herpes, and cryptosporidiosis. The average interval from initial infection to the onset of AIDS in an adult is 10 years in those not receiving potent antiviral therapy.

Pregnancy does not appear to accelerate the course of HIV infection. Pregnant women may, however, be at increased risk for developing infectious complications during pregnancy. These infections include opportunistic infections, postpartum infections, antepartum urinary tract infections, and sexually transmitted diseases. No direct detrimental effect on perinatal outcome has been documented. Studies to date have not shown an increased risk of growth restriction, preterm labor, or premature rupture of the membranes. In children, the disease progresses more rapidly. Of infants infected with HIV, half develop AIDS in the first year of life and 85% develop AIDS by age 3 years. Children have an extremely poor prognosis, the average survival time from diagnosis being 3 years.

Vertical Transmission

The risk of vertical transmission of HIV from an infected mother to her infant is between 20% and 30%. Such transmission accounts for 99% of cases of HIV infection in children. Vertical transmission may occur (1) in utero (transplacental), (2) intrapartum, and (3) postpartum. It is suspected that more than 50% of transmission occurs near the time of or during labor and delivery. Maternal-fetal transmission as a result of invasive procedures such as amniocentesis, chorionic villus sampling, umbilical blood sampling, or scalp electrode placement is theoretically possible, but the exact risk is unknown. Breastfeeding may increase the risk of transmission by 10% to 20%. There is no confirmed evidence that fetal HIV infection can result in structural anomalies. It appears that women with advanced disease, recent HIV infection, and/or preterm delivery have an increased risk of vertical transmission to their infants.

About 10 years ago, the administration of zidovudine, a nucleoside reverse-transcriptase inhibitor, to the mother during labor and to the infant for 6 weeks was shown to reduce the maternal transmission to the newborn from about 30% to 8% to 10%. More recently, potent antiretroviral therapy, which reduces the maternal plasma HIV RNA levels to less than 1000 copies per milliliter, has been shown to reduce the vertical transmission rate to only 1% to 2%. The current management for pregnant women involves the use of multiple agents to minimize the development of drug resistance. Because the risk of vertical transmission increases with maternal plasma HIV RNA concentrations, the therapeutic goal is to keep the maternal viral load either nil or less than 1000 copies per milliliter. Resistance testing should be considered for acute HIV infections, viral rebound, or persistent viremia in women already on a potent antiretroviral regimen, although whether such testing leads to better maternal or infant outcomes remains to be determined. In general, pregnant women should be maintained on the same antiretroviral therapy they received in the nonpregnant state, unless these drugs have an increased risk, such as delavirdine, efavirenz, or hydroxyurea.

Invasive fetal diagnostic procedures, such as amniocentesis and chorionic villus sampling, pose a theoretical risk of infecting the fetus, although the actual risk is unknown. Such procedures should either be avoided or performed only in gravidas on antiretroviral therapy with undetectable levels of HIV RNA.

Vaccinations, which are a concern in these patients, may be given under certain circumstances. For example, vaccinations for hepatitis B, influenza, and pneumococcus may be given to those on antiretroviral therapy provided the viral load is undetectable. Pregnant women on protease inhibitors should be screened for gestational diabetes at the initial visit in addition to the usual time at 24 to 28 weeks because these drugs can cause hyperglycemia.

Pregnant women should receive counseling on the risk of newborn infection and the delivery choices available. **Women who have viral loads greater than 1000 should be offered a cesarean delivery, which may reduce vertical transmission under these conditions.** Such cesarean deliveries should be scheduled at about 38 weeks of gestation to reduce the chance of labor or rupture of membranes. Amniocentesis for lung maturity should not be performed because of the possibility that the needle might transmit HIV from maternal blood to the fetus. **Women on antiretroviral therapy with viral loads less than 1000 HIV RNA copies per milliliter are at very low risk (1% to 2%) of passing the virus on to the fetus/newborn.** Vaginal delivery should be offered to such patients. All procedures should be avoided that may increase the risk of fetal HIV infection, such as artificial rupture of membranes, invasive fetal heart rate monitoring, fetal blood sampling, assisted delivery (forceps or vacuum), or episiotomy. **Once the membranes have ruptured, labor should be augmented with oxytocin to reduce the interval between membrane rupture and delivery.**

Regardless of the mode of delivery, all women should continue to receive antiretroviral medications as prescribed. Zidovudine (2 mg/kg over 1 hr, followed by 1 mg/kg/hr until delivery) should be infused intravenously to the gravida after the onset of labor or rupture of membranes or at least 3 hours before cesarean delivery.

Screening for HIV Infection in Pregnancy

All pregnant women should be offered HIV testing. Such voluntary testing requires that the patient give informed consent, with adequate counseling before and after testing. When counseling a newly identified HIV-positive pregnant woman, it is necessary to discuss the risk of perinatal transmission. Counseling on disease prevention, including a discussion of safe sexual practices, information on AZT therapy, and avoidance of breastfeeding, is imperative. Reproductive options with respect to the present pregnancy and future family planning need to be addressed.

RUBELLA (GERMAN MEASLES)

Rubella results from infection with a single-stranded RNA togavirus transmitted via the respiratory route, with highest attack rates occurring between March and May. It is highly contagious, with 75% of those infected becoming clinically ill. The incubation period is 14 to 21 days.

Diagnosis

The diagnosis of rubella is best made by serologic testing. **The IgM response is a rapid one** that begins at the onset of the rash and then declines and disappears by 4 to 8 weeks. **IgG response also begins at the onset of the rash and remains elevated for life.** The diagnosis can be made by the presence of a fourfold rise in the hemagglutination-inhibiting (HAI) antibody titer in paired sera obtained 2 weeks apart or by the presence of IgM. Rubella can also be diagnosed by culture and isolation of the virus during the acute phase of infection, although this technique is slow. The presence of IgM in cord blood or IgG in an infant after 6 months of age supports the diagnosis of perinatal rubella infection.

Impact on Pregnancy

Between 10% and 15% of adult women are susceptible to rubella. The disease course is unaltered by pregnancy, and the mother may or may not exhibit the full clinical disease. **The severity of the mother's illness does not have an impact on the risk of fetal infection.** Rather, it is the trimester in which infection occurs that has the greatest impact on fetal risk. Fetal infection may result in a normal baby, spontaneous

---

Box 17-5. Congenital rubella syndrome

Symmetric intrauterine growth restriction
Congenital deafness (detected after age 1 yr)
Cardiac malformations
  Patent ductus arteriosus
  Pulmonary artery hypoplasia
Eye lesions
  Cataracts
  Retinopathy
  Microphthalmia
Hepatosplenomegaly
Central nervous system involvement
  Microcephaly
  Panencephalitis
  Brain calcifications
  Psychomotor retardation
Hepatitis
Thrombocytopenic purpura

---

abortion, or the congenital rubella syndrome (CRS). Specifically, **infection in the 1st trimester carries a 25% risk of development of the congenital rubella syndrome (50% risk in the first 4 weeks),** whereas the risk of CRS drops to less than 1% if infection occurs in the 2nd or 3rd trimesters. Components of CRS are outlined in Box 17-5.

Routine rubella susceptibility testing should be performed in all pregnant women with a single IgG level. Those who are nonimmune should be vaccinated in the immediate postpartum period. Follow-up antibody titers should then be obtained, because up to 20% will fail to develop an antibody response. Rubella is not a contraindication to breastfeeding. There is no specific treatment for rubella, and routine prophylaxis with γ-globulin after exposure is not recommended because it has not been shown to change the risk of fetal involvement.

CYTOMEGALOVIRUS

Cytomegalovirus (CMV) is a DNA virus and a member of the herpes virus family and thus has the ability to establish latency. The virus is transmitted in a number of ways, including blood transfusion, organ transplant, sexual contact, breast milk, urine, or saliva; transplacentally; or at delivery by direct contact. **Between 30% and 60% of school-aged children are seropositive for CMV, as are 50% to 85% of all pregnant women,** which suggests that a prior infection occurred. Infection may be expressed as a mononucleosis-like illness, although subclinical infection is more common. Viral excretion may continue for months, and the virus may establish latency in lymphocytes, salivary glands, renal tubules, and the endometrium. Reactivation may occur years after primary infection, and reinfection with a different strain of the virus is also possible.

Diagnosis

The virus may be isolated on urine culture or by culture of other body secretions or tissues. Serologic testing is possible, with an elevation in IgM that peaks 3 to 6 months after infection and resolves by 1 to 2 years. IgG elevates rapidly and persists for life. Problems with serologic testing include (1) the prolonged elevation in levels of IgM, making delineation of timing of infection difficult, and (2) a 20% false-negative rate in IgM testing. In addition, the presence of IgG does not rule out the presence of persistent disease.

Impact on Pregnancy

CMV is the most common congenital viral infection in the United States, affecting 0.5% to 2.5% of all live-born infants per year. Placental infection may occur without fetal infection, and fetal infection can occur when the mother does not exhibit symptoms. The risk of transmission is constant across trimesters, with a 40% to 50% maternal-infant transmission rate. **Approximately 10% to 20% of infected infants are symptomatic at birth, exhibiting nonimmune hydrops, symmetric intrauterine growth restriction (IUGR), chorioretinitis, microcephaly, cerebral calcifications, hepatosplenomegaly, and hydrocephaly. Approximately 80% to 90% are asymptomatic at birth but later exhibit mental retardation, visual impairment, progressive hearing loss, and delayed psychomotor development** (Box 17-6). How severely an infant will be affected is unrelated to the point in pregnancy at which maternal infection occurred. Recurrent CMV infection is associated with a much lower fetal risk, with a 0.15% to 1% maternal-fetal transmission rate. Only three cases of severely affected infants have ever been reported.

There is no effective treatment available for CMV infection in pregnancy. Preventive measures include good hygiene in high-risk settings, such as the

> ## Box 17-6. Problems associated with congenital cytomegalovirus infection
>
> Nonimmune hydrops
> Symmetric growth restriction
> Chorioretinitis
> Microcephaly
> Cerebral calcifications
> Hepatosplenomegaly
> Hydrocephaly
> Later problems
>   Visual impairment
>   Hearing loss
>   Delayed psychomotor development

neonatal intensive care unit, day-care centers, and dialysis units. Maternal transfusion with CMV-positive blood should be avoided. Aids to making the diagnosis of fetal infection in a suspected case include ultrasonography (to identify symmetric IUGR, nonimmune hydrops or ascites, or central nervous system [CNS] abnormalities), and amniotic fluid CMV culture.

VARICELLA-ZOSTER

Acute varicella infection, or chickenpox, is caused by the varicella-zoster virus, which is a DNA herpes virus transmitted by direct contact or via the respiratory route. The attack rate in susceptible individuals is over 90%. The incubation period is 10 to 21 days. Infection is believed to be more severe in adults, and potential complications include encephalitis and pneumonia. **Because it is a herpes virus, the varicella virus has the ability to establish latency in nerve ganglia. Reactivation of the virus results in herpes zoster (shingles).**

Diagnosis

The diagnosis of chickenpox is usually determined by the patient's clinical presentation, although the virus may be cultured from vesicles during the first 4 days of the rash. On serologic testing, varicella-zoster IgM will rise in 2 weeks on ELISA or complement fixation. Paired sera for IgG obtained 2 weeks apart may also detect infection.

Fluorescent antibody membrane antigen (FAMA) is the most useful test to determine whether or not a woman is immune.

Impact on Pregnancy

Between 5% and 10% of adult women are susceptible to the varicella virus. Acute varicella infection complicates 1 in 7500 pregnancies. **Potential maternal complications include preterm labor, encephalitis, and varicella pneumonia.** Maternal management should be symptomatic, but a chest x-ray should be obtained to rule out pneumonia. Varicella pneumonia complicates 16% of cases and carries a mortality rate of up to 40%. If pneumonia is confirmed or suspected, the patient requires immediate hospital admission and institution of antiviral therapy, because rapid respiratory decompensation is not uncommon.

A congenital varicella syndrome has been described. Diagnosis of the syndrome is based on IgM-positive cord blood and clinical findings in the newborn, which include limb hypoplasia, cutaneous scars, chorioretinitis, cataracts, cortical atrophy, microcephaly, and symmetric IUGR. The risk of this fetal syndrome is 2% if maternal infection occurred between 13 and 30 weeks and 0.4% if maternal infection occurred before 13 weeks of gestation. No cases have been identified as a result of maternal infection past 30 weeks' gestation. In the presence of fetal infection, ultrasound may reveal hydrops, organ calcifications, limb deformities, microcephaly, or growth restriction. However, **no reliable methods of definitive prenatal diagnosis are available.**

If maternal infection occurs within 3 weeks of delivery, the fetus has a 24% risk of developing infection after delivery. If maternal infection occurs 5 to 21 days before delivery and the infant develops infection, it is typically mild and self-limited. However, **if maternal infection occurs between 4 days before delivery and 2 days after delivery, the infant is at great risk of developing a fulminant infection with a 30% mortality rate.** Varicella-zoster immune globulin (VZIG) should be given to these infants within 72 hours of birth, and they should be placed in contact isolation. The placenta and fetal membranes should be considered infectious.

For the exposed gravid woman who has no knowledge of a prior infection, a varicella IgG titer should be obtained immediately. If results are delayed or if the patient proves to be nonimmune, VZIG should be administered within 6 days of exposure, although it is unclear whether or not this therapy will modify the disease course and risk to the fetus. Administration of VZIG is also recommended after exposure to zoster. Varicella vaccine is composed of a live attenuated virus and, therefore, is contraindicated in pregnancy. **Herpes zoster does not occur more frequently in pregnancy. If it does occur it poses no risk to the fetus.** If zoster develops close to delivery, varicella may be transmitted through contact with a lesion, so this should be avoided.

HEPATITIS B AND C

The hepatitis B virus is a DNA virus that is transmitted via blood, saliva, vaginal secretions, semen, and breast milk and across the placenta. The population at greatest risk for contracting the virus includes intravenous drug abusers, homosexuals, individuals of Asian descent, and health care workers. Infection with the virus is either asymptomatic or expressed as acute hepatitis. Ten percent of individuals go on to develop chronic active or persistent hepatitis.

Impact on Pregnancy

The course of acute hepatitis is unaltered in pregnancy. Fetal infection may occur and is most likely if maternal infection occurs in the 3rd trimester. **Chronic active hepatitis is associated with an increased risk of prematurity, low birth weight, and neonatal death.** Maternal prognosis is very poor if the disease is complicated by cirrhosis, varices, or liver failure.

The incidence of hepatitis B surface antigen (HBsAg) positivity (chronic carrier state) in pregnancy in the United States is 6 to 10 per 1000 pregnancies. Women who are asymptomatic HBsAg carriers are at no higher risk for antepartum complications than are the general population. However, **newborns delivered to mothers positive for HBsAg have a 10% risk of developing acute infection at birth. This is in contrast to those delivered to mothers positive for both HBsAg and hepatitis Be antigen (HBeAg), in which the infant's risk increases to 70% to 90%.** Infection in the infant may be fulminant and lethal. **If the infant survives, it has an 85% to 90% chance of becoming a chronic hepatitis carrier and a 25% chance of developing liver cirrhosis, hepatocellular carcinoma, or both.** Therefore, it is recommended that all pregnant women be screened for HBsAg carriage during

---

Box 17-7. High-risk groups for HBsAg carriage

Birth in Haiti or Africa
Asian, Pacific Island, or Eskimo descent (immigrant or born in the United States)
Work or treatment in a hemodialysis unit
Work or residence in institutions for the mentally handicapped
History of repeated transfusions
Occupational exposure to blood
Repetitive episodes of sexually transmitted diseases
Intravenous drug abuse
Prostitution
Household contact with a hepatitis carrier
Household contact with a hemodialysis patient

---

pregnancy. Women in high-risk groups (Box 17-7) should be rescreened in the third trimester if the initial screen is negative.

If a pregnant woman is found on screening to be HBsAg-positive, liver function tests and a complete hepatitis panel should be performed. Household members and sexual contacts should be tested and offered vaccination if they are susceptible. Transmission to the infant is believed to occur by direct contact during delivery. Therefore the newborn is given hepatitis immune globulin and hepatitis vaccine soon after delivery, which reduces the risk of infection to less than 10%. **Pregnant women at high risk for becoming infected with hepatitis B who test negative for the HBsAg should be offered vaccination.** Available vaccines are produced by recombinant DNA technology and are therefore safe for use in pregnancy. The Centers for Disease Control and Prevention has recommended that all children receive vaccination against hepatitis B as well.

About 8% of pregnant women who are hepatitis C virus-positive transmit the virus to their offspring. Unfortunately, antibodies to hepatitis C do not protect against the disease and vertical transmission cannot be prevented at this time. Breastfeeding is associated with a 2% to 3% risk of viral transfer to the infant.

HERPES SIMPLEX

The herpes simplex virus (HSV) is a member of the DNA herpes virus family and is transmitted by intimate mucocutaneous contact. Because the virus has the ability to establish latency in sensory ganglia, it is an incurable sexually transmitted disease and is highly contagious. The clinical manifestations of herpes genitalis and its diagnosis are discussed in Chapter 23.

Impact on Pregnancy

Primary genital herpes. Patients who acquire primary herpes in pregnancy have an increased risk of obstetric and neonatal complications. **Maternal infection has been associated with an increased risk of spontaneous abortion, IUGR, and preterm labor.** Fifty percent of infants born vaginally to mothers with a primary infection at delivery have HSV infection.

Recurrent genital herpes. Complications from a recurrence in pregnancy are rare. However, 4% of infants born to mothers with recurrent infection at the time of delivery have HSV infection.

Neonatal herpes. The incidence of neonatal herpes is 0.01% to 0.04% of all deliveries, with infection acquired by the infant via passage through an infected birth canal or via an ascending infection in 90% of cases. Transplacental infection has also been documented as a route of transmission, as has close contact with an infected individual after delivery. **Premature infants are at the greatest risk for contracting infection, and they account for more than two-thirds of reported cases.** Symptoms typically present on day 2 to 3 of life, with rapid progression of disease thereafter. **Sixty percent of infected infants die in the neonatal period, and 50% of survivors have significant sequelae, including microcephaly, mental retardation, seizures, and microphthalmos.**

Management in Pregnancy

Because of lack of correlation with cervical shedding at the time of delivery, antepartum surveillance cultures are of little clinical use and are not recommended. Women with a prior history of herpes should be allowed to deliver vaginally if no genital lesions are present at the time of labor. **Patients with active lesions, either recurrent or primary, at the time of labor should be delivered by cesarean section.** Those with active lesions at sites distant from the genital area may be delivered vaginally if the lesions are covered. Once delivered, isolation of the mother from her infant is not necessary as long as direct contact with lesions is avoided. **Mothers may breast-feed so long as no lesions are present on the breasts.**

BACTERIAL INFECTIONS
URINARY TRACT INFECTIONS

Urinary tract infections occur more frequently in pregnancy and the puerperium and are among the most common medical complications of pregnancy. This increased incidence appears to be a result of both hormonal (progesterone) and mechanical factors that increase urinary stasis.

Urinary tract infections in pregnancy may be either asymptomatic or symptomatic (e.g., cystitis, pyelonephritis). **By definition, asymptomatic bacteriuria is the presence of ≥100,000 organisms/mL in a clean urine specimen from an asymptomatic patient.** The incidence of asymptomatic bacteriuria in pregnancy is the same as in the nonpregnant sexually active population, ranging from 2% to 10%. Highest rates are found in inner city populations and in patients with sickle cell disease or trait. *Escherichia coli* **is the organism most frequently isolated (60%).** Other organisms encountered are *Proteus mirabilis*, **enterococci,** *Klebsiella pneumoniae*, **and group B streptococci. If the condition is left untreated, roughly 20% of pregnant women develop either acute cystitis or pyelonephritis later in pregnancy.** Treatment consists of a 7- to 10-day course of either an **ampicillin** or a first-generation **cephalosporin. Nitrofurantoin** has also been safely used in pregnancy. After treatment, it is wise to follow with urine cultures because up to 25% of patients have a recurrence later in the pregnancy.

Acute cystitis complicates 1% to 2% of pregnancies and is characterized by dysuria, frequency, urgency, and hematuria. Systemic signs and symptoms, such as flank pain or fever, are absent. Urinalysis reveals bacteriuria, pyuria, and often hematuria. As in patients with asymptomatic bacteriuria, treatment is instituted on an outpatient basis while awaiting the results of sensitivity tests. Follow-up surveillance cultures are indicated.

Acute pyelonephritis occurs in approximately 2% of pregnancies, most frequently in the 3rd trimester. It is characterized by flank pain, fever, rigors, and the urinary complaints of cystitis. A rare associated complication is septic shock and adult respiratory distress syndrome. Often, nausea and vomiting may be present and the patient may be markedly dehydrated. Physical examination reveals fever and costovertebral angle tenderness. **As a result of sepsis, premature uterine contractions are frequent.** Urinalysis reveals the same findings as are found with acute cystitis, and blood cultures are positive in 10% of cases. Organisms responsible are the same as those causing asymptomatic bacteriuria and cystitis.

Hospitalization, intravenous antibiotic therapy, monitoring for preterm labor, and close observation of fluid status are indicated when a diagnosis of pyelonephritis is made. Usually, ampicillin or cefazolin therapy is initiated, with cefazolin gaining a great deal of popularity in areas in which resistance to ampicillin is prominent. Most patients (>80%) become asymptomatic and afebrile within 48 hours of initiation of antibiotic therapy and may be discharged at this point, continuing oral antibiotics for a 10-day course. Serial urine cultures are indicated because 10% to 25% of patients have a recurrence later in the pregnancy. Those with recurrent pyelonephritis should receive chronic antibiotic suppression and have an intravenous pyelogram performed 6 weeks postpartum to rule out urinary tract abnormalities.

GROUP B STREPTOCOCCI

Group B streptococci (GBS) are considered part of the normal flora of humans. The gastrointestinal tract is the major reservoir, although the organism has been isolated from the vagina, cervix, throat, skin, urethra, and urine of healthy individuals. **GBS may be transmitted to the genital tract by fecal contamination or sexual transmission from a colonized partner. Vaginal carriage rates vary from 15% to 40%,** but they are the same in pregnant women as in sexually active nonpregnant women. Carriage rates do not appear to be affected by age, race, socioeconomic status, or parity. The majority (two-thirds) of pregnant women who carry GBS do so intermittently or transiently, and only one-third of all pregnant GBS carriers have the organism chronically.

Diagnosis

Group B streptococci grow readily on routine bacteriologic media and are easy to isolate from clinical specimens. A number of rapid assays for the detection of GBS have been developed over recent years. These include assays based on GBS antigen detection and a GBS-DNA probe. These assays are specific when compared with culture, although their sensitivity is low (60% to 70%).

Impact on Pregnancy

GBS may be transferred from a colonized mother to her infant via vertical transmission at delivery. **Transmission rates of 35% to 70% have been reported, with the highest transmission rates occurring in women with heavy vaginal colonization. Other risk factors for transmission are preterm labor or delivery, preterm rupture of membranes, low birth weight, prolonged rupture of membranes (greater than 12 to 18 hours before delivery), intrapartum fever, and a history of previously delivering an infected infant.**

GBS sepsis is the most common cause of neonatal sepsis in the United States, with 1 to 2 cases per 1000 live births per year reported. Neonatal infection with GBS is of two clinically distinct types: early-onset and late-onset disease. **Late-onset GBS infection** has been linked to a nosocomial source in the nursery, occurs after the first week of life (mean onset, 4 weeks), and usually **is exhibited as meningitis (80%) or another type of focal infection. Early-onset GBS infection is characterized by its rapid onset and fulminant course,** with presentation typically within the first 48 hours of life. Pathogenesis of this form of GBS sepsis is best explained by direct maternal-infant transmission at delivery. **The infant presents with respiratory distress and pneumonia, and 30% develop meningitis. Septicemia, shock, and death may result even when antibiotics are begun expediently.** The overall infant mortality rate from early-onset disease is 50%. Preterm infants in whom bacterial colonization has occurred have an 8% to 10% risk of developing sepsis and account for more than 90% of deaths reported. The risk of sepsis developing in a full-term infant with bacterial colonization is 1% to 2%.

GBS is the second most common cause of bacteriuria in pregnancy and is a major cause of puerperal infection. Infection with GBS accounts for 20% of cases of endomyometritis and is unique in its acute onset (within the first 48 hours postpartum) and typically fulminant course.

Treating carriers in labor will reduce the rate of transmission to the infant. Therefore, most management protocols are focused on intrapartum therapy. Second- or third-trimester antepartum cultures generally have a poor positive predictive value with respect to culture status at delivery. Laboring gravidas are given antibiotic prophylaxis if they have high risk factors, such as intrapartum fever (≥38°C), preterm delivery (<37 weeks of gestation), or prolonged membrane rupture (≥18 hours).

A culture-based approach may be more effective than the risk-based approach in preventing early-onset group B streptococcal disease in the newborn. Thus, both the Centers for Disease Control and Prevention (CDC) and the Committee on Obstetric Practice of the American College of Obstetricians and Gynecologists (ACOG) now support a screening program in which **vaginal and rectal group B streptococci cultures are obtained at 35 to 37 weeks of gestation for virtually all gravidas.** The exceptions would be those who have GBS bacteriuria during the current pregnancy or a previous infant with invasive GBS disease. **Intrapartum antibiotic prophylaxis** would be indicated for pregnant women with (1) **a previous infant with invasive GBS disease, (2) GBS bacteriuria during the current pregnancy, (3) positive GBS screening culture during current pregnancy,** or (4) **unknown GBS status with one of the high-risk factors** of preterm delivery, prolonged membrane rupture, or intrapartum fever. Antibiotic prophylaxis is not indicated for those undergoing a scheduled cesarean delivery in the absence of labor or amniotic membrane rupture.

TUBERCULOSIS

Although the incidence of active tuberculosis (TB) in the United States is very low (0.6% to 1%), **approximately 10% of all women of child-bearing age test positive on PPD testing.** A positive PPD test indicates that the patient has been infected with tuberculosis in the past. It does not indicate active disease. Tuberculin skin testing is not a routine component of prenatal screening, but it is performed in high-risk populations. High-risk groups include lower-socioeconomic-status minority women and women who live in areas in which large numbers of immigrants from Southeast Asia, Central America, or South America reside. HIV-positive patients should also have a PPD test.

Pregnancy does not alter the course of active tuberculosis nor does it place the known PPD-positive woman at greater risk of disease reactivation. Tuberculosis can, however, **be passed to the fetus by a hematogenous route** across the placenta **or as a result of the fetus's swallowing infected amniotic fluid.** The risk of pregnancy wastage is increased, and congenital tuberculosis may be evident at birth. An affected infant exhibits low birth weight, failure to thrive, fever, respiratory distress, adenopathy, and hepatosplenomegaly and is at high risk of dying without rapid treatment. Treatment of the mother with active disease during pregnancy eliminates the fetal risks.

The pregnant patient who tests positive for tuberculosis should have a chest x-ray (with abdominal shielding) to rule out active disease. If the chest x-ray is suspicious for active disease, three sets of sputum cultures should be obtained. If the cultures are positive, therapy should be instituted without delay. If the chest x-ray is normal, no further treatment is required, but the patient should be followed with an annual chest x-ray. Prophylactic treatment with single-agent therapy is recommended for patients who are recent PPD converters, those who live with someone with active TB, and those who are immunosuppressed and PPD-positive (e.g., AIDS sufferers and diabetic persons).

Several drugs are available for therapy, but all have potential maternal and fetal risks. Untreated TB is believed, however, to be of greater risk to both the mother and infant. **Isoniazid (INH) is considered the safest drug for use in pregnancy.** Fetal risks include potential CNS toxicity, but treating the mother with vitamin B_6 supplements eliminates this risk. The main risk to the mother is hepatitis, so monthly liver function tests should be performed. **Rifampin has been linked to limb reduction defects in the fetus and hepatitis in the mother. Ethambutol is safer than rifampin but is not as effective,** and it has been associated with a reversible maternal optic neuritis in 6% of patients. **Streptomycin is to be avoided in pregnancy** because of the risk of nephrotoxicity and permanent cranial nerve VIII damage in the fetus. **For women with active disease, current recommendations are for 9 months of therapy with INH and rifampin.** After delivery, newborns should be isolated from their mothers with active disease until the mothers are culture-negative. **INH prophylaxis of the infant is recommended because 50% of infants develop active TB by 1 year of age without it.** Once the mother is culture-negative, she may breastfeed because only small concentrations of the drugs pass into the milk.

SYPHILIS

All pregnant women should be screened for syphilis at the first prenatal visit with either a

venereal disease research laboratories (VDRL) test or a rapid plasma reagin (RPR) test. These tests carry a false-positive rate of between 0.5% and 14% because they are nonspecific for treponemes. Common causes of false-positive results are drug addiction, autoimmune disease, recent viral infection or immunization, or pregnancy itself. False-positive titers are usually 1:4. Specific treponemal tests, such as the fluorescent treponemal antibody absorption test (FTA-ABS), are performed to confirm the diagnosis.

Impact on Pregnancy

Maternal infection can result in transplacental transmission to the fetus at any gestational age. Mothers with primary and secondary syphilis are more likely to transmit the infection, with more severe manifestations occurring in the fetus. Transmission rates for primary and secondary disease are between 50% and 80%. There is a wide range of fetal responses to infection.

Components of early congenital syphilitic infection include nonimmune hydrops, hepatosplenomegaly, profound anemia and thrombocytopenia, skin lesions, rash, osteitis and periostitis, pneumonia, and hepatitis. The perinatal mortality rate from congenital syphilis is roughly 50%.

Late congenital syphilis (diagnosed after 2 years of age) is a multisystem disease characterized by dental abnormalities (Hutchinson's teeth, mulberry molars); saber shins; destruction of the nasal septum, resulting in a saddle-nose deformity; interstitial keratitis; eighth nerve deafness; and failure to thrive.

Treatment

Treatment of the condition in pregnancy is the same as that in the nonpregnant state. Penicillin G is the therapy of choice. Patients with primary, secondary, or latent syphilis of less than 12 months' duration are treated with a single dose of benzathine penicillin, 2.4 million U, IM. Those with syphilis of undetermined length or with latent infection for longer than 1 year receive this therapy weekly for 3 weeks. For patients with penicillin allergy, erythromycin therapy has been used but has been associated with an 11% failure rate. Therefore desensitization and use of penicillin is recommended. Patients with neurosyphilis require admission and prolonged intravenous penicillin therapy.

Women treated for syphilis during their pregnancy require careful follow-up with monthly VDRL or RPR titers to ensure that the treatment is successful. Patients with syphilis remain positive on FTA-ABS testing for the remainder of their lives. Patients' sexual contacts should be referred for treatment. Neonates are evaluated and treated as indicated.

PARASITIC INFECTIONS
TOXOPLASMOSIS

Toxoplasmosis is a systemic disease caused by the protozoan *Toxoplasma gondii*. Between 15% and 40% of women of reproductive age have antibodies (IgG) to toxoplasmosis and therefore are immune to future infection. Occasionally, toxoplasmosis presents as a mononucleosis-like syndrome, but most infections are subclinical. The organism is acquired by ingesting undercooked meat or unpasteurized goat's milk or by exposure to feces from an infected cat.

Impact on Pregnancy

The incidence of primary infection in pregnancy is 1 in 1000. Routine screening for toxoplasmosis is not recommended in pregnancy. The risk of transmission to the fetus is 15% in the 1st trimester, 25% in the 2nd trimester, and 65% in the 3rd trimester. However, the severity of fetal infection is greatest with first-trimester infection. The classic triad of hydrocephalus, intracranial calcifications, and chorioretinitis is rarely seen. Approximately 75% of infected infants are asymptomatic at birth. Between 25% and 50% exhibit the sequelae shown in Box 17-8. The presence of IgM in cord blood confirms the diagnosis. In addition, placental culture

---

Box 17-8. Manifestations of congenital toxoplasmosis infection

Hydrocephalus
Chorioretinitis
Microcephaly
Microphthalmia
Hepatosplenomegaly
Cerebral calcifications
Adenopathy
Convulsions
Delayed mental development

reveals the organism in more than 90% of cases of congenital infection. Because it is very often a subclinical infection, toxoplasmosis is rarely diagnosed during pregnancy. It should be considered in the differential diagnosis of anyone with a mononucleosis-like (Epstein-Barr) syndrome. Diagnosis by serologic testing for both IgG and IgM is by a positive finding of IgM or a fourfold rise in IgG titer in paired sequential samples obtained 2 to 3 weeks apart. IgM titers may remain elevated for 4 months. **It is possible to diagnose fetal infection by culture and serologic testing of amniotic fluid and fetal blood in conjunction with the ultrasonic findings.**

Treatment

Toxoplasmosis is a self-limiting infection. Owing to the fetal risk, spiramycin is utilized for treatment in the absence of fetal infection in Europe, but it is obtainable in the United States only through special permission from the Food and Drug Administration (FDA). **If fetal infection is identified, therapy with pyrimethamine and sulfadiazine plus folinic acid should be given and has been shown to reduce the severity of fetal damage.** To prevent infection, pregnant women should be advised to avoid contact with cat litter or feces, to wear gloves while gardening, and to avoid ingestion of raw meat or unpasteurized goat's milk.

SURGICAL CONDITIONS DURING PREGNANCY

Pregnancy substantially enhances the problems associated with surgery. Physiologic changes and the altered immunologic responses of pregnancy change the diagnostic parameters of surgical diseases. Reluctance to operate during pregnancy may add to critical delays and increase the morbidity for both the fetus and the mother.

Common surgical conditions complicating pregnancy include acute appendicitis, acute cholecystitis, acute pancreatitis, and ovarian neoplasms (Table 17-8). Cancer of the breast, cervix, bowel, and skin are occasionally diagnosed during pregnancy and may require relatively urgent surgery.

ACUTE CONDITIONS

The general approach to acute surgical conditions during pregnancy (e.g., acute appendicitis) is to manage the problem regardless of the pregnancy.

Table 17-8. Surgical conditions in pregnancy	
Acute	**Nonemergency**
Acute appendicitis	Adnexal tumors
Acute cholecystitis	Cervical cancer
Acute pancreatitis	Breast cancer
Abdominal trauma	Gastrointestinal cancer
Torsion of uterine adnexa	Melanoma, osteosarcoma
Pelvic abscess	
Peptic ulcer disease	
Bowel obstruction	
Intracranial hemorrhage	
Thromboembolic disease	

Because of the possible teratogenic risk of anesthesia and the possibility of surgery inducing an abortion in the 1st trimester, surgery for some semi-urgent conditions (e.g., an ovarian neoplasm) is better delayed until the more stable 2nd trimester. If the uterus is to be removed (e.g., stage Ib cervical cancer), surgery may be delayed in the interests of fetal maturity.

Acute nonobstetric surgical emergencies occur in all three trimesters of pregnancy. The overall incidence is approximately 1 in 500 pregnancies. The more common acute conditions resulting in a "surgical abdomen" necessitating immediate surgery are appendicitis, cholecystitis and cholelithiasis, pancreatitis, bowel obstruction, adnexal torsion, and abdominal trauma.

APPENDICITIS

The incidence of acute appendicitis in pregnancy is approximately 1 in 1500 gestations, and it is constant throughout the three trimesters. The usual symptoms of acute appendicitis, such as epigastric pain, nausea, vomiting, and lower abdominal pain, may be less apparent during pregnancy. Hence, **the diagnosis is often difficult, and the differential diagnosis may be especially confusing** (Box 17-9). Persistent vomiting with right-sided pain, tenderness, and guarding generally leads to the diagnosis. The enlarging uterus displaces the appendix superiorly and laterally as pregnancy progresses, so the point of maximal tenderness also rises and may be masked by the overlying uterus and broad ligament (Figure 17-1). **Tenderness and guarding are elicited more laterally than expected.** The somewhat increased white blood cell count seen in normal pregnancy further confuses the issue and

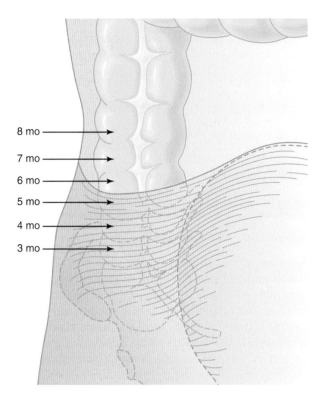

8 mo

7 mo

6 mo

5 mo

4 mo

3 mo

Figure 17-1. The changing position of the right colon and appendix as pregnancy progresses and the uterus enlarges.

makes the diagnosis notoriously difficult, frequently resulting in delayed surgery and an increased rate of premature labor, infant morbidity, and, rarely, maternal death.

Although acute appendicitis does not occur more often during the 3rd trimester, rupture occurs more frequently at that time, with a higher morbidity and mortality. The incidence of perfora-

| Box 17-9. | **Differential diagnosis of acute appendicitis in pregnancy** |

Ruptured corpus luteum
Pyelonephritis
Ectopic pregnancy
Acute mesenteric lymphadenitis
Regional enteritis (Crohn disease)
Salpingo-ovarian abscess
Acute mesenteric thrombosis

tion is 10% in the 1st trimester and increases to 40% in the 3rd trimester. The recent perinatal mortality rate associated with acute appendicitis is less than 5%.

If acute appendicitis cannot be ruled out in the face of reasonably definite signs and symptoms, laparotomy with or without appendectomy should be carried out. In the 1st trimester with a fairly certain diagnosis, a McBurney or a transverse or Rockey-Davis incision is employed. If the diagnosis is equivocal, a right paramedian incision should be made to allow a more extensive exploration. If acute appendicitis is encountered late in pregnancy, appendectomy should be carried out without a concurrent cesarean section. Appropriate antibiotics, along with the judicious use of tocolytics, should be employed postoperatively. If labor occurs with a recent laparotomy incision, it can be managed quite well with epidural anesthesia and shortening of the second stage of labor with a low forceps delivery.

ACUTE CHOLECYSTITIS AND CHOLELITHIASIS

An increase in serum cholesterol and lipid levels in pregnancy, along with biliary stasis, leads to a higher incidence of cholelithiasis, biliary obstruction, and cholecystitis. The high levels of estrogens in pregnancy increase the saturation of cholesterol in the bile. Virtually all of the gallstones associated with pregnancy are composed of crystallized cholesterol. The incidence of hospitalization for cholecystitis in pregnancy is 1% to 2%, but only 1 in 2000 pregnant women require cholecystectomy. In more recent years, ultrasonography has revealed a fairly high incidence of cholelithiasis in pregnancy (4%), and the incidence of cholecystectomy in pregnancy has appreciably increased.

Nausea and vomiting, along with right upper quadrant tenderness and guarding, generally suggest biliary tract disease. In the 3rd trimester, the large uterus may make it difficult to evaluate any tenderness and guarding. An increasing white blood cell count with slightly elevated alkaline phosphatase and bilirubin levels, jaundice in the presence of stones, or increased thickness of the gallbladder wall on ultrasonography serves to authenticate the diagnosis. Fifty percent of patients with cholelithiasis are asymptomatic, and the severity of biliary colic varies considerably.

The nausea and vomiting, leukocytosis, and somewhat increased alkaline phosphatase level of normal pregnancy serve to make the diagnosis more difficult. **Pernicious nausea and vomiting of pregnancy and viral hepatitis must be considered in the differential diagnosis.** Markedly elevated aspartate transaminase and alanine transaminase levels (>200 U/L), especially without leukocytosis, should suggest viral hepatitis and mitigate against a diagnosis of acute cholecystitis.

Generally, cholecystitis can be managed medically in pregnancy. Parenteral fluids, gastric decompression, and dietary measures should be the primary approach to management. If symptoms and signs persist with progressive peritonitis, cholecystectomy is indicated. **Although laparoscopic cholecystectomy has been performed in pregnancy, this approach is not generally recommended.**

ACUTE PANCREATITIS

Generally, pancreatitis is associated with cholecystitis, cholelithiasis, or alcoholism, but there are other associations (Box 17-10). The incidence in pregnancy varies from 1:1000 to 1:4000. The incidence of acute pancreatitis increases somewhat in the 3rd trimester.

Acute pancreatitis is seen less often in pregnancy, probably because the age-related contributing factors of alcoholism and cholelithiasis are more common later in life, but **mortality from pancreatitis is significantly higher when it does occur in pregnancy.** As noted in Box 17-11, some drugs not uncommonly prescribed in pregnancy are associated with acute pancreatitis.

The prime symptom of pancreatitis is severe, noncolicky epigastric pain radiating to the high back, which is relieved somewhat by leaning

---

Box 17-11. Drugs associated with acute pancreatitis

Thiazide diuretics
Furosemide
Acetaminophen
Clonidine
Isoniazid
Rifampin
Tetracycline
Propoxyphene
Steroids

---

forward. Nausea and vomiting generally are present but may not be prominent initially. Upper abdominal guarding may be difficult to assess in late pregnancy because of the enlarging uterus. **An elevated serum amylase level** (>200 U/dL, or urinary amylase excretion exceeding 300 U/hour) **generally confirms the diagnosis,** although cholecystitis, peptic ulcer, and diabetic ketoacidosis may also be associated with less marked elevations of serum amylase. On rare occasions, a technetium scan may aid in the diagnosis by outlining the biliary tree with minimal irradiation to the fetus.

Generally, the disease is self-limiting and responds within 1 to 10 days to bed rest, parenteral fluids, pain relief, and nasogastric suction. Any complications must be managed as they arise. Occasionally the disease becomes severe and protracted, with extensive pancreatic edema and autodigestion, massive ascites, hemoperitoneum, fever, and paralytic ileus. In such cases, mortality is high, and peritoneal lavage, operative drainage, partial pancreatic resection, or some combination of these procedures may be required.

BOWEL OBSTRUCTION

Bowel obstruction in pregnancy is most often associated with postoperative adhesions, although volvulus and intussusception are rare causes. It generally occurs in late pregnancy and is associated with traction on adhesions as the uterus enlarges. The nausea and vomiting often seen in early pregnancy may confuse the issue, but the more colicky character of the pain, along with abdominal tenderness, distention, and abnormal peristalsis, is very helpful in making the diagnosis. **An upright x-ray film of the abdomen showing characteristic dilated loops of**

Box 17-10. Risk factors associated with acute pancreatitis

Alcohol abuse
Cholecystitis/cholelithiasis
Abdominal trauma
Infectious diseases: mumps, hepatitis
Elevated lipid levels
Drugs (e.g., isoniazid, diuretics, steroids)
Familial pancreatitis
Rare: ischemic vascular disease, systemic lupus erythematosus (SLE)
Idiopathic

bowel and air-fluid levels serves to confirm the obstruction.

Management does not differ from that in the nonpregnant patient. Nasogastric suction should be instituted and fluid and electrolyte balance carefully monitored. **If the obstruction does not resolve after 48 to 96 hours, an exploratory laparotomy should be carried out through an appropriate incision (usually a right or left paramedian incision).** The appropriate surgical procedure should be carried out without disturbing the uterus. If uterine contractions occur postoperatively, tocolytics may be employed.

ADNEXAL TORSION

Torsion of the uterine adnexa tends to occur somewhat more commonly in pregnancy, possibly because the supporting ligaments elongate as the gestation progresses. Ovarian tumors (e.g., cystic teratomas, corpus luteum cysts) may become ischemic if their vascular pedicles undergo torsion. Such ischemic events are usually heralded by the sudden onset of severe abdominal pain, which may radiate to the flank and down the anterior thigh.

During the 1st and early 2nd trimesters, a mass is usually felt on pelvic examination or is visualized by ultrasonography. Later in the pregnancy it may be impossible to palpate a mass clinically. Low-grade fever and leukocytosis may be present, and serum creatine phosphokinase levels may be elevated, depending on the extent of the infarction. The most likely differential diagnoses include ectopic pregnancy and hemorrhagic corpus luteum, both of which seldom occur beyond 10 to 12 gestational weeks.

Although the pain may diminish somewhat after 24 hours, removal of the infarcted organ is indicated. If the excised ovary contains the corpus luteum, progesterone supplementation is generally necessary prior to 8 weeks' gestation.

ABDOMINAL TRAUMA

By far, the most common abdominal trauma in pregnancy occurs in automobile accidents. Abruptio placentae, uterine contusions, and fetal skull fractures may result. Abruptio placentae is treated expectantly unless fetal monitoring indicates fetal distress, in which case immediate abdominal delivery is in order if the fetus is at a reasonably safe gestational age (28 weeks or greater). Abdominal exploration may be necessary to stop bleeding and repair uterine lacerations. Lap-shoulder harness seat belts, rather than lap belts, are advisable for pregnant women after 12 weeks' gestation.

Gunshot wounds of the abdomen are treated as in nonpregnant patients, with measures taken to stop bleeding and repair visceral or uterine injuries. So long as the pregnancy is intact, the uterus should not be disturbed. Careful monitoring of fetal well-being should be maintained before and after the operation.

OVARIAN TUMORS

Adnexal masses are not at all uncommon in pregnancy and can best be identified by pelvic examination early in the pregnancy. Most of these ovarian masses are functional cysts (e.g., corpus luteal cysts) that regress as the gonadotropin levels fall during the second trimester. All adnexal masses should be evaluated by ultrasonography. **Solid ovarian tumors larger than 5 cm or complex cystic tumors larger than 8 cm deserve exploration without undue delay,** preferably early in the 2nd trimester. The incidence of ovarian carcinoma in pregnancy is 1 in 2000.

Suggested Reading

American College of Obstetricians and Gynecologists Committee Opinion: Zidovudine for the prevention of vertical transmission of human immunodeficiency virus. Bulletin No. 148. Washington, DC, ACOG, December 1994.

American College of Obstetricians and Gynecologists: Guidelines for hepatitis B virus screening and vaccination during pregnancy. Technical Bulletin No. 111. Washington, DC, ACOG, 1992.

American College of Obstetricians and Gynecologists: Perinatal herpes simplex virus infections, Technical Bulletin No. 122. Washington, DC, ACOG, 1988.

American College of Obstetricians and Gynecologists: Perinatal viral and parasitic infections. Technical Bulletin No. 177. Washington, DC, ACOG, 1993.

American College of Obstetricians and Gynecologists: Rubella and pregnancy. Technical Bulletin No. 171. Washington, DC, ACOG, 1992.

American College of Obstetricians and Gynecologists: Trauma during pregnancy. Technical Bulletin No. 161. Washington, DC, ACOG, November 1991.

Watts, HD. Drug therapy: management of human immunodeficiency virus infection in pregnancy. N Engl J Med 346:1879–1891, 2002.

18

Obstetric Procedures

Ramen H. Chmait and Thomas R. Moore

As the fetus has become more accessible via technological advances in prenatal and antenatal surveillance, the desire to intervene on behalf of the fetus has led to the development of a number of obstetric diagnostic and therapeutic procedures. Any procedure that is performed during pregnancy has inherent risk to both the mother and the fetus. Appropriate nondirective counseling that details the potential benefits and risks of all options is of the utmost importance prior to embarking on any procedure.

PRENATAL DIAGNOSTIC AND THERAPEUTIC PROCEDURES
ULTRASOUND

Prenatal transvaginal and transabdominal ultrasound plays a pivotal role in modern-day obstetrical care, with ultrasound imaging being done in approximately 70% of pregnancies in the United States today. Human data have shown no adverse fetal effects of ultrasound.

Transvaginal Ultrasound

Transvaginal ultrasound is useful in the 1st trimester of pregnancy because it allows for better resolution of the pelvic organs and developing pregnancy. This is the case because the uterus remains a pelvic organ until the 2nd trimester. Transvaginal ultrasound is commonly used in the first trimester to determine accurate **dating of the pregnancy,** as well as **fetal location and number. The nuchal translucency measurement,** a sonographically derived assessment of the subcutaneous fluid collection at the level of the fetal neck, is a screening test for chromosomal and structural abnormalities that is being performed

between 11 and 14 weeks' gestation, typically via transvaginal ultrasound. **Transvaginal sonographic measurement of cervical length in the midtrimester can be utilized to identify patients at risk for preterm delivery.** The median length of the cervix at 24 to 28 weeks is 3.5 cm. Patients with a cervical length less than 2.5 cm are at significantly increased risk of preterm birth (threefold to fivefold). **Finally, transvaginal ultrasound imaging of the lower uterine segment allows for very precise identification of placental location in relation to the internal cervical os.** In a patient with vaginal bleeding, excluding placenta previa is important in management.

Transabdominal Ultrasound

After 16 weeks' gestation, transabdominal ultrasound is utilized to evaluate the fetus for structural abnormalities and to provide information regarding fetal well-being. The ability of a 2nd trimester scan to identify a fetus with an anomaly ranges from 17% to 74%. The reason various studies show such a wide range in the sensitivity is probably due to variations in patient population and operator skill. The specificity, or the ability of ultrasound to correctly identify a normal fetus, approaches 100% in all studies. Thus **ultrasound is useful in ruling out fetal anomalies,** but it is not as reliable in detecting them. Box 18-1 lists common abnormalities that may be identified prenatally with ultrasound.

In the 3rd trimester, transabdominal ultrasound is useful in assessing fetal growth. Serial biometric measurements of the fetal head, abdomen, and limbs provide longitudinal information regarding the fetal growth trajectory. Software packages integral to the ultrasonic machines allow calculation of a fetal

Box 18-1. Examples of fetal abnormalities detected by prenatal ultrasound

CENTRAL NERVOUS SYSTEM
- Hydrocephalus
- Anencephaly
- Spina Bifida

FACE
- Cleft lip and/or palate

NECK
- Cystic hygroma
- Goiter
- Nuchal skin thickening

HEART
- Atrial septal defect
- Ventricular septal defect
- Tetralogy of Fallot
- Transposition of the great vessels
- Arrhythmias

LUNGS
- Congenital cystic adenomatoid malformation (CCAM)
- Lung sequestration
- Diaphragmatic hernia

ABDOMINAL WALL
- Gastroschisis
- Omphalocele

GASTROINTESTINAL TRACT
- Bowel atresia or obstruction

URINARY SYSTEM
- Renal agenesis
- Polycystic kidney disease
- Hydronephrosis
- Posterior urethral valves

SKELETAL DYSPLASIA

weight estimate from these measurements; this estimate is often utilized clinically. However, understanding that these estimates may have an error of ±15% (a variation of ±1 lb or 450 g in a 7 lb or 3400 g estimate) limits the utility of ultrasonic fetal weight, especially in larger (>8 lb or 4000 g) fetuses.

Ultrasound visualization of aspects of fetal behavior (body movement, breathing) provides highly predictive information regarding fetal oxygenation and well-being. The **biophysical profile,** which combines a **fetal heart rate evaluation** (nonstress test) with real-time sonographic observations over a 30 minute span, consists of allotting 2 points each for **fetal breathing activity** (30 seconds of rhythmic movement of the fetal thorax), **fetal movement** (at least three movements of the body or limb), **fetal tone** (one extension and flexion of a limb joint), and the **amniotic fluid** (single deepest vertical pocket of amniotic fluid greater than 2 cm).

Doppler Sonography

Doppler sonography, which can precisely measure the velocity profile of blood flowing through fetal vessels, **allows for characterization of vascular impedance.** The umbilical artery, which normally has high-velocity flow during cardiac diastole, may have low, absent, or even reversed diastolic flow in a compromised fetus with high resistance placental vascularity. Similarly, because the peak flow velocity through a blood vessel is inversely proportional to the viscosity of the liquid flowing through it, Doppler studies of the fetal middle cerebral artery are now used as a noninvasive marker of severe fetal anemia in pregnancies complicated by isoimmunization.

Finally, **ultrasound is utilized to assist in performing invasive obstetric procedures.** Amniocentesis, chorionic villus sampling, and percutaneous umbilical blood sampling (cordocentesis) are examples of procedures that require continuous ultrasonic guidance.

AMNIOCENTESIS

Amniocentesis, which involves removing a sample of fluid from the amniotic cavity, is the most common invasive prenatal diagnostic procedure. Using direct ultrasonic guidance, a 22-gauge needle is advanced into a clear pocket of amniotic fluid under sterile conditions, taking care to avoid maternal bowel and vessels, as well as the placenta if possible. Approximately 20 cc of amniotic fluid is withdrawn for genetic procedures. **Rh immune globulin (Rh$_O$-GAM) must be given to the Rh-negative gravida** because of the small risk of procedure-related isoimmunization.

Genetic Diagnosis

Amniocentesis for prenatal diagnosis of chromosomal anomalies is performed at **16 to 20 weeks of**

gestation. The procedure-related **risks are an approximately 0.5% pregnancy loss rate and a 1% postprocedure measurable amniotic fluid leakage rate.** Early amniocentesis done before the 13th week of gestation is associated with a higher miscarriage rate (3% to 4%), higher postprocedure leakage rate (3%), and an additional risk of clubfoot (1%). Amniotic cells require approximately 2 weeks of culture before chromosomal analysis is possible, although florescent in-situ hybridization (FISH) can be used with chromosome-specific probes (e.g., trisomy 21, 18, and 13) which can give preliminary results in 3 days.

Single gene defects that have been characterized at the molecular level are amenable to prenatal diagnosis via amniocentesis. **Using polymerase chain reaction, fetal DNA in the amniocytes can be amplified rapidly to allow for direct or indirect molecular analysis of genetic disorders.** Examples of common prenatally diagnosed genetic disorders include cystic fibrosis, Tay-Sachs disease, sickle cell disease and fragile X syndrome. As the human genome mapping project advances, an increasing number of genetic disorders will be prenatally diagnosed in this manner.

Biochemical Testing

An example of biochemical testing which can be performed on amniotic fluid is **determination of the level of alpha-fetoprotein (AFP).** AFP is a fetal serum protein that should, under normal circumstances, be detectable in the amniotic fluid in only trace amounts. **In the event that the fetal dorsal or ventral wall is open (e.g., neural tube defect or gastroschisis), amniotic fluid AFP will be elevated,** allowing detection of these defects even if ultrasonic imaging is equivocal or nondiagnostic.

Other Diagnostic Testing

Amniocentesis is also commonly utilized in the third trimester to determine the risk of neonatal lung immaturity in the case of impending premature birth or prior to elective delivery. This is performed by measuring the **pulmonary phospholipids,** which enter the amniotic fluid from the fetal lungs. **The presence of phosphatidylglycerol and a lecithin-to-sphingomyelin (L/S) ratio greater than 2.0 are associated with minimal risk of respiratory distress in the neonate.** In a case of suspected premature rupture of the membranes when the diagnosis is unclear using standard tests, infusion of 2 to 3 cc of indigo dye into the amniotic fluid may be performed. If the dye is then noted on vaginally placed gauze, rupture of the membranes is confirmed. **Finally, amniotic fluid Gram stain, white blood cell count, glucose level, interleukin-6 level, and culture have been used to diagnose preterm chorioamnionitis.**

Therapeutic Amniocentesis

The primary role of a therapeutic amniocentesis has been in the management of polyhydramnios and twin-twin transfusion syndrome. Polyhydramnios, defined as a single deepest vertical pocket of amniotic fluid greater than 8 cm on ultrasound, can cause maternal respiratory embarrassment or premature labor. Excessive amniotic fluid volume may arise from lack of fetal swallowing, or from excessive fetal urination. The latter condition occurs in the twin-twin transfusion syndrome because of an unbalanced vascular connection in the placenta of monochorionic twins (see Chapter 14). Serial amniocenteses to remove large volumes of excessive amniotic fluid from the sac of the recipient twin have been associated with improved perinatal outcome.

CHORIONIC VILLUS SAMPLING

Another method to access fetal cells for prenatal diagnosis is via chorionic villus sampling (CVS). The indications for CVS are similar to amniocentesis. **The advantage of CVS is that it is performed earlier (typically between the 10th and 12th week of gestation) than amniocentesis, allowing for earlier prenatal diagnosis.** Although technically feasible, CVS is not performed before the 9th week, as it has been associated with an increase risk of oromandibular/limb dystrophy, presumably from a vascular insult.

CVS may be performed under sterile conditions transcervically or transabdominally. In transcervical CVS, the distal 3 to 5 cm of a catheter is inserted through the cervix and into the placenta under sonographic guidance. A 20-mL syringe with nutrient medium is attached and negative pressure applied to obtain fragments of placental villi. Transabdominal CVS approach utilizes an 18- to 20-gauge needle inserted into the placenta transabdominally. With either approach, Rh immune globulin (Rh$_O$-GAM) should be administered to Rh negative patients. Both methods have equivalent low complication rates. **The procedure related loss rate is <1%.**

Direct visual inspection of dividing villi cells obtained with CVS allows for detection of chromosomal abnormalities within 3 days, and tissue culture yields cytogenetic results in 6 to 8 days. **The diagnostic precision of CVS is somewhat less than the standard amniocentesis due to a 1% risk of chromosomal mosaicism, which is often due to confined placental mosaicism.** A disadvantage of CVS is that amniotic fluid AFP levels cannot be assessed with this technique, and thus patients at risk for neural tube defects must be deferred to amniocentesis in the second trimester.

CORDOCENTESIS

Cordocentesis (percutaneous umbilical blood sampling) is a procedure in which fetal blood is obtained directly from the umbilical vein at the placental cord insertion site under direct ultrasonic guidance. Confirmation of the fetal origin of the blood specimen is obtained by measuring the fetal MCV, which is typically greater than 120 fL (maternal MCV is usually <100 fL).

Historically, the most common indication for cordocentesis was to determine fetal hematocrit in the hemolytic disease, Rh-isoimmunization. With the recent advent of fetal anemia assessment via Doppler of the fetal middle cerebral artery, cordocentesis for this indication has waned over the last few years. **Today, cordocentesis is often performed for rapid fetal karyotype evaluation.** Unlike amniocytes, fetal leukocytes may be cultured rapidly, and results are typically available in 3 days.

The fetal loss rate is about 1% per procedure. In the case of a hydropic fetus, the risk of fetal loss may approach 7%. The cause of pregnancy loss may be due to chorioamnionitis, rupture of membranes, bleeding from the puncture site, bradycardia, or thrombosis of the vessel.

OPERATIVE DELIVERY

The incidence of an operative obstetric delivery in the United States today is approximately 35% to 40%, of which 10% to 15% are operative vaginal deliveries using either a forceps or vacuum device. **Approximately 25% of all deliveries are cesarean sections.** Each operative procedure has inherent benefits and risks.

OBSTETRIC FORCEPS

Forceps are instruments designed to provide traction and/or rotation of the fetal head when the expulsive efforts of the mother are insufficient to accomplish safe delivery of the fetus. Currently used forceps are shown in Figure 18-1. There are two classes of

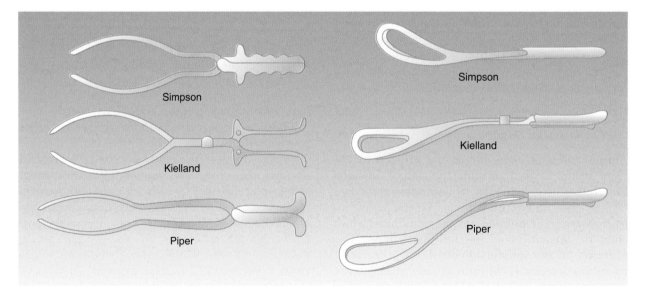

Figure 18-1. Types of obstetric forceps in use. Kielland forceps (for midforceps rotation) are used infrequently.

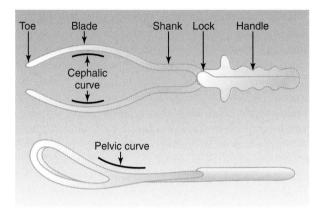

Figure 18-2. Components of classic forceps.

obstetric forceps: classical forceps and specialized forceps. Forceps selection depends on the obstetric indication.

Classic or standard forceps are used to effect delivery by applying traction to the fetal skull. The components of each blade are illustrated in Figure 18-2. The blades have a **cephalic curve** designed to conform to the curvature of the fetal head. Simpson

forceps have a tapered cephalic curve that is designed to fit on a molded fetal head, whereas Elliot forceps have a more rounded cephalic curve that is suited for an unmolded fetal head. The **pelvic curve** of classic forceps approximates the shape of the birth canal.

Indications

In general, there are four indications for an operative vaginal delivery:

1. **Prolonged second stage of labor**. In nulliparous women this is defined as lack of continuing progress for 2 hours without regional anesthesia or 3 hours with regional anesthesia. In multiparous women it is defined as lack of continuing progress for 1 hour without regional anesthesia and 2 hours with regional anesthesia
2. **Suspicion of immediate or impending fetal compromise.**
3. **To stabilize the aftercoming head during a breech delivery** (Figure 18-3).
4. **To shorten the second stage of labor for maternal benefit**. Maternal conditions such as hypertension, cardiac disorders, or pulmonary disease, in which strenuous pushing in the

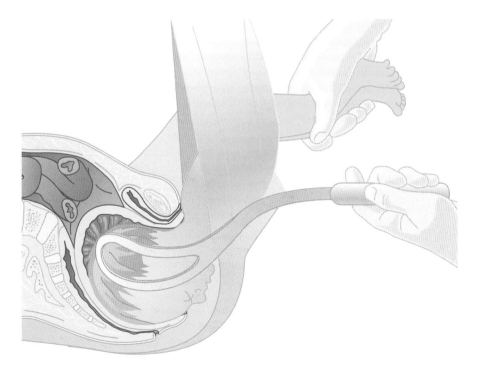

Figure 18-3. Delivery of the aftercoming head, using Piper forceps.

second stage of labor is considered hazardous, may be indications for forceps delivery. Epidural analgesia, which also decreases strenuous pushing during the second stage of labor, may also be recommended for this purpose.

Types of Forceps Operations

Forceps application is classified according to the station and position of the presenting part at the time the forceps are applied. The American College of Obstetricians and Gynecologists (ACOG) has proposed the following classification:

1. **Outlet forceps:** Scalp visible at the introitus without separating the labia, fetal head at perineum, fetal skull at pelvic floor, sagittal suture in anteroposterior or right/left occiput anterior or posterior position, and rotation of the fetal head does not exceed 45 degrees.
2. **Low forceps:** The leading part of the fetal skull is at station +2 cm or more. Low forceps have two subdivisions: rotation of 45 degrees or less and rotation of more than 45 degrees.
3. **Mid forceps:** Fetal head is engaged but the leading point of the skull is above station +2 cm.

Prior to performing a forceps-assisted vaginal delivery, appropriate consent from the patient regarding potential risks and benefits should be obtained. The indication for the procedure should be clearly outlined to the patient and in the medical record. **The cervix must be fully dilated, membranes ruptured, and the fetal head engaged into the pelvis.** Clinical assessment to determine the level of the presenting part, estimation of the fetal size, and adequacy of the maternal pelvis is mandatory. **There must be no doubt regarding the position of the fetal head.** This evaluation is performed by palpation of the sutures and fontanelles in comparison to the maternal pelvis. **Anesthesia must be adequate** via either pudendal nerve block with local infiltration (for outlet forceps only) or regional anesthesia. **The bladder should be emptied** to prevent damage to that structure and to provide more room to effect delivery.

Forceps Technique

The forceps blades are inserted sequentially into the vagina such that the sagital suture of the fetal head is directly between and perpendicular to the shanks.

Damage to maternal tissues may be avoided by placing one operator hand into the vagina to guide the toe of the blade along the natural pelvic curve of the birth canal. With the next maternal pushing effort, the forceps are locked and traction is applied. The direction of pull should be parallel to the axis of the birth canal at that level, such that typically there is downward traction initially, followed by ever-increasing upward traction as delivery of the fetal head occurs. With complete delivery of the head, the shanks are nearly perpendicular to the floor. **If progress of the fetal head is not obtained with appropriate traction, cephalopelvic disproportion should be suspected and the procedure should be abandoned (failed forceps) in favor of a cesarean section.**

Potential complications of forceps delivery to both the mother and the fetus are addressed after the following section on vacuum delivery.

VACUUM EXTRACTION

The vacuum extractor is an instrument that utilizes a suction cup that is applied to the fetal head. Because of relative ease of use compared to forceps, vacuum delivery has become more prevalent in the United States. After confirming that no maternal tissue is trapped between the cup and the fetal head, the vacuum seal is obtained from a suction pump. Traction is then applied using similar principles described above for a forceps delivery. **Flexion of the fetal head must be maintained to provide the smallest diameter to the maternal pelvis by placing the posterior edge of the suction cup 3 cm from the anterior fontanelle squarely over the sagital suture.** This is illustrated in Figure 18-4. With the next maternal pushing effort, traction is applied parallel to the axis of the birth canal. Detachment of the suction cup from the fetal head during traction is termed a "pop-off." If progress down the birth canal is not obtained with appropriate traction or if two "pop-offs" occur, cephalopelvic disproportion should be suspected and the procedure should be discontinued in favor of a cesarean delivery. **The indications for vacuum delivery are the same as for forceps delivery.**

The requirements for the use of the vacuum extractor are also the same, with few exceptions. The vacuum extractor is contraindicated in preterm delivery, because the preterm fetal head and scalp are more prone to injury from the suction cup. The vacuum extractor is suitable for all vertex presentations, but

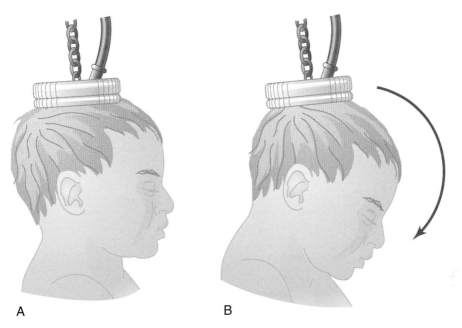

Figure 18-4. Application of the vacuum extractor. *A,* Incorrect application, which deflexes the fetal head, thereby increasing the presenting diameter. *B,* Correct application over the posterior fontanelle, which flexes the fetal head when traction is applied.

unlike forceps, it must never be used for delivery of fetuses presenting by the face or breech.

COMPARISON OF FORCEPS AND VACUUM DELIVERY

Understanding the potential advantages and disadvantages of each operative vaginal delivery instrument allows the operator to counsel the mother appropriately and choose the device that is best suited for the particular clinical situation.

Forceps have a higher overall success for vaginal delivery. **The failure rate for forceps is 7%, whereas the rate for vacuum extraction is 12%. In general, forceps deliveries cause higher rates of maternal injury**, and **vacuum extraction causes higher rates of fetal morbidity**. Forceps have an increased risk of trauma to vaginal and perineal tissues and damage to the maternal anal sphincter. In contrast, neonates delivered by vacuum have more cephalohematomas (accumulation of blood beneath the periosteum) and exclusively have subgaleal hematomas (blood in the space above the periosteum that has a large potential space and can allow significant blood loss) and retinal hemorrhages. **Sequential use of one instrument followed by the other has been associated with a disproportionately high fetal morbidity rate** and should be avoided or approached with extreme caution. Long-term retrospective studies of adolescents delivered by normal vaginal delivery, forceps, vacuums, and cesarean delivery have shown little difference in physical and cognitive impairment.

CESAREAN DELIVERY

Cesarean delivery is delivery of the fetus through an incision in the maternal abdomen and uterus. Hospitals that offer obstetric services must have the personnel and equipment to perform an emergent cesarean delivery within 30 minutes.

Cesarean delivery is the most common major operation performed in the United States today. **The rate of cesarean deliveries has increased fivefold, from 5% of births in 1970 to nearly 25% of births today**. This dramatic increase in the cesarean delivery rate has been attributed to many factors, including assumed benefit for the fetus, relatively low maternal risk, societal preference, and fear of litigation.

The perinatal benefits of cesarean section are largely based on unquantified and scanty evidence. There has been over a 10-fold decrease in the perinatal mortality in the United States over the last 40 years with the advancement in perinatal and neonatal care. How much of this improvement is due to the increased utilization of cesarean delivery is debatable. An exception to this uncertainty is with respect to term breech delivery. **Perinatal and neonatal mortality and significant neonatal morbidity has been shown to decrease from 5.0% for those delivered vaginally to 1.6% for those delivered by cesarean.**

The overall mortality rate from cesarean delivery is currently less than 1 in 1000, but this is about five times greater than that from vaginal delivery. However, **recent studies have shown that the maternal mortality rate for an elective cesarean approximates that of vaginal delivery.** This is due to advances in surgical techniques, anesthetic care, blood transfusions, and antibiotics.

The morbidity of cesarean delivery is increased compared to vaginal delivery, due to increased postpartum infections, hemorrhage, and thromboembolic disease. The relative risk of endomyometritis is substantially higher in cesarean delivery patients compared to those delivered vaginally, although that rate is halved with prophylactic antibiotics. Hemorrhage may be due to obstetric causes, such as uterine atony, and surgical causes, such as bleeding from the uterine incision site or a severed vessel. Cesarean delivery is associated with a significant increase in thromboembolic events compared to vaginal delivery.

Indications

Four indications for cesarean delivery account for 90% of the dramatic increase in this procedure over the past forty years: dystocia (30%), repeat cesarean section (25% to 30%), breech presentation (10% to 15%), and fetal distress (10% to 15%). **An absolute indication for a cesarean delivery is a previous incision through the myometrium of the uterus.** This occurs in all classical cesarean deliveries and some myomectomy surgeries. **All pregnancies complicated by placenta previa should also be delivered by cesarean.**

Types of Cesarean

Cesarean deliveries are classified by the uterine incision (Figure 18-5) not the skin incision. **The low transverse cesarean delivery (LTCD) uterine incision is transverse in the lower uterine segment.** The advantages of this approach include decreased

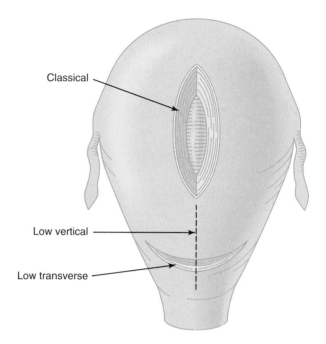

Figure 18-5. Types of cesarean delivery incisions.

rate of rupture of the scar in a subsequent pregnancy and a reduced risk of bleeding, peritonitis, paralytic ileus, and bowel adhesions.

An alternative approach is the classic cesarean section. This operation employs a vertical incision in the upper segment of the uterus through the myometrium of the uterus. A vertical incision may be made in the lower segment, in which case the procedure is referred to as a **low vertical cesarean,** although the incision invariably extends into the upper segment of the uterus. **The common indications for a classical cesarean section include the preterm breech with an undeveloped lower uterine segment, transverse back down fetal position, poor access to the lower segment due to myomas or adhesions, or in the case in which a cesarean hysterectomy is planned.**

The type of uterine incision has important implications regarding risk of uterine rupture in future pregnancies. Uterine rupture, defined as separation of the uterine incision, may cause significant maternal complications due to massive hemorrhage and fetal damage or death. **A LTCD incision is associated with less than a 1% risk of symptomatic uterine rupture in the subsequent pregnancy,** although this risk may be higher if an induction is carried out. **A classic cesarean delivery carries a 4% to 7% risk** of uterine rupture. Patients with a classical uterine incision are destined to have repeat cesareans for all subsequent deliveries.

Prevention

Two clinical interventions have been shown to reduce cesarean section rates: external cephalic version (ECV) and vaginal birth after cesarean section (VBAC).

External cephalic version. ECV converts a malpresenting fetus to the vertex position to avoid a cesarean delivery for breech presentation. This procedure is performed in labor and delivery, after the 36th or 37th week of gestation, under ultrasonic guidance. A tocolytic may be given to decrease uterine tone. Using external manipulation, the fetus is gently guided to the vertex presentation. **Fetal risks due to umbilical cord entanglement and placenta abruption are low (<1%).**

The success rate of ECV is about 60%. Parity, gestational age, placental location, and dilation/station affect this success rate. An ECV program can decrease the rate of cesarean section in this group of patients by more than half, and an obstetric service's overall cesarean section rate by approximately 2%.

Vaginal birth after cesarean delivery. Women with a prior cesarean represent the second most common overall cause of cesarean delivery (25% to 30%). In fact about 10% to 15% of pregnant women have had a previous cesarean delivery.

A trial of labor may be offered if one or two previous LTCDs were performed and the uterine incision did not extend into the cervix or uterine upper segment and there is no history of uterine rupture. An adequate maternal pelvic size should be noted by clinical examination. Personnel and equipment should be readily available in case of emergent cesarean.

The overall success rate of VBAC is approximately 70%, although this value ranges from 60% (dystocia) to 90% (malpresentation) depending on the indication for the previous cesarean. Numerous reports attest to its relative safety. Compared with repeat cesarean, a successful vaginal delivery is associated with less maternal morbidity without an increase in perinatal morbidity. However, if uterine rupture does occur, there may be a 10-fold increase in perinatal mortality and substantial maternal morbidity as well.

Suggested Reading

American College of Obstetricians and Gynecologists: External cephalic version. Practice Bulletin No. 13. Washington, DC, ACOG, 2000.

American College of Obstetricians and Gynecologists: Operative vaginal delivery, Practice Bulletin No. 17. Washington, DC, ACOG, 2000.

American College of Obstetricians and Gynecologists: Vaginal birth after previous cesarean section, Practice Bulletin No. 5. Washington, DC, ACOG, 1999.

Canadian Collaborative CVS/Amniocentesis Clinical Trial Group: Multicentre randomized clinical trial of chorionic villus sampling and amniocentesis. Lancet 1:1, 1989.

Towner D, Castro MA, Eby-Wilkens E, et al: Effect of mode of delivery in nulliparous women on neonatal intracranial injury. N Engl J Med 341:1709–1714, 1999.

PART THREE | Gynecology

Anita L. Nelson

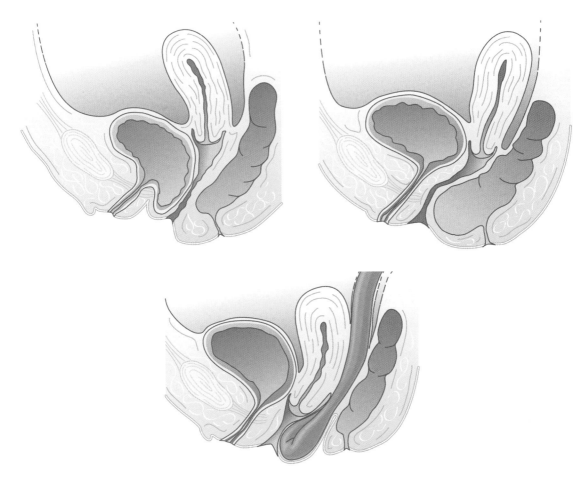

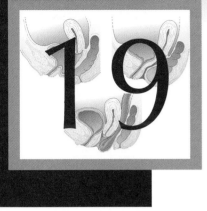

19

Congenital Anomalies and Benign Conditions of the Vulva and Vagina

Anita L. Nelson and Joseph C. Gambone

Vulvovaginal problems are among the 10 leading disorders encountered by primary care clinicians. Definitive diagnosis may be delayed even though the woman may complain of pruritus and irritation. There is a strong tendency for both patients and providers to treat the symptom without a thorough clinical examination or laboratory analysis. **It is important to establish a specific diagnosis before initiating therapy.**

In this chapter, benign lesions of the vulva and vagina will be described in the broad categories of congenital anomalies, benign neoplastic conditions, dermatologic changes, trauma, and functional disorders.

VULVA
CONGENITAL ANOMALIES OF THE VULVA

Congenital anomalies of the external genitalia are quite variable. Ambiguous genitalia can present with clitoromegaly, bifid clitoris, or midline fusion of labioscrotal folds. Clitoral agnesis is also possible as a result of failure of the genital tubercle to develop. Many of these defects are associated with other problems such as bladder extrophy. Incomplete development of the genitalia can result in a cloaca with no definite separation of the bladder and vagina. Hernial sacs may present in the newborn as vulvar masses. Similarly, any of the cells types normally found in the vulva can present at birth with overexuberant development, such as a hemangioma or neuroma.

The problems of sexual identification posed by ambiguous genitalia are particularly important at birth. Caution, sensitivity, and the avoidance of hasty decisions and confusing terminology should **be the rule when dealing with anxious parents and relatives.** Careful physical examination, pelvic ultrasonography, hormonal studies, examination of a buccal smear for sex chromatin, karyotyping, and consultation with specialists may be necessary before the sex of rearing is assigned. The assignment of sex will determine the need for any corrective surgery or hormonal manipulation and the manner in which the parents rear the child. These factors are all critical to the child's proper gender identification.

Female pseudohermaphroditism is caused by masculinization occurring in utero, the infant presenting with ambiguous genitalia. Masculinization of the genetically female fetus occurs secondary to the endogenous hormonal milieu, **as in congenital adrenal hyperplasia** (Figure 19-1), **or as a result of exogenous hormonal ingestion by the mother.** Androgen-producing tumors of the ovary or adrenal gland, although rarely, also cause this problem. **Enlargement of the clitoris is the most conspicuous abnormality.** Fusion of the labioscrotal folds also occurs in various degrees, producing a hypospadiac urethral meatus and a malpositioned vaginal orifice. Internal genital development is normal.

However, **when the genetic sex is male (46 XY), there may be complete external phenotypic development along female lines. This occurs in the testicular feminization syndrome (androgen insensitivity syndrome),** a genetic abnormality most commonly inherited as an x-linked recessive disorder. Because of a genetic deficiency of androgen receptors, the external genital development occurs along female lines. Testes are usually undescended and are located

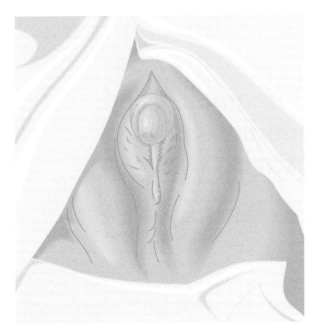

Figure 19-1. Illustration of ambiguous genitalia in an infant with congenital adrenal hyperplasia. This female exhibits clitoromegaly and an obscure vaginal orifice.

in the inguinal canals or the labial areas. After puberty, external genitalia are generally normal on examination, with the exception of scanty or absent pubic hair. Sufficient vaginal development to allow adequate coital activity is present in many cases. Müllerian inhibiting substance is produced, which is the reason for the lack of müllerian duct development.

Male pseudohermaphroditism may occur with varying degrees of virilization and müllerian development. This is most commonly the result of genetic mosaicism, such as 45 XO/46 XY. Many factors must be taken into account in the determination of gender role in these cases, and a full discussion of this problem is beyond the scope of this book. In a phenotypic female with a Y chromosome, localization and removal of the gonadal tissue and subsequent hormonal management are necessary (as with androgen insensitivity syndrome) because malignant neoplastic transformation commonly occurs in these gonads.

In true hermaphroditism, which is rare, dual gonadal development occurs, either in the form of an ovotestis or as a separate ovary and testis. Although some of these cases represent mosaicism of the normal female and male chromosomal complement, the usual chromosomal pattern is 46 XX. Most true hermaphrodites have some degree of both female and male development internally and externally. The extent to which masculinization occurs depends on the relative amount of testicular tissue and its relative contribution of testosterone. Confirmation of the diagnosis requires laparotomy.

BENIGN CONDITIONS OF THE VULVA

Box 19-1 lists significant noninfectious conditions that may affect the vulva. Infectious conditions of the vulva are discussed in Chapter 23.

Structural and Benign Neoplastic Conditions

Young girls can develop **labial agglutination,** which is easily treated by estrogen cream and massage to separate the labia majora. **Fox-Fordyce disease** is characterized by a series of pruritic, raised, yellowish retention cysts (often inflamed) in the axilla, mons, or labia, which result from keratin-plugged apocrine glands.

Other cysts can also develop in the vulva, reflecting the variety of dermoid structures present. The most common are **epidermal inclusion cysts** and **sebaceous cysts** located below the epidermis, which are mobile, non-tender, spherical, and slow growing. Sebaceous cysts are slightly firmer than other inclusion cysts; they are filled with dry caseous material. Most such inclusion cysts require no treatment if they are asymptomatic. The mucous glands of the vestibule and periurethral areas can become obstructed and form cystic structures. The milk line extends from the axilla to the vulva, and postpartum women can form **galactoceles** in the labia. **Vulvar varicosities** can enlarge, especially in pregnancy, to cause discomfort and pose possible risks of rupture or thrombosis.

Urethral caruncles appear as small, fleshy outgrowths of the distal edge of the urethra (Figure 19-2). In children, this results from spontaneous prolapse of the urethral mucosa. On the other hand, in postmenopausal women, the caruncle occurs when the hypoestrogenic vaginal epithelium contracts and everts the urethral mucosa.

Vulvar vestibulitis (vestibular adenitis) is a relatively rare condition in which one or more of the minor vestibular glands becomes inflamed. This condition is characterized by severe introital dyspareunia and, occasionally, vulvar pain. On examination, the lesions may be visualized as 1 to 4-mm erythematous dots that are exceedingly tender when gently touched with a cotton-tipped swab. Although

Box 19-1. Benign noninfectious vulvar abnormalities

STRUCTURAL AND BENIGN NEOPLASTIC CONDITIONS
Labial agglutination
Fox-Fordyce disease
Cysts
    Epidermal inclusion
    Sebaceous
    Galactocele
Vulvar varicosities
Urethral caruncles
Vulvar vestibulitis (vestibular adenitis)
Lentigo (freckles)
Nevi (moles)
Fibromas
Lipomas
Hidradenoma (apocrine gland tumor)
Syringoma (eccrine gland tumor)
Granular cell myoblastoma (Schwann cell tumor)
Neurofibroma (associated with von Recklinghausen's
    disease)
Cherry angiomata
Clitoromegaly

TRAUMATIC LESIONS
Blunt trauma
Genital mutilation
Obstetric lacerations

EPITHELIAL DISORDERS (NONNEOPLASTIC)
Squamous hyperplasia (formerly hyperplastic dystrophy)
Lichen sclerosis
Lichen planus
Pemphigus
Behçet's syndrome
Crohn disease
Aphthous ulcers
Decubitus ulcers
Acanthosis nigricans

FUNCTIONAL DISORDER
Vulvodynia

described as an "itis," vestibulitis is not an infectious process and will not respond to antibiotic therapy. Topical estrogen creams or hydrocortisone may be tried, but surgical therapy to remove the glandular area may ultimately be required. Other interventions may be necessary to deal with the associated sexual dysfunction.

The external genitalia can also be the site of benign growths. Both **lentigo** (freckles) and **nevi** (moles) (Figure 19-3) can be found on the labia and must be

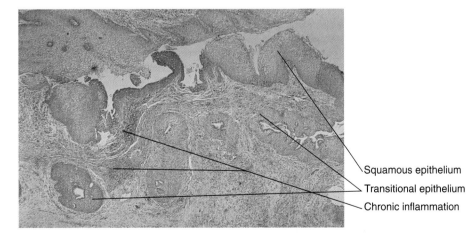

Figure 19-2. Urethral caruncle. This lesion usually presents as a small, painful, red lump at the urethral meatus. In this example, transitional epithelium can be recognized and there is a papillomatous pattern involving small, neighboring glands. A little chronic inflammation is seen.

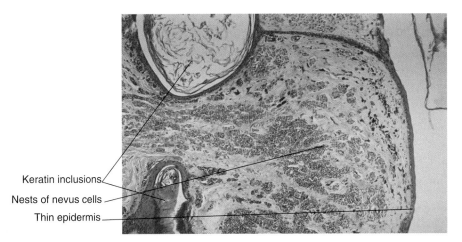

Keratin inclusions

Nests of nevus cells

Thin epidermis

Figure 19-3. Benign intradermal nevus. Nevi may occur on the vulva, usually on the labia majora. The covering epidermis is seen to be thinned and nests of nevus cells, some of which are pigmented, can be seen in the dermis.

clearly distinguished from melanomas. Often excisional biopsy is needed. **Fibromas** are the most common benign solid tumors that form in the deeper connective tissue of the vulva. Although fibromas are slow growing and most are 1 to 10 cm, they can become gigantic (>250 lb). **Lipomas** are also slow-growing tumors of the vulva, composed of adipose cells. Other tumors derive from tissue found in the external genitalia, such as **hidradenoma** (the apocrine gland tumor), **syringoma** (eccrine gland tumor), **granular cell myoblastoma** (neural sheath Schwann cell tumor) and **neurofibroma** (from von Recklinghausen's disease). These lesions should be removed surgically if they cause any problems. Small cherry **angiomata** can develop in the fourth and fifth decade and appear as multiple red lesions 2 to 3 mm in diameter.

Clitoromegaly may develop after birth in response to excessive androgen exposure. In the nonerect state, the clitoris usually is 0.5 cm wide and 1 to 1.5 cm long. **Clitoromegaly is a sign of virilization** and is diagnosed when the product of the external clitoral length times the width at the base of the clitoris exceeds 35 mm^2 (in a non-erect state) in an adult woman, or the width at the base is >1 cm.

TRAUMATIC LESIONS

Blunt trauma to the female genitalia from falls, moving vehicle accidents, or sexual assault (see Chapter 29) most commonly results in vulvar bruising, lacerations, and hematomas. Close observation and surgical exploration may be necessary to determine the full extent of the injuries and to repair them appropriately.

Genital body piercing and tattoos can cause infection or skin irritation. The area around the piercing can develop localized skin thickening and even trauma after sexual activity.

Female genital mutilation has been performed on a great many women worldwide and continues to be a very common practice, especially in some African countries. There are four different procedures performed ranging from simple clitoridectomy (the Sunna procedure) to clitoridectomy, labia minor excision, and fusion of the labia majora (total infibulation). These anatomic changes have a profound impact on infection risk, sexual function, and vaginal delivery.

Women who have suffered **obstetric lacerations** or episiotomies posteriorly into the rectum, anteriorly into the urethra, or laterally into the labia will have scarring that reflects these injuries or their repairs.

EPITHELIAL CONDITIONS

Squamous cell hyperplasia is a local thickening of the epithelium that may result from a prolonged itch-scratch cycle. Women may note pruritus and pain. Examination reveals a white or reddish, thickened, leathery raised surface. The effects of scratching may be evident as linear excoriations. The lesions tend to be discrete but may be multiple and coexist with other vulvar pathology. Histologically, the rete ridges deepen and there is hyperkeratosis of the superficial

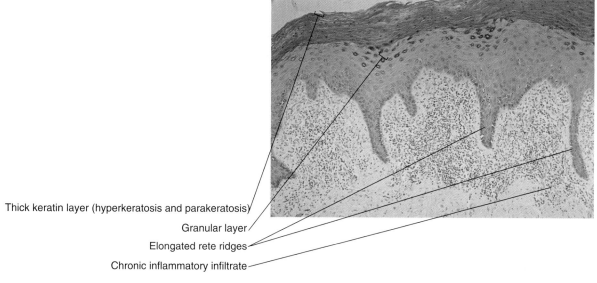

Thick keratin layer (hyperkeratosis and parakeratosis)
Granular layer
Elongated rete ridges
Chronic inflammatory infiltrate

Figure 19-4. Squamous cell hyperplasia. Microscopy shows marked hyperkeratosis and parakeratosis with a prominent granular layer. Acanthosis, with prolongation of rete ridges, is also seen and there is a dense infiltrate of chronic inflammatory cells, mainly lymphocytes, in the superficial dermis.

layer of the epidermis (Figure 19-4). Treatment includes moderate-strength steroid ointments with antipruritic agents.

Lichen sclerosis often causes intense pruritus, dyspareunia, and burning pain. Although it can develop in any body area in any age person, it is most prevalent on the vulva of menopausal women. On examination, the skin is thin, inelastic, and white, with a crinkled, "tissue paper" appearance. Ultimately, lichen sclerosis can involve all the genital area from the mons to the anal area in a keyhole pattern. **Biopsy will reveal a thin epithelium with loss of rete ridges and inflammatory cells lining the basement membrane** (Figure 19-5). Diagnosis is important

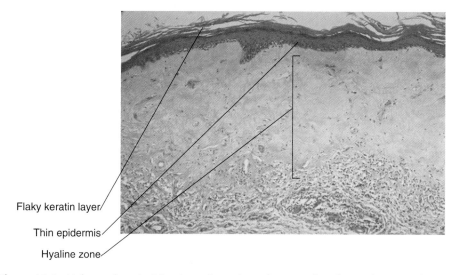

Flaky keratin layer
Thin epidermis
Hyaline zone

Figure 19-5. Lichen sclerosis. Histology shows hyperkeratosis but the epidermis is thinner than normal. The most striking feature of lichen sclerosis is the presence of a hyaline zone in the superficial dermis. This is the result of edema and degeneration of the collagen and elastic fibers of the dermis.

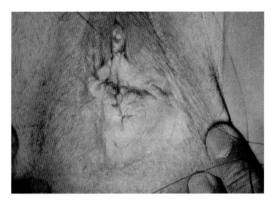

Figure 19-6. Vulva with lichen sclerosis.

because this is a chronic, progressive disease with the potential to constrict and destroy the normal genital architecture. In the long run, the labia minora are lost, the labia majora flatten, the introitus becomes severely constricted, and the clitoris becomes inverted and trapped (Figure 19-6). Treatment involves the use of potent topical steroids such as 0.05% clobetasol. Eighty percent of lesions will respond, and long-term therapy with lower-potency steroids or topical emollients may be necessary.

Lichen planus presents as purplish, polygonal papules that may appear in their erosive form. Lichen planus may involve the vagina and the mouth as well as the vulva. Topical and systemic steroids are recommended for treatment. It is possible that many dermatologic changes coexist. Combinations of lichen sclerosis and dysplasia, hyperplasia, or carcinoma are possible. Multiple biopsies may be necessary to characterize completely all the pathologies present in one woman.

The epithelium of the vulva is susceptible to dermatologic disorders found elsewhere on the body surface, although the clinical manifestations of those disorders may be slightly different because of the vulva's moist environment. A correct diagnosis is critical, and tissue punch biopsy may be required (Figure 19-7). **Psoriasis** generally appears velvety but may

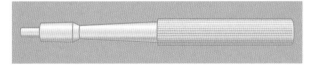

Figure 19-7. A disposable cutaneous punch biopsy instrument.

lack the characteristic scaly patches found on the flexor surfaces (e.g., knees and elbows). **Eczema** has a more erythematous presentation and may be difficult to diagnose unless lesions that are more characteristic can be found on the scalp, umbilicus, or extremities. Even in these circumstances, diagnostic biopsy may be needed to rule out conditions that are more serious. **Pemphigus** is an autoimmune blistering disease involving the vulvovaginal and conjunctival areas. **Behçet's syndrome** classically involves ulcerations in the genital and oral area as well with superficial ocular lesions. The genital lesions are distinctive and can result over time in a scarred, fenestrated vulva. The etiology is unknown as is an effective treatment. Diagnosis is based on the concurrence of vulvar, oral and ocular involvement, the recurrent nature of the disease, and the exclusion of other conditions, such as syphilis or Crohn disease.

Crohn disease is primarily a gastrointestinal (GI) disorder, but vulvar ulcers can precede the development of GI ulcerations. The vulvar ulcers are slitlike "knife-cut" ulcers with prominent edema. Draining sinuses and fistulae to the rectum may occur. **Aphthous ulcers,** which are superficial and painful, can be found not only on the labia but also in the mouth. **Decubitus ulcers** can develop in frail women over the bony prominences of their ischial tuberosities or sacrococcygeal region or in areas susceptible to friction from indwelling catheters.

Acanthosis nigricans is most commonly found in the intertriginous area, in the axilla or on the nape of the neck. It is recognizable with its darkly pigmented velvety or warty surface. **Acanthosis nigricans** is related most closely to insulin resistance but can be linked to malignancy or other benign conditions.

The labia are exposed to a wide range of chemicals and other foreign materials that can induce **contact dermatitis** (erythema and burning) or irritative changes. A careful history may identify the use of a specific irritant, such as harsh soaps, perfumed toilet paper, deodorant spray, panty liners, or latex condoms. Physical examination may reveal erythema, edema, and occasionally excoriation or ulceration. In the more chronic state, the epidermis can thicken. Biopsy of any thickened or suspicious area is imperative at the initial examination, and later biopsy of unresponsive areas may be necessary. In the acute phase, management involves stopping all exposure to potential irritants and keeping the area dry. The use of topical mild to moderate potency corticosteroids for 1 to 4 weeks may calm the inflammatory response. Antihistamines, cold packs, and bland emollients may provide relief from the pruritus.

Vulvar intraepithelial neoplasia, Paget's disease of the vulva, and invasive tumors of the vulva are discussed in Chapter 41.

FUNCTIONAL

Vulvodynia is a term used to describe chronic vulvar discomfort or pain with no obvious pathology. Vulvodynia can be localized but generally is described as a burning, aching, stinging sensation involving isolated areas or the entire external genital area. Other pathology must be ruled out before the diagnosis can be applied. Many women who suffer vulvodynia share a history of prior vulvar treatments with laser, loop electrosurgical excision procedure (LEEP), or multiple topical medications. Others have a history of herpes simplex virus infection. It is thought that these women maybe suffering from peripheral neuropathy. Treatment is challenging but starts by removing all irritants and providing a trial of low-dose tricyclic antidepressants to treat peripheral neuropathy. Pruritus may be addressed with a variety of agents including doxepin 5% cream.

VAGINA
CONGENITAL ABNORMALITIES

Many variations and combinations of anomalies of the vagina occur. The more common anomalies of the vagina include canalization defects such as imperforate hymen, longitudinal and transverse vaginal septa, partial development (vaginal atresia), and double vagina. Congenital absence of the vagina (agenesis) is less common.

Imperforate hymen represents the mildest form of these canalization abnormalities. It occurs at the site where the vaginal plate contacts the urogenital sinus. After birth, a bulging, membrane-like structure may be noticed in the vestibule, usually blocking egress of mucus (Figure 19-8). If not detected until after menarche, an imperforate hymen may be seen as a dark bluish membrane blocking menstrual flow at the introitus. A similar anomaly, the **transverse vaginal septum,** is most commonly found at the junction of the upper and middle thirds of the vagina. At times, a transverse vaginal septum will have a sinus tract or perforation that allows menstruation. Thus, the septum may become apparent only after intercourse is impeded. Patients with an imperforate hymen or

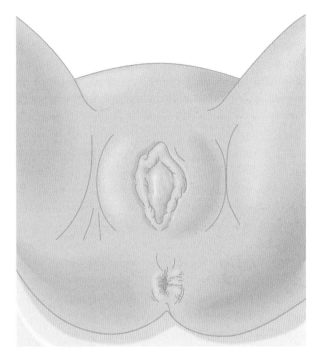

Figure 19-8. Illustration of female infant with a bulging introital mass, a tense imperforate hymen blocking the egress of mucus (mucocolpos) or blood (hemocolpos) from the vagina.

transverse vaginal septum usually have normal development of the upper reproductive tract.

Atresia of the vagina generally represents a more substantial lack of canalization at the caudal or cranial end of the vaginal plate. If cranially placed, the upper vagina and cervix may be absent, but the uterine fundus and fallopian tubes are unaffected.

A midline longitudinal septum may be present, creating a double vagina. The longitudinal septum may be only partially present at various levels in the upper and middle vagina, either in the midline or deviated to one side. In addition, a longitudinal septum may attach to the lateral vaginal wall, creating a blind vaginal pouch with or without a communicating sinus tract. These septa are usually associated with a double cervix and one of the various duplication anomalies of the uterine fundus, although the upper tract is often entirely normal.

Vaginal agenesis represents the most extreme instance of a vaginal anomaly, with total absence of the vagina. If the uterus is absent but the fallopian tubes are spared, the defect is **müllerian agenesis or Rokitansky-Kuster-Hauster syndrome.** Isolated vaginal agenesis with normal uterine and fallopian tube development is rare and is thought to be the end result of isolated vaginal plate malformation.

Adenosis of the vaginal wall consists of islands of columnar epithelium in the normal squamous epithelium. It is often located in the upper one-third of the vagina. The incidence of this finding is much higher in women exposed in utero to diethylstilbesterol (DES) (Figure 19-9, A and B).

Dysontogenic cysts of the vagina are generally thick-walled, soft cysts resulting from embryonic remnants. **Gartner's duct cysts** are the most common of these. They arise from the remnant of the wolffian

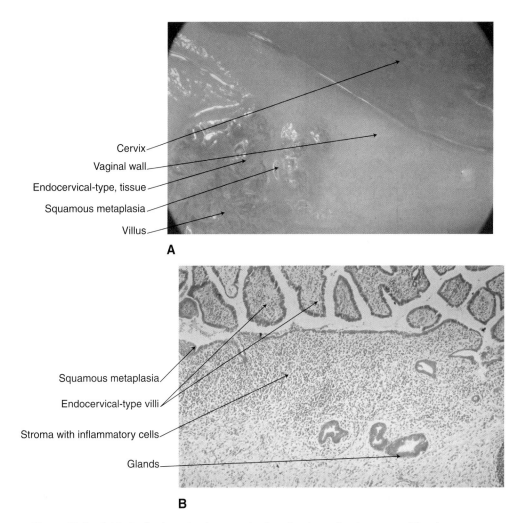

Cervix

Vaginal wall

Endocervical-type, tissue

Squamous metaplasia

Villus

A

Squamous metaplasia

Endocervical-type villi

Stroma with inflammatory cells

Glands

B

Figure 19-9. *A,* Vaginal adenosis photographed at the time of colposcopy. Glands are not normally present in the vagina and columnar epithelium should not be seen. In vaginal adenosis, endocervical-type glands with columnar epithelium on the surface are seen in the vaginal wall. This illustration shows part of the posterior lip of the cervix, in the upper right-hand corner, and the vaginal wall occupies the lower left part of the photograph. In the lower left-hand corner are irregular areas of endocervical tissue, showing the villous pattern usually seen on the cervix. Tongues of squamous metaplasia are seen separating smaller islands of endocervical-type tissue. *B,* Vaginal adenosis. Biopsy of the area shown in *A.* The papillary nature of the surface lesion is apparent and endocervical-type glands are present in the lamina propria. There is a little superficial inflammation, and at the extreme left hand end of the surface epithelium, a zone of squamous metaplasia can be recognized.

duct (mesonephros). They vary in size from 1 to 5 cm and are found on the anterior-lateral walls in the upper half of the vagina and more laterally in the lower vagina. Most are asymptomatic and require no intervention.

BENIGN CONDITIONS OF THE VAGINA

Common infectious conditions of the vagina are discussed in Chapter 23.

Structural and Benign Neoplastic Conditions

Urethral diverticula are small (0.3 to 3-cm) saclike projections that can be found in the anterior vagina along the posterior urethra. As obstructed periurethral glands they may or may not communicate with the urethra. Urethral diverticula can cause recurrent urinary tract infections, dysuria, dyspareunia, and, occasionally, urinary dribbling. **Most women with urethral diverticula have symptoms of chronic urinary tract infection.** Urethral dilation or surgical excision of the diverticula may be necessary.

Inclusion cysts are common lesions that result from an infolding of the vaginal epithelium. They are usually located in the posterior or lateral wall of the lower one-third of the vagina. They are most frequently associated with lacerations from childbirth or gynecologic surgery.

Bartholin's cyst is the most common vaginal-vulvar tumor. It presents as a swelling posterolaterally in the introitus, usually unilaterally. The cyst is usually less than 3 cm in diameter. Careful examination of the base of the cyst is necessary (especially in a woman over 40 years of age) to rule out an underlying Bartholin carcinoma (see Chapter 41). Another cystic structure that may be found in the upper one-third of the vagina is an implant of endometriosis. **Endometriosis** presents as steel gray or black cysts that may bleed slightly at the time of menstruation.

Structural changes that develop with time generally result from the loss of pelvic support. Cystoceles, rectoceles, and enteroceles are more thoroughly discussed in Chapter 24. **Ureterovaginal, vesicovaginal, and rectovaginal fistulae** may result from infection, complications of surgery or radiation therapy, obstetric injury, or invasive carcinoma. They cause chronic vaginal discharge and considerable vulvovaginal irritation.

TRAUMA

The most common cause of vaginal trauma is sexual assault, although some superficial vaginal abrasions can occur with consensual intercourse. Focal abrasions may result from tampons (especially when used on low-flow days), a poorly fitted diaphragm, or prolonged pessary use. A lost or forgotten tampon or retained vaginal packing material most often presents with a foul-smelling vaginal discharge. Vaginal trauma can also result from other foreign objects, straddle injuries, childbirth, and gynecologic surgery. Lacerations and hematomas from vaginal trauma pose significant and immediate challenges, but potential damage to surrounding bladder and bowel structures must also be evaluated.

DERMATOLOGIC

Erosive lichen planus with its characteristic erythematous papules can involve the vagina as well as the vulvar vestibule. Condylomata acuminata and flat warts from human papilloma virus (HPV) can be found in the vaginal vault, as can herpes simplex infections.

FUNCTIONAL

Vaginismus is an involuntary contraction of the vaginal introital and levator ani muscles. Vaginismus may preclude or render very painful vaginal penetration during coitus, pelvic examination, or tampon use. Often a history of sexual abuse or phobias about vaginal trauma are associated with vaginism; these may respond to education and desensitization.

Suggested Reading

Foster DC: Vulvar disease. Obstet Gynecol 100:145–163, 2002.

Nunns D: Vulvar pain syndromes. Br J Obstet Gynecol 107:1185–1193, 2000.

Toubia N: Female circumcision as a public health issue. New Engl J Med 331(11): 712–716, 1994.

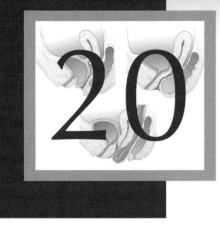

20 Congenital Anomalies and Benign Conditions of the Uterine Corpus and Cervix

J. George Moore and Anita L. Nelson

Benign conditions of the uterine corpus and cervix are commonly encountered in gynecologic practice, because they affect a woman's fertility and can cause abnormal uterine bleeding or pelvic pain. In this chapter, congenital anomalies, benign neoplasms, epithelial changes, and functional disorders of the uterus (corpus and cervix) are discussed.

CONGENITAL ANOMALIES OF THE UTERINE CORPUS AND CERVIX

The upper vagina, cervix, uterine corpus, and fallopian tubes are formed from the paramesonephric (müllerian) ducts. **The absence of a Y chromosome and the resultant absence of müllerian inhibiting substance lead to the development of the paramesonephric system, with the regression of the mesonephric system.** The paramesonephric ducts first arise at 6 weeks lateral to the cranial pole of the mesonephric duct and expand caudally. By 9 to 10 weeks, they fuse in the midline at the urogenital septum to form the uterovaginal primordium. Later, dissolution of the septum between the fused paramesonephric ducts leads to the development of a single uterus and cervix.

The most common anomalies of the uterus result from either incomplete fusion of the paramesonephric ducts, incomplete dissolution of the midline fusion of those ducts, or formation failures. Figure 20-1 shows variations of the uterine and cervical development and demonstrates that communication between the dual systems can exist at several levels. Failure of fusion is most evident in **uterus didelphys,** which presents with two separate uterine bodies, each with its own cervix and attached fallopian tube and vagina. **A bicornuate uterus with a rudimentary horn** also represents a fusion failure. Less complete fusion failure is seen in the **bicornuate uterus with or without double cervices.** Incomplete dissolution of the midline fusion of the paramesonephria explains the **septate uterus.** Failure of formation can be seen in the **unicornuate uterus. In müllerian agnesis, there is complete lack of development of the paramesonephric system.** The affected woman generally has an incomplete development of the fallopian tubes associated with the absence of the uterus and most of the vagina. All of these conditions occur in normal karyotypic and phenotypic females but can be associated with important anomalies of the urinary system.

The most common congenital cervical anomalies are the result of malfusion of the paramesonephric (müllerian) ducts with varying degrees of separation, as seen in the didelphys cervix or septate cervix.

These different anatomies may have a significant effect on a woman's risk of infertility and early pregnancy loss and may also cause dysmenorrhea and dyspareunia. Women with fusion anomalies may present with menstrual blood trapped in a noncommunicating uterine horn or vagina.

In addition to these macroscopic differences, subtle anomalies may exist within the uterine vascular system, such as an **arteriovenous malformation,** rupture of which may cause life-threatening hemorrhage.

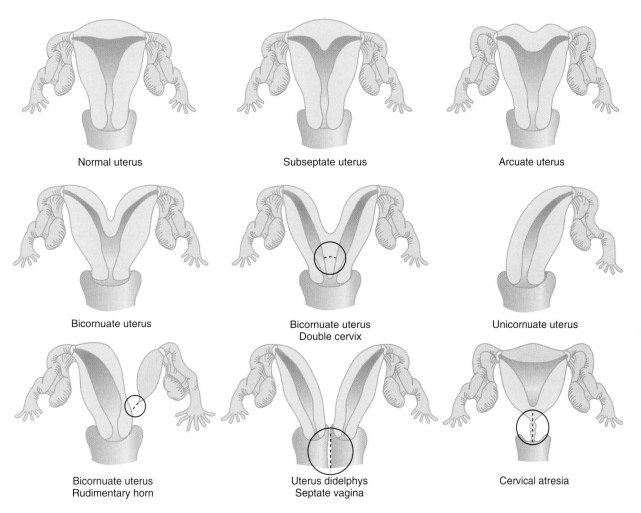

Normal uterus   Subseptate uterus   Arcuate uterus

Bicornuate uterus   Bicornuate uterus
Double cervix   Unicornuate uterus

Bicornuate uterus   Uterus didelphys   Cervical atresia
Rudimentary horn   Septate vagina

Figure 20-1. Variations in uterine development. The dotted lines within circles represent potential sites of communication or obstruction.

Although all of these anomalies can occur spontaneously, they may also be caused by early maternal exposure to certain drugs. The most notable of these drugs is diethylstilbestrol (DES). A **DES-exposed female infant has an increased risk for a small, T-shaped endometrial cavity (Figure 20-2A) or cervical collar deformity (Figure 20-2B).** DES exposure in utero can also produce fallopian tube abnormalities although it does not appear to cause abnormalities of the urinary tract.

STRUCTURAL AND BENIGN NEOPLASTIC CONDITIONS
UTERINE LEIOMYOMAS

Uterine leiomyomas ("fibroids") are benign tumors derived from the smooth muscle cells of the myometrium. They are the most common neoplasm of the uterus. Estimates are that more than 45% of women have leiomyomas by the fifth decade of life, but most are asymptomatic. However, **leiomyomas can cause excessive uterine bleeding, pelvic pressure and pain, as well as infertility.** They are the primary indication for 200,000 to 300,000 hysterectomies in the United States each year. Although leiomyomas have the potential to grow to impressive sizes, **their malignant potential is minimal.** Sarcomatous changes occur in less than 1 per 1000 uteri with fibroids.

Risk factors for developing leiomyomas include increasing age during the reproductive years, ethnicity (African-American women have at least a 2- to 3-fold increased risk compared to Caucasian women), nulliparity, and family history. The data are suggestive

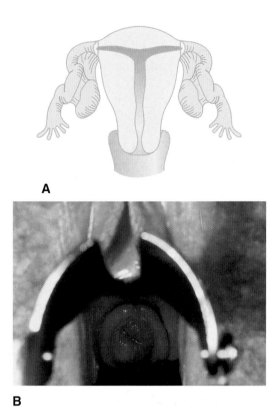

A

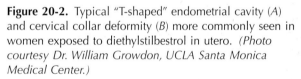

B

Figure 20-2. Typical "T-shaped" endometrial cavity (*A*) and cervical collar deformity (*B*) more commonly seen in women exposed to diethylstilbestrol in utero. *(Photo courtesy Dr. William Growdon, UCLA Santa Monica Medical Center.)*

that higher body mass index is associated with a greater risk of leiomyomata. Oral contraceptive pills and depot medroxyprogesterone acetate (DMPA) injections may be associated with reduced risk.

Pathogenesis

Factors that initiate leiomyomata are not known, but ovarian sex steroids are important for their growth. Leiomyomas rarely develop before menarche and seldom develop or enlarge after menopause, unless stimulated by exogenous hormones. **Leiomyomas can also enlarge dramatically during pregnancy.** Leiomyomas have increased levels of estrogen and progesterone receptors compared to other smooth muscle cells. Estrogen stimulates the proliferation of smooth muscle cell, whereas progesterone increases the production of proteins that interfere with pro-

grammed cell death (or apoptosis). Leiomyomas also have higher levels of growth factors that stimulate the production of fibronectin and collagen, major components of the extracellular matrix that characterizes these lesions.

Characteristics

Leiomyomas are usually spherical, well-circumscribed, white, firm lesions with a whorled appearance on cut section. Although the leiomyoma appears discrete, it does not have a true cellular capsule. Compressed smooth muscle cells on the tumor's periphery provide the false impression of such a capsule. **Few blood vessels and lymphatics traverse the pseudocapsule,** leading to degenerative changes as the tumors enlarge. **The most commonly observed degenerative change is that of hyaline acellularity,** in which the fibrous and muscle tissues are replaced with hyaline tissue. If the hyaline substance breaks down from a further reduction in blood supply, **cystic degeneration may occur. Calcification may occur in degenerated fibroids,** particularly after the menopause. **Fatty degeneration may also occur** but is rare. **During pregnancy, 5% to 10% of women with fibroids undergo a painful red or carneous degeneration** caused by hemorrhage into the tumor.

Leiomyomas arise within the myometrium (**intramural**), but some migrate toward the serosal surface (**subserosal**) or toward the endometrium (**submucosal**) as depicted in Figure 20-3). Individual tumors may migrate further by developing large pedicles. The submucosal leiomyomas can extend through the endometrial canal and about from the cervical os. An aborting leiomyoma causes significant bleeding and cramping pain. A subserosal leiomyoma on a long pedicle can present as a mass that feels separate from the uterus. Rarely, pedunculated subserosal myomata attach to the blood supply of the omentum or bowel mesentery and lose their uterine connection to become **parasitic leiomyomas.** Leiomyomas can also arise in the cervix, between the leaves of the broad ligament (intraligamentous), and in the various supporting ligaments (round or uterosacral) of the uterus.

Symptoms

The majority of uterine leiomyomas cause no symptoms. On occasion, the patient may become aware of a lower abdominal mass if it protrudes above

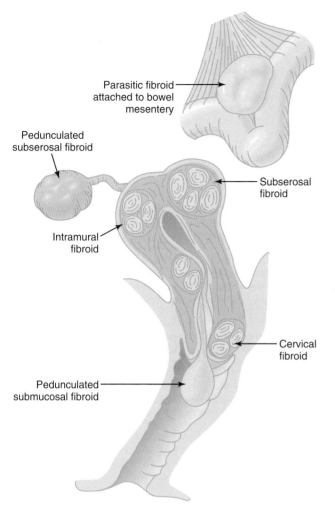

Figure 20-3. Uterine leiomyomas (fibroids) in various anatomic locations.

Labels in figure:
Parasitic fibroid attached to bowel mesentery
Pedunculated subserosal fibroid
Intramural fibroid
Subserosal fibroid
Cervical fibroid
Pedunculated submucosal fibroid

the pelvis. Quite often, the discomfort develops insidiously and the symptoms are difficult for a patient to define. **She may complain of pelvic pressure, congestion, bloating, a feeling of heaviness in the lower abdomen, or lower back pain.** She may note frequency of urination. Urinary retention and hydronephrosis are rare but result from the fact that the bladder and large leiomyomas compete for space within the pelvis.

Menorrhagia may be associated with intramural or submucosal tumor. Metrorrhagia has been associated with submucous myomas ulcerating through the endometrial lining. Excessive bleeding may result in anemia, weakness, dyspnea, and even congestive heart failure.

Fibroids are not generally painful, but **severe pain may be associated with red degeneration (acute infarction) within a fibroid.** This most commonly occurs during pregnancy. In addition, pressure pains may occur in the lower abdomen and pelvis if a myomatous uterus becomes incarcerated within the pelvis. Dyspareunia is also common with incarceration. There is an increased incidence of secondary dysmenorrhea in women with uterine myomas, generally caused by the increased blood loss. Although many women with uterine myomas become pregnant and carry their pregnancies to term, **these lesions may be associated with an increased incidence of infertility** because of placentation challenges.

Signs

Very large fibroids can be palpated abdominally. Those smaller than a 12- to 14-week gestational size are usually confined to the pelvis. The bladder should be emptied before examination to avoid the confusion of urinary retention. Although submucous fibroids may not be palpable, **on bimanual pelvic examination a firm, irregularly enlarged uterus with smoothly rounded or bosselated protrusions may be felt if the tumors are subserosal or intramural.** The tumors are usually nontender. Their consistency may vary from rock hard, as in the case of a calcified postmenopausal leiomyoma, to soft or even cystic, as in the case of cystic degeneration of the tumor. In general, the myomatous masses are in the midline, but sometimes a large portion of the tumor lies in the lateral aspect of the pelvis and may be indistinguishable from an adnexal mass. **If the mass moves with the cervix, it is suggestive of a leiomyoma.** Often the presence of a leiomyoma precludes a proper evaluation of the adnexa, but ultrasound imaging can help to distinguish adnexal masses from laterally placed myomas.

Differential Diagnosis

The differential diagnosis of a leiomyoma is extensive and includes other uterine pathology, such as uterine sarcoma, and other processes, such as inflammation, that can cause pelvic masses. **The most common differential diagnoses are an ovarian neoplasm, a tubo-ovarian inflammatory mass, a pelvic kidney, a diverticular or inflammatory bowel mass, or cancer of the colon.** Ultrasonography may visualize

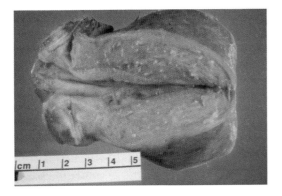

Figure 20-4. Enlarged uterus cut open to demonstrate homogeneous enlargement secondary to adenomyosis. A diagnosis of leiomyomata may be incorrectly made at the time of pelvic examination. *Courtesy Dr. Sathima Nataratan, UCLA Medical Center.*

the fibroids and identify normal ovaries apart from the leiomyomas. Adenomyosis (see Chapter 26) usually results in a uniformly enlarged uterus (Figure 20-4) but may on occasion be diagnosed as leiomyoma.

Management

In general, if a small asymptomatic fibroid is detected, a repeat ultrasonic examination within 6 months is prudent to rule out a rapidly growing uterine sarcoma. The need for other interventions is determined by the clinical concerns presented by the leiomyoma. If menorrhagia is the chief complaint, it is imperative that an endometrial aspiration or a fractional dilatation and curettage (D&C) be performed to rule out related pathology.

Medical Management

Menorrhagia caused by fibroids may be managed hormonally in many cases. **Progestin-only therapies** (oral or injected medroxyprogesterone acetate, progestin-only oral contraceptive pills, or levonorgestrel-releasing intrauterine devices) **or combination hormonal contraceptive methods** (oral contraceptive pills, vaginal rings, or patches) **are usually a first therapeutic option.** The goal may be to reduce monthly menstrual blood loss with cyclic hormonal methods or to eliminate menses with extended or continuous use of these methods.

GnRH agonists have demonstrated considerable efficacy in blocking ovarian steroidogenesis, which halts endometrial proliferation. Simultaneously, GnRH agonists reduce the volume of the

myometrium and the leiomyomas. This allows for correction of anemia and reduces intraoperative blood loss. **The effects of GnRH-agonist therapy disappear soon after the drug is stopped.** However, because of the intense vasomotor symptoms and the deleterious effect the GnRH-agonists may have on bone mineral density, only short courses of these agonists can be administered, usually in preparation for myomectomy or hysterectomy. Intermittent GnRH-agonist administration has been shown to reduce side effects while achieving therapeutic goals longer term. **Combining GnRH agonists with hormonal agents, such as low-dose progesterone or estrogen/progestin combinations, may minimize some adverse effects of hypoestrogenism (such as osteoporosis), but long-term data are not available.**

Clinical trials using the selective antiprogesterone receptor antagonist, mifepristone (RU 486), to reduce the size of uterine myomas have shown a reduction of 50% over a 3-month period. Doses of 5, 25, or 50 mg/day for up to 6 months have been used to ablate endometriosis and to reduce the size of uterine myomas without producing the changes in bone density noted with GnRH agonists and without untoward glucocorticoid effects.

Surgical Management

Medical therapy is of limited value in treating the other problems posed by leiomyoma. Surgical interventions are important to treat these problems as well as to treat leiomyoma that are not responsive to medical management. Table 20-1 lists the surgical indications for patients with leiomyoma. **Myomectomy is the preferred surgical procedure for women with a limited number of tumors who desire uterine preservation.** Myomectomy occasionally can be performed hysteroscopically for submucous masses or transabdominally (either laparoscopically or with laparotomy) for other leiomyomas. Pretreatment for 3 months with GnRH agonists and the use of vasoconstrictive agents intraoperatively may improve surgical outcomes whatever surgical approach is used.

Myomectomy may not be successful in avoiding hysterectomy. Not all the tumors may be removed, and new leiomyomata may grow in the future. About 25% of women will require a subsequent operation. **If the endometrial cavity is entered during myomectomy, future deliveries must be by cesarean.**

Table 20-1. Intervention for patients with leiomyomata not amenable to medical therapy*

Clinical Presentation	Nonmedical Options	Comments
Desired fertility	Embolization or myomectomy	Usually used for a limited number of leiomyomata
Desires uterine preservation or poor surgical risk	Endometrial ablation or embolization	Embolization only for a limited number of leiomyomata
No desired fertility or uterine preservation	Endometrial ablation or hysterectomy	Hysterectomy is definitive therapy
Rapidly growing uterus (double in size in 6 months)	Exploratory laparotomy, abdominal hysterectomy	More extensive surgery if malignancy discovered

*Generally failed medical therapy or large (>12–14 weeks' gestational size) uterus.

Hysterectomy provides definitive therapy. If the uterus is large (>12 to 14 cm), laparotomy is generally the preferred approach. **Vaginal hysterectomy is generally preferred if the uterus is not bulky** and the vagina is not constricted. Laparoscopically assisted vaginal hysterectomy permits excellent visualization of the adnexae and controlled dissection from above without a large abdominal incision. Rapid growth of a uterus caused by leiomyoma (doubling in size in <6 months) may be the result of leiomyosarcoma, and hysterectomy is generally recommended.

Other therapies are emerging, especially for women who desire uterine preservation. **Embolization of the uterine arteries supplying the leiomyomas has been found to be effective,** at least in the short term, for controlling leiomyoma-induced bleeding and to shrink the myomas. **Endometrial ablation with hysteroscopic resection, laser ablation, or roller ball may be technically difficult if the leiomyomata distort the cavity,** but the newer thermal balloon methods may be successful. This approach may be appropriate for women who are poor candidates for more extensive surgery.

ENDOMETRIAL POLYPS

Endometrial polyps form from the endometrium to create abnormal protrusions of friable tissue into the endometrial cavity. They can cause menorrhagia and spontaneous bleeding during the reproductive years and postmenopausal bleeding after menopause. On ultrasound, endometrial polyps may appear as a focal thickening of the endometrial stripe. **They can be recognized on sonohysterography** or **by sonohysteroscopy.** Endometrial polyps may evade detection by endometrial aspiration or D&C because they are too large to be aspirated through the sampling orifice

and are very flexible and can fold out of the path of the sharp curette. Histologic evaluation of the polyp is imperative, because although most are benign, endometrial hyperplasia, endometrial carcinoma, and carcinosarcomas may also present as polyps.

NORMAL CERVIX

At birth, a pale pink squamous epithelium covers the outer rim of the cervix. The inner aspect of the ectocervix is covered with the taller columnar cells. The junction between the two is called the original squamocolumnar junction (Figure 20-5). The columnar epithelium appears redder because of the closer proximity of its underlying blood vessels to the surface. **With acidification of the vagina at menarche, the ectocervix undergoes an accelerated rate of squamous metaplasia in a radial pattern, from the squamocolumnar junction inward, which produces the transformation zone.** A new squamocolumnar junction is formed, that moves progressively up the endocervical canal (see Figure 39-1). Younger women are often found to have a reddish ring of tissue surrounding the os, which is sometimes called a **cervical ectropion,** but in reality, this is an area of columnar epithelium that has not yet undergone squamous metaplasia.

Under the influence of estrogen (birth control pills, pregnancy), the columnar epithelium of more mature women may evert and present a similarly appearing ectropion. The columnar cells produce mucus and are more vulnerable to trauma and infection with chlamydia. Therefore **women with a cervical ectropion may notice more vaginal secretions and, occasionally, postcoital spotting.** Once other etiologies have been ruled out, no treatment is needed for the friable tissue.

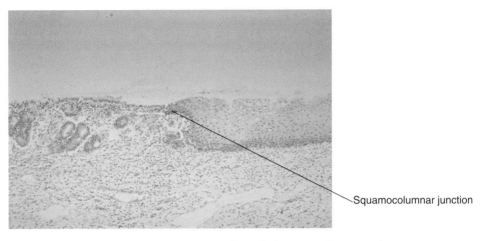

Squamocolumnar junction

Figure 20-5. Squamocolumnar junction. In the "ideal" cervix, the original squamous epithelium abuts the columnar epithelium. The squamocolumnar junction thus formed may be situated at the external cervical os, but in most women of childbearing age, the original squamocolumnar junction is located on the vaginal portion of the cervix.

Nabothian cysts on the cervix are so common that they are considered a normal variant. They result from the process of squamous metaplasia. A layer of superficial squamous epithelium entraps an invagination of columnar cells beneath its surface. The underlying columnar cells continue to secrete mucus, and a mucous retention cyst is created. Nabothian cysts are opaque, with a yellowish or bluish hue. They vary generally in size from 0.3 to 3 cm (Figure 20-6), although larger Nabothian cysts have been reported.

CERVICAL POLYPS

Ectocervical and endocervical polyps are the most common benign neoplastic growths of the cervix.

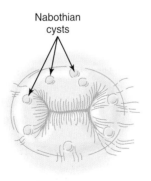

Nabothian cysts

Figure 20-6. Cervix of a multiparous woman with Nabothian cysts.

A polyp is a localized proliferation of cells (usually columnar) located in the endocervix. Endocervical polyps tend to the more beefy red in color and arise from the endocervical canal on a long, pedunculated stalk. Ectocervical polyps are less common, are generally pale, and arise from the ectocervix to create a broad-based protrusion. Cervical polyps may be isolated or multiple and vary in diameter from a few millimeters to several centimeters. **If symptomatic, they most commonly cause coital bleeding or menorrhagia.** Narrow-based polyps are removed by twisting the polyp off at its base. Broader-based polyps may be better removed with cautery or other modalities that can control bleeding after removal. **Although the incidence of malignancy is very low (1% or less), both squamous cell carcinomas and adenocarcinomas can present as polyps.** All specimens must be sent for pathologic examination.

TRAUMA OF THE UTERINE CORPUS AND CERVIX

Most trauma to the uterus has an obstetric basis, such as uterine rupture from prolonged labor, caused by a Bandl's ring, or rupture along a previous uterine scar. However, uterine perforation is also possible with operative procedures such as D&C, endometrial aspiration, or intrauterine device (IUD) placement.

Most trauma to the cervix occurs with vaginal delivery. The cervix can tear if the os is incom-

pletely dilated prior to delivery. Lacerations can also occur with an instrumental delivery. Trauma may also occur during gynecologic operations, such as cervical conization, hysteroscopy, abortion or other intrauterine procedures. Trauma to the cervix can occur with sexual assault.

EPITHELIAL CONDITIONS OF THE UTERINE CORPUS AND CERVIX
ENDOMETRIAL HYPERPLASIA

Endometrial hyperplasia represents an overabundant growth of the endometrium generally caused by persistent levels of estrogen unopposed by progesterone. **Hyperplasia is most frequently seen at the extremes of a woman's reproductive years when ovulation is infrequent.** It also occurs in association with unopposed estrogenic stimulation, such as the following:

1. **Polycystic ovarian syndrome (PCOS)**
2. Estrogen-producing tumors such as **granulosa-theca cell tumors**
3. **Obesity** because of peripheral conversion of androgens to estrogen in adipose cells
4. Prolonged use of **exogenous estrogens** without progestins
5. Use of **tamoxifen.**

A spectrum of histologic variations exists. **There are two categories (simple hyperplasia and complex hyperplasia) and two subcategories (with and without atypia).** Complex atypical hyperplasia has the greatest malignant potential; about 20% to 30% of cases progress to endometrial carcinoma, if untreated.

Diagnosis

Endometrial hyperplasia should be suspected when at-risk women develop menorrhagia or intermenstrual bleeding. Endometrial sampling is necessary to obtain a histologic diagnosis. Other procedures, such as fractional D&C or hysteroscopically directed biopsy, may be needed to rule out carcinoma or other pathology. **In postmenopausal women, a thin (<4 mm) endometrial stripe on transvaginal ultrasound is reassuring.**

Treatment

Treatment of hyperplasia without atypia generally consists of a thorough, coordinated sloughing of the hyperplastic endometrium and therapies directed at preventing recurrence. **Simple hyperplasia without atypia should be treated initially with medroxyprogesterone acetate (MPA) 5 to 10 mg per day for 10 days each month for 3 months,** then biopsy should be repeated to confirm normalization of the endometrium. **Complex hyperplasia must be evaluated with a fractional D&C and should be initially treated with daily progestin therapy for 3 to 6 months. Test of cure with another biopsy is then neede.** Estrogen-producing tumors should be extirpated. In the longer run, a source of progestin must be supplied either cyclically with MPA or, more continuously, with combination hormonal contraceptives, depot MPA or the levonorgestrel-releasing IUD. **Complex hyperplasia with atypia is best treated by hysterectomy** once carcinoma has been excluded. Complex hyperplasia with atypia may be treated medically as outlined above if the patient desires to preserve her fertility, but only if careful follow-up is likely. **Endometrial ablation is absolutely contraindicated in any of these situations until the endometrium normalizes.**

ASHERMAN'S SYNDROME

The endometrium is denuded and the endometrial cavity filled with adhesions in patients with Asherman's syndrome. Most commonly, the scarring results from curettage in high-risk settings, such as postpartum hemorrhage or septic abortion, although vigorous scraping under any circumstances can result in the loss of the endometrium and consequent adhesion of opposing myometrial surfaces. Endometrial ablation procedures are designed to deliberately destroy the endometrium and create such scarring.

FUNCTIONAL CONDITIONS OF THE UTERINE CORPUS AND CERVIX

Noncongenital cervical stenosis usually arises after trauma (endocervical curettage, conization) or **hypoestrogenism** (menopause, prolonged depot MPA use). Problems arise if blood from the endometrium cannot escape into the vagina, in which case the uterus becomes grossly distended **(hematometra).** Similarly, sperm may be unable to enter the upper genital tract. Cervical stenosis may also cause cervical sampling for microscopic evaluation to be incomplete.

Cervical incompetence is a condition in which the cervix is unable to maintain closure under the pressure of a progressively enlarging pregnant uterus and painlessly dilates, resulting in pregnancy loss, most commonly in the 2nd trimester (see Chapter 13). **Cervical incompetence may be intrinsic** (caused by poor ground substance in the cervix), **the result of cervical surgery** (especially loop electrosurgical excision procedure (LEEP) and cold knife conization) for cervical dysplasia, **or the result of DES exposure in utero.**

Suggested Reading

American College of Obstetricians and Gynecologists: Surgical alternative to hysterectomy in the management of leiomyomas. Practice Bulletin No.16, Washington, DC, ACOG, May 2000.

Management of uterine leiomyomata: What do we really know? Obstet Gynecol 100:8–17, 2002.

Spies JB, Ascher SA: Uterine artery embolization for leiomyomata. Obstet Gynecol 98:29–34, 2001.

Stewart EA: Uterine fibroids. Lancet 357:293–298, 2001.

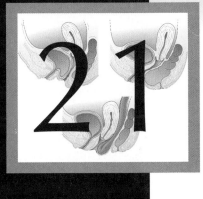

21

Congenital Anomalies and Benign Conditions of the Ovaries and Fallopian Tubes

J. George Moore and Anita L. Nelson

CONGENITAL ANOMALIES OF THE OVARIES AND FALLOPIAN TUBES

Abnormal embryologic development of the ovaries is uncommon. Congenital duplication or absence of ovarian tissue may occur, as may ectopic ovarian tissue and supernumerary ovaries. Although rare, the sexual bipotentiality noted in embryologic development can progress without the usual regression of one system, producing an ovotestis and subsequent intersex problems.

Genetic chromosomal disorders, such as **Turner syndrome (45 XO),** are associated with a lack of normal gonadal development, as evidenced by the rudimentary streaked ovaries that are a hallmark of the disorder. This provides evidence that two X chromosomes are required for normal ovarian development, testicular predominance occurs with the addition of a single Y chromosome, even in the face of multiple X chromosomes. Such predominance is seen in **Klinefelter syndrome (47 XXY),** in which testicular development occurs embryologically. In **testicular feminization (46 XY),** the lack of androgen receptors produces a phenotypic female in the face of a Y chromosome. The gonads in these women (functioning testes) should be removed (usually after puberty) because of their significant malignant potential.

Isolated anomalies of the fallopian tubes, the end result of abnormal development of the proximal unfused portions of the paramesonephric ducts, are rare. Aplasia or atresia, usually of the distal ampullary segment of the fallopian tube, is most commonly unilateral in the presence of otherwise normal development. Bilateral aplasia is noted in some cases of uterine and vaginal agenesis.

Complete duplication of the fallopian tubes is rarely seen, but distal duplication and accessory ostia are relatively common.

In addition, women exposed in utero to certain drugs, such as diethylstilbesterol (DES), may have abnormalities in the architecture of the fallopian tubes. With DES exposure, the tubes may be shortened, distorted, or clubbed.

BENIGN CONDITIONS OF THE OVARIES

Infectious conditions of the ovaries and fallopian tubes are discussed in Chapter 23.

FUNCTIONAL AND BENIGN OVARIAN TUMORS

The human ovary has a striking propensity to develop a wide variety of tumors, the majority of which are benign. As indicated in Table 21-1, ovarian tumors may be functional, inflammatory, metaplastic, or neoplastic. During the childbearing years, 70% of noninflammatory ovarian tumors are functional. The remainder is either neoplastic (20%) or endometriomas (10%). The management of ovarian tumors, whether functional, benign, or malignant, involves difficult decisions that may affect a woman's hormonal status or fertility. Only functional cysts and benign ovarian neoplasms are considered in this chapter.

Table 21-1. Differential diagnosis of ovarian tumors	
Pathogenesis	Specific Type
Functional	Follicular cysts
	Lutein cysts
	Polycystic sclerotic ovaries
Inflammatory	Salpingo-oophoritis
	Pyogenic oophoritis—puerperal, abortal, or IUD-related
	Granulomatous oophoritis
Metaplastic	Endometriomas
Neoplastic	Premenarchal years—10% are malignant
	Menstruating years—15% are malignant
	Postmenopausal years—50% are malignant

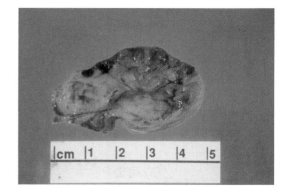

Figure 21-1. Ovary with multiple cysts lining the capsule consistent with polycystic ovarian syndrome. *Courtesy Dr. Sathima Natarajan, UCLA Medical Center.*

Functional Ovarian Cysts and Tumors

Pathogenesis. Dozens of ovarian follicles form each cycle. However, to be classified a "functional cyst," the mass must reach a diameter of at least 3 cm. Functional cysts may cause pelvic pain, a dull sensation, or heaviness in the pelvis.

If the ovarian follicle fails to rupture in the course of follicular development and ovulation, a **follicular cyst,** lined by one or more layers of granulosa cells, may develop. Similarly, **a lutein cyst** may develop if the corpus luteum becomes cystic, grows to over 3 cm, and fails to regress normally after 14 days. **Hemorrhagic cysts,** especially hemorrhagic corpus luteum cysts, are more likely to cause symptoms and are more vulnerable to rupture toward the end of the menstrual cycle. The hemorrhage within the cyst results from invasion of the ovarian vessels into the corpus luteum cyst 2 to 3 days after ovulation.

Other specific types of lutein cysts may occur with abnormally high serum levels of human chorionic gonadotropin (hCG) or increased ovarian sensitivity to gonadotropins. **Theca-lutein cysts** may develop in association with the high levels of hCG present in patients with a hydatidiform mole or choriocarcinoma. Patients undergoing ovulation induction with gonadotropins or clomiphene may also develop theca-lutein cysts. Theca-lutein cysts are usually bilateral, may become quite large (>30 cm), and characteristically regress slowly after the gonadotropin level falls. Rarely, when follicles are stimulated with gonadotropins, theca-lutein cysts can become so extensive as to cause massive ascites and dangerous problems with systemic fluid imbalance.

A **luteoma of pregnancy** is a related condition in which there is a hyperplasic reaction of ovarian theca cells, presumably from prolonged hCG stimulation during pregnancy. The luteomas characteristically appear as brown to reddish-brown nodules that may be cystic or solid. A luteoma of pregnancy may be associated with multifetal pregnancies or hydramnios. They can cause maternal virilization in 30% of women and, less often, ambiguous genitalia in a female fetus. Although ovarian enlargement may be impressive, surgical resection is not indicated, because luteomas regress spontaneously postpartum.

Polycystic ovarian syndrome, a functional disorder generally associated with chronic anovulation and hyperandrogenism, can also produce enlarged ovaries with multiple simple follicles (Figure 21-1). The hormonal aspects of this syndrome are discussed further in Chapter 33.

Clinical features. An ovarian follicular cyst is usually asymptomatic, unilocular ("simple"), and can reach 15 cm in diameter. It usually regresses during the subsequent menstrual cycles. In general, a lutein cyst is apt to be smaller but more firm or even solid in consistency and is more likely to cause pain or signs of peritoneal irritation. Because it may continue to produce progesterone, it is also more likely to cause delayed menses. On occasion, a functional ovarian cyst may undergo **torsion** (see below) or may **rupture,** which may produce acute lower abdominal pain and tenderness and significant hemoperitoneum.

Diagnosis. The presumptive diagnosis of a functional ovarian tumor is usually made when a 5 to 8-cm cystic adnexal mass is noted on bimanual examination; it is confirmed when the lesion regresses over the course of the next several cycles. In general, the cyst is mobile, unilateral, and not associated with ascites. On rare occasions, the mass may exceed 8 cm and be quite tender to palpation. On occasion, hemorrhagic lutein cysts may have a solid rather than a cystic consistency. A pelvic ultrasound will confirm the cystic nature of the mass, but it cannot differentiate with certainty between a functional and a neoplastic tumor. If the patient has delayed menses, abnormal uterine bleeding, or severe pelvic pain, the differential diagnosis must include ectopic pregnancy, pelvic abscess, or adnexal torsion of a neoplastic cyst. A pregnancy test (hCG), diagnostic laparoscopy, or, rarely, laparotomy, may be needed.

Management. When a reproductive-age patient who is asymptomatic or experiencing only mild symptoms presents with an adnexal cyst that is less than 6 cm in diameter, it is appropriate to wait and reexamine the patient after her next menses. Treatment with hormones (usually low-dose contraceptive agents) to suppress gonadotropin levels and to prevent development of another cyst that could confuse the clinical picture (Table 21-2) is appropriate. If the cystic mass is between 6 and 8 cm, or if it is fixed or feels solid, a pelvic ultrasound study should be obtained to determine that it is unilocular.

If the lesion does not fulfill the requirements for observation because it is painful, multilocular, or partially solid, surgical exploration is indicated. Laparo-scopic cystectomy to allow histologic evaluation may be needed to differentiate between a functional and a neoplastic ovarian cyst. Aspiration of the fluid alone as a diagnostic tool is inadequate because the false-negative rate for the cytologic examination is high and slow leakage of the fluid will disseminate cancer if the cyst is malignant.

Table 21-3, from a seminal series before the widespread use of ultrasound, demonstrates the outcome of a large group of patients with a cystic adnexal mass in their reproductive years who were started on gonadotropin suppression (using low-dose oral contraceptives) at the time of diagnosis, then followed up for 6 weeks. Spontaneous regression (confirming the functional nature of the cyst) occurred in approximately 70% of the patients. Operative intervention in these patients was avoided. However, the remaining 30% of women will need operative intervention.

When the patient is in her late 40s, the chances of an ovarian neoplasm are increased, and observational delays should be undertaken with caution.

Benign Neoplastic Ovarian Tumors

Ovarian neoplasms may be divided generally by cell type of origin into three main groups: epithelial, stromal, and germ-cell. Taken as a group, the epithelial tumors are by far the most common type of ovarian benign neoplasms, although the single most common benign ovarian neoplasm is the benign cystic teratoma (dermoid cyst), which is a germ-cell tumor (Table

---

Table 21-2. Management of a cystic adnexal mass

Age	Size of Cyst (cm)	Management
Premenarchal	>2	Exploratory laparotomy
Reproductive age	<6	Observe for 6 wk
	6–8	Observe if unilocular; surgically explore if multilocular or solid on ultrasonography
	>8	Resect at laparotomy/laparoscopy
Postmenopausal	>4	Resect at laparotomy/laparoscopy

Table 21-3. Adnexal cysts observed for 6 weeks in 286 patients aged 16 to 48 years

Type of Cyst	No. of Patients	%
Regressed under observation	205	72
Required exploratory laparotomy	81	28
Ovarian neoplasms	46	16
Benign epithelial	32	
Benign teratoma	9	
Malignant epithelial	4	
Dysgerminoma	1	
Endometriosis	28	10
Paraovarian cyst	4	1.4
Hydrosalpinx	3	1
Functional cysts	0	0

Data from Spanos WI: Preoperative hormonal therapy of cystic adnexal masses. Am J Obstet Gynecol 116:551, 1973.

21-4). Mixed tumors, as the name implies, are derived from more than one ovarian cell type.

Epithelial ovarian neoplasms. These tumors are believed to be derived from the mesothelial cells lining the peritoneal cavity and also lining the surface of the ovary in greater density. Similar tumors occasionally arise from the mesothelial lining of the pleural cavity. Because all müllerian structures are derived from the special mesothelium of the gonadal ridge and ultimately differentiate into several different histologic tissues (cervical epithelium, endometrium, ciliated endosalpinx, and serous ovarian surface), it is reasonable to postulate that the ovarian mesothelial cells retain the capability to change by metaplasia into any of these müllerian types of epithelium. Thus, the mucinous ovarian neoplasm cytologically resembles the endocervical epithelium (Figure 21-2A), the endometrioid ovarian neoplasm resembles the endometrium, and, occasionally, ovarian tumors are made up of what appears to be ciliated endosalpingial tissue. The most common epithelial ovarian tumors retain their serous cell type and are termed serous cystadenomas (Figure 21-2B).

Each of the epithelial ovarian neoplasms has characteristic clinical and histologic features. The serous tumors are bilateral in about 10% of cases. **Of all serous tumors, about 70% are benign, 5% to 10% have borderline malignant potential and 20% to 25% are malignant,** depending largely on the patient's age. Serous cystadenomas tend to be multilocular, although small unilocular serous cystomas are not uncommon. Histologically, serous tumors characteristically form psammoma bodies (from the Greek psammos, meaning sand), which are calcific, concentric concretions. Psammoma bodies occur occasionally in benign serous neoplasms and frequently in serous cystadenocarcinomas. Papillary patterns are also common (Figure 21-3).

The mucinous neoplasms of the ovary can attain a huge size, often filling the entire pelvis and abdomen. They are often multilocular, and benign mucinous tumors are bilateral in less than 10% of cases. **About 85% of mucinous tumors are benign.** Mucinous tumors are often associated with a mucocele of the appendix. **Rarely, a benign mucinous tumor may be complicated by pseudomyxoma peritonei,** a condition in which a great many benign implants are seeded onto the surface of the bowel and other visceral abdominal organs and produce large quantities of mucus.

The **Brenner tumor** is a small, smooth solid ovarian neoplasm, usually benign, with a large fibrotic component that encases epithelioid cells that resemble transitional cells of the bladder (Figure 21-4). In about 33% of cases, Brenner tumors are associated with mucinous epithelial elements.

Table 21-4. Incidence of primary ovarian neoplasms in the Denver metropolitan area

Type of Ovarian Neoplasm	No.	%
Benign cystic teratoma	103	26.5
Serous cystadenoma/cystadenofibroma	72	18.5
Mucinous cystadenoma/cystadenofibroma	48	12.5
Fibroma	39	10.0
Serous carcinoma	26	6.7
Endometrioid carcinoma	14	3.6
Mixed carcinoma	12	3.1
Serous borderline tumor	12	3.1
Brenner tumor, benign	11	2.8
Thecoma	11	2.8
Clear cell carcinoma	8	2.1
Mucinous carcinoma	6	1.6
Mucinous borderline tumor	6	1.6
Immature teratoma	3	0.8
Other	18	4.7

Data from Katsube Y, Berg JW, Silverberg SG: Epidemiologic pathology of ovarian tumors: A histopathologic review of primary ovarian neoplasms diagnosed in the Denver Standard metropolitan statistical area, July 1–December 31, 1969 and July 1–December 31, 1979. Int J Gynecol Pathol 1:5, 1982.

Sex cord-stromal ovarian neoplasms. These tumors include fibromas, granulosa-theca cell tumors, and Sertoli-Leydig cell tumors. Combinations of the latter two types are termed gynandroblastomas.

The tumors in this category derive from the sex cords and specialized stroma of the developing gonad. The embryologic origins of granulosa and theca cells as well as their counterparts in the testes, the Sertoli and Leydig cells, arise from cells that make up this specialized gonadal stroma. If the ultimate differentiation of cell types occurring in the tumor is feminine, the neoplasm becomes a granulosa-cell tumor, a theca-cell tumor, or in many instances, a mixed granulosa-theca cell tumor. Neoplasms containing cells that take on a masculine differentiation become Sertoli-Leydig cell tumors. This is far less common. The fibroma represents a stromal cell

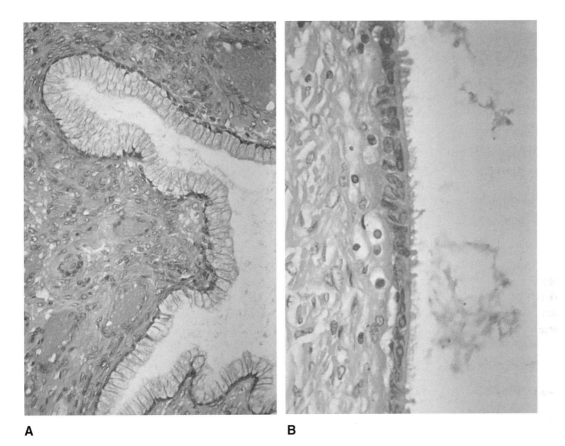

A   **B**

Figure 21-2. Histologic differences between a benign mucinous cystadenoma (*A*) and a benign serous cystadenoma (*B*). The mucinous tumor has taller columnar cells with basal nuclei and abundant mucin, whereas the serous tumor has smaller cuboidal cells lined by focal cilia. *Courtesy Dr. Sathima Natarajan, UCLA Medical Center.*

neoplasm developing from mature fibroblasts in the ovarian stroma.

The granulosa-theca cell neoplasms as well as their androgenic counterparts are generally referred to as functioning (not functional) ovarian tumors. They occur in any age group, from birth on, but more commonly in the postmenopausal years. Their functioning characteristics are responsible for a variety of associated presenting signs and symptoms. **The granulosa-theca cell tumors promote feminizing signs and symptoms,** such as precocious menarche, precocious thelarche, or premenarchal uterine bleeding during infancy and childhood. In the reproductive years, menorrhagia (with alternating amenorrhea), endometrial hyperplasia, and, not infrequently, endometrial cancer, breast tenderness, and fluid retention occur. Postmenopausal bleeding may occur in older women with granulosa theca cell

tumors. In contrast, **the less frequent Sertoli-Leydig cell tumors are responsible for virilizing effects,** such as hirsutism, recession of the frontal scalp hairline, deepening of the voice, clitoromegaly, and a defeminizing change in body habitus to a muscular build. Fifteen percent of these tumors have no such visible endocrinologic effects. **Except for the pure thecoma, all of these tumors have low malignant potential** and are discussed further in Chapter 40.

The **ovarian fibroma,** another ovarian stromal tumor, forms a solid, encapsulated smooth-surfaced tumor made up of interlacing bundles of fibrocytes. It is not hormonally active. It is glistening white on its cut surface (Figure 21-5), as opposed to the soft yellow appearance of the granulosa-theca cell or the smaller hilus cell tumor. On occasion, this tumor is associated with ascites caused by the transudation of fluid from the ovarian fibroid. The flow of this ascitic fluid

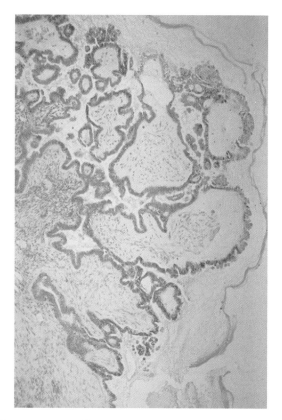

Figure 21-3. Papillary serous cystadenoma. This benign serous tumor is lined by a single layer of epithelium that covers the complex papillary excrescences that arise from the internal surface of the cyst. The papillary excrescences may sometimes be seen on the external surface of the cyst. This does not necessarily signify malignancy, however.

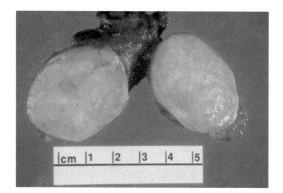

Figure 21-4. Gross appearance of a cut-open Brenner tumor. *Courtesy Dr. Sathima Natarajan, UCLA Medical Center.*

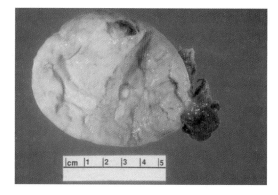

Figure 21-5. Gross appearance of an ovarian fibroma. *Courtesy of Dr. Sathima Natarajan, UCLA Medical Center.*

through the transdiaphragmatic lymphatics into the right pleural cavity may result in **Meigs' syndrome** (ascites and hydrothorax in association with an ovarian fibroma). The ovarian fibroma may be associated with theca-cell elements called a fibrothecoma.

Germ-cell tumors. Germ-cell neoplasms can occur at any age. They make up about 60% of ovarian neoplasms occurring in infants and children.

The most common ovarian neoplasm is the benign cystic teratoma, a germ-cell tumor that can take on a great variety of forms with virtually all adult tissues being represented. Ten percent to 15% of teratomas are bilateral. The benign cystic teratoma, commonly referred to as a dermoid cyst, is composed primarily of ectodermal tissue (such as sweat and sebaceous glands, hair follicles, and teeth), with some mesodermal and rarely endodermal elements. These are slow-growing tumors. Half are diagnosed in women between 25 and 50 years of age. Most are less than 10 cm in diameter. Because of the oily secretion of the sebaceous glands, the desquamated squamous cells, the presence of hair, and the presence of a dermoid tubercle (of Rokitansky), which often contains a hard, well-formed tooth, the dermoid cyst has a characteristic gross and histologic appearance (Figures 21-6, A and B). Other tissue components commonly found in benign cystic teratomas include mature brain, bronchus, thyroid, cartilage, intestine, bone, and carcinoid cells. As opposed to similar tissues found in a malignant immature teratoma, the tissues making up the benign (mature) teratoma are all of an adult, well-differentiated form.

Mixed ovarian neoplasms. The most common ovarian tumor in which the neoplastic elements are

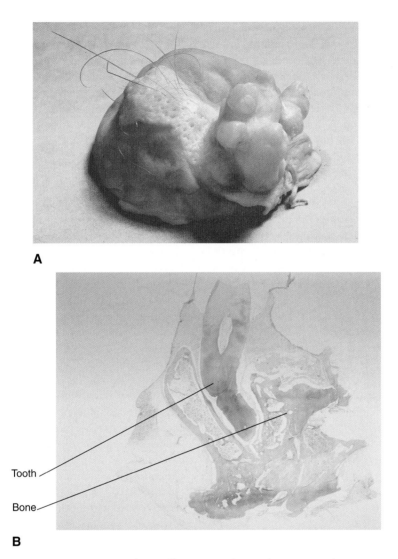

A

B

Tooth

Bone

Figure 21-6. Gross appearance of a small cut-open dermoid cyst. Note the presence of hair-bearing skin on the left and teeth on the right (A) and the histologic appearance of the tooth and bone (B).

composed of more than one cell type is the **cystadenofibroma,** or the fibrocystadenoma. These tumors generally take their characteristics from the epithelial component, although they tend to be more solid than the epithelial ovarian neoplasms.

The **gonadoblastoma** is a tumor composed of cells resembling those of a dysgerminoma and others resembling granulosa and Sertoli cells. Characteristically, calcific concretions are a prominent feature of this neoplasm. **Almost all patients with a gonadoblastoma have dysgenetic gonads, and a Y chromosome has been detected in more than 90%**

of cases. Although the gonadoblastoma is initially benign, about half of these tumors may predispose to the development of dysgerminomas or other malignant germ-cell tumors.

Diagnosis of benign ovarian tumors. The clinical features of benign ovarian tumors are often nonspecific. Except for the functioning ovarian neoplasms, most benign ovarian tumors are asymptomatic unless they undergo torsion (see below) or rupture. They usually enlarge very slowly, so that an increase in abdominal girth or pressure on surrounding organs is not perceived until the later stages of growth. Any pelvic pain is generally mild and intermittent, unless the tumor twists on its pedicle, when infarction may induce severe pain and tenderness. On rare occasions, an ovarian cyst may rupture spontaneously from internal hemorrhage or intracystic pressure, resulting in pain and peritoneal irritation. A cyst may also rupture occasionally during or following a bimanual pelvic examination or with intercourse. Depending on the cystic contents, pain of varying degrees of severity can result. The escape of thin serous fluid without hemorrhage may evoke little pain or tenderness, but the oily contents of a dermoid cyst or the thick mucinous fluid of a mucinous cystadenoma may be irritating to both the parietal and the visceral peritoneum, with the development of peritonitis and the subsequent formation of troublesome intraabdominal adhesions.

Bimanual pelvic examination generally indicates the presence of the tumor in the pelvis, but the tumor may be too small to be palpated. If the tumor is large enough, it may be detected by abdominal palpation. Examination may suggest a cystic mass or a solid tumor. Movement of the mass separate from the uterus supports the suspicion of an adnexal mass instead of a uterine leiomyoma. Percussion of the abdomen in a patient with a large ovarian cyst reveals dullness anteriorly with tympany in the flanks as the bowel is displaced laterally by the tumor.

If the tumor undergoes torsion and infarction or rupture, signs of peritoneal irritation may be present. If complete infarction has occurred, there may be abdominal rigidity. Paralytic ileus may also be present.

Pelvic ultrasonography, particularly **transvaginal ultrasonography,** with or without color Doppler, may be helpful. A pelvic ultrasound will be highly suggestive of a dermoid cyst, especially if it is found to include a tooth-like calcification.

Tumor markers, such as **serum CA 125,** may help to distinguish between benign and malignant masses, particularly in a postmenopausal patient. When clinical evaluation, pelvic ultrasonography, or tumor markers all indicate malignancy, the positive predictive value of the combination is high in postmenopausal women. Such patients should be referred to a gynecologic oncologist for surgical evaluation.

Laparoscopy is helpful in distinguishing between a uterine myoma, a quiescent hydrosalpinx, and an ovarian tumor, but it will not distinguish between a functional cyst, a benign neoplasm, or an encapsulated malignant ovarian neoplasm. On occasion, laparoscopy may identify endometriosis on the surface of the ovary. One cannot distinguish unequivocally, however, an ovarian endometrioma from an ovarian neoplasm by visualization alone. In general, laparotomy is preferable to laparoscopy in the ultimate evaluation of a suspicious adnexal mass unless the entire mass can be removed intact laparoscopically for histologic examination without rupture.

Management of Ovarian Neoplasms

No persistent ovarian neoplasm should be assumed to be benign until proven so by surgical exploration and pathological examination. The indications for exploratory laparotomy in a patient with a pelvic mass have been discussed under functional tumors. If laparotomy is indicated, any ascitic fluid should be collected on opening the peritoneal cavity and sent for cytologic examination. A frozen-section histologic diagnosis should be obtained intraoperatively to exclude malignancy. The definitive treatment will depend on the type of neoplasm, the patient's age, and her desire for future childbearing.

Benign epithelial ovarian neoplasms are generally treated by unilateral salpingo-oophorectomy. The contralateral ovary must be carefully inspected to exclude a bilateral lesion. Because of the possible coexistence of an appendiceal mucocele with a mucinous cystadenoma, appendectomy is also indicated in such patients. If the patient is young and nulliparous, the ovarian neoplasm is unilocular, and there are no excrescences within the cyst, an ovarian cystectomy with preservation of the ovary may be performed. **In an older woman, a total abdominal hysterectomy and bilateral salpingo-oophorectomy (TAH-BSO) may be appropriate,** particularly if there is any suspicion of malignancy.

Stromal-cell neoplasms of the ovary are generally treated by unilateral salpingo-oophorectomy when future pregnancies are a consideration. Ovarian fibromas, even when associated with ascites and a right hydrothorax (Meigs syndrome), are almost always benign and might even be treated by resection from the ovary in a young woman.

Cystic teratomas ("dermoids") can be treated by ovarian cystectomy. Because 15% to 20% are bilateral, the contralateral ovary should be carefully evaluated and any cysts resected. **In a patient with a gonadoblastoma, dysgenetic ovaries are usually present, necessitating bilateral salpingo-oophorectomy**, particularly in the presence of a Y chromosome. With the possibility of embryo transfer now becoming available to these patients, the uterus should be left in situ if future fertility is desired, even when both ovaries have been removed.

BENIGN CONDITIONS OF THE FALLOPIAN TUBES

Most benign tumors of the fallopian tubes are infectious/inflammatory (hydrosalpinx, Figure 21-7A, and pyosalpinx, Figure 21-7B). Benign neoplasms of the oviducts are rare. Although the tubes, uterine corpus, and uterine cervix are from the same müllerian anlage (primordial tissue), the tubes have less of a tendency toward neoplastic transformation.

Tubal neoplasms that do occur are **epithelial adenomas and polyps, myomas** from the tubal musculature, **inclusion cysts** from the mesothelium, or **angiomas** from the tubal vasculature.

It is quite difficult to differentiate a tubal neoplasm from other adnexal masses on examination, and operative exploration is generally necessary to confirm the diagnosis. Salpingectomy represents the definitive treatment, although if pathologic evaluation confirms

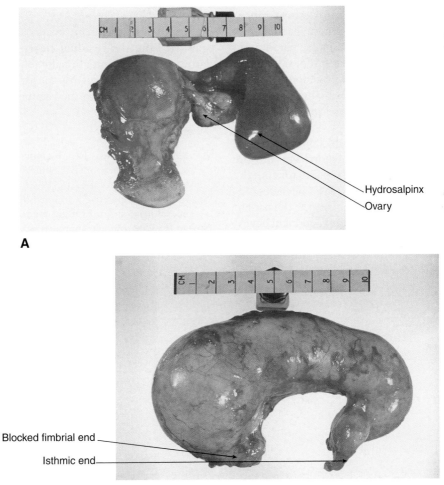

Figure 21-7. Hydrosalpinx (*A*). A gross photograph of a hydrosalpinx of the right fallopian tube. In this example, the ovary is not involved in the inflammatory process. Sometimes the acute inflammation may spread to the ovary from the tube, giving rise to a tubo-ovarian abscess. Pyosalpinx (*B*). In this gross photograph, the isthmic end of the tube is at the right and the blocked fimbrial end is on the left.

the benign nature of the neoplasm, normal portions of the tube may be preserved for fertility reasons in selected cases.

As the name parovarian (beside the ovary) implies, parovarian neoplasms are generally located within the broad ligament between the tube and the ovary. These tumors are generally small compared with ovarian cysts, measuring less than 8 cm in diameter. Histologically, most appear to be derived from paramesonephric (müllerian) structures or occasionally from mesonephric (wolffian) remnants. Although the malignancy rate is less than 10%, it is necessary to resect the cystic mass to obtain a pathologic assessment.

Torsion either of the ovary alone or of both the ovary and fallopian tube (adnexal torsion) represents an acute surgical emergency. Torsion is a complication of benign ovarian tumors, paraovarian cysts, and tubal ligation remnants. Adnexal torsion causes severe acute, unilateral lower abdominal pain, which starts often as less severe pain alternating with a dull soreness. This pattern results from intermittent twisting and untwisting of the mass. With torsion, the venous blood supply is occluded, which increases pressure in the mass and can cause hemorrhage into the mass. With more prolonged and extensive torsion, the arterial supply is occluded and the mass necroses.

The diagnosis may be confusing because the patient may also have fever, nausea, vomiting, and leukocytosis suggestive of appendicitis. Ultrasonic studies, including Doppler color flow studies, can help pinpoint the diagnosis preoperatively, but prompt surgical intervention, usually with unilateral salpingo oophorectomy, is required. If the mass has not necrosed, it may be untwisted. Cystectomy or other procedures to remove the underlying pathology will be necessary. In some cases, the ovary may be sutured to the pelvic side wall to prevent reccurrence. If the tube has undergone necrosis, a unilateral salpingectomy or salpingo-oophorectomy may be necessary.

Ovarian remnant syndrome may be the cause of cyclic pelvic pain and deep dyspareunia in women who have previously undergone hysterectomy with salpingo-oophorectomy. A residual part of the ovary may be left inadvertently and adhere to the vaginal cuff or the retroperitoneum space near a ureter. Surgical excision of the small mass is required to relieve the pain.

The ovarian remnant syndrome must be distinguished from the **residual ovary syndrome.** In the latter, an ovary is intentionally left at the time of hysterectomy but subsequently causes deep dyspareunia if it becomes adherent to the vaginal cuff.

Suggested Reading

Kahn MA, Demopoulas RI: Mucinous ovarian tumors with pseudomyoma peritonei: A clinicopathological study. Int J Gynecol Pathol 11:15, 1992.

Spanos WJ: Preoperative hormonal therapy of cystic adnexal masses. Am J Obstet Gynecol 116:551, 1973.

Steege JF: Laparoscopic approach to the adnexal mass. Clin Obstet Gynecol 37:392, 1994.

Trimbos B, Hacker NF: The case against aspirating ovarian cysts. Cancer 72:828, 1993.

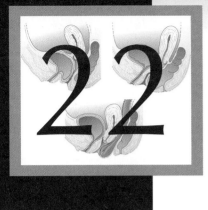

22 Dysmenorrhea and Chronic Pelvic Pain

Andrea J. Rapkin and Joseph C. Gambone

Painful menstruation, or dysmenorrhea, may be primary or secondary to organic pelvic disease. Dysmenorrhea is referred to as primary when no readily identifiable cause exists. **About 50% of menstruating women are affected by dysmenorrhea,** and 10% have severe symptoms necessitating time off from work or school. The typical age range of occurrence for primary dysmenorrhea is between 17 and 22 years, whereas secondary dysmenorrhea becomes more common as a woman ages.

PRIMARY DYSMENORRHEA
PATHOPHYSIOLOGY

Primary dysmenorrhea occurs during ovulatory cycles and usually appears within 6 to 12 months of the menarche. The etiology of primary dysmenorrhea has been attributed to uterine contractions with ischemia. Women with dysmenorrhea have increased uterine activity, which results in increased resting tone, increased contractility, and increased frequency of contractions. During menstruation, prostaglandins are released as a consequence of endometrial cell lysis with instability of lysosomes and release of enzymes, which break down cell membranes.

The evidence that prostaglandins are involved in primary dysmenorrhea is convincing. Menstrual fluid from women with this disorder have higher than normal levels of prostaglandins (especially $PGF_{2\alpha}$ and PGE_2), and these levels can be reduced to below normal with nonsteroidal anti-inflammatory drugs (NSAIDs), which are effective treatments. Infusions of $PGF_{2\alpha}$ or PGE_2 reproduce the discomfort and many of the associated symptoms such as nausea, vomiting, and headache. Secretory endometrium contains much more prostaglandin than proliferative endometrium. **Anovulatory endometrium (without progesterone) contains little prostaglandin, and these menses are usually painless.**

Figure 22-1 summarizes the relationships among endometrial cell wall breakdown, prostaglandin synthesis, uterine contractions, ischemia, and pain.

CLINICAL FEATURES

The clinical features of primary dysmenorrhea are summarized in Box 22-1. Cramping usually begins a few hours before the onset of bleeding and may persist for hours or days. It is localized to the lower abdomen and may radiate to the thighs and lower back. The pain may be associated with altered bowel habits, nausea, fatigue, dizziness, and headache.

TREATMENT

NSAIDs are highly effective in the treatment of primary dysmenorrhea (Box 22-2). Typical examples include **ibuprofen** (400 mg every 6 hours), **naproxen sodium** (250 mg every 6 hours), and **mefenamic acid** (500 mg every 8 hours). Decreasing prostaglandin production by enzyme inhibition is the basis of all NSAIDs. **Women who experience gastrointestinal upset with NSAIDs may benefit from a new class of drugs called cyclo-oxygenase (COX) inhibitors.** There are two forms of this enzyme inhibitor, COX-1 and COX-2. The COX-2 enzyme inhibitor has been shown to be effective for the treatment of dysmenorrhea with fewer gastrointestinal side effects. **Oral contraceptive pills (OCs) reduce menstrual flow and inhibit ovulation and are also effective therapy**

Box 22-1. Features of primary dysmenorrhea

INITIAL ONSET
90% experience symptoms within 2 yr of menarche (i.e., when ovulation begins)

DURATION AND TYPE OF PAIN
Dysmenorrhea begins a few hours before or just after the onset of menstruation and usually lasts 48–72 hr
Pain is described as cramplike and is usually strongest over the lower abdomen and may radiate to the back or inner thighs

ASSOCIATED SYMPTOMS
Nausea and vomiting
Fatigue
Diarrhea
Lower backache
Headache

PELVIC EXAMINATION FINDINGS
Normal

Box 22-2. Treatment of primary dysmenorrhea

GENERAL MEASURES
Reassurance and explanation

MEDICAL MEASURES
Nonsteroidal anti-inflammatory drugs (NSAIDs)
Cyclo-oxygenase inhibitors (COX-2)
Oral contraceptive pills (OCs)
Progestins
Tocolytics
Analgesics

OTHER MEASURES
Psychotherapy
Hypnotherapy
Transcutaneous nerve stimulation (acupuncture)

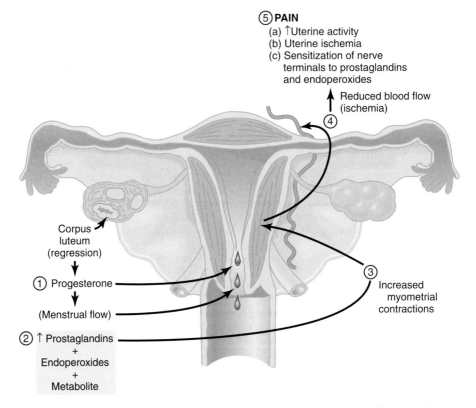

Figure 22-1. Postulated mechanism in the generation of pain in primary dysmenorrhea. Factors affecting central nervous perception of pain are not depicted. Modified from Dawood MY: Hormones, prostaglandins and dysmenorrhea. *In* Dawood MY (ed): Dysmenorrhea. Baltimore, Williams & Wilkins, 1981.

for primary dysmenorrhea. Extended cycle use of OCs or the use of injectable contraceptives minimizes the number of withdrawal bleeding episodes that users have. Some patients may benefit from using both oral contraceptive pills and NSAIDs.

Resistant cases may respond to tocolytic agents (e.g., salbutamol) or a calcium blocker (e.g., nifedipine), progestogens (especially medroxyprogesterone acetate or dydrogesterone), psychotherapy, or hypnotherapy. Surgical presacral neurectomy and uterosacral ligament section has been largely abandoned.

If a patient fails to respond to combined oral contraceptive pill and NSAID therapy, the diagnosis of primary dysmenorrhea should be questioned and consideration given to a secondary cause. Laparoscopy, ultrasonic imaging, and hysteroscopy with directed biopsy should be performed to exclude pelvic disease.

SECONDARY DYSMENORRHEA
PATHOPHYSIOLOGY

The mechanism of pain in secondary dysmenorrhea depends on the underlying (secondary) cause and in most cases is not well understood. Prostaglandins may also be involved in this type of dysmenorrhea.

CLINICAL FEATURES

The clinical features of some of the underlying causes of secondary dysmenorrhea are summarized in Box 22-3. In general, secondary dysmenorrhea is not limited to the menses and can occur before as well as after the menses. In addition, secondary dysmenorrhea is less related to the first day of flow, develops in older women (in their 30s or 40s), and is usually associated with other symptoms such as dyspareunia, infertility, or abnormal uterine bleeding.

TREATMENT

Management consists of the treatment of the underlying disease. The treatments used for primary dysmenorrhea are often helpful. Other specific treatments are discussed in the chapters dealing with the underlying causes.

CHRONIC PELVIC PAIN

Chronic pelvic pain (CPP) refers to pelvic pain of more than 6 months' duration. Purely cyclic uterine pain (dysmenorrhea) has been discussed above. CPP includes uterine and nonuterine pelvic pain that is primarily acyclic. Although CPP is an enigmatic entity, it is one of the most common presenting complaints in a gynecologic practice. As a health problem, it results in great cost to society in terms of hospital services, loss of productivity, and human misery.

Obviously, not all lower abdominal and low back pain is of gynecologic origin. **Careful evaluation is needed to distinguish gynecologic pain from that of orthopedic, gastrointestinal, urologic, neurologic, and psychosomatic origin.** The relationship between pelvic pain and the underlying gynecologic pathology is often inexplicable and frequently thought to be psychosomatic. The discovery of the role of prostaglandins in primary dysmenorrhea, however, formerly believed to be a neurotic affectation, calls for caution when making a diagnosis of psychosomatic pelvic pain. There is still much to be learned about the mechanisms involved in the production and perception of pelvic pain.

Box 22-3. Characteristics of some causes of secondary dysmenorrhea

ENDOMETRIOSIS
Pain extends to premenstrual or postmenstrual phase or may be continuous; may also have deep dyspareunia, premenstrual spotting, and tender pelvic nodules (especially on the uterosacral ligaments); onset is usually in the 20s and 30s but may start in teens

PELVIC INFLAMMATION
Initially pain may be menstrual, but often with each cycle it extends into the premenstrual phase; may have intermenstrual bleeding, dyspareunia, and pelvic tenderness

FIBROID TUMORS, ADENOMYOSIS
Dysmenorrhea is associated with a dull pelvic dragging sensation; uterus is generally clinically enlarged and may be mildly tender

OVARIAN CYSTS (ESPECIALLY ENDOMETRIOSIS AND LUTEAL CYSTS)
Should be clinically evident

PELVIC CONGESTION
A dull, ill-defined pelvic ache, usually worse premenstrually, relieved by menses; often a history of sexual problems

ANATOMY AND PHYSIOLOGY

The pain fibers to pelvic organs are shown in Table 22-1. Painful impulses that originate in the skin, muscles, bones, joints, and parietal peritoneum travel in somatic nerve fibers, whereas those originating in the internal organs travel in visceral nerves.

Visceral pain is more diffusely spread than somatic pain because of a phenomenon called *viscerosomatic convergence* **and the lack of a well-defined projection area in the sensory cortex for its identification.** Viscerosomatic convergence occurs in all second-order neurons in the dorsal horn of the spinal cord that receive visceral input. No second-order neurons in the dorsal horn receive only visceral input. The viscerosomatic neurons have larger receptive fields than do the somatic second-order neurons, and the number of somatic second-order neurons vastly exceeds the number of viscerosomatic neurons. Visceral pain is therefore usually referred to the skin, which is supplied by the corresponding spinal cord segment (referred pain). For example, the initial pain of appendicitis is referred to the epigastric area, as both structures are innervated by the thoracic cord segments T8, T9, and T10.

The structures of the female genital tract vary in their sensitivity to pain. The skin of the external genitalia is exquisitely sensitive. Pain sensation is variable in the vagina, as the upper segment is somewhat less sensitive than the lower. **The cervix is relatively insensitive to small biopsies but is sensitive to deep incision or to dilatation.** The uterus is quite sensitive. The ovaries are insensitive to many stimuli, but they are sensitive to rapid distension of the ovarian capsule or compression during physical examination.

PATIENT EVALUATION
HISTORY

The history should include a description of the localization, quality, radiation, intensity, and duration of the pain, together with any aggravating or alleviating factors. The relationship of the pain to the menstrual cycle (including the presence of abnormal uterine bleeding), bowel movements, urination, sexual intercourse, and physical activity should be noted. A history of similar painful episodes in the past should be sought, as should the presence of other somatic complaints, such as anorexia, weight loss, or gastrointestinal or urologic symptoms. It should be established whether complaints are solely musculoskeletal, such as low or radicular back pain, or whether these accompany the patient's pelvic pain.

The degree to which the pain disrupts the patient's everyday activities should be ascertained. Prominent events in the patient's life that may have occurred concurrent with the onset of pain

Organ	Spinal Segments	Nerves
Perineum, vulva, lower vagina	S2–4	Pudendal, inguinal, genitofemoral, posterofemoral cutaneous
Upper vagina, cervix, lower uterine segment, posterior urethra, bladder trigone, uterosacral and cardinal ligaments, rectosigmoid, lower ureters	S2–4	Pelvic parasympathetics
Uterine fundus, proximal fallopain tubes, broad ligament, upper bladder, cecum, appendix, terminal large bowel	T11–12, L1	Sympathetics via hypogastric plexus
Outer two thirds of fallopian tubes, upper ureter	T9–10	Sympathetics via aortic and superior mesenteric plexus
Ovaries	T9–10	Sympathetics via renal and aortic plexus and celiac and mesenteric ganglia
Abdominal wall	T12–L1	Iliohypogastric
	T12–L1	Ilioinguinal
	L1–2	Genitofemoral

Table 22-1. Nerves carrying painful impulses from the pelvic organs

should also be discussed. For example, the pain may have begun after intercourse with a new partner (possible infectious etiology), rape (possible psychologic trauma), or lifting a heavy object (possible hernia). It should be established what pain medications the patient is taking and whether any compensation or litigation issues are pending.

Symptoms of stress (e.g., palpitations, headaches) or depression (e.g., sleep disorders, loss of memory) **should be elicited.** Other psychologic aspects to be investigated include the attitudes of both the patient and her significant others toward the pain, the illness, and her behavior resulting from the illness. **The possibility of secondary gain or other psychological benefits should be explored, as should concurrent upheavals in the patient's life.** A history of physical, sexual, or emotional abuse in the past or present should be queried. Psychologic evaluations should not preclude further diagnostic studies.

Gynecologic history should include inquiry regarding infertility, pelvic inflammation, history of pelvic surgery, gonococcal or chlamydial infection, endometriosis, and the date of the last pelvic examination. Details of abortion, childbirth, contraception, and sexual history should be sought. Surgical history should include all pelvic, orthopedic, urologic, and neurologic procedures. The medical history should focus on conditions that may impinge on the diagnosis of pelvic pain, such as irritable bowel syndrome, ulcerative colitis, Crohn disease, and interstitial cystitis.

PHYSICAL EXAMINATION

The examination of the abdomen should be performed gently so as to prevent involuntary guarding, which may obstruct the findings. The patient should be asked to point to the exact location of the pain and its radiation, and an attempt should be made to duplicate the pain by palpation of each abdominal quadrant. The severity of the pain should be quantified on a 0 to 10 scale (0 = no pain, 10 = hitting thumb with a hammer).

A gentle but thorough pelvic examination should be performed with an attempt to reproduce and localize the patient's pain. The examination may be suggestive of specific pelvic pathology. For example, patients with endometriosis may have a fixed retroverted uterus with tender uterosacral nodularity. Chronic salpingitis may be suggested by bilateral, tender, irregularly enlarged

adnexal structures. A prolapsed uterus may account for pelvic pressure, pain, or low backache.

The abdominal wall should be examined for evidence of myofascial trigger points and for iliohypogastric (T12, L1), ilioinguinal (T12, L1), or genitofemoral (L1, L2) nerve entrapment. Each dermatome of the abdominal wall and back is palpated with a fingertip and points of motion tenderness or "jump signs" are marked with a pen. The patient is asked to tense the abdominal muscles by performing a straight-leg raising maneuver or a partial sit-up. Points that are still tender or more tender or that reproduce the patient's pain should be injected with 2 to 3 ML of 2.5% bupivacaine. Chronic abdominal wall pain is confirmed if the pain level is reduced by at least 50% and outlasts the duration of the local anesthetic.

FURTHER INVESTIGATIONS

Psychological evaluation should be requested if an obviously traumatic event has occurred with the onset of pain; if there is obvious neurosis, psychosis, or secondary gain; or to aid in the planning of pain management sessions. The latter may involve cognitive behavioral and stress reduction therapy.

Laboratory studies are of limited utility in the diagnosis of CPP, although a complete blood cell count, erythrocyte sedimentation rate (ESR), and urinalysis are indicated. The ESR is nonspecific and will be increased in any type of inflammatory condition, such as subacute salpingo-oophoritis, tuberculosis, or inflammatory bowel disease. If bowel or urinary signs and symptoms are present, an endoscopy, abdominal and pelvic computed tomography (CT) scan, cystoscopy, or CT urogram may be useful. Similarly, if there is clinical evidence of musculoskeletal disease, a lumbosacral x-ray film, CT scan, magnetic resonance imaging (MRI) scan, or orthopedic consultation may be in order.

If no obvious cause for the pain is uncovered, pelvic ultrasonography may be helpful, particularly in obese patients or those who are unable to relax for the complete examination. **Diagnostic laparoscopy is the ultimate method of diagnosis for patients with CPP of undetermined etiology.** Laparoscopic examination and bimanual examination may differ in 20% to 30% of cases. Laparoscopy should only be performed if no etiology for the pain can be identified.

DIFFERENTIAL DIAGNOSIS
ORGANIC CAUSES OF CHRONIC PELVIC PAIN

Of women with CPP who are subjected to diagnostic laparoscopy, approximately a third have no apparent pathology, a third have endometriosis, a quarter have adhesions or stigmata of chronic pelvic inflammatory disease (PID), and the remainder have other causes (Box 22-4).

Endometriosis

Endometriosis may be missed visually at the time of diagnostic laparoscopy in as many as 20% to 30% of women who have the disease proven histologically, so it is justifiable to initiate treatment based on a presumptive diagnosis of the disease once other etiologies have been ruled out.

The size and location of the endometriotic implants do not appear to correlate with the presence of pain, and the reasons for the pain are not fully understood.

Chronic Pelvic Inflammatory Disease

Chronic pelvic inflammatory disease (PID) may cause pain because of recurrent exacerbations that require active antibiotic therapy or because of hydrosalpinges and adhesions between the tubes, ovaries, and intestinal structures. **Before ascribing symptoms to adhesions, one must have specifically noted adhesions in the area of pain localization,** because some patients with extensive pelvic adhesions discovered incidentally during surgery for other reasons are asymptomatic.

> **Box 22-4. Gynecologic causes of chronic pelvic pain**
>
> Endometriosis
> Salpingo-oophoritis (pelvic inflammatory disease)
> Ovarian remnant syndrome
> Pelvic congestion syndrome
> Cyclic pelvic (uterine) pain
> Myomata uteri (degenerating)
> Adenomyosis
> Adhesions

Ovarian Pain

Ovarian cysts are usually asymptomatic, but episodic pain may occur secondary to rapid distention of the ovarian capsule. **An ovary or ovarian remnant may occasionally become retroperitoneal secondary to inflammation or previous surgery, and cyst formation in these circumstances may be painful.** Some women, for unknown reasons, may develop multiple recurrent hemorrhagic ovarian cysts that seem to cause pelvic pain and dyspareunia on an intermittent basis.

UTERINE PAIN

Adenomyosis (or endometriosis interna) may cause dysmenorrhea and menorrhagia, but rarely does it cause chronic intermenstrual pain. **Uterine myomas usually do not cause pelvic pain unless they are degenerating, undergoing torsion (twisting on their pedicles), or compressing pelvic nerves. On occasion, a submucous leiomyoma may attempt to deliver via the cervix, which may cause considerable pelvic pain akin to childbirth.** Uterine myomas may cause pain from rapid growth or infarction during pregnancy.

Pelvic pain is not likely to be caused by variations in uterine position, but **deep dyspareunia may occasionally be associated with uterine retroversion,** especially when the uterus is fixed in place by scarring. The pain has been ascribed to irritation of pelvic nerves by the stretching of the uterosacral ligaments as well as to congestion of pelvic veins secondary to retroversion. The dyspareunia is typically worse during intercourse in the missionary position and is improved in the female superior position. A tender uterus that is in a fixed retroverted position usually signifies other intraperitoneal pathology, such as endometriosis or PID, and diagnosis rests on laparoscopic findings.

Pelvic Congestion Syndrome

The concept of a pelvic congestion syndrome still has many proponents. **This entity has been described in multiparous women who have pelvic vein varicosities and congested pelvic organs.** The pelvic pain is worse premenstrually and is increased by fatigue, standing, and sexual intercourse. Many women with this condition are noted to have a uterus that is mobile, retroverted, soft, boggy, and slightly enlarged. **There may be associated menorrhagia** and urinary frequency. Dilated veins may be seen on venographic studies. Factors other than venous congestion may be involved, however, because most women with pelvic varicosities have no pain. Surgery for this condition, consisting of hysterectomy and oophorectomy, may be beneficial for women who have completed their families, as is ovarian hormone suppression and cognitive behavioral therapy.

Genitourinary Pelvic Pain

A variety of genitourinary problems result in pelvic pain. **Urinary retention, urethral syndrome, trigonitis, and interstitial cystitis are prime examples. Urinary urgency, frequency, nocturia, and pelvic pain may suggest early interstitial cystitis.** A thorough genitourinary evaluation is an important part of the workup for CPP. As many as one in five women have interstitial cystitis.

Gastrointestinal Pain

Gastrointestinal sources of CPP include penetrating neoplasms of the gastrointestinal tract, irritable bowel syndrome, partial bowel obstruction, inflammatory bowel disease, diverticulitis, and hernia formation. Because the innervation of the lower intestinal tract is the same as that of the uterus and fallopian tubes, the patient's complaint of pelvic pain may be confused with pain of gynecologic origin.

Neuromuscular Pain

Pain of neuromuscular origin, which is experienced as low back pain, usually increases with activity and stress. **Chronic low back pain without lower abdominal pain is seldom of gynecologic etiology.** On occasion, neuromuscular symptoms are accompanied by a pelvic mass, and surgical exploration may reveal a neuroma or bony tumor.

PSYCHOLOGIC FACTORS

A pathologic diagnosis may not be made in approximately a third of patients with CPP, even after laparoscopy, which has led to the postulation that **psychological factors** may be etiologic. The patients have been assumed to be anxious, neurotic, anorgasmic, and insecure in their roles as women or as mothers. **When subjected to the Minnesota Multiphasic Personality Inventory (MMPI), these patients have shown a greater degree of anxiety,** hypochondriasis, and hysteria than control subjects. The profiles are similar, however, in patients who have chronic pain with organic pathology, indicating that chronic pain per se engenders a complex, debilitating, psychologic response. Chronic pain patients with and without pathology tend to feel depressed, helpless, and passive. They withdraw from social and sexual activity and are preoccupied with pain and suffering. These women are also at risk for chronic fatigue syndrome.

Pain Perception Factors

Chronic pain is characterized by physiologic, emotional, and behavioral responses that are different from those of acute pain. Although both acute and chronic pain consist of a stimulus and a psychic response, for acute pain these may be adaptive and appropriate, whereas for chronic pain this may not be the case. In fact, **the response to chronic pain may be greatly affected by learning. The patient's reaction to pain and the reaction of significant others to the patient and her pain may be so reinforcing that the behavior may persist even after the painful stimulus has resolved.** Figure 22-2 illustrates the possible levels of agreement between sensory input, the pain sensation or perception, the patient's suffering, and the patient's pain behavior. In acute pain, the pain perception, suffering, and behavior are *usually* commensurate with the degree of sensory input. **In chronic pain, the**

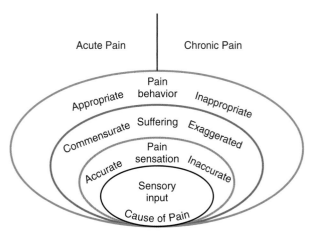

Figure 22-2. A model to illustrate the *usual* characteristics of acute vs. chronic pain in terms of the interplay between pain and sensation and the way pain may be experienced. Modified from Reading AE: Psychological Aspects of Pregnancy. New York, Longman Press, 1983, p 73.

suffering and behavioral responses to a given sensory input may be quite exaggerated and may persist even after the stimulus has remitted.

Modulation of Sensation

Pain impulses are subjected to a large amount of modulation en route to the central nervous system. **The first synapse in the dorsal horn is an important focus of enhancement, inhibition, or facilitation. Modulation of sensations may also occur within the spinothalamic system, the descending inhibitory neurosystems, and the frontal cortex.** Various neurotransmitters and neuromodulators are present in the dorsal horn and at other higher levels of the neuraxis. Excitatory modulators include substance P, glutamate, aspartate, calcitonin gene-related peptide (CGRP), and vasoactive intestinal peptide (VIP). Inhibitory neuromediators include endogenous opioid peptides, norepinephrine, serotonin, and ρ-aminobutyric acid (GABA).

Within this context, anxiety and other psychological states may be considered to be facilitators or inhibitors of neurologic transmission. It is possible that many forms of CPP, in particular those without pathology, may result from modulation of afferent impulses or abnormality of descending inhibition in the dorsal horn, spinal cord, or cerebral cortex.

MANAGEMENT

In dealing with patients with CPP, a therapeutic, supportive, and sympathetic (but structured) physician-patient relationship should be established. The patient should be given regular follow-up appointments and should not be told to call only if the pain persists. This reinforces pain behavior as a means of procuring sympathy and medical attention.

A negative evaluation or the finding of pathology not amenable to therapy (e.g., dense pelvic adhesions) does not mean that the patient should be discharged from care without therapy directed toward her symptoms. **After initial reassurance that there is no serious underlying pathology, symptomatic therapy should be undertaken. The symptoms of pain should be approached with the seriousness and direction afforded to any other condition.**

TEAM MANAGEMENT

The most productive strategy for the management of patients with CPP is referral to a multidisciplinary pain clinic. The personnel at such a facility should include a gynecologist, a psychologist who also has expertise in sexual and marital counseling, an anesthesiologist, and, occasionally, an acupuncturist. It is the role of the psychologist to provide cognitive behavioral pain management and stress reduction, assertiveness training, and adaptive coping strategies. Marital and sexual counseling may be needed as well. This aspect of therapy is crucial, because many of these patients have become interpersonally, sexually, and sometimes even occupationally withdrawn. **Relaxation, cognitive, and behavioral therapies are employed to replace the pain behavior and its secondary gain with effective behavioral responses. Multidisciplinary management has been shown to be more effective than traditional gynecologic management.** When a designated multidisciplinary pain clinic is not available, it is important to involve other specialists by referral.

MEDICAL AND SURGICAL MANAGEMENT

The gynecologist continues to assess progress, coordinate care, and provide periodic gynecologic examinations. **In the initial stages of therapy, a trial of ovulation/menstrual suppression with the birth control pills, high-dose progestins or a gonadotropin-releasing hormone agonist (GnRH-a) may be helpful.** This is especially so in patients who have midcycle, premenstrual, or menstrual exacerbation of pain, or in those who have ovarian pathology, such as periovarian adhesions or recurrent functional cyst formation. **NSAIDs, such as ibuprofen or naproxen, are also useful.** Pharmacologic approaches to increase inhibitory neuromodulators such as norepinephrine, serotonin (5-HT), and GABA are frequently used in the form of tricyclic antidepressants or other GABA-ergic agents.

Surgical procedures that have not proved to be effective for CPP without pathology include unilateral adnexectomy for unilateral pain or total abdominal hysterectomy, presacral neurectomy, or uterine suspension for generalized pelvic pain. Lysis of adhesions is also usually nonproductive, unless the site of adhesions, visualized by the laparoscope, specifically coincides with the localization of pain. Pelvic adhesions often recur following surgical lysis. **Without proof of organic pathology or a reasonable functional explanation for the pelvic pain, a thorough psychosomatic evaluation should be carried out before a surgical corrective procedure is considered.**

ANESTHESIA

Acupuncture, nerve blocks, and trigger-point injections of local anesthetics may provide prolonged pain relief. Acupuncture has been used successfully for dysmenorrhea, and trigger-point injections and nerve blocks with local anesthetics have been used successfully for pelvic pain. Acupuncture probably increases spinal cord endorphins. In patients who complain of pelvic pain, trigger points are usually found either on the lower abdominal wall, lower back, or the vaginal and vulvar areas. **A significant percentage of patients with pelvic pain have abdominal wall trigger points or nerve entrapments that respond to biweekly injections of a local anesthetic (usually up to five injections is sufficient).** Anesthesia of trigger points may abolish pain by lowering the impulses from the area of referred pain, thereby diminishing the afferent impulses reaching the dorsal horn to a level below the threshold for pain transmission.

Suggested Readings

American College of Obstetricians and Gynecologists: Chronic pelvic pain. Technical Bulletin No. 223. Washington, DC, ACOG, 1996.

American College of Obstetricians and Gynecologists: Medical management of endometriosis. Clinical management guidelines for obstetricians and gynecologists. Practice Bulletin No. 11, Washington, DC, ACOG, 1999.

Gambone JC, Mittman BS, Munro MG, et al: Consensus statement for the management of chronic pelvic pain and endometriosis: Proceedings of an expert panel consensus process. Fertil Steril 78:961–972, 2002.

Reiter RC: A profile of women with chronic pelvic pain. Clin Obstet Gynecol 33:130–136, 1990.

Reiter RC, Gambone JC: Nongynecologic somatic pathology in women with chronic pelvic pain and negative laparoscopy. J Reprod Med 36:253–259, 1991.

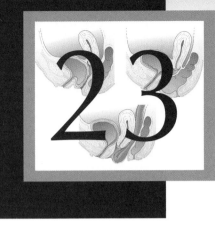

23 Pelvic Infections: Vulvovaginitis, Sexually Transmitted Infections, and Pelvic Inflammatory Disease

James A. McGregor, Janice I. French, and Joel B. Lench

Pelvic infections in women affecting the vulva, vagina, and cervix (lower reproductive tract) and the uterine corpus, fallopian tubes, and ovaries (upper reproductive tract) are common gynecologic problems. Many but not all of these infections are sexually transmitted and require partner treatment for effective immediate and preventive care. Recently the term *sexually transmitted infection (STI)* has replaced *sexually transmitted disease (STD)* to emphasize the infectious nature of these frequently asymptomatic disorders and the need for screening, early recognition, and treatment. The most common STIs are *Chlamydia*, genital herpes (GH), human papillomavirus infection (HPV), and gonorrhea. Trichomoniasis is the one form of vulvovaginitis that is considered to be an STI. Upper reproductive tract infection in the form of pelvic inflammatory disease (PID) is a serious consequence of unrecognized or inadequately treated lower tract disease. The diagnosis and management of common female pelvic infections is covered in this chapter.

NORMAL PHYSIOLOGY AND MICROECOLOGY OF THE VAGINA

The vagina is lined by nonkeratinized stratified squamous epithelium, which is powerfully influenced by estrogen and progesterone. **The vagina of the newborn is colonized by aerobic and anaerobic bacteria acquired while passing through the birth canal.** The newborn's vaginal epithelium is strongly estrogenized and rich in glycogen, which supports growth of lactic acid producing lactobacilli. This results in a low pH (<4.7), which promotes further growth of acidophilic-protective microflora. **Within days of birth, estrogen decreases** and the vaginal epithelium becomes thin, atrophic, and largely devoid of glycogen. In this environment, the pH rises and acidophilic organisms no longer have a selective advantage. **As a consequence, the predominant vaginal microflora become diverse Gram-positive cocci and bacilli.**

With the onset of puberty and ovarian steroidogenesis, the vagina again becomes estrogenized, and the glycogen content increases. **Lactic acid and hydrogen peroxide (H_2O_2) producing lactobacilli again predominate** resulting in a vaginal pH of between 3.5 and 4.5. Even so, a wide variety of aerobic and anaerobic bacteria can be cultured from the normal vagina. Most women harbor at least three to eight types of bacteria at any given time. Lactic acid, H_2O_2, and other substances produced by "healthy" lactobacilli provide some protection in the lower reproductive tract from STIs, including human immunodeficiency virus (HIV).

Multiple factors may alter this protective microflora. Antibiotics suppress growth of commensal organisms, which can allow pathogenic strains (e.g. yeasts) to predominate. **Douching with water or nonbuffered solutions** may transiently alter the pH or selectively suppress endogenous bacteria. **Sexual intercourse with introduction of semen** raises the pH to as high as 7.2 for 6 to 8 hours, making the vaginal milieu receptive to STI pathogens. During coitus, vaginal transudate increases vaginal fluid and serves as lubrication. Vaginal transudate has the same pH as blood (7.4), which also favors attachment of abnormal microflora. **The presence of a foreign body** (e.g., forgotten diaphragm or tampon in adults or various small objects in children) dramatically disrupts normal vaginal cleansing mechanisms and may lead to secondary infection.

PHYSIOLOGIC VAGINAL FLUIDS

Vaginal fluid is a mixture consisting of cervical mucus (the major component), endometrial and oviductal fluid, exudates from the Bartholin's and Skene's glands, transudate from the vaginal squamous epithelium together with exfoliated squamous cells, and metabolic products of the microflora. Vaginal fluid is composed of proteins, polysaccharides, amino acids, enzymes, and immunoglobulins. Physiologic increases in vaginal and endocervical fluid occur during pregnancy, at mid menstrual cycle, and during intercourse. In postmenopausal women (not using estrogens), vaginal fluid may become markedly decreased, which predisposes to infection with various exogenous microflora (e.g., *Escherichia coli*, staphylococcus, and streptococcal species).

INVESTIGATION OF VAGINAL DISCHARGE

Patients with a vaginal infection frequently complain of a nonbloody vaginal discharge. The characteristics of the discharge (e.g., color, texture, viscosity, and odor) are helpful in making the correct diagnosis. Normal vaginal fluid pH is <4.7 in ovulatory women. Vaginal pH can be easily determined by using pH paper with an appropriate pH range (3.5 to 7.0). New self-care over-the-counter (OTC) tests, such as "pH on a stick" and "pH glove," are available to test vaginal pH.

 Testing for the presence of an amine odor (referred to as a positive whiff test) **is performed by putting a few drops of 10% potassium hydroxide (KOH) in the spoon of a vaginal speculum** after it is removed from the vagina. With healthy vaginal fluid no odor is noted. **An "amine," or "fishy," odor suggests infection with trichomoniasis or bacterial vaginosis.**

 A wet-mount preparation of the discharge should be evaluated. Using a cotton-tipped applicator, a sample of vaginal discharge from the posterior fornix is suspended in 2 mL of normal saline. A drop of this solution is placed on a glass slide, covered with a coverslip, and examined under the microscope. **Motile trichomonads may be seen on this type of wet mount (Figure 23-1).** Also, epithelial cells with irregular, granular edges **(clue cells)** are indicative of clumped bacteria on the cell wall and are **highly**

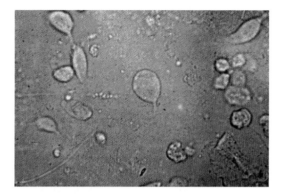

Figure 23-1. Microscopic view (high power) of a Trichomonad in a saline wet-mount preparation. The organisms are usually motile in this type of preparation.

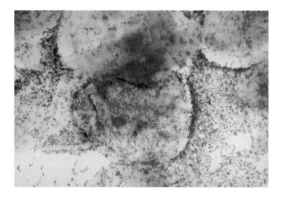

Figure 23-2. Microscopic view of clue cells in a saline wet-mount preparation. Note the irregular or serrated cell walls.

suggestive of bacterial vaginosis if present in >20% of epithelial cells (Figure 23-2). If the cells are not sufficiently separated, **an aliquot of fluid is placed in a drop of 10% to 20% KOH** (to eliminate cellular and other debris while leaving mycelia) and examined microscopically, to visualize the pseudohyphae or spores of *Candida* infection. In complicated or atypical cases, bacterial and/or yeast cultures are required.

VAGINAL DISCHARGE ETIOLOGY

Vaginitis and complaints referable to the vagina (e.g., discharge, pruritus, burning, and "late" dysuria) are very common. A correct diagnosis can be difficult because symptoms and signs may be nonspecific, patients frequently self-medicate with OTC products, there may be multiple causes adding some diagnostic confusion, and accurate diagnostic tools are either not available or are not employed properly.

Up to 90% of cases of vaginitis appear to be caused by three conditions. **Bacterial vaginosis (BV) accounts for 40% to 50%, vulvovaginal candidiasis (VVC) for 20% to 25%, and trichomoniasis for 15% to 20% of cases.** Mucopurulent cervicitis ("mucopus" or MCP) caused by *chlamydia, N. gonorrhoeae*, mycoplasma, or BV-associated bacteria may also cause vaginal irritation and discharge (Figure 23-3). Less common types include **atrophic vaginitis** (overgrowth with aerobic/anaerobic microflora in the absence of lactobacilli and with hypoestrogenized tissues), **foreign-body vaginitis, genital ulcer diseases** such as herpes and syphilis, **desquamative vaginitis** (most commonly group B streptococcal overgrowth), and **lichen planus.**

Standard clinic or office diagnosis of vaginitis requires a working microscope, pH paper, KOH, saline solution, slides, coverslips, and the ability to recognize an amine odor (whiff test). In many settings, these rudimentary tools are not available. Newer, inexpensive "point of care" products can detect vaginal sialidase, amines, and prolineaminopeptidase and other biomarker substances. In difficult or refractory cases, additional tests for vaginal agents may be used such as culture for *T. vaginalis, Candida* mycoplasmas,

or predominant vaginal aerobic bacterial. Table 23-1 lists the common causes, characteristics, and treatments for vulvar and vaginal infections.

BACTERIAL VAGINOSIS

Bacterial vaginosis (BV) is the most common cause of vaginal discharge, but is often without other symptoms. Bacterial vaginosis occurs subsequent to a significant disruption of "healthy" vaginal microflora, (typically *L. jensenii* and *L. crispatus*) by a characteristic set of "BV complex" microorganisms: *G. vaginalis*, genital mycoplasmas (*M. hominis, U. urealyticum*) and vaginal anaerobic bacteria, including *Prevotella, Bacteriodes*, and *Mobiluncus species.* Risk factors for acquisition of BV include a new sexual partner, smoking, intrauterine device (IUD) use, and frequent douching.

Classic features of BV discharge include "profuse," "milky," non-adherent discharge that demonstrates an amine or fishy odor after alkalization with a drop of KOH (positive whiff test).

The presence of BV heightens a nonpregnant woman's risk for pelvic inflammatory disease (PID), postoperative infections (e.g., after hysterectomy or pregnancy termination), and HIV transmission. Partner treatment is generally not recommended.

Table 23-1. Common causes of vulvovaginitis			
Infection	Symptoms/Findings	Diagnosis	Treatment†
Yeast	Vaginal burning, itching, irritation; curdy white discharge	Wet prep and/or KOH microscopic examination shows pseudohyphae, or budding yeast	Butoconazole 2% cream* 5 g intravaginally for 3 days or Fluconazole 150 mg orally in a single dose†
Bacterial vaginosis	Asymptomatic, or vaginal odor; odor after intercourse, or increased discharge	Wet prep "clue cells"; release of amine odor; positive whiff test with KOH; vaginal fluid pH >4.5	Metronidazole 500 mg orally twice a day for 7 days or Clindamycin cream 2%, one applicator (5 g) intravaginally at bedtime for 7 days†
Trichomoniasis	Asymptomatic, or increased thin or thick, green or yellow foul smelling discharge; frothy in 2% to 3% of cases; strawberry cervix in 2% to 3% of cases	Motile trichomonads on microscopic examination of wet mount	Metronidazole 2 g orally in a single dose†

*Over-the-counter (OTC) preparation.
†See Centers for Disease Control (CDC) website for a more complete list of recommended and alternative treatments at www.cdc.gov.

VULVOVAGINAL CANDIDIASIS

Vulvovaginal candidiasis (VVC) is the second most common cause of vulvovaginal-related symptoms. Wide use of over-the-counter antifungal products for self-diagnosed candidiasis has resulted in a decreased frequency of doctor visits, but women who do present are less likely to present with "textbook" findings. *Candida albicans* formerly caused over 90% of VVC, but **now less azole-susceptible species, such as *Candida glabrata*, are recognized as causative agents in 15% of cases.** These less susceptible yeasts necessitate prolonged or alternative treatments. Because of *Candida's* requirement for estrogenated tissues, VVC becomes more common after menarche and less common after menopause. An estimated 75% of women acquire VVC at some time in their life, and 5% suffer frequent symptomatic recurrences. VVC is considered recurrent when at least four episodes occur within 1 year. **Risk factors for recurrent VVC include high-dose oral contraceptives, diaphragm use with a spermicide, diabetes mellitus, antibiotic use, pregnancy, immunosuppression from any cause** (HIV/AIDS, transplantation, alcoholism), and possibly **tight occlusive clothing.**

The classic presentation of VVC includes vaginal itching, burning, irritation, and possibly postvoiding dysuria. The discharge is usually odorless, has a pH of <4.7, and is thick or curdy with the appearance of cottage cheese (Figure 23-3). Examination often shows vulvovaginal erythema, often with evidence of acute or chronic excoriation.

Microscopic examination of a wet mount preparation is positive for budding yeast cells, pseudohyphae, or mycelial tangles (Figure 23-4) in 50% to 70% of cases. **Women with suggestive clinical findings but absent wet preparation evidence may benefit from fungal culture.** First line treatments include topical or oral antifungal (imidazole) agents. Documented cases of recurrences can be effectively treated by: confirming the diagnosis and treating with weekly suppressive doses of topical imidazoles. Boric acid (600 mg vaginal gelatin capsules) three times daily for 1 week is an effective treatment for imidazole-resistant species. Although VVC is not thought to be sexually transmitted in most cases, male partners with diabetes sometimes reinfect their partners.

TRICHOMONIASIS

Trichomoniasis (exocervicitis, vaginitis, and urethritis) is caused by the protozoan *Trichomonas vaginalis*, which

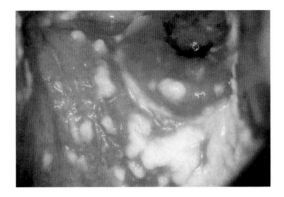

Figure 23-3. Cottage cheese or "curd-like" appearance of vaginal discharge is typical of vulvovaginitis due to yeast.

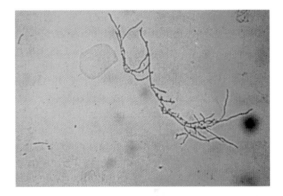

Figure 23-4. Mycelial tangles of yeast pseudohyphae in KOH wet-mount preparation.

occurs worldwide. **About 50% of cases in women and men are asymptomatic.** Symptomatic infection is classically manifested by green-yellow, frothy vaginal discharge (Figure 23-5), "musty" odor, dyspareunia, vulvovaginal irritation, and occasionally dysuria. **Male partners are often "asymptomatic" even though they demonstrate nongonococcal urethritis (NGU) on direct examination.** The diagnosis of trichomoniasis in patients and their sexual partners should be followed by screening for other prevalent STIs and empiric treatment of partners. Diagnosis is usually made on clinical findings and can be confirmed by seeing the characteristic motility of trichomonads on a saline wet mount. Much more sensitive techniques, including culture, polymerase chain reaction (PCR), and antigen testing, are available although none is FDA approved.

In addition to vulvovaginitis and urethritis, trichomoniasis is associated with upper reproductive

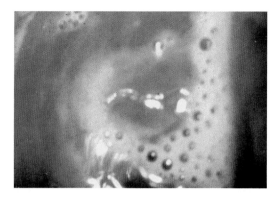

Figure 23-5. Purulent "bubbly" cervical-vaginal fluid characteristic of trichomoniasis.

tract symptoms, an increased risk of adverse pregnancy outcomes (prematurity, low birth weight), and increased transmission of HIV infection.

Metronidazole (2 g single oral dose) **is the recommended treatment** (Table 23-1). Other nitroimidazoles (tinidazole, ornidazole) may be available outside of the US. These agents are equally effective and are reported to be better tolerated. Patients should not consume alcohol for 2 days after treatment. Metronidazole is not teratogenic in recommended dosages but has been traditionally avoided during the first 12 weeks of pregnancy. Prompt early treatment during pregnancy relieves symptoms, reduces the risk of HIV transmission, and may improve pregnancy outcomes. Trichomoniasis should be treated prior to vaginal surgical procedures.

Metronidazole resistance is increasing and may be overcome by using tinidazole (made available for compassionate use by the Food and Drug Administration) **or using higher doses of metronidazole** (2 g daily for 7 days). Reversible side effects of metronidazole toxicity include an "antabuse reaction" with alcohol exposure, neutropenia, and peripheral neuropathy. Higher-dose treatment for resistant trichomoniasis in pregnancy should be prescribed with caution.

ATROPHIC VAGINITIS

Atrophic vaginitis is the most common cause of vaginal irritation among climacteric patients. As the term indicates, **the atrophy of the vaginal epithelium results in secondary infection.** The vulva and introitus quickly become involved because of the associated discharge, and the situation may be exacerbated by a foreign body (such as a pessary). Patients complain of vulvar irritation and discharge, which may be

clear or yellow but occasionally will be blood-tinged. Associated symptoms of frequency, urgency, and stress incontinence may occur.

Examination of the external genitalia may reveal a watery discharge with generalized vulvar erythema, often with excoriation. Speculum examination reveals a pale epithelium with patches of erythema. Superficial blood vessels are visible and may bleed easily on contact. If bleeding is present, the examiner must consider the possibility of a coexistent neoplasm. The discharge has a pH of 5.5 or higher. **A simple evaluation of the epithelial cells using a saline wet mount preparation or Papanicolaou smear will confirm the diagnosis, with immature basal cells and parabasal cells replacing superficial vaginal epithelial cells.**

The treatment of choice is topical estrogen available in vaginal creams, suppositories, or rings. If systemic hormonal treatment is desirable, oral tablets, transdermal patches, and gels are available. If a yellow or green discharge is present, indicating an associated infection, intravaginal sulfa cream may be useful. Aerobic cultures for predominant microorganisms should be obtained in refractory cases.

FOREIGN-BODY VAGINITIS

When a mother states there is discharge on the baby's diaper or the child has vulvar itching, infection, or a bloody vaginal discharge, a foreign body should be suspected in addition to sexual abuse. In adults, forgotten or lost tampons, diaphragms, or condoms may be the cause of vaginitis. With removal of the foreign body and vaginal application of some form of sulfa cream (or estrogen cream in children), rapid improvement usually occurs.

OTHER COMMON SEXUALLY TRANSMITTED INFECTIONS (STIs)

GENITAL HERPES

Genital herpes (GH) is the most prevalent STI in the US, with an estimated 50 million adults infected (active or latent) with herpes simplex virus (HSV) and about 1.5 million new cases occurring every year. It is a chronic life-long viral infection with the potential for rare to frequent recurrences. This infection may have devastating emotional and social consequences. Unfortunately, **only 10% to 20% of infected persons know that they are infected, and 70% of transmissions are from asymptomatic viral shed-**

ding from infected partners with no visible lesions. Individuals who are infected with HSV are at increased risk of acquiring and transmitting HIV. HSV has two serotypes, HSV-1 and HSV-2. HSV-1 is most commonly associated with oral lesions (cold sores), but about 30% of primary GH is due to HSV-1. HSV-2 is the cause of 70% of primary GH and 95% of recurrent GH. The frequency of recurrences is much higher after a primary infection with HSV-2 than HSV-1. The virus enters the body through mucosa or microabrasions in the skin and follows the sensory nerves to the dorsal spinal ganglion where it remains dormant until reactivated. Transmission occurs through intimate genital, oral or anal contact. An infected mother can transmit the virus to her infant during delivery resulting in significant fetal mortality and morbidity (see Chapter 17). Regular condom use decreases transmission by about 50%, especially from men to women.

Primary GH infection occurs when the infected person has no HSV-2 or HSV-1 antibodies. The usual clinical presentation is multiple, bilateral, and painful anogenital vesicles or ulcers with an erythematous base. Systemic symptoms may also be present such as fever, headache, malaise, and lymphadenopathy. Acute cervicitis may be present. The lesions heal without scarring in 14 to 21 days.

Recurrent GH infection occurs when the infected person has HSV antibodies to the same serotype. The lesions are fewer, unilateral, and less painful. Systemic symptoms and lymphadenopathy are rare. The lesions heal without scarring in 5 to 7 days in immunocompetent individuals.

Laboratory tests that are used to confirm the diagnosis include: (1) viral culture that requires live cells from a lesion is expensive and time-consuming but has a relatively low sensitivity (50% to 80%); (2) polymerase chain reaction (PCR), which is expensive and very accurate, is not used routinely on genital lesions but is very useful for testing cerebrospinal fluid; and (3) type-specific serologic tests for HSV-1 and HSV-2 antibodies are highly sensitive and specific tests that can identify individuals who are asymptomatic.

The goals of treatment for GH are symptom relief, acceleration of lesion healing, and a decrease in frequency of recurrences. Education and supportive counseling are also important. The antiviral agents (acyclovir, famciclovir, and valacyclovir) are safe and effective for treating primary and episodic outbreaks, and suppressive therapy for patients with chronic disease. No treatment, however, completely eradicates

the latent virus from the dorsal ganglia of the spinal cord. Work is underway to develop an HSV vaccine.

HUMAN PAPILLOMAVIRUS (HPV)

Genital **human papillomavirus (HPV)** is a common viral STI with an estimated 20 million infected persons in the US and 5 million new cases every year. It is believed that about 75% of sexually active adults will be infected sometime in their life. **The large majority of HPV cases are latent infections with no visible lesions and are only diagnosed by DNA hybridization testing performed in the evaluation of an abnormal pap smear.** Subclinical infections have lesions that are only visible during colposcopy. Clinical infections are characterized by readily visible "warty" growths called condylomata acuminata on the vulva, vagina, cervix, urethra, and perianal area. There are about 1 million new cases of these external genital (venereal) warts every year in the US. HPV infection usually clears spontaneously within 2 years, but recurrences are common. **There are about 200 HPV genotypes. Some have been strongly associated with genital neoplasia and cancers, especially cervical (see Chapter 39).** Biopsies of atypical or persistent lesions are needed to rule out neoplastic disease. Because these growths may also mimic condylomata lata, syphilis must be excluded if the lesions are atypical or do not respond to treatment. Transmission of HPV can occur even when there are no visible lesions. Regular condom use may provide some degree of protection. During pregnancy, condylomata may increase in number and size. **However, transmission from mother to infant is very rare.** HPV vaccine research is ongoing, but no vaccine is commercially available.

The reasons for treating visible genital warts are to relieve symptoms (pain and/or bleeding) and sometimes for cosmetic concerns of the patient. Multiple therapeutic modalities are available to treat these lesions and all are comparable. Provider-applied topical therapies include (1) podophyllin resin 10% to 25% in tincture of benzoin and (2) trichloroacetic acid (TCA) or bichloracetic acid (BCA) 80% to 90%. Patient-applied topical therapies include (1) podofilox 0.5% solution or gel and (2) imiquimod 5% cream. Surgical therapies include (1) cryotherapy, (2) manual excision, (3) electrocautery, (4) laser vaporization, and (5) intralesional interferon. **Podophyllin, podofilox, and imiquimod should not be used during pregnancy.**

CHLAMYDIA

Chlamydia has the highest incidence of any bacterial STI in the US, with 3 million new cases every year. The majority of cases (75%) are found in individuals who are <25 years old and about half of the cases are in teenagers. *Chlamydia trachomatis* is an obligate intracellular bacteria that grows in vitro only in tissue culture and in women infects the columnar epithelium of the endocervix, urethra, endometrium, fallopian tubes, and the rectum. This organism can persist for long periods in an asymptomatic carrier state. There is no vaccine available and even though *Chlamydia* antibodies are produced, they do not protect against reinfection. Because **about 70% of infected females and 50% of infected males have no symptoms,** it is very difficult to diagnose and treat this "hidden" infection. In those cases where symptoms are present, the clinical manifestations of lower genital tract *Chlamydia* infection are (1) mucopurulent cervicitis or mucopus, which is a yellow discharge coming from a swollen, red, friable cervix that bleeds easily (see Figure 23-3) and (2) acute urethritis and dysuria with minimal frequency/urgency and a negative urine culture.

Various laboratory tests are used to confirm the diagnosis of *Chlamydia*: (1) tissue culture, which requires live cells is expensive; (2) antigen tests are inexpensive and rapid with a high sensitivity and specificity; and (3) DNA hybridization tests and nucleic acid amplification tests (PCR and ligase chain reaction) are more expensive and rapid. **These newer tests can be done on urine specimens instead of cervical swabs, and therefore they are very convenient for screening purposes.** Selective screening should be performed at least annually on sexually active females <25 years old. Also test individuals with risk factors (unmarried, multiple partners, inconsistent use of barrier contraceptive methods, previous history of any STI) and all pregnant women. **It is estimated that 30% of untreated chlamydial cervicitis will progress to PID. Aggressive screening and appropriate early treatment has been shown to decrease the incidence of PID.**

General treatment guidelines for lower genital tract *Chlamydia* infection include the following: (1) presumptive treatment with appropriate antibiotics (e.g., azithromycin 1 g orally in a single dose or doxycycline 100 mg twice a day for 7 days); (2) treatment of all sexual contacts within the past 60 days prior to diagnosis; (3) testing for other STIs, including gonorrhea, syphilis, hepatitis B, and HIV; and (4) abstinence from sexual contact for 7 days after last partner has started antibiotic therapy. Test of cure is not necessary; however, rescreening in 3 to 4 months to check for reinfection is recommended.

Chlamydia infection during pregnancy can cause adverse outcomes for both mother and infant. These include preterm labor, chorioamnionitis and postpartum endometritis. Intrapartum transmission to the infant can cause neonatal conjunctivitis and/or pneumonia.

GONORRHEA

Neisseria gonorrhoeae is the second most common bacterial STI in the United States with 600,000 new cases annually. The organism is a gram negative diplococcus and it infects the same columnar epithelium as *Chlamydia*. Additionally, it can infect the pharynx in about 10% of the cases. It can also survive in the host as an asymptomatic carrier. There is no vaccine available and no immunity is conferred even though antibodies are produced. **Most infected women, but only 5% of infected men, have no symptoms.** If symptoms are present, the clinical manifestations of lower genital tract gonococcal infections are the same as for *Chlamydia* and include mucopurulent cervicitis, which involves a swollen, red, friable cervix, contact bleeding, and acute urethritis, producing dysuria with minimal frequency/urgency and a usually negative urine culture.

Laboratory tests that can be used to confirm the diagnosis include Gram's stain of the discharge or cervix, which is rapid and inexpensive. The presence of gram-negative diplococci in the leukocytes is very sensitive for men; however, in women, the sensitivity is only 50%. Thayer-Martin or Transgrow media culture is inexpensive, but takes longer with a sensitivity of 90% and a specificity of 97%. DNA hybridization test is inexpensive and rapid with a high sensitivity and specificity, and nucleic acid amplification tests (PCR and LCR) are more expensive and rapid with very high sensitivity and specificity. These tests can be done on urine and/or cervical swabs. **Because most women with gonococcal cervical infection are asymptomatic, selective screening of high risk persons is essential in attempting to control the progression and spread of this disease. It is estimated that about 15% of untreated gonococcal cervical infection will progress to PID.**

Resistant strains of gonorrhea include penicillinase-producing *N. gonorrhoeae* (PPNG), chromosomal mediated–resistant *N. gonorrhoeae* (CMRNG), tetracycline-resistant *N. gonorrhoeae* (TRNG), and quinolone-resistant *N. gonorrhoeae* (QRNG). It is important to avoid using quinolones for the treatment of gonorrhea in California or in cases where the disease may have been acquired in Asia or the Pacific Islands.

General treatment guidelines for lower genital tract gonorrhea infection include: (1) treatment with appropriate antibiotics (e.g., cefixime 400 mg orally in a single dose or ceftriaxone 125 mg IM in a single dose); (2) simultaneous treatment for *Chlamydia* (i.e., 1 g of azithromycin orally in a single dose) because 20% to 40% of gonococcal cervical infections also have *Chlamydia*; (3) treatment of all sexual contacts within the past 60 days prior to diagnosis; (4) abstinence from sexual activity for 7 days after the start of antibiotic therapy; (5) testing for other STIs, including *Chlamydia*, syphilis, hepatitis B, HIV. Test of cure is not necessary, however, rescreening in 3 to 4 months to check for reinfection may be helpful.

Gonococcal infection during pregnancy can cause adverse outcomes for both the mother and infant. These include preterm labor and delivery, chorioamnionitis, and postpartum endometritis. Intrapartum transmission to the infant can cause neonatal conjunctivitis *(ophthalmia neonatorum)*.

PELVIC INFLAMMATORY DISEASE

PID is a morbid and costly sexually transmitted bacterial upper-reproductive-tract infection affecting nonpregnant and occasionally pregnant women. Studies demonstrate the importance of pathogenic lower-reproductive-tract microorganisms ascending from the endocervix to mediate endometritis, salpingitis, and sometimes peritonitis.

EPIDEMIOLOGY AND PATHOGENESIS

More than 10% of reproductive-age women report a history of PID. PID is an expensive public health problem. It has been estimated that the direct costs of treating PID in the US exceed $6 billion annually. These costs do not include the indirect costs for treating sequelae such as infertility, ectopic pregnancy, and preterm birth.

The most important "single agent" causes of PID include *C. trachomatis*, *N. gonorrhoeae*, and genital mycoplasmas *(M. hominis, U. urealyticum, and M. genitalium)*. Each of these is an STI with inoculation occurring most commonly during intercourse. *M. hominis, U. urealyticum,* and *M. genitalium* are widely recognized causes of nongonococcal urethritis (NGU) in males and females. Both *C. trachomatis* and *N. gonorrhoeae* have well-defined molecular virulence factors that mediate genital attachment and cell damage. Unlike gonorrhea, which occurs more frequently within inner-city and minority populations, chlamydial infections are broadly distributed among most racial, ethnic, and economic groups.

PID develops in 15% to 30% of women with inadequately treated gonococcal or chlamydial cervicitis. There are an estimated 3 million chlamydial genital infections yearly in the United States. The highest rates of chlamydial cervicitis occur in sexually active adolescents and young adults between the ages of 20 and 25 years. The largely asymptomatic nature of chlamydial cervicitis in women and urethritis in men makes routine screening and treatment for *Chlamydia* necessary for the prevention of PID.

The most common microbial isolates recovered from patients at laparoscopy or at drainage of pelvic abscesses are endogenous lower-reproductive-tract or gastrointestinal microflora, including *E. coli, Bacteriodes* and *Prevotella* species, *G. vaginalis,* and anaerobic streptococci. These common sexually transmitted and endogenous agents should be "covered" during antibiotic treatment for PID.

COMPLICATIONS

The sequelae of PID are much more common and long standing than previously recognized. A seminal study of PID was performed in Lund, Sweden, where 2500 women were followed with their disease from 1960 to 1984. **Women with clinical PID were six times more likely to have an ectopic pregnancy and 14 times more likely to have tubal factor infertility than women without PID.** Women with a history of PID were 6 to 10 times more likely than healthy controls to have the diagnosis of endometritis, suffer from chronic pelvic pain, or require a hysterectomy.

SYMPTOMS

Women with symptomatic PID commonly have lower abdominal pain and tenderness (especially when walking or during coitus), abnormal vaginal discharge,

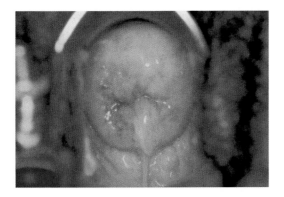

Figure 23-6. Uterine cervix at the time of speculum examination with mucopus protruding from the os.

chills, and fever. Less common symptoms include irregular vaginal bleeding, dysuria, nausea, and vomiting. No specific combination of symptoms is consistently associated with PID. Some women are asymptomatic.

SIGNS

Clinical signs in women with laparoscopically confirmed PID most frequently include **lower abdominal tenderness,** with or without rebound tenderness; **uterine and adnexal tenderness** to palpation and motion; and findings of **mucopurulent cervicitis** (Figure 23-6). Fever is the least common finding. A pregnancy test should be performed when symptoms or signs of pregnancy are present.

INVESTIGATIONS

Nucleic acid, antigenic, or culture tests should be done to detect chlamydial and gonococcal infections. Confirmatory laboratory evidence includes **leukocytosis, increased erythrocyte sedimentation rate or C-reactive protein level,** and microscopic or leukocyte esterase test evidence of purulent cervical discharge (mucopus). **Pelvic ultrasonic studies** may show enlarged fallopian tubes that are tender when approached with a vaginal probe, as well as cul-de-sac fluid (approximately 50% sensitivity).

Laparoscopy is no longer considered clinically necessary for diagnosis of PID or tubo-ovarian abscess (TOA) because it is invasive and costly, and safer, effective antimicrobial regimens are now available. Laparoscopy is generally not performed unless

differentiation from other processes (e.g., appendicitis) is required. **Positive findings on endometrial biopsy** (presence of plasma cells and polymorphonuclear cells) **are also confirmatory,** but they are not commonly performed because of discomfort.

DIAGNOSIS

PID should be diagnosed and treated empirically in sexually active young women and women with risk factors who have uterine/adnexal or cervical motion tenderness. The CDC cautions that PID is unlikely if the patient does not have a mucopurulent cervical discharge or white blood cells on her vaginal wet mount. Abnormal findings that make the diagnosis more secure include fever, elevated erythrocyte sedimentation rate, elevated C-reactive protein, and documented cervical infection with gonorrhea or chlamydia.

TREATMENT

Therapeutic goals for treating PID are elimination of reproductive tract infection and inflammation, improvement of symptoms and physical findings, prevention or minimization of long-term sequelae, and eradication of causal agents from the patient and her sexual partner(s).

Empiric antibiotic regimens should be aimed at treating likely causative agents, that is, *N. gonorrhoeae, C. trachomatis,* genital mycoplasmas, and bacterial vaginosis–associated endogenous microflora. The latter include anaerobic (*Bacteroides* and *Prevotella* species and anaerobic streptococci) as well as aerobic organisms (*G. vaginalis, E. coli,* and facultative streptococci). Except for *N. gonorrhoeae* and some anaerobes, resistance is not yet a clinical problem.

The need for hospitalization is an important treatment decision (Box 23-1). **Women with severe infections or an inability to take and absorb oral antibiotics** (nausea, vomiting, possible peritonitis, and ileus) **should be hospitalized** and treated until clinical improvement is evident. Similarly, women with a questionable diagnosis, pregnancy, or inability to be treated on an outpatient basis, should be admitted initially and treated with parenteral agents so as to ensure compliance and treatment efficacy, as should those who fail to respond to outpatient therapy.

Table 23-2 lists antibiotic regimens for inpatient and outpatient management, as recommended

Table 23-2. Centers for Disease Control and Prevention recommended treatments for pelvic inflammatory disease, 2002*

Regimen A	Regimen B
INPATIENT TREATMENT	
Cefoxitin 2 g IV q6h	Clindamycin 900 mg IV q8h
or	*plus*
Cefotetan 2 g IV q12h	gentamicin 2 mg/kg IV once, followed by 1.5 mg/kg IV q8h until
plus	improved, followed by doxycycline, 100 mg orally bid, to complete
doxycycline 100 mg IV q12h until improved, followed by doxycycline 100 mg orally bid, to complete 14 days	14 days
OUTPATIENT TREATMENT	
Ofloxacin 400 mg orally bid for 14 days	Ceftriaxone 250 mg IM single dose
or	*or*
Levofloxacin 500 mg q day for 14 days	Cefoxitin 2 g IM single dose and probenecid 1 g orally,
With or without	*plus*
metronidazole 500 mg bid orally for 14 days	doxycycline 100 mg bid, to complete 14 days
	With or without
	Metronidazole 500 mg orally bid for 14 days

* See Centers for Disease Control (CDC) for a more complete list of recommended and alternative treatments at www.cdc.gov.

Box 23-1. Pelvic inflammatory disease: Clinical criteria for hospitalization/parenteral treatment

1. Surgical emergencies (e.g., appendicitis) not ruled out
2. Pregnancy (decrease fetal wastage from preterm birth)
3. Failed oral treatment (no improvement with short-term treatment)
4. Compliance questionable (i.e., patient unable to follow or tolerate outpatient regimen)
5. Severe illness (toxicity: nausea, vomiting, high fever)
6. Tubo-ovarian abscess shown or suspected

by the Centers for Disease Control (CDC). Other recommended and alternative treatments are listed on their website, www.cdc.gov.

Outpatient treatments may be selected for the majority of women who will return promptly if no improvement is seen within 24 to 48 hours and who are likely to be compliant. Direct observation of initial oral treatment is preferred. Adjunctive anti-inflammatory agents to reduce peritubal fibroblastic proliferation and scarring have been proposed (short-term anti-inflammatory agents, including low-dose corticosteroids and nonsteroidal anti-inflammatory agents) but none has proved consistently beneficial in animal or human studies.

Patients should be reevaluated 3 to 4 weeks after treatment. Pelvic examination should be done at that time to ensure adequacy of treatment. Counseling regarding preventative strategies for STIs and HIV infection, as well as contraceptive advice, should be repeated at the follow-up visit.

PREVENTION OF PELVIC INFLAMMATORY DISEASE

Developments in diagnostic testing for prevalent STIs and the use of single-dose antibiotic treatments for gonococcal and chlamydial infections, trichomoniasis, and BV have led to new opportunities to prevent PID. The practice of routine screening, treatment, and prevention for chlamydial infections has already dramatically reduced rates of PID and sequelae in US studies.

Use of sensitive and specific nucleic acid diagnostic techniques such as polymerase chain reaction (PCR) and ligase chain reaction (LCR) for common STIs allows for relatively inexpensive screening and diagnosis in both high- and low-prevalence populations. Although direct cervical or urethral sampling is preferable, both females and males may now submit either urine samples or self-collected swabs for accurate and inexpensive nucleic acid–based testing. **Use of urine-based testing greatly facilitates identification of infected asymptomatic carriers.**

Single-dose regimens, such as azithromycin, 1 g orally (for chlamydial infections), and cefixime, 400 mg, or ofloxacin, 400 mg orally (for nonresistant gonorrhea), **simplify treatment** and ensure greater compliance. Directly observed therapy also ensures compliance.

To minimize the risk of reinfection, partners for the last 60 days should be identified, diagnosed and given specific treatment or treated empirically for both chlamydial infection and gonorrhea. The majority of infected male partners are asymptomatic. This practice should minimize recurrence and reinfection that can lead to permanent agglutinative adhesions (Figure 23-7).

OTHER INDICATIONS FOR STI TESTING

Recent studies are reassuring with respect to a lack of an association between PID and IUD use. However, these devices are intended only for couples who are in stable, mutually monogamous relationships. It is prudent however to screen patients for common STIs

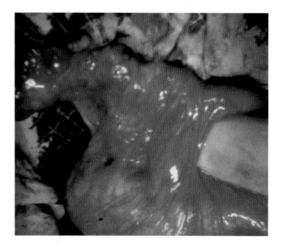

Figure 23-7. View of agglutinated adhesions of the female reproductive organs at the time of laparotomy typical of recurrent episodes of pelvic inflammatory disease (PID).

and to treat for BV prior to insertion to minimize the risk of endometrial contamination.

TUBO-OVARIAN ABSCESS

Tubo-ovarian abscess (TOA) involving fallopian tubes, ovaries, bowel, and possibly other pelvic structures is a potentially lethal complication of PID. Inflammatory complexes (adnexal structures that are agglutinated) also represent severe infection but do not contain significant amounts of pus and are more easily treated with antibiotics.

TOAs occur in approximately 10% of women hospitalized for PID. A TOA in the course of the initial episode of PID represents severe infection in which the host is unable to localize tissue damage. Some TOAs are caused by reactivation of past infection or repeated infections or occur as a result of postpartum or postoperative infections.

Rupture of a TOA causes spreading peritonitis, which can be rapidly lethal in the absence of expeditious surgical drainage, antimicrobial treatment, and systemic vital organ support. TOAs may cause considerable long-term morbidity from irreversible tubal and ovarian damage, with subsequent infertility, chronic pain, and gonadal failure. Rarely, death results from uncontrolled sepsis.

A TOA is distinguished from uncomplicated endometritis/salpingitis by the presence of a tender inflammatory adnexal mass. Confirmation of the diagnosis may require the use of imaging techniques such as ultrasonography, computed tomography (CT), or magnetic resonance imaging (MRI) as depicted in Figure 23-8. Drainage of a TOA under ultrasound guidance can be both diagnostic and therapeutic. Laparotomy or laparoscopy may also be required to distinguish TOAs from inflammatory complexes, twisted or infected adnexal structures, or pelvic abscesses from other sources (e.g., appendicitis or diverticulitis). **If there is doubt regarding the diagnosis, laparoscopy should be performed promptly.** If laparoscopy or laparotomy is performed, the TOA or pyosalpinx should be drained (extraperitoneally if possible), followed by copious irrigation.

Broad-spectrum intravenous antibiotic treatment, including coverage for endogenous pelvic microorganisms (*E. coli*, *B. fragilis*, and aerobic and anaerobic cocci) and *N. gonorrhoeae*, **should be started promptly after obtaining microbiologic**

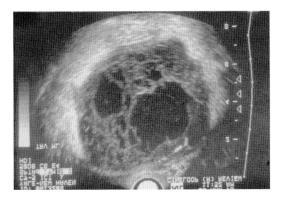

Figure 23-8. Magnetic resonance imaging (MRI) of a tubo-ovarian abscess (TOA).

tests from the cervix. Intensive antibiotic treatment for TOAs should consist of **broad coverage, multi-agent regimens**.

Such regimens are associated with curative response rates of approximately 85%. Some meta-analyses have found improved results if clindamycin is included in a multiagent regimen. **Empiric oral antibiotic treatment** (e.g., oral doxycycline, 100 mg, twice daily), amoxicillin/clavulanic acid (250 mg, three times a day), or metronidazole (500 mg, twice a day) **is traditionally given for at least 7 days after response to parenteral treatment.**

In the face of clinical deterioration or the absence of obvious clinical improvement after 24 to 48 hours of antibiotic treatment, other modalities should be utilized. Interventional radiographic procedures can be performed using vaginal, abdominal, or rectal ultrasound guidance with aspiration. For women desiring future fertility or when uterine and ovarian preservation is a goal, incision and drainage of infected abscess cavities and possibly salpingectomy are the usual treatments. Total abdominal hysterectomy and bilateral salpingo-oophorectomy may be necessary in refractory cases. Laparotomy is usually performed, although laparoscopy also facilitates differentiation of other causes of pelvic abscess, such as diverticular disease.

LESS COMMON SEXUALLY TRANSMITTED INFECTIONS

Chancroid is caused by *Haemophilus ducreyi*. The lesions, called "soft chancres," are painful and are usually accompanied by pelvic adenopathy. Diagnosis is made clinically and confirmed with cultures. Treatment is with azithromycin 1 g in single oral dose or ceftriaxone 250 mg IM in a single dose.

Granuloma inguinale (Donovanosis) is caused by *Calymmatobacterium granulomatis*. The lesions are red and raised. Treatment is with doxycycline 100 mg twice a day for a minimum of 3 weeks.

Lymphogranuloma venereum (LGV) is caused by *Chlamydia trachomatis*. Vesicles progress to bubo formation. A complement fixation test is available for diagnosis. Treatment is with doxycycline 100 mg twice a day for at least 3 weeks.

Molluscum contagiosum is caused by *Poxviridae*. The raised papules with waxy cores are desiccated or treated with cryotherapy or topical imiquimod.

Syphilis is relatively uncommon in the US. It is particularly important, however, for the obstetrician to recognize this infection in the pregnant patient (see Chapter 17) or in women who may become pregnant. Syphilis is caused by *Treponema pallidum*. Treatment is with parenteral penicillin G.

HIV/AIDS AND REPRODUCTIVE-TRACT INFECTIONS IN WOMEN

Lower- and upper-reproductive-tract infections may increase HIV risk in multiple ways. The presence of vaginal, cervical, and endometrial infection may amplify both the susceptibility to HIV infection as well as its transmission to sexual partners. Both ulcer- and nonulcer-causing STIs appear to increase the susceptibility to HIV by damaging host defenses or increasing the number and efficiency of HIV viral receptors. Conversely, genital tract inflammation increases local release of HIV virus, which potentiates transmission to sexual partners and vaginally delivered babies. Screening and treatment for STIs provides an opportunity to reduce the risks of HIV acquisition and transmission.

Suggested Reading

CDC: Sexually transmitted diseases: Treatment Guidelines 2002; MMWR 51:1–77, 2002.

Haefner HK: Current evaluation and management of vulvovaginitis. Clin Obstet Gynecol 42:182–195, 1999.

Korn AP: Gynecologic care of women infected with HIV. Clin Obstet Gynecol 44:226–242, 2001.

Koumans EH, Markowitz LL, Hogan V: CDC Working Group. Indications for therapy and treatment recommendations for bacterial vaginosis (BV) in non-pregnant and pregnant women: A synthesis of data. CID 35(Suppl 2):157–172, 2002.

Ross J: Pelvic inflammatory disease (PID). BMJ 322:658–659, 2001.

Ross JDC. An update on pelvic inflammatory disease. Sex Transm Infect 78:18–19, 2002.

Simms I, Stephenson JM: Pelvic inflammatory disease epidemiology: What do we know and what do we need to know? Sex Transm Infect 76:80–87, 2000.

Sobel J: Current concepts: Vaginitis. N Engl J Med 337:1896–1903, 1997.

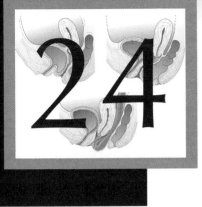

24 Genitourinary Dysfunction: Pelvic Organ Prolapse, Urinary Incontinence, and Infections

Narender N. Bhatia

Detailed knowledge of female pelvic anatomy facilitates understanding and management of pelvic relaxation defects and urinary incontinence.

NORMAL PELVIC ANATOMY AND SUPPORTS

Anatomically, the pelvic organs, including the vagina, uterus, bladder, and rectum, are maintained within the pelvis by the bilaterally paired and posteriorly fused levator ani muscles. **The anterior separation between the levator ani is called the levator hiatus. Inferiorly, the levator hiatus is covered by the urogenital diaphragm. The urethra, vagina, and rectum pass through the levator hiatus and urogenital diaphragm as they exit the pelvis. The endopelvic fascia is a visceral pelvic fascia that invests the pelvic organs and forms bilateral condensations referred to as ligaments (i.e., pubourethral, cardinal, and uterosacral ligaments).** These ligaments attach the organs to the fascia of the pelvic side walls and bony pelvis (see Chapter 3). Damage to the vagina and its support system allows the urethra, bladder, rectum, and small bowel to protrude into the vaginal canal.

The **perineal body** is a central point for the attachment of the perineal musculature. **Although the contents of the abdominal cavity bear down on the pelvic organs, they remain suspended in their relation to each other and to the underlying levator sling and perineal body.**

PELVIC ORGAN PROLAPSE

Pelvic organ prolapse refers to protrusion of the pelvic organs into or out of the vaginal canal. They may occur singly but are more commonly combined (Box 24-1).

UTERINE PROLAPSE

Although vaginal prolapse can occur without uterine prolapse, the uterus cannot descend without carrying the upper vagina with it.

Complete procidentia represents failure of all the genital supports. Hypertrophy, elongation, congestion, and edema of the cervix may sometimes cause a large protrusion of tissue beyond the introitus, which may be mistaken for a procidentia.

VAGINAL PROLAPSE

The bulging or descent of the bladder into the upper anterior vaginal wall is called a **cystocele** (Figure 24-1). Upper posterior vaginal wall prolapse is nearly always associated with herniation of the pouch of Douglas, and, because this is likely to contain loops of bowel, it is called an **enterocele.** Lower posterior vaginal wall prolapse is called a **rectocele.**

Vaginal vault prolapse or inversion of the vagina may be seen after vaginal or abdominal hysterectomy and represents failure of the supports around the upper vagina.

Box 24-1. Types of pelvic organ prolapse

ANTERIOR VAGINAL PROLAPSE
Cystourethrocele
Cystocele

APICAL VAGINAL PROLAPSE
Uterovaginal
Vaginal vault (posthysterectomy)

POSTERIOR VAGINAL PROLAPSE
Enterocele
Rectocele

ETIOLOGY OF PROLAPSE

The pelvic fascia, ligaments, and muscles may become attenuated from excessive stretching during pregnancy, labor, and difficult vaginal delivery, especially with forceps or vacuum extraction. Asian and black women are less likely than white women to develop prolapse.

Increased intraabdominal pressure resulting from a chronic cough, ascites, repeated lifting of heavy weights, or habitual straining as a result of constipation may predispose to prolapse. Atrophy of the supporting tissues with aging, especially after menopause, also plays an important part in the initiation or worsening of pelvic relaxation.

Iatrogenic factors include failure to adequately correct all pelvic support defects at the time of surgery.

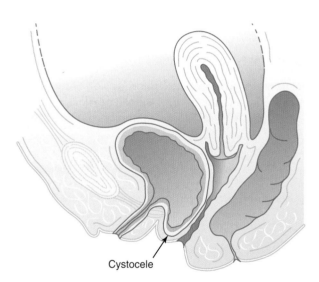

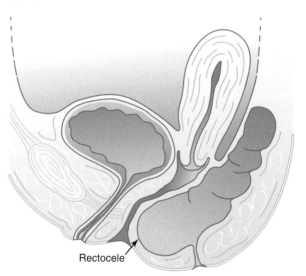

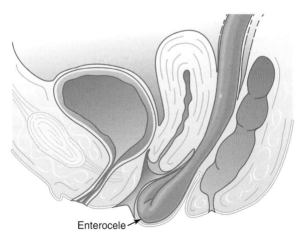

Figure 24-1. Diagrammatic representation of the various types of vaginal prolapse.

SYMPTOMS

Often there is a feeling of heaviness or fullness in the pelvis. Patients may describe "something falling out" or a bearing-down discomfort and backache. **The characteristic of nearly all symptoms is that they are worse after prolonged standing, worse late in the day, and immediately and completely relieved by lying down.**

Neglected cases of procidentia (uterine prolapse through the vaginal introitus) may be complicated by excessive purulent discharge, decubitus ulceration, bleeding, and, rarely, carcinoma of the cervix.

Symptoms of urinary frequency and urgency, urinary incontinence, and occasionally, urinary retention may be seen in patients with anterior vaginal wall prolapse. Patients with a rectocele may have difficulty emptying the rectum and complain of constipation and the need to splint.

DIAGNOSIS

Vaginal examination should be performed by using a single-blade speculum. While depressing the posterior vaginal wall, the patient is asked to strain down. This demonstrates the descent of the anterior vaginal wall consistent with cystocele and urethral displacement. Similarly, retraction of the anterior vaginal wall during straining demonstrates an enterocele and rectocele. **Rectal examination is often useful to demonstrate a rectocele and to distinguish it from an enterocele.** The clinical grading of pelvic organ prolapse is shown in Table 24-1.

MANAGEMENT

Prophylactic measures include diagnosis and treatment of chronic respiratory and metabolic disorders, correction of constipation and intraabdominal disorders that may cause chronic increases in intraabdominal pressure, and administration of estrogen to menopausal women. **Failure to recognize and treat significant support defects at the time of concomitant gynecologic surgery may lead to progression of prolapse** and associated conditions, including urinary incontinence or retention and urinary tract infections (UTIs).

Nonsurgical Treatment

When only a mild degree of pelvic relaxation is present, perineal exercises may improve the tone of the pelvic floor musculature. Pessaries (Figure 24-2) may be used to correct prolapse in the following situations: (1) if the patient is medically unfit for surgery, (2) during pregnancy and the postpartum period, and (3) to promote healing of a decubitus ulcer before surgery.

Pessaries may cause vaginal irritation and ulceration. Periodically (e.g., every 6 to 12 weeks) vaginal pessaries should be removed, cleaned, and reinserted. Failure to do so may result in serious consequences, including fistula formation, impaction, bleeding, and infection.

Surgical Treatment

The main objectives of surgery are to relieve symptoms, restore normal anatomic relationships, restore normal visceral function, allow satisfactory coital function, and attain a durable result.

Anterior colporrhaphy corrects cystocele and urethral displacement. It involves plication of the pubocervical fascia to support the bladder and urethra. **Posterior colporrhaphy corrects a rectocele. Perineorrhaphy repairs** a deficient perineal body.

Repair of an enterocele. The repair of an enterocele follows the general principles of hernia repair. The contents are reduced, the neck of the peritoneal sac is ligated, and the defect is repaired by approximating the uterosacral ligaments and levator ani muscles.

Manchester operation. This operation combines anterior colporrhaphy, amputation of the elongated cervix, posterior colpoperineorrhaphy, and suturing of the cardinal ligaments in front of the cervical stump to antevert the uterus.

Table 24-1. Clinical grading of pelvic organ prolapse	
Grade	Description
0	No descent
1	Descent between normal position and ischial spines
2	Descent between ischial spines and hymen
3	Descent within hymen
4	Descent through hymen

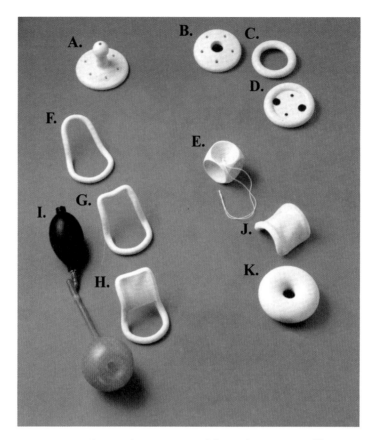

Figure 24-2. Some types of vaginal pessaries used for prolapse. (A) Gellhorn, (B) Shaatz, (C) Ring, (D) ring with support, (E) Cube, (F) Smith, (G) Hodge, (H) Hodge with support for cystocele, (I) Inflatoball, (J) Gehrung, and (K) Donut.

Vaginal hysterectomy. This may be performed alone or in conjunction with anterior and posterior colporrhaphy.

LeFort's partial colpocleisis involves suturing the partially denuded anterior and posterior vaginal walls together in such a way that the uterus is supported above the partially occluded vagina.

Complete colpocleisis involves total obliteration of the vagina.

Vaginal vault suspension (colpopexy) can be accomplished vaginally or abdominally by suspending the vaginal vault to the sacrum or sacrospinous ligaments, or the uterosacral ligaments.

Paravaginal repair. Abdominal or vaginal paravaginal repairs are performed primarily for the correction of cystourethrocele, with or without associated stress urinary incontinence (SUI). Following exposure of the retropubic space, interrupted permanent sutures are used to reattach bilaterally the anterior superior vaginal sulci to the arcus tendineus fasciae pelvis ("white line") extending from the ischial spine to the lower edge of the pubic ramus. In the presence of SUI, additional measures should be taken to achieve suspension of the bladder neck and proximal urethra.

URINARY INCONTINENCE

Urinary incontinence is defined as the involuntary loss of urine that is objectively demonstrable and is a social or hygienic problem. Urinary incontinence has been reported to affect 10% to 25% of women younger than 65 years, 15% to 30% of non-institutionalized women older than 65 years, and more than 50% of nursing home residents. **Recent estimates suggest the direct financial costs of urinary incontinence in the United States are between $10 and $15 billion per year.**

ANATOMY AND PHYSIOLOGY OF THE LOWER URINARY TRACT

In the adult female, the urethra is a muscular tube, 3 to 4 cm in length, lined proximally with transitional epithelium and distally with stratified squamous epithelium. It is surrounded mainly by smooth muscle. **The striated muscular urethral sphincter, which surrounds the distal two-thirds of the urethra, contributes about 50% of the total urethral resistance and serves as a secondary defense against incontinence.** It is also responsible for the interruption of urinary flow at the end of micturition.

The two posterior pubourethral ligaments provide a strong suspensory mechanism for the urethra and serve to hold it forward and in close proximity to the pubis under conditions of stress. They extend from the lower part of the pubic bone to the urethra at the junction of its middle and distal third.

INNERVATION

The lower urinary tract is under the control of both parasympathetic and sympathetic nerves. **The parasympathetic fibers originate in the sacral spinal cord segments S2 through S4.** Stimulation of the pelvic parasympathetic nerves and administration of cholinergic drugs cause the detrusor muscle to contract. Anticholinergic drugs reduce the vesicle pressure and increase the bladder capacity.

The sympathetic fibers originate from thoracolumbar segments (T10 through L2) of the spinal cord. The sympathetic system has α- and β-adrenergic components. The β fibers terminate primarily in the detrusor muscle, whereas the α fibers terminate primarily in the urethra. α-Adrenergic stimulation contracts the bladder neck and urethra and relaxes the detrusor. β-Adrenergic stimulation relaxes the urethra and detrusor muscle. **The pudendal nerve (S2 through S4) provides motor innervation to the striated urethral sphincter.**

FACTORS INFLUENCING BLADDER BEHAVIOR
Sensory Innervation

Afferent impulses from the bladder, trigone, and proximal urethra pass to S2 through S4 levels of the spinal cord by means of the pelvic hypogastric nerves. The sensitivity of these nerve endings may be enhanced by acute infection, interstitial cystitis, radiation cystitis, and increased intravesical pressure. The last may occur in the standing or bending-forward position or in association with obesity, pregnancy, or pelvic tumors.

Inhibitory impulses, probably relayed by the pudendal nerve, also pass to S2 through S4 following mechanical stimulation of the perineum and anal canal. Their passage may explain why pain in this region can cause urinary retention.

Central Nervous System

In infancy, the storage and expulsion of urine is automatic and controlled at the level of the sacral reflex arc. Later, connections to the higher centers become established, and by training and conditioning, this spinal reflex becomes socially influenced so that voiding can be voluntarily accomplished. Although organic neurologic diseases may interrupt the influence of the higher centers on the spinal reflex arc, micturition patterns may also be profoundly altered by mental, environmental, and sociologic disturbances.

CONTINENCE CONTROL

The normal bladder holds urine because the intraurethral pressure exceeds the intravesical pressure. The pubourethral ligaments and surrounding fascia support the urethra so that abrupt increases in intraabdominal pressure are transmitted equally to the bladder and proximal third of the urethra, thus maintaining a pressure gradient between the two. In addition, a reflex contraction of the levator ani compresses the mid-urethra.

STRESS URINARY INCONTINENCE

SUI is the involuntary loss of urine through an intact urethra, secondary to a sudden increase in intraabdominal pressure and in the absence of a bladder contraction.

Grade I: Incontinence only with severe stress, such as coughing, sneezing, or jogging.

Grade II: Incontinence with moderate stress, such as rapid movement or walking up and down stairs.

Grade III: Incontinence with mild stress, such as standing. The patient is continent in the supine position.

ETIOLOGY

Pregnancy, labor, and delivery may damage the normal supports of the bladder neck and proximal urethra. In addition, continence deteriorates with increasing age and onset of menopause. **The most commonly accepted theory for the pathogenesis of SUI is that the bladder neck/proximal urethra drops below the pelvic floor because of pelvic relaxation defects.** Therefore, the increase in intraabdominal pressure induced by coughing is not transmitted equally to the bladder and proximal urethra. The urethral resistance is overcome by the increased bladder pressure, and leakage of urine results.

PELVIC EXAMINATION

Inspection of the vaginal walls should be performed with a single-blade speculum, which allows optimal visualization of the anterior vaginal wall and urethrovesical junction. Scarring, tenderness, and rigidity of the urethra from previous vaginal surgeries or pelvic trauma may be reflected by a scarred anterior vaginal wall. Because the distal urethra is estrogen-dependent, the patient with atrophic vaginitis also has atrophic urethritis.

DIAGNOSTIC TESTS
Stress Test

The patient is examined with a full bladder in the lithotomy position. While the physician observes the urethral meatus, the patient is asked to cough. SUI is suggested if short spurts of urine escape simultaneously with each cough. A delayed leakage, or loss of large volumes of urine, suggests uninhibited bladder contractions. If loss of urine is not demonstrated in the lithotomy position, the test should be repeated with the patient in a standing position.

The Q-Tip (Cotton Swab) Test

This test determines the mobility and descent of the urethrovesical junction on straining. With the patient in the lithotomy position, the examiner inserts a lubricated Q-tip into the urethra to the level of the urethrovesical junction and measures the angle between the Q-tip and the horizontal. The patient then strains maximally, which produces descent of the urethrovesical junction. Along with the descent, the Q-tip moves, producing a new angle with the horizontal. **The normal change in angle is up to 30 degrees. In patients with pelvic relaxation and SUI, the change in Q-tip angle is in the range of 50 to 60 degrees or more (Figure 24-3).**

Urethrocystoscopy

Urethrocystoscopy allows the physician to examine inside the urethra, urethrovesical junction, bladder walls, and ureteral orifices. Urethroscopy is useful to detect bladder stones, tumors, diverticula, or sutures from prior surgeries.

Cystometrogram

Cystometry consists of distending the bladder with known volumes of water or carbon dioxide and observing pressure changes in the bladder function during filling (Figure 24-4). **The most important observation is the presence of a detrusor reflex and the patient's ability to control or inhibit this reflex.**

The first sensation of bladder filling should occur at volumes of 150 to 200 mL. The critical volume (400 to 500 mL) is the capacity that the bladder musculature tolerates before the patient experiences a strong desire to urinate. At this point, if the patient is asked to void, a terminal contraction may appear and is seen as a sudden rise in intravesical pressure. At the peak of the contraction, the patient is instructed to inhibit this reflex (indicated by *arrows* in Figures 24-4A and B). A normal person should be able to inhibit this detrusor reflex and thereby bring down intravesical pressure (see Figure 24-4A). In a urologically or neurologically abnormal patient, the detrusor reflex may appear without the specific instruction to void, and the patient cannot inhibit it (see Figure 24-4B); this observation is referred to as an **uninhibited detrusor contraction.** Other terms for this disorder include overactive bladder, detrusor dyssynergia, detrusor hyperreflexia, irritable bladder, hypertonic bladder, unstable bladder, and uninhibited neurogenic bladder.

These cystometric procedures allow differentiation between patients who are incontinent as a result of uninhibited detrusor contraction and those who have SUI. Conversely, the hypotonic bladder accommodates excessive amounts of gas or water with little increase in intravesical pressure, and the terminal detrusor contraction is absent when the patient is asked to void (see Figure 24-4C).

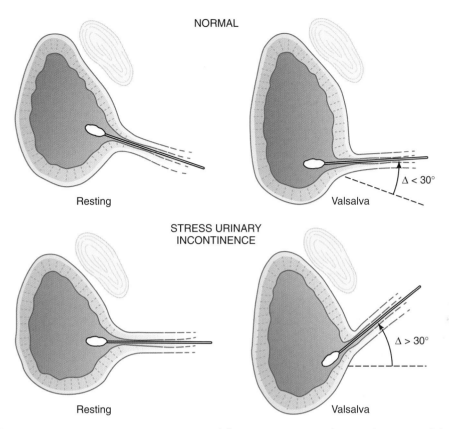

Figure 24-3. Diagrammatic representation of the Q-tip (cotton swab) test, showing mobility of the urethrovesical junction in a continent patient and a patient with SUI.

Urethral Pressure Measurements

A low urethral pressure may be found in patients with SUI, whereas an abnormally high urethral closing pressure may be associated with voiding difficulties, hesitancy, and urinary retention.

The urethral closing pressure profile (UCPP) is a graphic record of pressure along the length of the urethra. The urethral closing pressure normally varies between 50 and 100 cm H_2O. A Valsalva maneuver and/or abdominal leak point pressure of less than 60 cm H_2O or urethral closure pressure of <20 cm H_2O are suggestive of the diagnosis of **intrinsic sphincteric deficiency (ISD).**

Uroflowmetry

Uroflowmetry records rates of urine flow through the urethra when the patient is asked to void spontaneously.

Voiding Cystourethrogram

In this radiologic investigation, fluoroscopy is used to observe bladder filling, the mobility of the urethra and bladder base, and the anatomic changes during voiding. The procedure provides valuable information regarding bladder size and the competence of the bladder neck during coughing. It may detect any bladder trabeculation, vesicoureteral reflux during voiding, funneling of the bladder neck, bladder, and urethral diverticula, and outflow obstruction.

Ultrasonography

Employing real-time or sector ultrasonography, information can be obtained about the inclination of the urethra, flatness of the bladder base, and mobility and funneling of the urethrovesical junction, both at rest and with a Valsalva maneuver. In addition, bladder or urethral diverticula may be identified.

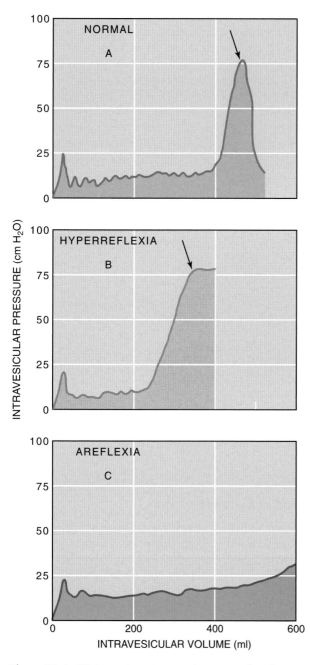

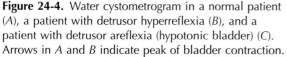

Figure 24-4. Water cystometrogram in a normal patient (*A*), a patient with detrusor hyperreflexia (*B*), and a patient with detrusor areflexia (hypotonic bladder) (*C*). Arrows in *A* and *B* indicate peak of bladder contraction.

Video-urodynamics incorporate fluoroscopy with concurrent measurement of bladder and urethral pressures. **Magnetic resonance imaging (MRI)** studies are being increasingly employed to study pelvic floor and relaxation defects in incontinent patients.

SUMMARY

For about 90% of patients with SUI, a good history and physical examination, uroflowmetry, cystourethroscopy, the Q-tip test, the stress test, and the cystometrogram are adequate investigations. Additional urodynamic, electromyographic, electrophysiologic, and radiologic studies may be necessary in patients with a history of multiple previous surgeries for urinary incontinence and for patients with associated neurologic disease.

TREATMENT
Medical Therapy

In postmenopausal incontinent women, **estrogens improve urethral closing pressure, vaginal epithelial thickness and vascularity, and possible reflex urethral functions.** α-Adrenergic stimulants, such as phenylpropanolamine or pseudoephedrine, may enhance urethral closure and improve continence. Early trials of Duloxetine have been encouraging for treatment of SUI.

Physical Therapy

Pelvic floor exercises (Kegel exercises) are known to improve or cure mild forms of stress incontinence. Kegel exercises require diligence and willingness to practice at home and at work. Many women find them difficult, fatiguing, or time-consuming. Kegel exercises before and after delivery may help patients with postpartum urinary incontinence.

Intravaginal Devices

Large pelvic diaphragms, tampons, weighted vaginal cones, and various types of vaginal pessaries have been used to elevate and support the bladder neck and urethra. **The pessary may provide an acceptable alternative for patients unfit for surgery. A bladder neck prosthesis (Introl), adhesive patch (Miniguard), urethral cup (FEM-ASSIST), and urethral catheter (Reliance)** have been marketed with suboptimal outcomes.

Surgical Therapy

Surgery is the most commonly employed treatment of SUI. The aim of all surgical procedures is to correct the pelvic relaxation defect and to stabilize and restore the normal intraabdominal position of the bladder neck and proximal urethra. The approach may be vaginal, abdominal, or combined abdominovaginal.

Vaginal approach. Anterior vaginal repair (Kelly's plication) is an excellent procedure for correction of cystocele but less effective for correction of stress incontinence. In patients with large cystoceles, over-correction of the cystocele may result in postoperative stress incontinence in a previously continent patient. Such patients may require prophylactic urethral plication or retropubic urethropexy in addition to anterior colporrhaphy.

Abdominal retropubic urethropexy has a long-term success rate of 85% to 95%. **The retropubic urethropexy is performed extraperitoneally (in the space of Retzius) by placing sutures in the fascia lateral to and on each side of the bladder neck and proximal urethra and elevating the vesicourethral junction by attaching the sutures to the symphysis pubis (Marshall-Marchetti-Krantz procedure) or to Cooper's ligament (Burch procedure).**

Though recent popularity of operative laparoscopy for various gynecologic procedures has stimulated use of the **laparoscope for bladder neck suspension procedures,** their **long-term success rates have been disappointing.**

Postoperatively, a transurethral or suprapubic catheter is left in the bladder for continuous bladder drainage for 48 to 72 hours before instituting spontaneous voiding. Some patients (20% to 30%) may need prolonged postoperative bladder drainage (more than 7 days). An occasional patient may develop osteitis pubis after the Marshall-Marchetti-Krantz procedure.

Needle suspension procedures such as the Pereyra, the Raz, and the Stamey have fallen into disfavor as their long-term success rates have been less than 50%.

Recently, the tension-free vaginal tape (TVT) has been gaining wide acceptance as a minimally invasive procedure for treatment of SUI. The TVT type procedures utilize a synthetic prolene mesh placed at the level of the mid-urethra through small vaginal or abdominal incisions.

SPECIAL PROCEDURES

Conventional incontinence surgical procedures sometimes fail in patients with the diagnosis of intrinsic urethral sphincter dysfunction. These patients may be treated by use of a suburethral **sling procedure, periurethral bulking injections (with GAX-collagen or Teflon paste) to improve urethral coaptation, or placement of an artificial urinary sphincter.** The best approach for intrinsic urethral sphincter dysfunction with hypermobility is the suburethral sling procedure; for intrinsic urethral sphincter dysfunction without hypermobility, use of injections or an artificial sphincter is recommended. These operations may be associated with a high risk of postoperative complications, especially urinary retention, voiding dysfunction, and mechanical failure.

Suburethral slings may be performed using autologous material, such as fascia lata or rectus fascia, a dermal graft, or synthetic materials. However, synthetic materials are more prone to infection or rejection. **Cure rates for suburethral sling procedures are reported to be 70% to 95%.**

Because of the significant risk of urinary retention necessitating prolonged catheter use, women who are unwilling or unable to perform intermittent self-catheterization may not be good candidates for a sling procedure.

Periurethral injections of GAX-collagen are a reasonable alternative to a suburethral sling procedure in women with a well-supported but poorly functioning intrinsic urethra, with short-term cure rates approaching 70%.

The critical operation for SUI is the first one performed, and the cure rate declines more or less proportionately to the number of subsequent operations performed. Every effort should be made to use all necessary resources for a proper preoperative evaluation before embarking on any kind of surgical procedure for incontinence.

TOTAL INCONTINENCE—URINARY FISTULA

Pelvic surgery, irradiation, or both now account for 95% of the vesicovaginal fistulas in the United States. More than 50% occur following simple abdominal or vaginal hysterectomy. Obstetric injuries, once the leading cause of urinary fistulas, have almost disappeared in developed countries. They usually result from operative deliveries (e.g., forceps) rather than from neglected labor and pressure necrosis. Approximately 1% to 2% of radical hysterectomies are followed in 10 to 21 days by a urinary fistula, usually ureterovaginal. These fistulas are usually due to devascularization of the ureter rather than direct injury.

Urethrovaginal fistulas generally occur as complications of surgery for urethral diverticula, anterior vaginal wall prolapse, or SUI.

DIAGNOSIS OF FISTULAS

The usual history of painless and continuous vaginal leakage of urine soon after pelvic surgery is strongly suggestive of this problem. **Instillation of methylene blue dye into the bladder will discolor a vaginal pack if a vesicovaginal fistula is present. Intravenous indigo-carmine is excreted in the urine and will discolor a vaginal pack in the presence of a vesicovaginal or ureterovaginal fistula.** In addition, cystourethroscopy should be performed to determine the site and number of fistulas. The majority of posthysterectomy vesicovaginal fistulas are located just anterior to the vaginal vault. **An intravenous pyelogram and/or retrograde pyelogram should be undertaken to localize a ureterovaginal fistula.**

FISTULA REPAIR

Most of the obstetric fistulas can be repaired immediately on detection. For postsurgical fistulas, it is usual to wait some weeks to allow the inflammation to settle and the tissues to attain good vascularity and pliability. During this waiting period, UTI should be treated and estrogen therapy instituted in postmenopausal women. **Steroids have been advocated to hasten resolution of inflammatory changes and allow early surgical intervention. Their use in this circumstance is controversial.**

Vesicovaginal Fistula

The vaginal approach (**Latzko's operation**) is the procedure of choice. **A bulbocavernosus muscle flap or fat pad (Martius graft) may be interposed between the bladder and vagina to provide support, vascularity, and strength to the suture line, especially in patients who have had multiple previous attempted repairs and in those with a postradiation fistula.** Large radiation-induced fistulas may necessitate urinary conduit for urinary diversion.

Ureterovaginal Fistula

Treatment of a ureterovaginal fistula depends on its size and location. **Small fistulas usually close spontaneously after placement of a ureteric stent (double J), provided the tissues have not been irradiated.**

If the fistula is close to the ureterovesical junction, the ureter proximal to the fistula can be reimplanted into the bladder (**ureteroneocystostomy**). If the fistula is several centimeters from the bladder, a **Boari flap** may be useful, a **segment of ileum may be interposed** between the proximal ureter and the bladder, or rarely a **transureteroneoureterostomy,** may be employed.

URGE INCONTINENCE

Urge incontinence is characterized by the presence of involuntary and uninhibited detrusor contractions of 15 cm H_2O or more during cystometric evaluation.

The incidence of bladder instability in the general population varies from 10% to 15%. **In most patients, the exact etiology of bladder instability remains unknown.** Clinical symptoms may include urinary urgency, frequency, urge incontinence, and nocturia.

TREATMENT

In treating urge incontinence, it is important to exclude significant outflow obstruction to avoid precipitating acute urinary retention.

Pharmacologic Treatment

It is reasonable to try several drugs, increasing the dose up to the maximum tolerated, until the most effective drug for a particular patient is found.

Anticholinergic drugs. These are the most frequently employed agents. **Propantheline (Pro-Banthine),** 15 to 30 mg three times daily, and **oxybutynin chloride (Ditropan),** 5 mg three times daily. Ditropan XL and tolterodine (Detrol LA), both single-dose, slow-release medications, act by inhibiting the cholinergically innervated detrusor muscle.

β-Sympathomimetic agonists. The detrusor-relaxing action of β-adrenergic receptors forms the basis for the use of drugs like **metaproterenol (Alupent),** 20 mg twice daily. They enhance the effect of propantheline.

Musculotropic drugs. Flavoxate (Urispas), 200 mg three times daily, acts by causing direct relaxation of the detrusor muscle. **Diazepam (Valium)** acts by a combination of direct smooth muscle relaxation, anticholinergic effect, and central nervous system sedation.

Tricyclic antidepressants. Imipramine (Tofranil), 25 to 50 mg two to three times a day, relaxes the detrusor muscle by virtue of its anticholinergic action, and it helps to enhance continence by its α-adrenergic stimulation of the urethra, so it is very useful in patients with mixed incontinence.

Dopamine agonists. Bromocriptine (5 mg three times daily) has been shown to be beneficial in detrusor instability, probably as a result of both central and peripheral actions.

Bladder Training

Bladder training represents a behavioral modification designed to repeat the process of toilet training. The essential aim is to increase bladder capacity day by day and to prolong the intervals between voiding. Supportive treatment may be provided by the use of various pharmacologic agents.

Functional Electrical Stimulation

Functional electrical stimulation offers an alternative for treating stress or urge incontinence. A vaginal or rectal probe is inserted, usually twice daily for 15 to 30 minutes, to provide electrical stimulation to the pelvic muscles or to the nerves to these structures. Stimulation of the afferent fibers of the pudendal nerve can produce contractions of the pelvic floor and periurethral skeletal muscles, which augment their tone in women with stress incontinence.

Additionally, stimulation inhibits involuntary detrusor contractions. **These devices may be efficacious in women when more traditional treatment approaches have failed.**

OVERFLOW INCONTINENCE

Urinary retention and overflow incontinence may result from detrusor areflexia or a hypotonic bladder, as is seen with lower motor neuron disease, spinal cord injuries, or autonomic neuropathy (diabetes mellitus). These patients are best managed by intermittent self-catheterization.

Overflow incontinence may also occur when there is an outflow obstruction. Straining to void,

poor stream, retention of urine, and incomplete emptying may indicate an obstructive disorder. Overdistention of the bladder because of unrecognized urinary retention may occur in the postoperative period. This is a temporary problem related to postoperative pain and may be managed by continuous bladder drainage for 24 to 48 hours.

URETHRAL SYNDROME

The urethral syndrome occurs in a patient with various lower urinary tract symptoms, in the absence of obvious bladder or urethral abnormality, and with no evidence of UTI. **Any combination of symptoms may be present, the most common being urinary frequency, urgency, dysuria, postvoid fullness, incontinence, and dyspareunia.** The true incidence is unknown, although it is estimated to occur in up to 20% to 30% of all adult females.

Possible causes include psychogenic factors, atrophic urethritis in postmenopausal patients, bacterial infection, nonbacterial infection with *Chlamydia* and *Mycoplasma* organisms, urethral stenosis and spasm, allergy, neurogenic factors, and trauma during sexual intercourse.

Diagnosis is based on a detailed history and physical examination, negative urine cultures, dynamic cystourethroscopy, and urodynamic studies.

TREATMENT

Application of vaginal estrogen cream is effective in patients with atrophic urethritis. Some patients may improve with use of tetracycline for 10 to 14 days. Internal urethrotomy and urethrolysis have also been employed with variable success.

URINARY TRACT INFECTION

UTI is one of the most frequently diagnosed infectious diseases in medical practice. More than 5 to 7 million episodes of UTI are estimated to occur in the US with an annual cost in excess of $1 billion.

Approximately 20% to 30% of women will have at least one UTI during their lifetime, 20% of whom will develop recurrent infections. Ninety-five percent of UTIs are symptomatic, and three-quarters of these symptomatic episodes show positive urine cultures. Almost all asymptomatic patients have negative cultures.

TERMINOLOGY

The terminology surrounding UTIs is rather complex and requires some definition.

Bacteriuria means the presence of bacteria in the urine.

Significant bacteriuria is generally accepted as a bacterial colony count of 10^5 or more per milliliter of urine in a properly collected "clean catch" specimen in an asymptomatic patient. Lower colony counts may be accepted in symptomatic patients.

Asymptomatic bacteriuria is significant bacteriuria with or without pyuria in a patient without symptoms of UTI.

Pyelonephritis is a bacterial infection of the renal parenchyma and the renal pelvicaliceal system. Acute pyelonephritis is commonly associated with chills and fever, flank pain, costovertebral tenderness, urinary frequency, urgency, and dysuria. Chronic pyelonephritis denotes histologic changes of patchy interstitial nephritis, destruction of tubules, cellular infiltration, and inflammatory changes in the renal parenchyma.

Chronic pyelonephritis is not synonymous with chronic UTI, which means only prolonged presence of bacteria.

Cystitis is an inflammation of the urinary bladder. Patients with cystitis usually have symptoms of lower urinary tract irritation, such as dysuria (burning on urination), urgency, frequency with small amounts of voided urine, nocturia, suprapubic discomfort, and, at times, urinary incontinence and hematuria.

Persistence of bacteriuria is the presence of microorganisms that were isolated at the start of treatment and continue to be isolated while the patient is receiving therapy. Persistence may be caused by several factors, including the presence of resistant organisms, inadequate drug therapy, and poor patient compliance.

Superinfection is the appearance of a different organism while a patient is still receiving therapy. The new organism may be a different strain or a different serologic type.

Relapse occurs with the recurrence of significant bacteriuria with the same species and serologic strain of organism. Relapse usually appears within 2 to 3 weeks of completion of therapy and most likely represents perineal colonization by the infecting organism.

Reinfection is an infection occurring after cessation of therapy with a different strain of microorganism or a different serologic type of the original infecting strain. Typically, reinfection occurs 2 to 12 weeks after a previous episode of infection and indicates recurrent bladder bacteriuria.

Recurrent UTI is diagnosed with two UTIs within 6 months or 3 or more during 1 year in which the initial episode is resolved and subsequently followed by another UTI. Women of blood group B or AB have an increased risk of recurrent UTIs.

INCIDENCE AND PREVALENCE

After the age of 1 year and throughout adulthood, females are affected more frequently than males (10:1 ratio). Asymptomatic bacteriuria increases from an incidence in preschool children of 1% to 5% to a peak of about 10% in postmenopausal women. Urologic abnormalities are found in up to 70% of children with a UTI.

PATHOGENESIS

Bacteria may gain entry to the urinary tract by three pathways: the ascending route, the descending or hematogenous route, and the lymphatic route.

Ascending Infection

The female is more susceptible because of the short length of the urethra, urethral contamination by rectal pathogens, introital and vestibular colonization by pathogenic bacteria, and decreased urethral resistance after menopause. Sexual intercourse is a major source of bacteriuria within 24 hours, and the relative risk is proportional to the frequency of intercourse in the past 7 days (honeymoon cystitis). Additional sources of infection include diaphragm use, vulvovaginitis, urethral diverticula, poor hygiene, and indiscriminate urethral catheterization. Infrequent and incomplete voiding resulting in large bladder volumes increases the susceptibility to chronic urinary infection.

Hematogenous Infection

Urinary infection via the hematogenous route is very uncommon, but it is seen occasionally in elderly, debilitated, or immunosuppressed patients with overwhelming infections in whom kidney infection is only part of the multisystemic involvement. Renal tuberculosis is almost always acquired via the hematogenous route.

Lymphatic Infection

Experimental evidence suggests that bacterial infection spreads along lymphatic channels that connect the bowel and the urinary tract.

HOST DEFENSE MECHANISMS

Entrance of bacteria into the urinary tract does not necessarily result in infection. Natural barriers for invasion, such as the "washout" effect of normal periodic voiding, the antiseptic properties of the bladder tissues, and the high concentration of organic acids in normal urine, prevent bacterial invasion. Other factors, such as a pH <5 and urea ammonium and organic acid content of the urine, all affect bacterial growth. If invasion takes place, the bacteria may remain in the bladder or may ascend to the kidney. **Transient vesicoureteral reflux seen in association with severe lower UTIs may allow the infected urine to reach the kidneys.**

PERPETUATING FACTORS

The following factors encourage and perpetuate UTIs:
1. **Mechanical urinary obstruction.** Ureteropelvic junction obstruction, ureteral stricture, urethral stenosis, and calculi are common to patients with recurrent or chronic UTIs.
2. **Functional urinary obstruction abnormalities.** Incomplete bladder emptying and vesicoureteric reflux also encourage stasis of urine and bacterial growth. Pregnancy produces transient functional ureteral obstruction both mechanically and hormonally. Hypospadias may result in repeated infections after coitus (honeymoon cystitis).
3. **Systemic factors.** Diabetes mellitus, gout, sickle cell trait, cystic renal disease, and metabolic disorders, such as nephrocalcinosis, chronic potassium deficiency, and renal tubular defects, increase susceptibility to pyelonephritis.

CLINICAL CLASSIFICATION

From the point of view of pathogenesis and management, UTIs in nonpregnant females can be considered to be either uncomplicated or complicated. **Uncomplicated cases account for 95% of UTIs in women and seldom produce renal damage.** They are either the first episode of infection or an episode far removed in time from a previous urinary infection. Ninety percent of first infections are due to *Escherichia coli*. Seventy-five percent of these infective episodes do not recur for several years. **Complicated UTIs occur in patients with neurologic or obstructive abnormalities or in those with underlying parenchymal disease.**

INVESTIGATIONS
Urinalysis

Microscopic examination of an uncentrifuged, unstained specimen (a drop of urine on the slide covered with a coverslip) provides better than 90% accuracy in detecting significant bacteriuria when one or more bacteria are seen per high-power field. A positive Gram stain almost always correlates with a positive quantitative culture. A negative Gram stain virtually eliminates significant bacteriuria.

Pyuria is arbitrarily defined as the presence of five or more white blood cells per high-power field in the centrifuged specimen. The presence of white blood cells (pyuria) and red blood cells along with bacteriuria suggests infection. **Pyuria without significant bacteria may indicate a nonbacterial inflammation or a urinary tract foreign body or tumor. It is a classic finding in urinary tuberculosis. Casts, when present, indicate renal parenchymal disease.**

URINE CULTURE/MICROBIOLOGY

A quantitative urine culture is the most important laboratory test in the diagnosis and management of complicated or uncomplicated UTIs. *Escherichia coli* is the predominant organism in 80% to 85% of patients. The remaining less common organisms are *Klebsiella-Enterobacter*, *Proteus* species, *Enterococcus*, *Staphylococcus*, and group D *Streptococcus*. Anaerobic fecal bacteria do not grow well in urine and are rarely seen in urinary infections. Yeast, such as *Candida albicans* (Funguria), may be seen in patients with diabetes mellitus or in individuals receiving immunosuppressive therapy, especially in the presence of foreign bodies or indwelling catheters.

There are three techniques for urine collection: (1) the midstream "clean-catch" method, (2) urethral catheterization, and (3) suprapubic aspiration. The midstream clean-catch method has an 80% reliability, which increases to 95% if two consecutive specimens show a colony count of 100,000 or more of the same organism. In routine cases of uncomplicated infections, the presence of two or more species of organisms in the same specimen normally suggests contamination. Urethral catheterization provides an optimal urine specimen. A positive culture has a 95% accuracy, and false-positive cultures are rare.

Suprapubic aspiration, although providing the most reliable specimen, is reserved for those in whom contamination is difficult to avoid (e.g., young children and elderly people).

RADIOLOGIC STUDIES

An intravenous pyelogram is critical in the evaluation of patients whose recurrences are due to bacterial persistence (e.g., stones or infected congenital anomalies), but it is of almost no value in the 99% of patients with reinfections. Cystography and voiding urethrocystography may help to detect ureteric reflux, diverticulae, or fistulous tracts in patients with persistent bacteriuria.

ENDOSCOPIC STUDIES

Endoscopic studies such as urethroscopy and cystoscopy may be necessary to detect chronic trigonitis, urethritis, urethral or bladder diverticulae, fistulas, foreign bodies, or bladder wall trabeculation.

RENAL FUNCTION TESTS

Renal function tests are not required in a patient with an initial uncomplicated UTI. **If episodes recur, blood urea nitrogen and serum creatinine levels should be obtained.** If renal insufficiency is present, a creatinine clearance is helpful.

URINARY TRACT INFECTION LOCALIZATION STUDIES

The clinical presentation does not always allow differentiation between renal infections and lower UTIs. The clinical usefulness of localization lies in planning patient management, because the presence of renal infection usually necessitates a more vigorous and extended therapeutic approach than does the presence of lower UTI alone.

Indirect methods of localization include (1) **special staining of urinary sediment** to detect polymorphonuclear leukocytes originating in the kidney ("glitter cell" stain), (2) **examination of urinary sediment after intravenous injection of bacterial pyrogens or adrenocorticosteroids,** (3) measurement of the excretion of various **urinary enzymes,** (4) tests of maximal **urinary concentrating ability,** (5) determination of the immunologic response by estimating **serum antibody titers against type-specific organisms** in the urine, and (6) **urine examination for bacteria that are antibody-coated.** The latter test is based on the observation that unlike bladder bacteriuria, renal infection produces a systemic antibody response.

Direct methods of localization, although invasive, are more accurate and include (1) selective ureteral catheterization via cystoscopy, (2) the bladder washout technique, and (3) examination of renal tissue for bacteria or bacterial antigen by the fluorescent antibody technique.

MANAGEMENT

Unless physical examination and urinalysis (bacteriuria) clearly indicate urinary infection, it is advisable to withhold definite antimicrobial therapy until culture and sensitivity reports are available. **As a general rule, bacteriuria should be treated, and not pyuria.** General measures in the management of UTIs involve the following:

1. **Rest and hydration.** Hydration promotes dilution of bacterial counts, frequent bladder emptying, and reduction of medullary osmolality, which assists phagocytosis.
2. **Acidification of the urine.** Ascorbic acid (500 mg twice daily), ammonium chloride (12 g/day in divided doses), or apricot, plum, prune, or cranberry juices have been employed to increase the antibacterial activity of urine and to inhibit bacterial multiplication. Grapefruit juice and carbonated drinks, particularly those containing citrates, turn the urine alkaline and should be avoided.
3. **Urinary analgesics.** Agents such as phenazopyridine hydrochloride (Pyridium), 100 mg twice daily for 2 to 3 days, are often helpful in relieving dysuria.

Basic Principles of Antimicrobial Therapy

The drug selected should be readily available, of low cost, rapidly absorbed from the upper gastrointestinal tract with minimal irritation, and selectively excreted in the urinary tract. **A high serum level of antibiotics is undesirable in the treatment of acute** cystitis because it tends to alter normal bacterial flora (Table 24-2). Nitrofurantoin (Macrodantin) produces low serum levels with a half-life of only 19 minutes, thereby minimizing the chances of alteration of intestinal and vaginal bacterial flora. Treatment with nitrofurantoin is effective against all uropathogens except Proteus species.

Single-dose therapy is an effective alternative to a 3- to 7-day course, especially in patients with acute cystitis (Table 24-3). Single-dose therapy fails in more than 50% of patients with an upper tract infection; however, as many as 40% of women with only lower tract symptoms also have upper tract infections.

For pyelonephritis, an antibiotic should be selected that will attain a significant serum level, because the badly infected renal tissue is poorly perfused. The cephalosporins are more effective and cause fewer side effects and relapses. Cephalosporins (e.g., Keflex, Duricef) are slowly and effectively excreted in urine, thereby reducing the frequency of daily drug administration (500 mg to 1000 mg twice daily).

Antibiotics such as ampicillin, tetracycline, and trimethoprim-sulfamethoxazole (e.g., Septra, Bactrim) alter the intestinal flora, destroy the normal vaginal and periurethral flora, and may result in a relapse of the UTI. Quinolones, both first- and second-generation (e.g., ciprofloxacin, norfloxacin) have been found to be very effective against uropathogens.

The high pH of urine associated with Proteus infection results from the splitting of urea and the subsequent liberation of ammonia. The urine has a characteristic "fishy" smell. If the urine is very alkaline (pH > 8.0), trimethoprim-sulfamethoxazole should be prescribed.

For patients with renal insufficiency, ampicillin, trimethoprim-sulfamethoxazole, and doxycycline have been shown to reach adequate levels in the urine without toxic levels in serum. Nitrofurantoin should be avoided, as high serum levels may lead to peripheral neuropathy. Similarly, tetracycline may lead to severe hepatic damage. **Dosages of aminoglycosides should be adjusted in accordance with creatinine clearance, and the serum levels should be monitored.**

Antimicrobial agents commonly used in the management of UTIs and their relative effectiveness against various organisms are shown in Table 24-4.

Symptoms without bacteriuria. Treatment should be symptomatic, such as increased fluid intake, the administration of phenazopyridine, and warm sitz baths.

Asymptomatic bacteriuria. Although this condition may be ignored in many patients who have no evidence of mechanical obstruction or renal insufficiency, **children and pregnant women should be given aggressive antimicrobial therapy.** As many as 40% of pregnant women with asymptomatic bacteriuria later develop symptomatic UTIs, usually pyelonephritis.

Acute symptomatic infections. Patients with evidence of bacteremia (e.g., shaking chills) or endotoxemia (e.g., hypotension or respiratory alkalosis) should be hospitalized. It is almost always prudent to hospitalize the febrile diabetic. **In the acutely ill patient with suspected bacteremia, aminoglycosides should be employed.** The patient's temperature should be monitored. If the fever persists longer than 72 to 96 hours, a complication of infection, such as perinephric abscess, or of treatment, such as drug fever, should be contemplated and investigated.

Table 24-2. Commonly used drug regimens for oral treatment of bacterial cystitis (3- to 7-day course)		
Drugs	Dosage (mg)	Interval
TMP-SMX	160/800	Every 12 hr
Nitrofurantoin	50–100	Every 6–8 hr
Norfloxacin	400	Every 12 hr
Ciprofloxacin	250	Every 12 hr
Lomefloxacin	400	Once daily
Ofloxacin	200	Every 12 hr
Cefadroxil	500	Every 12 hr
Cefixime	400	Once daily
Amoxicillin	250	Every 8 hr
Ampicillin	250–500	Every 6 hr
Tetracycline	250–500	Every 6 hr

TMP, Trimethoprim; SMX, Sulfamethoxazole.

Table 24-3. Suggested drugs for single-dose therapy	
Drugs	Dosage
TMP	600 mg
TMP-SMX	1.92 g
Norfloxacin	800 mg
Lomefloxacin	400 mg
Ciprofloxacin	500 mg
Fosfomycin-trometamol	3 g

TMP, Trimethoprim; SMX, Sulfamethoxazole.

Table 24-4. Antimicrobial agents used in the management of urinary tract infections and their usual effectiveness against common pathogens

Agent	Serum Levels	Urine Levels	E. coli	Klebsiella	Pseudomonas	Enterococcus	Proteus
Trimethoprim-sulfamethoxazole	±	++	++	++	−	−	++
Nitrofurantoin	−	++	++	±	−	±	−
Ampicillin	+	++	++	−	−	++	++
Cephalothin	++	++	++	++	−	±	++
Tetracycline	±	+	±	±	−	++	−
Kanamycin	++	++	++	++	−	−	++
Gentamicin	++	++	++	++	++	−	++
Carbenicillin	++	++	++	−	++	−	++

++, Good; +, adequate; ±, occasionally effective; −, not effective.

RECURRENT URINARY TRACT INFECTIONS

Patients with recurrent infections demonstrate abnormal vaginal biologic factors. Colonization of vaginal and urethral mucosa usually precedes bacteriuria. Bacterial adherence to squamous cells and lack of vaginal antibody to *E. coli* probably lead to vaginal colonization. Women resistant to *E. coli* carry specific antibodies to their own **E. coli.**

The benefit of long-term administration (6 to 18 months) of antimicrobials in women with recurrent UTIs has been demonstrated. Trimethoprim-sulfamethoxazole has been found to be effective and is the only antibacterial agent known to be excreted in vaginal fluid. Sulfonamides, tetracycline, and ampicillin are not effective prophylactically because of the rapid emergence of resistant fecal strains. Recurrent infections tend to occur in clusters. Prolonged remissions often occur between these clusters, and the timing of the clusters cannot be predicted. **Prophylactic therapy should be initiated when the patient has had two infections within 6 months, because she faces a 65% chance of another infection within the next 6 months.**

For women who are able to relate the frequently recurring infections to sexual activity, a single dose of an antimicrobial drug immediately after coitus has been shown to prevent bacteriuria and symptomatic infection.

Prevention of hospital-acquired UTIs in patients is important.

Sixty percent of hospital-acquired infections in gynecologic patients overall involve the urinary tract,

Box 24-2. Principles for bladder drainage

Avoid nonessential catheterization
Remove catheters promptly
Use correct sterile procedure for catheterization to avoid introducing bacteria
Maintain closed drainage
Disconnect the drainage system only when there is an obstruction
Avoid prophylactic antibiotics
Use suprapubic catheterization for prolonged bladder drainage

particularly in association with catheterization. The principles shown in Box 24-2 should be employed when drainage of the urinary bladder is performed.

Suggested Reading

American College of Obstetricians and Gynecologists: Urinary incontinence. Technical Bulletin No. 213. Washington, DC, ACOG, October 1995.

American College of Obstetricians and Gynecologists: Pelvic organ prolapse. Technical Bulletin No. 214. Washington, DC, ACOG, October 1995.

Bhatia NN, Bradley WE: Neuroanatomy and neurophysiology of the lower urinary tract: Female incontinence. *In* Raz S (ed): Female Urology. Philadelphia, WB Saunders, 1983, pp 12–32.

Ribeiro RM, Rossi P, Guidi HGC, et al: Symposium: Urinary tract infections in women. Int Urogyn J 13:198–203, 2002.

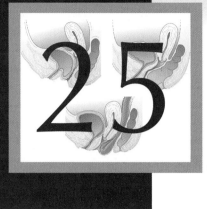

Ectopic Pregnancy

Anita L. Nelson, Catherine Marin DeUgarte, and
Joseph C. Gambone

An ectopic pregnancy is a gestation that implants outside of the endometrial cavity. It represents a serious hazard to a woman's health and her reproductive potential, and it requires prompt recognition and early appropriate intervention. **An ectopic pregnancy is estimated to occur in 1 of every 80 spontaneously conceived pregnancies.** More than 95% of ectopic pregnancies implant in various anatomic segments of the fallopian tube, including the interstitial (2%), isthmic (12%), ampullary (80%), and infundibular and fimbrial portions (6%). Other less common sites of ectopic implantation are the ovary, uterine cervix, or a rudimentary uterine horn. Rarely, an ectopic may be intraligamentous or in the peritoneal cavity. With in vitro fertilization (IVF) and other assisted reproductive technologies (ART), the risk of ectopic pregnancy increases substantially, and the location of those ectopic implantations changes (Figure 25-1).

EPIDEMIOLOGY AND ETIOLOGY

From the early 1970s to the early 1990s, the incidence of ectopic pregnancy in the United States tripled. Currently, this condition causes 6% of maternal deaths in the United States and is the most common cause of maternal mortality in the 1st trimester. Several factors contributed to this increased incidence:

1. Improved technology, which has allowed for earlier and more complete recognition of ectopic pregnancies that would previously have gone undetected.
2. The rising incidence of acute and chronic salpingitis, especially related to *Chlamydia trachomatis*.
3. An increasing number of tubal surgeries, such as tubal ligation and tubal reconstruction,

resulting in histologic and structural damage to the tubes.
4. Increasing use of conservative management of tubal pregnancy, which does not remove damaged tissue.

The key to the successful management of ectopic pregnancy is early diagnosis. Today, fewer women are seen in a state of hemorrhagic shock after tubal rupture. As a result, **mortality from ectopic pregnancies has steadily declined for the past 10 years.** This decrease is evidence that a high index of suspicion and vigorous efforts at early diagnosis are effective. **"Think ectopic!"** is a sign that should be in every emergency room.

The etiology of ectopic pregnancy is not always clear. As many as 50% of cases result from an alteration of tubal transport mechanisms because of damage to the ciliated surface of the endosalpinx caused by infections such as chlamydia and gonorrhea. Other etiologies include delayed fertilization, possible transmigration of the oocyte to the contralateral tube, and slowed tubal transport, which delays passage of the morula to the endometrial cavity. Chromosomal abnormalities of the fetus are not a cause of ectopic pregnancy.

NATURAL HISTORY OF UNTREATED ECTOPIC PREGNANCY

Tubal pregnancies rapidly invade the tubal mucosa, eroding into the tubal vessels, which become enlarged and engorged. The segment of the affected tube distends as the pregnancy grows and as blood from the eroded vessels dissects along the tubal wall. Possible outcomes of such abnormal gestations include the following:

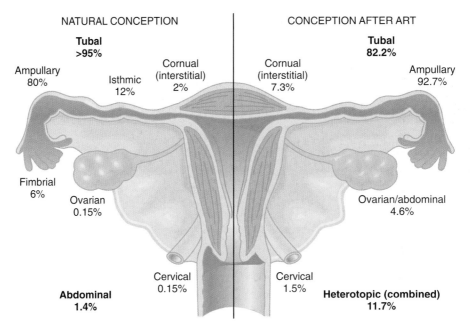

NATURAL CONCEPTION

CONCEPTION AFTER ART

Tubal
>95%

Ampullary
80%

Isthmic
12%

Cornual
(interstitial)
2%

Fimbrial
6%

Ovarian
0.15%

Tubal
82.2%

Cornual
(interstitial)
7.3%

Ampullary
92.7%

Ovarian/abdominal
4.6%

Cervical
0.15%

Cervical
1.5%

Abdominal
1.4%

Heterotopic (combined)
11.7%

Figure 25-1. Possible locations of ectopic pregnancy with spontaneous conception versus pregnancies that result from assisted reproductive technologies (ART) such as in vitro fertilization (IVF). *Modified from Pisarska MD et al: Clin Obstet Gynecol 42:3, 1999.*

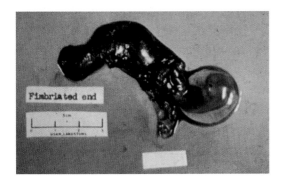

Figure 25-2. Ruptured fallopian tube with aborted ectopic pregnancy.

1. **Tubal rupture,** with resulting intraperitoneal hemorrhage (Figure 25-2).
2. **Pregnancy resorption,** as a result of the restricted blood supply.
3. **Tubal abortion into the peritoneal cavity.**
4. **Abdominal pregnancy,** a rare event in which the pregnancy is expelled from the tube, seeds onto a site in the abdominal cavity (e.g., the omentum, the small or large bowel, or the parietal peritoneum), and continues to grow. The pregnancy is usually not viable.

SYMPTOMS AND CLINICAL DIAGNOSIS

The classic triad of symptoms of ectopic pregnancy consists of amenorrhea, vaginal bleeding, and lower abdominal pain. For any individual woman, there are three possible clinical presentations: (1) acutely ruptured ectopic pregnancy, (2) probable ectopic pregnancy in a symptomatic woman, and (3) possible ectopic pregnancy.

ACUTELY RUPTURED ECTOPIC PREGNANCY

The patient who has experienced rupture of her ectopic pregnancy will most likely have intraperitoneal hemorrhage and will present with severe abdominal pain and dizziness. She may also complain of ipsilateral shoulder pain from phrenic nerve irritation from the blood in her abdomen. There may be signs of hemodynamic instability with tachycardia, diaphoresis, hypotension, and even loss of consciousness. Her entire abdomen may be distended and acutely tender with guarding and rebound tenderness. The patient will usually have cervical motion tenderness and a slightly enlarged, globular uterus. However, she may not have a palpable adnexal mass.

The diagnosis is facilitated by a positive urine pregnancy test, which detects human chorionic gonadotropin (hCG). **This clinical scenario represents a surgical emergency.** Although other tests are often not necessary, an ultrasound would reveal an empty uterus and free fluid (blood) in the peritoneal cavity. It is critical to establish large-bore intravenous lines and to start fluid resuscitation. Transfusion is important but should not delay emergency surgical intervention (usually by laparotomy).

PROBABLE ECTOPIC PREGNANCY

Women who present with lower pelvic pain and vaginal spotting or bleeding, with or without amenorrhea, can be rapidly tested for pregnancy. There are generally other clinical signs present such as tenderness of the abdomen along with adnexal or cervical motion tenderness. **The diagnosis of ectopic pregnancy may be confirmed by the absence of intrauterine pregnancy (IUP) on ultrasound in a woman with a level of hCG sufficient to identify an IUP** (see below and Figure 25-3). In symptomatic women, even though they have reasonably stable vital signs, surgical evaluation and therapy are generally indicated.

POSSIBLE ECTOPIC PREGNANCY

The most common clinical presentation is that of a possible ectopic pregnancy. **Patients with an ectopic pregnancy may be seen several times by a physician before the correct diagnosis is made.** The delayed diagnosis is related to a low index of suspicion by the clinician, often confused by a lack of typical symptoms. An awareness of the risk factors is important for a prompt diagnosis. Known risk factors are summarized in Box 25-1.

Lower abdominal pain is present in most cases. Amenorrhea or a history of an abnormal last menstrual period is obtained in 75% to 90% of ectopic pregnancies. Abnormal vaginal bleeding is seen in over half the patients, ranging from spotting to the equivalent of a normal menstrual period. This spotting or bleeding results from an abnormally low production of hCG by the ectopic trophoblastic tissue.

On physical examination, most patients are afebrile, and less than half have a discernable adnexal mass on pelvic examination. Often, the mass is palpated on the opposite side to the ectopic pregnancy and represents a corpus luteum in the contralateral ovary. The uterus

---

> **Box 25-1. Risk factors for ectopic pregnancy**
>
> 1. History of tubal infection
> 2. Cigarette smokers (increased relative risk (RR) = 1.26)
> 3. Prior ectopic pregnancy (increased RR = 1.15–1.5)
> 4. History of tubal sterilization within the past 1 to 2 years (higher incidence if cauterization was used)
> 5. History of tubal reconstructive surgery
> 6. Pregnancy with current IUD, depot medroxyprogesterone acetate, or emergency contraceptive pill use
> 7. Infertility due to tubal factors
> 8. Use of assisted reproductive technology (ART)

---

is soft and is either of normal size or slightly enlarged. On ultrasound, there is a thickened endometrial stripe, while histologically, there is almost always a localized hyperplasia of the uterine lining (Arias-Stella reaction).

DIAGNOSTIC TESTS

Two pivotal technologies have been introduced over the last three decades, which have revolutionized the diagnosis of early ectopic pregnancy: (1) blood and urine testing for hCG and (2) transvaginal ultrasonography. Older techniques, such as office dilatation and curettage (D&C), can also be utilized.

HUMAN CHORIONIC GONADOTROPIN TESTING

Human chorionic gonadotropin (hCG) is a glycoprotein consisting of two linked subunits, α and β. The α subunit consists of 92 amino acids and is similar in luteinizing hormone (LH), follicle-stimulating hormone (FSH), and thyroid-stimulating hormone (TSH). The β subunit is larger with 145 amino acids, is different for each glycoprotein hormone, and provides for unique biologic activity. Before the development of sensitive and specific assays for the entire hCG molecule, tests for only the β-subunit of hCG were routinely used for assessment in early pregnancy and especially to rule out ectopic pregnancies. This was because of the increased likelihood of "false-positive" results due to the cross-reactivity with other glycoprotein hormones (e.g., LH and FSH), which have similar α-subunits. Although the possibility of false positive results still exists due to circulating factors in the serum that may interact with hCG antibody, the more common laboratory test performed today is for the entire hCG molecule.

There are several different hCG-related moieties that circulate in the serum and concentrate in the urine, such as the biologically active hCG (nonnicked hCG), nicked hCG, free α-hCG, nicked and nonnicked free β-hCG, and β-core fragment. In different clinical situations, the relative concentrations of each of these molecules differ. For example, in early pregnancy, the concentration of biologically active hCG (nonnicked hCG) rises exponentially, but there is greater variability in pregnancies affected by Down syndrome and trophoblastic disease, allowing for some diagnostic suspicion of these conditions based on measured levels.

There are many different assays available today, most of which use at least two separate antibody binding sites to detect the presence or measure the concentration of hCG. **Until there is greater standardization of laboratory testing, it is important to compare over time only titers that are obtained from the same laboratory.** Technically, the **correct test to order today is hCG,** but many institutions use the designation β-hCG to determine serial titers of the pregnancy hormone. It is expected that in the near future, there will be new international standards and more precision in testing for the different components of hCG relevant to different clinical settings. For the remainder of this chapter and for clinical situations involving the assessment of early pregnancies, we will refer to hCG titers to assess normal and ectopic gestations.

The rapidly-dividing fertilized egg begins production of hCG even before pregnancy occurs, but communication with the maternal system starts with implantation. The sensitivity of the current methods for detection of hCG in the maternal serum allows for the confirmation of pregnancy before a missed period. The commercially available urinary hCG home testing kits, based on monoclonal antibodies, are sensitive to 25 mIU/mL and should reliably detect pregnancy by 1 week after a missed menses.

An accurate diagnosis of ectopic pregnancy requires knowledge of the dynamics of hCG. In the 1st trimester of normal pregnancies, serum titers of hCG increase exponentially following a nonlinear model. The doubling time of hCG in the serum varies from 1.2 days shortly after implantation to 3.5 days at 2 months after the last menstrual period. Healthy,

normally developing pregnancies generally can be detected by a normal rate of increase of maternal serum hCG levels. Over 66% of normal pregnancies show doubling of hCG levels every 48 hours in the first several weeks of pregnancy.

The discriminatory zone, or DZ, is defined as the titer of hCG at which an intrauterine sac should reliably be seen with transvaginal ultrasonography in a normal pregnancy (Figure 25-3A). DZ titers differ among institutions, but on average are equal to 1500 to 2000 mIU/mL of hCG (Figure 25-3).

Abnormalities in serial hCG determinations fall into two patterns: (1) titers plateauing or decreasing more slowly than the rates seen after spontaneous abortion or (2) titers that are not rising at a rate appropriate for a healthy intrauterine pregnancy. If the hCG titers in these cases are sufficiently high, ultrasound will provide a more definitive diagnosis. If, however, the hCG levels are increasing abnormally but are too low for ultrasonic detection, the patient can be told that the pregnancy is most likely abnormal and a diagnostic dilatation and curettage (D&C) may be offered. If no products of conception are found on pathologic examination, the diagnosis of ectopic pregnancy can be made and treatment initiated.

Serum progesterone levels greater than 25 ng/mL can very reliably indicate a normal IUP, and levels less than 5 ng/mL are consistent with an abnormal pregnancy. However, the value of progesterone testing for ectopic pregnancy is limited by the fact that it requires almost 24 hours to obtain a result and most of the progesterone levels obtained in this situation fall into the gray zone between 5 and 25 ng/mL.

TRANSVAGINAL ULTRASONOGRAPHY

Ultrasound has become the standard for the nonsurgical diagnosis of ectopic pregnancy, alone or in combination with hCG testing. Transvaginal ultrasonography can detect an intrauterine gestational sac as early as 5 weeks of amenorrhea (about 3 weeks after conception). The coexistence of an IUP and an ectopic pregnancy (heterotopic gestation) occurs only once in 10,000 to 30,000 spontaneous gestations but may occur as frequently as 1 in 100 pregnancies that result from IVF.

The date of conception is often not known, so serum hCG levels are used to determine when transvaginal ultrasonography can be helpful. If the sac

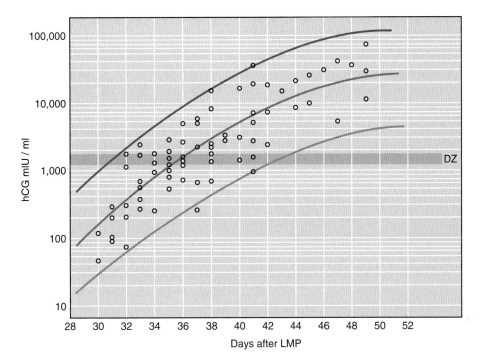

Figure 25-3. Distribution curve of hCG in normal pregnancies with an example of a discriminatory zone (DZ) in shaded area. The range of levels in the DZ (usually 1500–2000 mIU/mL, using the Third International Standard) represents the DZ level above which ultrasound evidence of an intrauterine pregnancy (IUP) should be seen. Each institution should establish this level based on variation in laboratory measurement and the interpretive skill of the ultrasonographer. *Modified from Pittaway DE,Reisch RL, Wentz AC: Doubling times of human chorionic gonadotropin increase in early variable intrauterine pregnancies. Am J Obstet Gynecol 152:299, 1985.*

is not visualized at that discriminatory level of hCG, the likelihood of an ectopic pregnancy is greater than 90%. **Multifetal pregnancies may produce more hCG and not have visible sacs when their collective titers first surpass the DZ.** Special caution is also needed to differentiate on ultrasonographic imaging between a true sac and a pseudosac. A pseudosac is a ring-like structure produced on ultrasound by a prominent decidual echo and not a true ectopic gestation. **The ultrasound can also detect a hemoperitoneum, which may be inferred by the sonographic finding of "free fluid in the cul-de-sac."**

OTHER TESTS

Culdocentesis is a technique by which a needle attached to a syringe is inserted transvaginally through the posterior vaginal fornix into the pouch of Douglas to detect any fluid within the peritoneal cavity. Although the procedure is simple, inexpensive, and rapid, it is quite uncomfortable for the patient and is of limited use in an unruptured ectopic pregnancy. Culdocentesis has been virtually replaced by transvaginal sonography and rapid hCG testing. Because it may be of value in a rare clinical situation in which immediate ultrasonography and hCG testing are not available, a well-trained gynecologist should be able to perform it.

DIFFERENTIAL DIAGNOSIS

Many gynecologic and nongynecologic disorders have symptoms in common with ectopic pregnancy and are listed in Box 25-2.

Box 25-2. Differential diagnosis for ectopic pregnancy

GYNECOLOGIC PROBLEMS
1. Threatened or incomplete abortion
2. Ruptured corpus luteum cyst
3. Acute pelvic inflammatory disease
4. Adnexal torsion
5. Degenerating leiomyoma (especially in pregnancy)

NONGYNECOLOGIC PROBLEMS
1. Acute appendicitis
2. Pyelonephritis
3. Pancreatitis

MANAGEMENT

The management of ectopic pregnancy has changed dramatically in recent years. Internationally, the gold standard is still laparoscopic therapy, because it allows for rapid diagnosis as well as treatment (Figure 25-4). Under certain circumstances, laparotomy may be necessary. When the patient is clinically stable and able to assure compliance with multiple return visits, medical therapy may be an option. The algorithm displayed in Figure 25-5 outlines a reasonable approach to diagnosis and management.

SURGICAL MANAGEMENT

Laparotomy is the preferred surgical approach for women who are hemodynamically unstable because rapid access to the bleeding site is critical. Laparotomy is also appropriate whenever it is anticipated that laparoscopy would not be successful, such as when the patient has significant intraperitoneal adhesions from prior surgeries, infection, or endometriosis. Also, the laparoscopic approach is not appropriate when laparoscopic equipment is not readily available and when there are no surgeons skilled in the procedure.

For hemodynamically stable patients, laparoscopy is the preferred surgical approach because patients require fewer days of postoperative hospitalization, suffer less postoperative pain, and recover more quickly. Laparoscopy also offers the potential to reduce overall treatment costs. If it is determined intraoperatively that laparoscopy is not possible, the surgery can always be converted to laparotomy. Laparoscopy is discussed further in Chapter 31.

Salpingectomy (removal of the entire fallopian tube) is recommended when there has been significant damage to the tube, when removal of the damaged elements would leave less than 6 cm of functional tube, or when a patient who previously has been sterilized verifies that she still does not desire future fertility. **Partial salpingectomy** (removal of a portion of the tube) is generally done only if the ectopic pregnancy is implanted in the ampullary portion. The remnants of the tube may be reapproximated in the future.

Salpingotomy and **salpingostomy** are both procedures in which the ectopic pregnancy site is identified and vasoconstrictive agents are injected beneath the implantation site. An incision is made parallel to the axis of the tube along its antimesenteric border over the site of implantation. The products of conception are removed by gentle dissection or hydrodissection. Bleeding is controlled by judicious use of electrocoagulating instruments. The tube and pelvis are copiously irrigated. In salpingotomy, the incision is closed, whereas it remains open in salpingostomy. **Most studies have shown that salpingostomy results in better long-term tubal function.**

There is a 10% to 20% risk of residual trophoblastic tissue whenever the products of conception are separated from the tube (i.e., when salpingostomy or salpingotomy are performed). Women who do not have resection of the affected tubal areas should have repeat hCG titers 3 to 7 days postoperatively to confirm that no hormone-producing cells remain behind to reinvade the tube. **If repeat hCG titers fail to decline appropriately, methotrexate (MTX) therapy can be started** (see below). The risk of incomplete trophoblastic tissue removal is greatest when the ectopic is "milked" through the tube to extrude through the fimbria. This technique should never be used, even when it appears that the pregnancy is spontaneously aborting through the fimbria.

MEDICAL MANAGEMENT WITH METHOTREXATE

In recent years, ambulatory diagnosis of women with early, unruptured ectopic pregnancies has replaced surgical diagnosis in many institutions. The early diagnosis of ectopic pregnancy also affords an opportunity to provide medical management with MTX on an ambulatory basis. Because of the side effects of MTX and the potential for tubal rupture, careful guidelines for patient selection are required, as shown in Table 25-1.

A suitable patient may be administered MTX in divided doses of $50 \, mg/m^2$ intramuscularly (half of the dose into each buttock—see PDA for dose calculator). She should return on days 4 and 7 for repeat hCG

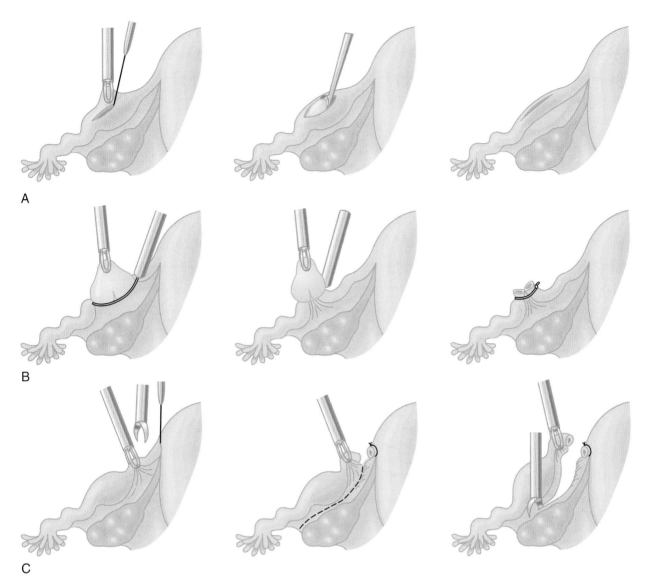

Figure 25-4. Methods of laparoscopic management of tubal pregnancy. *A,* Linear salpingostomy for an ampullary ectopic pregnancy. *B,* Partial salpingectomy with Endoloop. *C,* Salpingectomy using Endoloop and cautery scissors for isthmic tubal pregnancy.

determinations. If the titers fall at least 15% between those days, the patient can be followed at weekly intervals to verify at least a 15% decline every 7 days until the titers are undetectable (usually <5 mIU/mL). If the titers plateau or fall too slowly, another divided dose of MTX may be given if all the other criteria continue to be met. **If the patient becomes more symptomatic or if hCG titers increase during therapy, surgical intervention is required.** Some centers routinely recommend multiple doses of MTX. After injection, patients should be instructed to abstain from intercourse and to avoid folate-containing vitamins,

nonsteroidal anti-inflammatory agents, and alcoholic beverages. Effective contraception should be initiated once the decrease in hCG titers is observed.

EXPECTANT MANAGEMENT

Selected patients may qualify for expectant management if they are stable and the diagnosis of ectopic pregnancy is not yet certain. They must be carefully followed with serial hCG testing and monitoring. As many as 80% of ectopic pregnancies with hCG levels of 1000 mIU/mL or less will not rupture

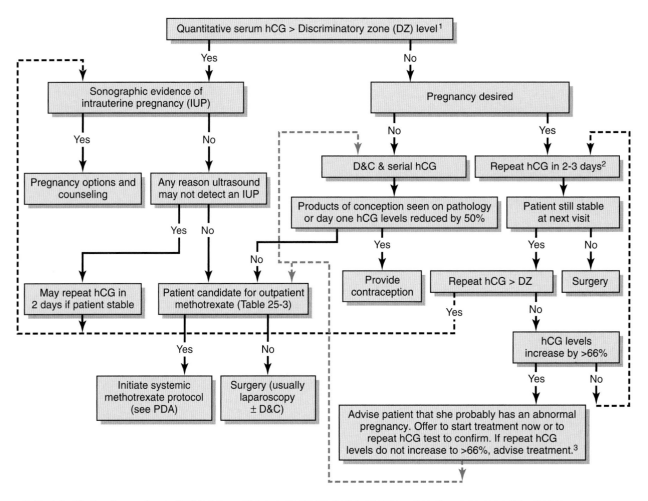

1. Each facility has its own level of hCG above which a normal intrauterine pregnancy can always be seen. Usually it is 1500-2000 mIU/mL.
2. Some clinicians recommend an ultrasonic study below the discriminatory zone (DZ). When ultrasound is performed below the DZ, however, results are frequently indeterminate.
3. Some clinicians recommend bypassing an outpatient D&C and evaluating the patient immediately for methotrexate therapy.

Figure 25-5. Algorithm for the diagnosis and treatment of ectopic pregnancy in a non-acute patient (stable vital signs and no obvious indication of ectopic pregnancy by symptoms or physical findings). *Modified from Nelson AL, Neinstein LS: Ectopic pregnancy. In Neinstein LS: Adolescent Health Care: A Practical Guide, 4th ed. Philadelphia, Lippincott Williams & Wilkins, 2002.*

spontaneously or bleed profusely but will undergo spontaneous resolution. Unfortunately, the 20% who will experience severe sequelae are not identifiable in advance. **Expectant management is generally reserved for reliable, relatively asymptomatic patients in whom the hCG titers are <200 mIU/mL and declining.**

OTHER ELEMENTS OF THERAPY

All Rh-negative, unsensitized women who have ectopic pregnancies should receive anti-Rh immunoglobulin (Rh$_O$-GAM). After an ectopic gestation, pregnancy should be avoided for at least 3 months to allow for the fallopian tube architecture to normalize. Contraception should be provided.

Table 25-1. Criteria for medical management of ectopic pregnancy

Criteria for Receiving Methotrexate (MTX)	Contraindications to Medical Therapy
ABSOLUTE INDICATIONS: 1. Hemodynamically stable without active bleeding or signs of hemoperitoneum 2. Nonlaparoscopic diagnosis 3. Patient desires future fertility 4. General anesthesia poses a significant risk 5. Patient is able to return for follow-up care 6. No contraindications to MTX	**ABSOLUTE CONTRAINDICATIONS:** 1. Breastfeeding 2. Overt or laboratory evidence of immunodeficiency 3. Alcoholism, alcoholic liver disease, or other chronic liver disease 4. Preexisting blood dyscrasias, such as bone marrow hypoplasia, leukopenia, thrombocytopenia or significant anemia 5. Known sensitivity to MTX 6. Active pulmonary disease 7. Peptic ulcer disease 8. Hepatic, renal, or hematologic dysfunction
RELATIVE INDICATIONS: 1. Unruptured mass ≤ 3.5 cm at its greatest dimension 2. No fetal cardiac motion detected 3. Patients whose hCG level does not exceed a predetermined value (6000–15,000 mIU/mL)	**RELATIVE CONTRAINDICATIONS:** 1. Gestational sac ≥ 3.5 cm 2. Embryonic cardiac motion

Data from American College of Obstetricians and Gynecologists: Medical management of tubal pregnancy. Practice Bulletin No. 3. Washington, DC, ACOG, December 1998.

TREATMENT OF UNCOMMON TYPES OF ECTOPIC PREGNANCIES

Ectopic pregnancy and tubal pregnancy are terms used interchangeably because other sites of ectopic implantation are rare. However, a pregnancy can implant on the surface of the ovary, producing identical symptoms to a tubal gestation. The treatment is aimed at removing the pregnancy and sacrificing as little as possible of the ovarian tissue. When this is deemed impossible, usually as a consequence of profuse bleeding, oophorectomy is indicated.

Cervical pregnancy usually presents with profuse vaginal bleeding, and attempts at removal of the pregnancy are often unsuccessful. **MTX and arterial embolization are used to manage cervical pregnancy if the patient is not actively bleeding.** Hysterectomy is reserved for large pregnancies not amenable to nonsurgical treatments and for actively bleeding pregnancies.

Pregnancies rarely implant in the abdominal cavity (e.g., on the omentum, bowel, or parietal or visceral peritoneum) but if they do so, they may rarely proceed to full term. **At the time of laparotomy in advanced gestations, the placenta presents a major technical difficulty.** Vital organs may be entirely or partially covered by the firmly attached placenta, and any attempt at removal may cause massive bleeding. Partial bowel resection may be required if the bowel is involved. **In most cases, it is best to leave the placenta attached,** especially if the pregnancy is in the 2nd or 3rd trimester, anticipating eventual spontaneous reabsorption. MTX treatment may also be useful to accelerate and enhance placental resorption.

IMPLICATIONS FOR FUTURE FERTILITY

Patients who have experienced an ectopic pregnancy are at risk for subsequent ectopic pregnancies and problems with infertility. Only 60% of women who have experienced an ectopic subsequently conceive. Having one ectopic pregnancy increases the risk of a future ectopic pregnancy by 7- to 13-fold. There is about a 50% to 80% chance that the next pregnancy will be intrauterine, and a 10% to 25% risk that it will be ectopic.

Suggested Reading

American College of Obstetricians and Gynecologists: Gynecologic ultrasonography. Technical Bulletin No. 215. Washington, DC, ACOG, November 1995.

American College of Obstetricians and Gynecologists: Medical management of tubal pregnancy. Practice Bulletin No. 3. Washington, DC, ACOG, December 1998.

Lemus J: Ectopic pregnancy: An update. Curr Opin Obstet Gynecol 12:369–375, 2000.

Lipscomb GH, Stoval TG, Ling FW: Primary care: Nonsurgical treatment of ectopic pregnancy. N Engl J Med 343(18):1325, 2000.

Endometriosis and Adenomyosis

J. George Moore and Joseph C. Gambone

ENDOMETRIOSIS

Endometriosis is a benign condition in which endometrial glands and stroma are present outside the uterine cavity and walls. Endometriosis is important in gynecology because of its frequency, distressing symptomatology, association with infertility, and potential for invasion of adjacent organ systems, such as the gastrointestinal or urinary tracts. Endometriosis often presents a difficult diagnostic challenge, and few gynecologic conditions can require such difficult surgical dissections.

INCIDENCE

The incidence of endometriosis in the general population is not known, but **it is estimated that 5% to 15% of women have some degree of the disease.** At least one-third of women with chronic pelvic pain have visualized endometriosis, as do a significant number of infertile women. Interestingly, endometriosis is noted in 5% to 15% of women undergoing gynecologic laparotomies, and it is an unexpected finding in approximately half of these cases.

The typical patient with endometriosis is in her 30s, nulliparous, and infertile. However, in practice, many women with endometriosis do not fit the classic picture. Occasionally, endometriosis may occur in infancy, childhood, or adolescence, but at these early ages, it is usually associated with obstructive genital anomalies. Although endometriosis should regress following the menopause unless estrogens are prescribed, 5% of new cases develop in that age group. In addition, the scarifying involution from preexisting lesions may result in obstructive problems, especially in the gastrointestinal and urinary tracts.

PATHOGENESIS

The pathogenesis of endometriosis is not understood. Genetic predisposition clearly plays a role. The following three hypotheses have been used to explain the various manifestations of endometriosis and the different locations in which endometriotic implants can be found:

1. **The retrograde menstruation theory** of Sampson proposes that endometrial fragments transported through the fallopian tubes at the time of menstruation implant and grow in various intraabdominal sites. Endometrial tissue, which is normally shed at the time of menstruation, is viable and capable of growth in vivo or in vitro. To explain some rare examples of endometriosis in distant sites, such as the lung, forehead, or axilla, it is necessary to postulate hematogenous spread.
2. **The müllerian metaplasia theory** of Meyer proposes that endometriosis results from the metaplastic transformation of peritoneal mesothelium into endometrium under the influence of certain, generally unidentified stimuli.
3. **The lymphatic spread theory** of Halban suggests that endometrial tissues are taken up into the lymphatics draining the uterus and are transported to the various pelvic sites where the tissue grows ectopically. Endometrial tissue has been found in pelvic lymphatics in up to 20% of patients with the disease.

Most authorities today believe that several factors are involved in the initiation and spread of endometriosis, including retrograde menstruation, coelomic metaplasia, immunologic changes and genetic predisposition. The fundamental question is why all menstruating women do not develop endometriosis. The amount of exposure to retrograde flow and the woman's immunologic response seem to be critical. Researchers have identified differences in the chemical composition and biologic pathways of endometrial cells from women with endometriosis compared with those of unaffected women. They have also found significant differences in the inflammatory factors and growth factors in the peritoneal fluid of affected women. A clearer understanding of the pathophysiology of endometriosis would provide insights into strategies for prevention and therapy.

SITES OF OCCURRENCE

Endometriosis occurs most commonly in the dependent portions of the pelvis. Specifically, implants can be found on the ovaries, the broad ligament, the peritoneal surfaces of the cul-de-sac (including the uterosacral ligaments and posterior cervix), and the rectovaginal septum (Figure 26-1). Quite frequently, the rectosigmoid colon is involved, as is the appendix and the vesicouterine fold of peritoneum. **Endometriosis is occasionally seen in laparotomy scars,** developing especially after a cesarean section or myomectomy when the endometrial cavity has been entered. It is probable that endometrial tissue is seeded into the surgical incision. **Two out of three women with endometriosis have ovarian involvement.**

PATHOLOGY

Islands of endometriosis respond cyclicly to ovarian steroidal hormone production. The implants proliferate under estrogenic stimulation and slough when support from estrogen and progesterone is removed with involution of the corpus luteum. The sloughed material induces a profound inflammatory response resulting immediately in pain and longer term in fibrosis. The macroscopic appearance of endometriosis depends on the site of the implant, activity of the lesion, day of the menstrual cycle, and the time since implantation.

Lesions may be raised and flat with red, black, or brown coloration; fibrotic scarred areas that are yellow or white in hue; or vesicles that are pink, clear, or red. The color of the implant is generally determined by its vascularity, the size of the lesion, and the amount of residual sloughed material. Newer implants tend to be red, blood-filled active lesions. Older lesions tend to be scarred with a puckered appearance.

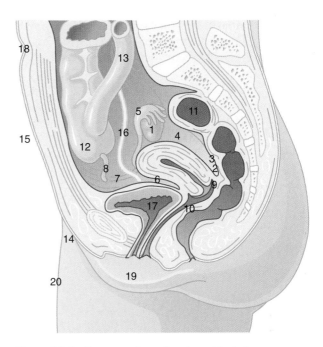

Figure 26-1. Common sites of endometriosis in decreasing order of frequency: (1) ovary, (2) cul-de-sac, (3) uterosacral ligaments, (4) broad ligaments, (5) fallopian tubes, (6) uterovesical fold, (7) round ligaments, (8) vermiform appendix, (9) vagina, (10) rectovaginal septum, (11) rectosigmoid colon, (12) cecum, (13) ileum, (14) inguinal canals, (15) abdominal scars, (16) ureters, (17) urinary bladder, (18) umbilicus, (19) vulva, and (20) peripheral sites.

Endometriomas of the ovary are cysts filled with thick, chocolate-colored fluid that sometimes has the black color and tarry consistency of crankcase oil. This characteristic fluid represents aged, hemolyzed blood and desquamated endometrium. Usually, endometrial glands and stroma are present in the cyst wall. Sometimes, however, the pressure of the enclosed fluid destroys the endometrial lining of the endometrioma, leaving only a fibrotic cyst wall infiltrated with large numbers of hemosiderin-laden macrophages. Generally, ovarian implants are associated with significant scarring of the ovary to the pelvic sidewall or broad ligament. Histologically, two of four characteristics must be found in the specimen to confirm the diagnosis—endometrial epithelium, endometrial glands, endometrial stroma, and hemosiderin-laden macrophages.

Although endometriosis is a benign process, it shares many characteristics with malignancy. It is locally infiltrative, invasive, and widely disseminated.

It is also curious that cyclic hormones induce growth, whereas continuous hormonal exposure, especially in high doses, induces regression.

STAGING

The American Society of Reproductive Medicine (ASRM) employs a staging protocol in an attempt to correlate fertility potential with a quantified stage of endometriosis. This staging, which was initially based on the allocation of points depending on the sites involved and extent of visualized disease (Figure 26-2), was modified to include a description of the color of the lesions and the percentage of surface involved in each lesion type, as well as a more detailed description of any endometrioma.

American Society for Reproductive Medicine
Revised Classification of Endometriosis

Patient's name _____ Date _____

Stage I (minimal)   — 1 – 5
Stage II (mind)   — 6 – 15
Stage III (moderate) — 16 – 40
Stage IV (severe)   — > 40

Laparoscopy_____ Laparotomy_____ Photography_____
Recommended treatment _____

Total _____ Prognosis _____

			<1 cm	1-3 cm	>3 cm
Peritoneum	Endometriosis				
		Superficial	1	2	4
		Deep	2	4	6
Ovary		R Superficial	1	2	4
		Deep	4	16	20
		L Superficial	1	2	4
		Deep	4	16	20
	Posterior cul-de-sac obliteration		Partial		Complete
			4		40
	Adhesions		<1/3 Enclosure	1/3 –2/3 Enclosure	>2/3 Enclosure
Ovary		R Filmy	1	2	4
		Dense	4	8	16
		L Filmy	1	2	4
		Dense	4	8	16
Tube		R Filmy	1	2	4
		Dense	4*	8*	16
		L Filmy	1	2	4
		Dense	4*	8*	16

*If the fimbriated end of the fallopian tube is completely enclosed, change the point assignment to 16. Denote appearance of superficial implant types as red [(R), red, red-pink, flamelike, vesicular blobs, clear vesicles], white [(W), opacifications, peritoneal defects, yellow- brown], or black [(B), black, hemosiderin deposits, blue]. Denote percent of total described as R__%, W__%, and B__%. Total should equal 100%.

Figure 26-2. Modified from the revised American Fertility Society classification of endometriosis. *Reprinted with permission from the American Society for Reproductive Medicine. Fertil Steril 67(5):819–820, 1996.*

SYMPTOMS

The characteristic triad of symptoms associated with endometriosis is dysmenorrhea, dyspareunia, and dyschezia. The pain that women suffer with endometriosis varies with the time since initiation. Early in the clinical course, women tend to have cyclic pelvic pain, which starts 1 to 2 days before the menstrual flow and resolves at the end of the menses. This secondary dysmenorrhea is thought to be related to the premenstrual swelling and extravasation of blood and menstrual debris, which induces an intense inflammatory reaction in the surrounding tissue mediated by prostaglandins and cytokines that are more directly responsible for triggering the pain sensation. Deep, infiltrating implants, especially those in the retroperitoneal space, are associated with more pain than are superficial lesions. Over time, the pain may become more chronic with exacerbations at the time of the menses. Interestingly, **there is no clear relationship between the stage of endometriosis and the frequency and severity of pain symptoms.**

Dyspareunia is generally associated with deep-thrust penetration during intercourse and occurs mainly when the cul-de-sac, uterosacral ligaments, and portions of the posterior vaginal fornix are involved. Deep thrust dyspareunia can also result from uterine immobility due to significant internal scarring caused by endometriosis. Endometriomas in these sites are usually exquisitely tender to touch.

Dyschezia is experienced with uterosacral, cul-de-sac, and rectosigmoid colon involvement. As the stool passes between the uterosacral ligaments, the characteristic dyschezia is experienced. **Premenstrual and postmenstrual spotting is a characteristic symptom of endometriosis.** Menorrhagia is uncommon, the amount of menstrual flow usually diminishing with endometriosis. If the ovarian capsule is involved with endometriosis, ovulatory pain and midcycle vaginal bleeding often occur. Rarely, as other organ systems are involved, menstrual hematochezia, hematuria, and other forms of endometriotic sloughing become evident.

The association between mild to moderate endometriosis and infertility is not clear. When endometriosis distorts the pelvic structures, its role in infertility is more predictable.

SIGNS

Endometriosis presents with a wide variety of signs varying from the presence of a small, exquisitely tender nodule in the cul-de-sac or on the uterosacral ligaments to a huge, relatively nontender, cystic abdominal mass. Occasionally, a small tender mulberry spot may be seen in the posterior fornix of the vagina. **Characteristically, a tender, fixed adnexal mass is appreciated on bimanual examination.** The uterus is fixed and retroverted in a substantial number of women with endometriosis. **Occasionally, no signs at all are appreciated on physical examination.**

DIFFERENTIAL DIAGNOSIS

The main differential diagnoses in the acute phase of endometriosis are (1) chronic pelvic inflammatory disease or recurrent acute salpingitis, (2) hemorrhagic corpus luteum, (3) benign or malignant ovarian neoplasm, and, occasionally, (4) ectopic pregnancy.

DIAGNOSIS

The diagnosis of endometriosis should be suspected in an afebrile patient with the characteristic triad of pelvic pain, a firm, fixed, tender adnexal mass, and tender nodularity in the cul-de-sac and uterosacral ligaments. The characteristic sharp, firm, exquisitely tender "barb" (from barbed wire) felt in the uterosacral ligament is the diagnostic sine qua non of endometriosis, but this finding is generally present only in severe cases. An ultrasonic evaluation may indicate an adnexal mass of complex echogenicity, with internal echoes consistent with old blood. Serum levels of the cancer antigen 125 (CA 125) are frequently elevated in women with endometriosis. However, the sensitivity of CA 125 in detecting endometriosis is only 20% to 30%, and it is not used to diagnose endometriosis.

The definitive diagnosis is generally made by the characteristic gross and histologic findings obtained at laparoscopy or laparotomy. Unfortunately, even the most experienced surgeon may fail to identify endometriotic implants because the older implants may have a very subtle appearance and the deeper infiltrating lesions may not be visible at the surface. Biopsy of suspicious lesions improves diagnostic accuracy.

MANAGEMENT

The management of endometriosis depends on certain key considerations: (1) the certainty of the diagnosis, (2) the severity of the symptoms, (3) the extent of the disease, (4) the desire for future fertility, (5) the age of the patient, and (6) the threat to the gastrointestinal or urinary tract or both.

Treatment is indicated for endometriosis associated pelvic pain, dysmenorrhea, dyspareunia, abnormal bleeding, ovarian cysts, and infertility due to gross distortion of tubal and ovarian anatomy. Surgical intervention is required for an endometrioma larger than 3 cm, gross distortion of pelvic anatomy, involvement of bowel or bladder, and adhesive disease. Surgery may improve fertility for women with severe endometriosis. Medical therapy is generally the first line to treat other symptomatic women. **There is no convincing evidence that treatment improves fertility in women with mild endometriosis.**

Surgical Treatments

The most comprehensive surgery includes total abdominal hysterectomy, bilateral salpingo-oophorectomy with destruction of all peritoneal implants, and dissection of all adhesions. Usually, an appendectomy is also preferred. Because of extensive adhesions, this surgery is often technically very challenging. If endometriosis involves the cul-de-sac or uterosacral ligaments, the proximity to the ureter, bladder, and sigmoid colon must be considered. If endometriosis obstructs the ureter, resection and ureteroplasty may be necessary to preserve renal function. **Nearly 25% of kidneys are lost when endometriosis blocks the ureter.** Obstruction of the rectosigmoid and even obstruction of the small intestine may require resection of the involved intestinal segment. The surgical risks must be carefully explained to the woman, as well as her subsequent need for treatment for loss of ovarian steroids. She also needs to understand that postoperatively, there is a 20% recurrence rate for endometriosis, usually involving the bowel.

Often the desire for future fertility precludes this surgical option. In this situation, laparoscopic or open surgery is designed to destroy all endometriotic implants and remove all adhesive disease. This usually involves excision (not lysis) of all adhesions and laser ablation or electrocautery of suspected implants. **Large endometriomas (>3 cm) are amenable only to surgical resection.** Because of extensive adhesive disease that generally surrounds these cysts, cystectomy is not always possible; oophorectomy may be necessary. Extensive tubal disease with or without

ovarian involvement may be treated with removal of the affected organs but with uterine preservation for in vitro fertilization (IVF). **Preoperative treatment with medical agents, such as gonadotropin-releasing hormone (GnRH) agonists for 3 to 6 months can improve surgical success.**

The role of medical therapy postoperatively remains controversial, although it is indicated to treat women who have known residual disease diagnosed at surgery. **There is a risk of recurrence of endometriosis throughout a woman's life**, so that measures should be taken to reduce her risk of retrograde menstruation or cyclic ovarian sex steroid production. Depot medroxyprogesterone acetate (DMPA), continuous oral contraceptives, and the levonorgestrel-releasing intrauterine device (IUD) are all attractive long-term options.

Medical Treatments

Therapy should be targeted toward relieving the patient's individual complaints and toward reducing the risk of disease progression. Asymptomatic women found incidentally to have endometriosis may not require any therapy. Dysmenorrhea due to endometriosis can be approached as outlined in Chapter 22, utilizing nonsteroidal anti-inflammatory drugs (NSAIDs) and menstrual minimization with hormonal regimens.

For relief of pelvic pain, short-term treatment may be used, and either a GnRH-agonist or danazol appears to be equally effective. Cost and potential side effects generally guide selection of one agent or the other.

Danazol is an androgenic derivative that may be used in a "pseudomenopause" regimen to suppress symptoms of endometriosis if fertility is not a present concern. It is given over a period of 6 to 9 months, and doses of 600 to 800 mg daily are generally necessary to suppress menstruation. Through its weak androgenic properties, danazol decreases the plasma levels of sex hormone–binding globulin (SHBG). The resulting increase of free testosterone may cause hirsutism and acne. **Three years after cessation of Danazol, 40% of patients will have recurrence of endometriosis. After a full course of danazol therapy, use of a cyclic oral contraceptive may help to delay or prevent such recurrence.**

GnRH-agonists effect a temporary medical castration, thereby bringing about a marked,

albeit temporary, regression of endometriosis. Treatment of women with endometriosis with GnRH-agonists usually produces relief of pain and involution of implants. The disadvantages of these agonists are related to cost, hot flashes, and side effects, including vaginal dryness. They also cause calcium loss from bone and an unfavorable lipid profile. If treatment with a GnRH agonist is effective in relieving chronic pelvic pain and surgery is not indicated, low-dose estrogen-progestin add-back therapy can permit longer-term use of GnRH agonists by eliminating the estrogen deficiency impacts without reducing the efficacy of GnRH agonists.

Oral contraceptives and oral medroxyprogesterone acetate are more effective in treating endometriosis-associated pelvic pain than placebos. The levonorgestrel-releasing IUD reduces dysmenorrhea and may be helpful in inducing regression of cul-de-sac implants without diminishing circulating estrogen levels in the serum.

PREVENTION OF ENDOMETRIOSIS

Whenever severe dysmenorrhea occurs in a young patient, the possibility of varying degrees of obstruction to the menstrual flow must be considered. The possibility of a blind uterine horn in a bicornuate uterus or an obstructing uterine or vaginal septum should be kept in mind. **In more than half the patients who are noted to develop endometriosis during childhood and adolescence, varying** degrees of genital tract obstruction may be found. Whenever a congenital abnormality of the urinary or intestinal tract is detected, the genital tract should be investigated for an obstructive lesion. Infants with genital tract obstruction have been noted to develop endometriosis even in the first year of life. **In all women, menstrual minimization and suppression of ovarian cycling can reduce the risk of endometriosis.**

ADENOMYOSIS

Adenomyosis is defined as the extension of endometrial glands and stroma into the uterine musculature more than 2.5 mm beneath the basalis layer. Often this is an incidental finding on pathologic examination when it is seen in up to 60% of women in their 40s. **About 15% of patients with adenomyosis have associated endometriosis.** Islands of adenomyosis do not participate in the proliferative and secretory cycles induced by the ovary.

PATHOLOGY

Generally, the gross appearance of the uterus consists of diffuse enlargement with a thickened myometrium containing characteristic glandular irregularities, with implants containing both glandular tissue and stroma (Figure 26-3). The endometrial cavity is also enlarged. Occasionally, the adenomyosis may be confined to one portion of the

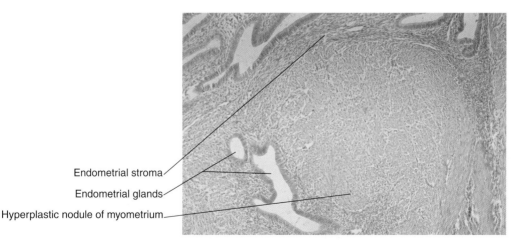

Endometrial stroma
Endometrial glands
Hyperplastic nodule of myometrium

Figure 26-3. Adenomyosis causing the enlargement of the uterus. A hyperplastic nodule of myometrium is seen. Note the endometrial glands and stroma.

myometrium and take the form of a fairly well-circumscribed adenomyoma. Contrary to the picture in a uterine myoma, no distinct capsular margin can be detected on cut section between the adenomyoma and the surrounding myometrium. The distinction between adenomyosis and uterine leiomyoma may not be clear on ultrasonic examination.

SYMPTOMS

Although many women are asymptomatic, those who suffer from this condition typically complain of severe secondary dysmenorrhea and menorrhagia. Even though the islands do not cycle in response to ovarian hormonal stimulation, there is still prostaglandin release and local inflammatory changes that can induce pain and tenderness and may disrupt the vasoconstriction of the arterial arcade supplying the endometrium. Deep thrust dyspareunia, especially premenstrually, can be caused by adenomyosis.

SIGNS

On pelvic examination, the uterus is generally symmetrically enlarged and somewhat boggy and tender if the examination is conducted premenstrually. Occasionally, it may enlarge asymmetrically, which makes it very difficult to distinguish adenomyosis from a myomatous uterus. The consistency of the enlarged adenomyomatous uterus is generally softer than that of a uterine myoma.

TREATMENT

The treatment of adenomyosis depends entirely on the symptoms and the possibility of other diagnoses. Any history of new onset or worsening menorrhagia, particularly in a woman with risk factors for endometrial cancer, should be investigated by endometrial biopsy or fractional dilatation and curettage and/or hysteroscopy to rule out malignancy. **Conservative management with NSAIDs and hormonal control of the endometrium are mainstays of therapy.** Combination oral contraceptives or hormone containing patches and vaginal rings may be used to reduce cyclic blood loss and menstrual pain. DMPA, Levonorgestrel IUD, and continuous oral contraceptive pills can be used to try to achieve amenorrhea. If the woman is not a candidate for any of these medical interventions or if medical treatments do not sufficiently control her symptoms, **hysterectomy may be indicated. Endometrial ablation to control the bleeding is another option.**

Suggested Reading

American College of Obstetrics and Gynecologists: Medical management of endometriosis. Practice Bulletin No. 11. Washington, DC, ACOG, December 1999.

Child TJ, Tan SL: Endometriosis: Aetiology, pathogenesis and treatment. Drugs 61:1735–1750, 2001.

Gambone JC, Mittman BS, Munro MG, et al: Consensus statement for the management of chronic pelvic pain and endometriosis: Proceedings of an expert-panel consensus process. Fertil Steril 78:961–972, 2002.

Olive DL, Pritts EA: Treatment of endometriosis. N Engl J Med 345:266–275, 2001.

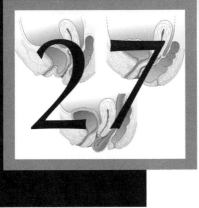

Family Planning: Contraception, Sterilization, and Abortion

Anita L. Nelson

Family planning enables sexually active couples to prepare for their pregnancies, in order to optimize both fetal and maternal outcomes. **Unplanned pregnancies constitute major public health problems.** The United Nations International Children's Emergency Fund (UNICEF) estimates that over 800,000 women worldwide die each year as a result of pregnancy and pregnancy-related causes and an additional 15 million women are severely disabled by pregnancy. Countries in which women utilize contraception have lower birth rates and the lowest rates of maternal mortality. Every method of birth control prescribed is safer than pregnancy.

Family planning is divided into three categories: (1) **contraception** (prevention of fertilization), (2) **interception** (prevention of implantation), and (3) **abortion** (interruption of an established pregnancy). Contraception methods can be either reversible or permanent (sterilization).

CONTRACEPTION
EFFICACY

The intrinsic effectiveness of birth control methods cannot be directly measured because many of the variables that contribute to fertility cannot be controlled in clinical trials. The only quantifiable event is failure, that is, the number of pregnancies that occur during contraceptive use. Failure rates that are determined during clinical trials are used as a basis for the Food and Drug Administration (FDA) product labeling. These estimates are often separated into two components. The **"perfect use failure rate"** represents the percentage of women who conceive in the first year of use when they use the method exactly as instructed, Unfortunately, the **"typical failure rates"** observed when couples use the method in the real world are significantly higher, (Table 27-1). Typical failure rates are the most accurate ones to quote when counseling patients, but the perfect use rates can be offered as an incentive.

Reversible contraceptive methods are best grouped by efficacy into three major groups—**the highly effective methods** (typical failure rates <3%), **very effective methods** (typical failure rates 3% to 10%), and **all others.** The first group is comprised of methods that require little patient involvement including implants, IUDs, and long-acting injections. The second tier methods include all the other hormonal methods, such as contraceptive pills, patches, and rings. The last group includes all the barrier and behavioral methods (Table 27-2).

COMBINATION HORMONAL METHODS OF CONTRACEPTION

In the United States (US), four different delivery systems are used to supply estrogen and progestin to provide contraception: oral contraceptive pills, vaginal rings, transdermal patches, and monthly injections.

Oral contraceptives (OCs) are the most extensively studied class of medications in history. Since the introduction of the first birth control pill (Enovid) in the US in 1960, the doses of the sex steroid hormones have decreased from nearly 10 mg of progestin and 150 μg of estrogen per tablet to about 1 mg of progestin and 20 to 35 μg of estrogen. Side effects and medical complications have diminished significantly as

Table 27-1.   Contraceptive failure rates comparing typical use and perfect use with continuation rates

Continuation (%)	% FAILURE WITHIN 1ST YR OF USE		Continuation Rate at 1 Yr
	Perfect Use	Typical Use	
No method	85	85	—
Male sterilization	0.10	0.15	100
Female sterilization	0.5	0.5	100
Copper ParaGard T 380A IUD	0.6	0.8	78
Levonorgestrel-releasing IUD	0.1	0.1	81
OC-combined	0.3	8.0	68
OC-progestin only	0.5	—	—
Diaphragm with spermicide	6	16	57
Condom male latex	2	15	53
Cervical cap—parous	26	32	46
Cervical cap—nulliparous	9	16	57
Spermicides	15	29	42
Rhythm (calendar)	19	25	—

OC, oral contraceptive.

Table 27-2.   Sterility status and contraceptive use among 54 million women age 15–44 years in the US

Status	Percentage Distribution
Sterile	29.7
Surgically sterile	23.6
Female	16.6
Male	7.0
Other causes	6.1
Contraceptive nonusers	33.6
Nonsurgical contraceptive users	36.7
Oral contraceptive users	18.5
Condom	8.8
Diaphragm	3.5
Intrauterine device	1.2
Rhythm	1.0
Sponge (spermicidal)	0.6
Other methods*	3.1
Total	100

*Coitus interruptus, emergency contraception, etc.
Data from the National Center for Health Statistics. Hyattsville, Md, 1990.

the doses have decreased. Today, **few healthy, reproductive-aged women have significant medical contraindications to oral contraceptive use.**

Different formulations are available containing estrogen, usually ethinyl estradiol, and a progestin, usually a 19-nortestosterone derivative with both progestogenic and androgenic effect. Preparations of oral contraceptives are either **monophasic** (each active pill contains the same dose of hormones) or **multiphasic** (the dose of hormones varies among the pills in the package) (see Table 21-3).

It is recommended that a woman take her first pill on the first day of her menses in order to avoid the need for a back-up method during the first cycle of use. A "quick start" routine has recently been recommended. The woman starts OCs on the first full day of her visit and uses a back-up method for 7 days. Traditionally, pills have been provided in packages with 21 active pills and 7 placebo (or iron) pills. Women who suffer dysmenorrhea or other menstrual-related problems (e.g., menstrual migraine) may use the active pills for all 28 days of a cycle to eliminate the artificial withdrawal bleeding and pain that may occur during the placebo pill interval.

Other delivery systems for estrogen and progestin have been introduced to reduce the possibility that daily pills may be forgotten.

Lunelle is a 0.5-cc injection with estradiol cypionate and depot medroxyprogesterone acetate (DMPA) administered intramuscularly once a month. It is no longer available in the US.

The Ortho-Evra patch is a transdermal system, which is placed on a woman's upper arm or torso (except her breasts). The patch slowly releases ethinyl estradiol and norelgestromin, which establishes steady serum levels for 7 days. A woman should apply one patch in a different area each week for 3 weeks, then have a patch-free week, during which she will have a withdrawal bleed.

Table 27-3. Hormonal content in OCs commonly available in the US

Brand Name	Estrogen*	Dose-μg/tablet (days on dose)	Progestin	Dose-mg/tablet (days on dose)
MONOPHASIC				
Alesse	E.E.	20 (21)	Levonorgestrel	1 (21)
Brevicon	E.E.	35 (21)	Norethindrone	0.5 (21)
Demulen	E.E.	50 (21)	Ethynodiol Diacotate	1 (21)
Demulen 1/35	E.E.	35 (21)	Ethynodiol Diacetate	1 (21)
Desogen	E.E.	30 (21)	Desogestrel	0.15 (21)
Genora 0.5/35	E.E.	35 (21)	Norethindrone	0.5 (21)
Genora 1/35	E.E.	35 (21)	Norethindrone	1 (21)
Levelen	E.E.	30 (21)	Levonorgestrel	0.15 (21)
Loestrin 1/20	E.E.	20 (21)	Norethindrone Acetate	1 (21)
Loestrin 1.5/30	E.E.	30 (21)	Norethindrone Acetate	1.5 (21)
Lo/Ovral	E.E.	30 (21)	Norgestrel	0.3 (21)
Modicon	E.E.	35 (21)	Norethindrone	0.5 (21)
Nordette	E.E.	30 (21)	Levonorgestrel	0.15 (21)
Norlestrin 1/50	E.E.	50 (21)	Norethindrone Acetate	1 (21)
Norlestrin 2.5/50	E.E.	50 (21)	Norethindrone Acetate	2.5 (21)
Norinyl 1 + 35	E.E.	35 (21)	Norethindrone	1 (21)
Norinyl 1 + 50	M	50 (21)	Norethindrone	1 (21)
Ortho-Cept	E.E.	30 (21)	Desogestrel	0.15 (21)
Ortho-Cyclen	E.E.	35 (21)	Norgestimate	0.25 (21)
Ortho-Novum 1/35	E.E.	35 (21)	Norethndrone	1 (21)
Ortho-Novum 1/50	M	50 (21)	Norethndrone	1 (21)
Ovcon	E.E.	35 (21)	Norethndrone	0.4 (21)
Ovral	E.E.	50 (21)	Norgestrel	0.5 (21)
Yasmin	E.E.	30 (21)	Drospironone	0.3 (21)
MULTIPHASIC				
Estrostep	E.E.	20 (5) 30 (7) 35 (9)	Norethindrone Acetate	1 (21)
Ortho-Novum 10/11	E.E.	35 (21)	Norethindrone	0.5 (10) 1 (11)
Ortho-Novum 7/7/7	E.E.	35 (21)	Norethindrone	0.5 (7) 0.75 (7) 1 (7)
Ortho Tri-Cyclen	E.E.	35 (21)	Norgestimate	0.18 (7) 0.215 (7) 0.25 (7)
Tri-Levlen	E.E.	30 (6) 40 (5) 30 (10)	Levonorgestrel	0.05 (6) 0.075 (5) 0.125 (10)
Tri-Norinyl	E.E.	35 (21)	Norethindrone	0.5 (7) 1.0 (9) 0.5 (5)
Triphasil	E.E.	30 (21)	Levonorgestrel	0.05 (6) 0.075 (5) 0.125 (10)
PROGESTIN ONLY				
Micronor			Norethindrone	0.35 (21)
Nor-QD			Norethindrone	0.35 (21)
Ovrette			Norgestrel	0.075 (21)

*E.E., Ethinyl estradiol; M, Mestranol.

NuvaRing is a flexible plastic ring made of an elastomer mixed with ethinyl estradiol and etonogestrel. Early in the menstrual cycle, the ring is placed into the upper vagina to release hormones for at least 21 days. The woman removes the ring after 3 weeks of use and waits a week to insert a new ring (during which time she should menstruate).

The pills, patches, and rings have all achieved comparable efficiency in comparative clinical trials, although consistent use was more commonly observed with the patch and the ring. The patch has a significantly higher failure rate when used in women who weigh more than 198 pounds.

Combination hormonal methods utilize two main mechanisms of contraceptive action: suppression of the LH surge (to prevent ovulation) and thickening of the cervical mucus (to prevent sperm entering the upper genital tract). Other mechanisms that have been suggested to contribute to efficacy include slowing of tubal transport and atrophy of the endometrium.

Table 27-4. Contraindications to the use of estrogen-containing contraceptives

ABSOLUTE		Relative Contraindications*
Venous thrombosis	Endometrial cancer	Complicated, prolonged diabetes
Pulmonary embolism	Hepatic tumor or abnormal liver function	Estrogen-dependent neoplasms
Coronary vascular disease	Unexplained abnormal uterine bleeding	Depression
Cerebrovascular accident	Age >35 and cigarette smoking	Severe varicose veins
Current pregnancy	Uncontrolled hypertension	Hypertriglyceridemia
Breast cancer within last 5 years	History of melanoma	

*Requires clinical judgment and informed consent.

Box 27-1. Complications of estrogen-containing contraceptives

Thromboembolism
Cerebrovascular accidents
Hypertension
Postpill amenorrhea
Increase in cholelithiasis
Benign hepatic tumors

Selection of appropriate candidates for combination hormonal contraception is the key to safe use (Table 27-4). Fortunately, serious complications are infrequent and are shown in Box 27-1.

Recent data are quite reassuring about OC use and the risk of breast cancer. Only the earlier, higher-dose OC formulations have been linked to a possible increased risk of breast cancer.

Although some women may be more sensitive than others to sex steroid hormones, side effects often attributed to hormonal use, such as headaches, breast tenderness, mood changes, gastrointestinal problems, cramping, and weight change, are no more frequent in low-dose OC users than in placebo pill users. **Breakthrough spotting and bleeding tend to resolve after 1 to 3 months of use.** Women who use medications that increase rates of hepatic metabolism (such as anticonvulsants or St. John's Wort) may need to use higher dose formulations to maintain adequate serum sex steroid levels. Antibiotics (except rifampin and possibly griseofulvin) do not significantly reduce circulating hormone levels or affect OC efficacy.

Oral contraceptives have been found to offer significant health benefits. **A woman's risk of developing ovarian and endometrial cancer is dramatically reduced by OC use** with an increase in protection with duration of use. For example, a woman who uses OCs for 12 years decreases her risk of developing epithelial ovarian carcinoma by about 80% and her risk of endometrial carcinoma by over 50%. Women using combination hormonal methods have a slightly higher risk of developing cervical intraepithelial neoplasia, but their **risks of developing pelvic inflammatory disease (PID), endometriosis, benign breast changes, and ectopic pregnancy are reduced.** Women lose less blood with menses and suffer less dysmenorrhea with cyclic OC use. Continuous OC use has the potential to eliminate menses altogether.

Return to fertility is delayed on average by 2 weeks after cessation of pills, patches or rings, and by about 4 weeks after stopping the combination contraceptive injection. Beyond that initial delay, fertility curves for most women are virtually identical to those who stop using the condom. Occasionally, a woman may have more prolonged ovulation suppression. The resulting **"postpill amenorrhea"** may persist for up to 6 months in some women but has no longer-term effect on fertility.

Male hormonal methods of birth control are currently under development. Safety and reversibility have been significant issues during the development of an effective hormonal method for men.

PROGESTIN-ONLY HORMONAL METHODS OF CONTRACEPTION

Progestin-only contraception is provided by implants, injections, pills, and intrauterine devices (IUDs). The hormonal IUD is discussed in the section on "Intrauterine Devices," but shares many characteristics of the other progestin-only delivery systems.

Efficacy varies by delivery system. **With the exception of the progestin-only pills, the progestin-only methods provide the greatest pregnancy**

protection of all reversible methods of female contraception.

The **Norplant** contraceptive system was composed of 6 silastic implants placed in the subcutaneous layer of the medial aspect of a woman's upper arm to release steady amounts of levonorgestrel. First-year pregnancy rates are 0.05%. This 6 implant system was FDA approved for 5 years of use, but in slender women (<154 lbs), the literature shows that use may be extended for an additional 2 years. The **Norplant II system** is composed of 2 rods, and was approved by the FDA in 1996 for up to 3 years of use. Neither of these systems is currently marketed in the US. A single implant system called **Implanon** has been tested internationally; no failures have been observed in over 70,000 women-cycles. It is hoped that this implant will be made available in the US. Implants have low circulating levels of progestin, but the constant serum levels of progestin provide consistent contraceptive effects on cervical mucus. Implanon also suppresses ovulation.

The **once-every-3-months intramuscular injection with 150 mg DMPA (Depo-Provera) is rarely associated with pregnancies,** except when the patient fails to return for reinjection. Serum levels of DMPA are considerably higher than with implants or IUDs. DMPA can suppress ovulation in addition to creating impenetrable cervical mucus. **DMPA is a preferred method for women using medications (such as anticonvulsants), which increase hepatic clearance of sex steroids.**

Progestin-only pills are most frequently used by breastfeeding women, although they can be used for other indications. In contrast to the convenience of progestin implants and injections, progestin-only pills require very strict adherence to every-24-hour administration and have failure rates of 3% to 9%.

Because progestins have little metabolic impact, virtually every woman can use at least one of these methods. For example, smokers of any age, women with a history of thrombosis, and breastfeeding women are all candidates for progestin-only methods.

The most common side effect associated with progestin-only methods is menstrual changes. Initially women experience unpredictable spotting and/or bleeding. With more prolonged use, especially of DMPA, the majority of women develop amenorrhea. This feature is appreciated by many women who suffer menstrual problems, such as dysmenorrhea or catamenial seizures, as well as by disabled or mentally retarded women for whom the hygiene issues of menstruation may be challenging. **The other side effects attributed to progestins include weight changes, headaches, and mood changes,** although causation has not been proven. Women using DMPA may have profound ovarian suppression; estrogen levels in these women may drop to the postmenopausal range. Reversible changes due to this hypoestrogenism, such as dry vagina and reduced bone mineral density, may develop. Return to fertility ranges from immediate with pills and implants to slow with DMPA; the average return to ovulation with DMPA is 10 months after the last injection.

INTRAUTERINE DEVICES

Worldwide, over 100 million women use IUDs. However, these devices are significantly underutilized in the US. Typical failure rates with IUDs are similar to the rates seen with sterilization. **Convenience, cost effectiveness and reversibility are all attractive features of the IUD.** Two IUDs are currently available in the US—the **Copper T380A (ParaGard)** IUD (Figure 27-1), which is approved for up to 10 years of use, and the **levonorgestrel-releasing intrauterine system (LNG-IUS, Mirena),** which is approved for up to 5 years.

The copper IUDs are functional spermicides. Sperm motility is severely compromised and the ability of the sperm to fertilize the egg is inhibited by the presence of copper ions. The inflammatory changes within the endometrium are also spermicidal. **The LNG-IUS prevents pregnancy primarily by maintaining thick, impenetrable cervical mucus.** Ovulation is rarely suppressed. The atrophic endometrial changes induced by the LNG over time may

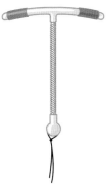

Figure 27-1. Copper T 380A-ParaGard IUD.

contribute to efficacy but primarily affects menstrual bleeding patterns.

IUDs are most appropriate for women who are in stable, mutually monogamous relationships at low risk for sexually transmitted infections (STIs). Appropriate nulliparous women can use IUDs, since long-term fertility is not affected. Women with history of PID who are currently at low risk for STIs may also be candidates if they have demonstrated their fertility subsequent to their tubal infections. IUDs are intended for women whose uterine cavities sound to 6 to 9 cm.

The main differentiating feature between the two different IUDs is the impact each has on menstrual bleeding. **The LNG-IUS generally induces unpredictable spotting and bleeding for up to 4 months, as the endometrial lining is thinning but subsequently results in a 70% to 90% reduction in menstrual blood loss.** On the other hand, **the copper IUD increases monthly blood loss by about 35%.** Therefore, women with heavy menses or dysmenorrhea are better served by the hormonal IUDs.

The insertion procedures are straightforward but require training. Insertion can be associated infrequently with complications, such as uterine perforation (1:1000). There is also a transient increased risk of upper genital tract infection (1:1000) due to endometrial contamination during device insertion. Copper IUDs may be associated with dysmenorrhea; however, continued utilization rates are high. Women need to check the IUD strings monthly to confirm that the IUD is still in place.

BARRIER METHODS

The advantage of barrier methods is that they are used only at the time of intercourse, so there is no requirement for continuous hormonal exposure or ongoing IUD use. However, the fact that intervention is required with every act of intercourse reduces spontaneity and significantly increases the gap between typical use failure rates and failure rates with consistent and correct use.

The male condom is the second most frequently used method of reversible contraception in the U.S. and is the method most commonly used with first coitus. Most male condoms are made of latex, polyurethane or sheep cecum. A variety of sizes, textures, and shapes enables virtually every man to find a condom he can utilize. **The latex male condom significantly reduces the transmission of STIs that** are fluid borne (such as human immunodeficiency virus [HIV], chlamydia, and gonorrhea), but it offers less protection against STIs that are spread by direct skin-to-skin contact (such as human papilloma virus [HPV] and herpes simplex virus [HSV]). Spermicidally-lubricated condoms are no longer recommended to add extra STI risk protection. The addition of spermicide to condoms has never been demonstrated to increase pregnancy protection.

Female barrier methods include the diaphragm, cervical cap, FemCap, and the female condom. For convenience, vaginal spermicides (foam, suppository, and film) are also included in this category. Female condoms (Reality) are disposable sacklike polyurethane devices. The leading edge of the condom is introduced high into the vagina and the ring at the base is placed against the labia around the introitus. The couple uses one female condom per act and must be attentive to ensure that the condom is correctly positioned throughout coitus. Vaginal diaphragms and the cervical cap (Prentif) need to be professionally fitted. **Diaphragms, cervical caps, and FemCaps are used in conjunction with spermicidal gel to block entry of the sperm into the upper genital tract.** Diaphragms, caps, and shields can be cleansed and reused for up to 12 months. Cervical caps can be used for multiple acts of intercourse for up to 48 hours.

Spermicides are available over-the-counter but are associated with relatively high failure rates. Spermicides with nonoxynol-9 (N-9) are available as foams, films, and suppositories. The foam is immediately active, but the films and suppositories require 10 to 15 minutes to melt in the vaginal vault. Vaginal sponges (not currently available in the US) also provide spermicide high in the vagina and have the added feature of absorbing the ejaculate. **Use of N-9 offers no protection against STIs.** Frequent N-9 use can cause chemical irritation of the vagina and may increase the risk of HIV transmission due to breaks in the epithelial lining. Spermicides should be used only once in 24 hours. Newer vaginal agents called microbicides are under development to reduce the risk of STIs and pregnancy.

BEHAVIORAL METHODS

Behavioral methods require self-discipline and often involve considerable time to master the techniques and collect information needed to make the method successful. **In natural family planning, a variety of methods, including basal body temperature, cer-**

vical mucus changes, and fertility monitors, are used to calculate a woman's fertile days each cycle. In **periodic abstinence** or natural family planing, couples avoid intercourse during the at-risk days, while in the **fertility awareness method,** couples use another method (usually condoms) during the woman's fertile days. The **Standard Days Method** uses an inexpensive necklace of colored beads **(Cycle-Beads)** to help women with 26- to 32-day menstrual cycles recognize the 12 days each month that they are potentially fertile. Newer tests and hand-held computer units are under development to more accurately determine an individual woman's fertile days.

Lactational amenorrhea can be used for the first 6 months postpartum by women who are exclusively breastfeeding their infants and who are amenorrheic. Pregnancy rates are low (2%), but after 6 months, breastfeeding women need additional protection because ovulation can precede their first menses.

Withdrawal or coitus interruptus requires that the man move his penis away from the woman's genitalia prior to ejaculation. Typical failure rates with withdrawal are comparable to the female barriers or natural family planning.

Other sexual practices that avoid genital contact reduce the risk of pregnancy. The range of practices is quite extensive, but the most common include oral genital stimulation and masturbation (either mutual or solo). Although these practices reduce the risk of pregnancy, some of them may not eliminate STI risks.

EMERGENCY CONTRACEPTION

One of the most important innovations in contraception has been the development of products specifically intended for postcoital contraception Approximately half of unintended pregnancies in the US occur in women not using contraceptives. These women and women who do not use contraception are candidates for emergency contraception (EC). **Two dedicated hormonal products are available in the US for EC: high-dose levonorgestrel (Plan B) and high-dose combined estrogen/progestin pills (Preven).** Labeling for each product requires two doses of pills to be taken 12 hours apart, starting as soon as possible after exposure. A more recent study of the levonorgestrel pills (Plan B) has demonstrated that combining the two pills in a single dose is just as effective.

It is recommended that emergency contraception be started within the first 72 hours, although there is still some benefit if it is started within 120 hours. **If the first dose of levonorgestrel pills is taken within the first 12 hours after exposure, the pregnancy rate is 0.5%,** whereas if the first dose is started 60 to 72 hours after exposure, the pregnancy rate increases to 4%. Therefore, physicians should provide women with EC in advance so that it is readily available when the need arises. Emergency contraception is not an abortifacient, but it has no teratogenic effect if inadvertently administered during pregnancy.

The levonorgestrel pills cause fewer side effects. Because virtually every woman can use them, most major medical organizations have recommended that levonorgestrel EC be made available over the counter. Various combinations of routine OCs can be offered if neither of the dedicated products is available (Table 27-5).

STERILIZATION

Permanent sterilization is the most common method of birth control used by US women over 30 years of age. Rates of sterilization in this country have stabilized in recent years, but the techniques used have changed, as has the ratio of male and female sterilizations.

Vasectomy (interruption of the vas deferens) can be done under local anesthesia in an office setting ("no scalpel" vasectomy) or as an outpatient surgical procedure using more conventional techniques. Infection and hematoma rates are lower with the former technique. No data are available about long-term efficacy

Table 27-5. Some prescription OCs that may be used for emergency contraception (EC)*	
Brand	Dose
Alesse	5 pink tablets
Levlen	4 light orange tablets
Lo/ovral	4 white tablets
Nordette	4 light orange tablets
Ovral	2 white tablets
Tri Levlen	4 light yellow tablets
Triphasil	4 light yellow tablets

*First dose within 72 hours of exposure (most effective within 24 hours) and same dose repeated in 12 hours.

of vasectomy. **Once a man has achieved azoospermia after 6 to 10 ejaculations after the procedure, he is considered sterile. There are no long-term hormonal, metabolic, or autoimmune effects** associated with vasectomy. Reversibility rates can approach 60% but decline over time.

Fallopian tube procedures are most commonly used for female sterilization (Table 27-6), although hysterectomy performed for other indications also sterilizes a woman. Tubal ligation can be done through a mini-laparotomy incision or it can be accomplished via the laparoscope. Usually, mini-laparotomy techniques with suture ligation and interruption of the tube (the Pomeroy technique, Figure 27-2) are performed through a small subumbilical incision immediately postpartum, when the fundus is just below the umbilicus. Laparoscopic approaches are usually performed as interval procedures (>6 weeks postpartum) in nonpregnant women when the woman's uterus lies in the pelvis. The fallopian tubes can be interrupted with cautery, clips, or rings (Figure 27-3).

Reversibility of the procedure varies by technique used and by the amount of the tube destroyed by the initial procedure. **The range of success of reversibility varies from 30% to 70%.** The convenience of tubal ligation is obvious, but the cost and the surgical and anesthetic risks (e.g., hemorrhage, infection, damage to intraperitoneal structures, and even death) need to be considered. Ten-year follow-up studies demonstrate that all sterilization methods are less effective in younger women compared to older women (up to 5.4% failure rates in women <28 years old), but that **postpartum sterilization procedures have the lowest 10-year failure rates.** Long-term complication rates are low—neither dysmenorrhea nor menstrual blood loss increases with sterilization. However, because at least 6% to 10% of women regret having been sterilized, it is critical to encourage women to consider all their reversible options prior to deciding to be sterilized.

Recently, transcervical tubal occlusion procedures have been developed to introduce occluding/fibrosing elements into the tubes hysteroscopically (Essure). Other medical approaches, with quinacrine placed into the endometrial cavity to destroy tubal epithelium, have been used to sterilize women. These approaches are not currently available in the US.

Table 27-6. Methods of tubal sterilization

Surgical Approach	Technique	Surgical Procedure
Laparotomy	Pomeroy	Ligature around a "knuckle" (or loop) of tube; excision distally
	Madlener	Crushing and ligature of loop of tube
	Irving	Double ligation, excision between; proximal end buried in myometrium; distal end buried in broad ligament
	Uchida	Tubal serosa stripped from muscular coat; tubal segment excised; proximal end ligated and buried in broad ligament
	Fimbriectomy	Ligation of distal end of tube and mesosalpinx; excision of fimbriated end
Laparoscopy	Electrocoagulation	Electrical "burn" of two adjacent segments with/without transection
	Falope ring	Loop of tube drawn into applicator tube; plastic ring placed around both limbs of loop
	Hulka clip	Plastic crushing clip placed across tube (not a loop); kept closed by steel spring
	Filshie clip	Titanium clip placed across the tube; associated with increased risk of infection
Minilaparotomy	Pomeroy ligation; electrocauterization	
Posterior colpotomy	Falope ring; Pomeroy ligation; Hulka clip	
Hysteroscopy	Insertion of tubal plug; electrocoagulation; chemical scarification	Cannulation of internal tubal ostia via a transcervical approach

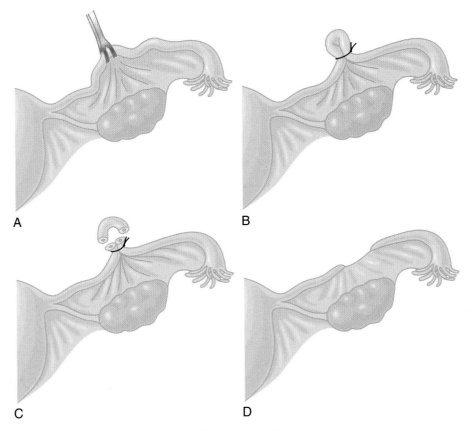

Figure 27-2. Pomeroy method of tubal ligation. *A,* Tube is grasped with Babcock forceps. *B,* A loop is ligated. *C,* The loop is excised. *D,* Several months later, the fibrosed ends of the tube separate.

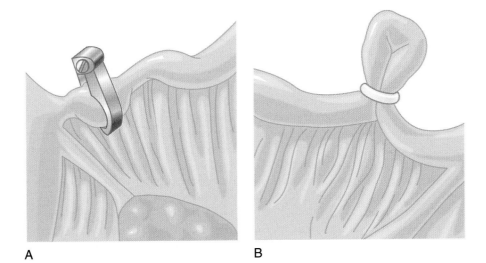

Figure 27-3. Tubal occlusion with *(A)* the Hulka clip and *(B)* the Falope ring. Cautery procedures use electric energy to destroy portions of each fallopian tube.

ABORTION

Abortion is the interruption (spontaneous or induced) of an established pregnancy before 20 weeks' gestational age. The term "miscarriage" is usually used by the lay public to describe the spontaneous loss. "Elective" or "therapeutic" abortions are terms used to describe induced pregnancy termination.

Under the 1963 *Roe v. Wade* US Supreme Court decision, induced abortion is a legal procedure until fetal "viability" is achieved, usually described as 24 weeks' gestational age unless a fetal anomaly inconsistent with extrauterine life is identified to permit later pregnancy interruption. Maternal mortality rates decrease significantly whenever abortion is legalized and provided by medically trained personnel. Tragically, UNICEF estimates that worldwide, 80,000 women die each year because of abortions, which are usually performed under desperate and unsanitary conditions.

Every woman who tests positive for an unplanned pregnancy needs to be made aware of all of her options, including continuing the pregnancy, abortion, and adoption. Decisions in these areas are extremely difficult and personal. In some states, women are required to wait 24 hours between the time consent is obtained and the time that the pregnancy termination can be performed. In some states, a teen's parental notification/approval is required prior to abortion. Access to abortion services may be difficult because over half of the counties in the US have no abortion providers.

Early in pregnancy (<49 days), both medical and surgical procedures can be offered. Mifepristone (an antiprogestin) can be administered and followed later by misoprostol (a prostaglandin) to induce uterine contractions to expel the products of conception. This approach has proven to be effective (96%) and safe. Other agents, such as methotrexate, can be used to induce abortion, but methotrexate generally requires a longer time to complete the process.

Manual vacuum aspiration is more than 99% effective in early pregnancy (<8 weeks from last menstrual period [LMP]). After that date, suction curettage can be used to evacuate the uterine contents after cervical dilation has been achieved with misoprostol or laminaria (Figure 27-4). These procedures can be performed under either local anesthesia (paracervical block) or with awake sedation. They all have

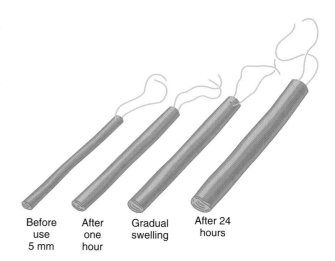

Before use 5 mm   After one hour   Gradual swelling   After 24 hours

Figure 27-4. Laminaria tents (osmotic dilators) used to gradually dilate a closed cervix.

very low complication rates, but the patient must understand the risk of hemorrhage, infection, uterine perforation, retained products of conception, and anesthetic complications. **In general, early pregnancy termination is medically safer than continuing the pregnancy or undergoing tonsillectomy.** There are no long-term adverse effects on reproductive health.

Second trimester abortions are generally performed because prenatal diagnosis has revealed a serious genetic abnormality or intrauterine fetal demise. Here, the role of medical abortion has been pivotal. **Antiprogestin or prostaglandin intravaginal suppositories are used to induce contractions, and the fetus is delivered vaginally.** Occasionally, follow-up curettage may be needed to remove an undelivered placenta. Some patients prefer surgical procedures such as dilation and evacuation (D&E) for elective termination, or this surgery may be needed to treat women with infected pregnancies (septic abortions). Surgical procedures beyond 90 days of gestation require more technical training and experience and have a higher complication rate.

Pregnancy loss under any circumstances (whether the pregnancy is desired or not) creates significant psychologic stress. Women often proceed through the same grieving steps as do people facing other significant losses. In addition, sometimes the approbation of their support system members can isolate women facing this crisis and complicate their recovery process. Empathy and understanding are important attributes of caregivers. **Although early abortion is an extremely safe procedure from a maternal medical safety perspective, most experts and patients would agree that pregnancy prevention is clearly preferable to pregnancy termination.**

Suggested Reading

Hatcher RA, Nelson AL, Zieman M, et al: A Pocket Guide to Managing Contraception, 6th ed. Tiger, GA, Bridging The Gap Foundation, 2003.

Hatcher RA, Trussell J, Stewart F, et al: Contraceptive Technology, 17th ed. New York, Ardent Media, 1998.

Speroff L, Darney PD: A Clinical Guide for Contraception, 3rd ed. Baltimore, MD, Lippincott Williams & Wilkins, 2001.

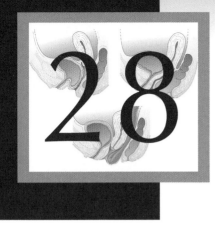

Human Sexuality

Catherine Marin DeUgarte and Martha J. Baird

The development of sexuality precedes puberty, but gender identity is sometimes not determined until age 3 or 4. Children that are unable to identify with the assigned gender at birth have **Gender identity disorder** (GID) or transgender issues later in life. **The diagnosis of GID can be made in an individual where there is a strong and persistent cross gender identity and a discomfort about the assigned gender.**

During puberty, many teens begin exploring their bodies as well as experiencing sexual activity with others. Many teens, especially males, have early intercourse and are not well educated about contraception, the risks of pregnancy or sexually transmitted diseases (STDs). Young girls often have intercourse because of feelings of love, while boys are usually driven by curiosity. It is especially important for physicians to discuss sexuality with teens and to educate them about contraception and STD prevention. Teens are often apprehensive about discussing these issues and may fear parental discovery. They are usually more receptive to "open-ended" questions.

The early reproductive years are often the time when sexuality is explored and reproduction or its prevention becomes a priority. Infertility may be an issue in this age group and many emotions may be evoked in infertile patients often leading to sexual problems.

With increasing age and especially after menopause, the frequency and satisfaction with intercourse may decline. Menopause is often accompanied by a significant decrease in estrogen production which in turn results in changes in the thickness and pliability of the vaginal epithelium and the acidity of the vaginal secretions. These changes may lead to decreased vaginal lubrication which predisposes women to infections and dyspareunia as well as more difficulty in achieving orgasm. In many older couples, the frequency of intercourse declines because of the male partner's inability to have erections. Illnesses or increased use of medications may also affect sexual functioning.

MODES OF SEXUAL EXPRESSION

Heterosexuals are individuals who engage in sexual activity with the opposite sex. Most individuals engage in heterosexual behavior, which is considered "normal." **Homosexuals are those who engage in sexual activities with members of the same sex.** Men who are homosexual are referred to as gay, and homosexual women are addressed as gay or lesbian. While gay men tend to engage in more physical relationships and may have multiple partners, lesbians are generally inclined to be monogamous. The reported incidence of homosexuality ranges from 6% to 20% in men and 3% to 18% in women. Several theories on homosexuality have been proposed including a genetic predisposition, the maternal use of prenatal hormones, and other environmental factors. A multifactorial cause is likely. **Many homosexuals feel a need to conceal their sexuality for fear of loss of family, friends, or jobs.** Familiarity with homosexuals has been shown to decrease the prejudice and recently many homosexuals have "come out," revealing their identities and demanding equal rights.

Bisexuals are those who engage in sexual activity with both men and women either concomitantly or at different phases of their life. The reported incidence of bisexuality is 1% to 7% of men and 1% to 2% of women, although many individuals briefly explore same sex activity at one time in their life and do not consider themselves bisexual.

Transgender or transsexual individuals are often confused with homosexuals. **They have a strong belief from childhood that they were born into a body with the wrong sex. Most are heterosexual to their identified gender** (i.e., men who believe they are women are attracted to men) and few are homosexual. Children with ambiguous genitalia who are assigned a particular gender may later show regret toward their assignment. Some experts recommend that these children be given a name that is appropriate to both genders to allow them to decide their gender later in life. Female-to-male transsexuals (FTM) are women that grow up as "tomboys" and often cross-dress. Male-to-female transsexuals (MTF) are men that grow up dressing as women. Transgender surgery is difficult to perform, especially FTM, and it is only performed in certain areas of the United States and the world. Box 28-1 lists variations in sexual preferences along with their definitions.

SEX WORKERS

Sex workers (often known as prostitutes or call girls) are individuals, usually women, who exchange sexual services for cash or other items of value. Prostitution is one of the world's oldest professions and is often done for economic survival, maintaining a drug habit, or for someone else's benefit. Prostitution is illegal in most countries.

THE SEXUAL RESPONSE CYCLE

The sexual response cycle was fully described by **Masters and Johnson** in 1966. Although other modifications have been published, it remains the classic description of human sexual response. The female cycle is divided into four phases while in men five phases are described.

FEMALE SEXUAL RESPONSE CYCLE
1. The Excitement Phase

This phase starts with physical or psychologic stimulation and may last minutes or hours. There is a chest sex flush accompanied with erect nipples and enlarged breasts. The uterus elevates and vaginal lubrication begins. The clitoris and labia enlarge and there is increased heart rate and blood pressure. Most muscles become tense (Figure 28-1).

2. The Plateau Phase

During this phase the breasts continue to enlarge and the clitoris may elevate and retract under its hood. The

---

Box 28-1. Sexual variations (paraphylias) and their definitions

Transvestism: Sexual excitement or gratification from wearing clothing of and enacting the opposite sex

Fetishism: Sexual excitement or gratification associated with an inanimate object (i.e., underwear) or body part (i.e., feet)

Pedophilia: Sexual excitement or gratification from children

Zoophylia: Sexual excitement or gratification through intercourse with animals

Exhibitionism: Sexual excitement or gratification from exposing one's body, especially the genitals

Voyeurism: Sexual excitement or gratification from watching others

Masochism: Sexual excitement or gratification from enduring physical or physiologic pain; may be self-inflicted

Sadism: Sexual excitement or gratification from inflicting physical or physiologic pain onto others; also cruelty not associated with sexual behaviors

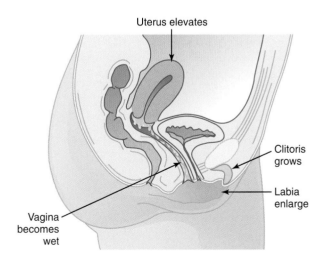

Figure 28-1. Female sexual response cycle: The excitement phase.

Bartholin's glands may secrete fluid near the vaginal opening and there is tenting of the uterus to allow easier sperm passage. The vagina and labia enlarge and there is increased blood pressure, heart rate, respiratory rate, and muscle tension (Figure 28-2).

3. The Orgasmic Phase

During this phase there is release of sexual tension. The orgasmic phase is possible without actual physical stimulation. This phase is concentrated in the clitoris, vagina, and uterus. There is contraction of vaginal, uterine, lower abdominal, and anal muscles. Usually there are 5 to 12 synchronized contractions 1 second apart. The first few contractions are the strongest and the closest together. Blood pressure, heart rate, and respiratory rate peak in this phase and there is usually loss of voluntary muscle tone (e.g., most women curl their toes at orgasm). Women can have multiple orgasms before they enter the resolution phase (Figure 28-3).

4. The Resolution Phase

During this phase the nipples and breasts decrease in size and the vagina, clitoris and uterus return to normal size. The sex flush disappears and the blood pressure, heart rate, and respiratory rate also return to normal (Figure 28-4).

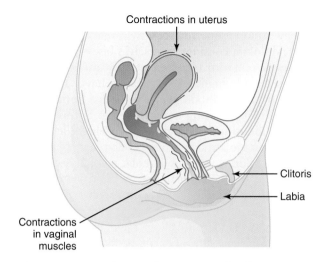

Figure 28-3. Female sexual response cycle: The orgasmic phase.

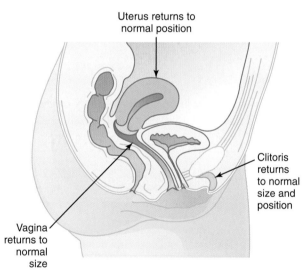

Figure 28-4. Female sexual response cycle: The resolution phase.

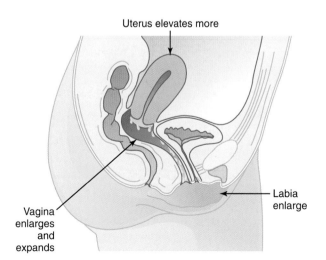

Figure 28-2. Female sexual response cycle: The plateau phase.

MALE SEXUAL RESPONSE CYCLE
1. The Excitement Phase

This phase begins with physical or psychologic stimulation and may last minutes or hours. The nipples and penis become erect and there is increased heart rate and blood pressure. The muscles become tense and there is blood pooling in the extremities with vasocongestion in the penis and scrotum with testicular swelling and elevation (Figure 28-5).

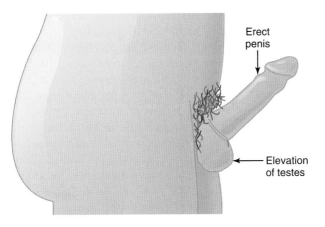

Figure 28-5. Male sexual response cycle: The excitement phase.

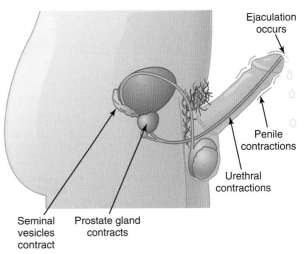

Figure 28-7. Male sexual response cycle: The orgasmic phase.

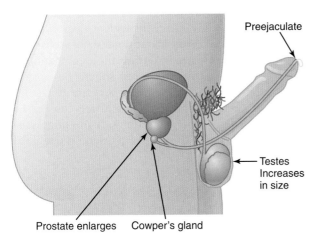

Figure 28-6. Male sexual response cycle: The plateau phase.

2. The Plateau Phase

The testicles enlarge by 50%, and the prostate and penis also enlarge. There is increased blood flow and the bulbourethral or Cowper's gland secretes preejaculatory fluid, which may contain sperm. There is increased blood pressure, heart rate, respiratory rate, and muscle tension. There is generally chest sex flushing (Figure 28-6).

3. The Orgasmic Phase

During the orgasmic phase there is release of sexual tension; this phase is possible without actual physical stimulation. There are rhythmic contractions of the seminal vesicles, vas deferens, and prostate. The ejaculatory ducts push semen into the urethra, and ejaculation occurs with urethral contractions. The first few contractions are the strongest and the closest together. During this phase the anal sphincter contracts. The **"point of imminence"** occurs a few seconds prior to ejaculation and refers to the point when a man knows an orgasm is inevitable (Figure 28-7).

4. The Resolution Phase

In the resolution phase the genitals and penis decrease in size and return to a flaccid state. The testes descend and the sex flush disappears. The blood pressure, heart rate, and respiratory rate return to normal (Figure 28-8).

5. The Refractory Phase

The refractory phase occurs only in men. Because of this phase, men are not able to have multiple orgasms. During this phase, no amount of stimulation will cause another ejaculation. This phase lasts minutes in young men and hours to days in older men.

The similarity between the male and female cycles is apparent. Although the average time spent in each phase may differ (due primarily to learned behaviors), the elements of each cycle are the same. Because different neuronal circuits mediate each of these phases,

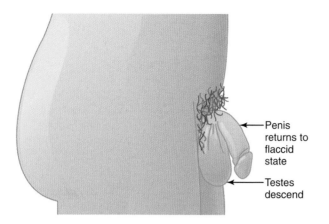

Penis returns to flaccid state

Testes descend

Figure 28-8. Male sexual response cycle: The resolution phase.

sexual dysfunction may affect some phases without affecting the others.

ASSESSMENT AND EVALUATION OF SEXUAL DYSFUNCTION

The assessment of sexual functioning should be an integral part of a complete medical evaluation, especially for the obstetrician-gynecologist. Skills for taking a sexual history are often overlooked in medical schools and sometimes ignored by physicians. It is more difficult to inquire about a patient's sexuality if the physician is uncomfortable with the topic or is judgmental about sexual orientation. Clinicians may also be concerned about a patient's answers, not knowing what to say or do if a history of sexual trauma is revealed. They may also feel untrained to deal with problems and solutions for sexual inadequacies. Often they worry that the patients will misunderstand or be offended by the questions.

In taking a history, it is helpful to follow a routine pattern of questioning: (1) age of menarche, (2) menstrual patterns, (3) pregnancy history, (4) contraception use, (5) STD prevention, (6) number of sexual partners, (7) sexual orientation and (8) difficulties with sexual relations. Domestic violence and sexual abuse questions can then follow. Some sample questions may include the following:

"Are you currently sexually active and if so, with men, women, or both?"

"Are you having any difficulties with sexual relations?"

"Have you ever been in a situation where you had unwanted or harmful sexual activity?"

There are several factors that may affect taking a sexual history. The physician's sexuality may influence the process. A gay physician may be more thorough or may be afraid to inquire about a patient's sexual orientation. At times, clinicians of both sexes may find themselves attracted to patients. In these instances, acceptance of the feelings as normal is appropriate as long as behavior is unaffected and a professional relationship is maintained. Some patients may be seductive or even make sexual advances. In such cases, the physician must make it clear to the patient that the relationship is professional and not personal.

Appropriate boundaries of behavior during a physical examination must be maintained, and caution should be used with inappropriate language or engaging in overly friendly conversations. Clinicians should realize that the patient might feel uncomfortable, especially with a doctor of the opposite sex, and fearful about potentially embarrassing discoveries, especially during the examination of the breasts and genitals. Drapes should be used to cover all the private body parts that are not being examined, and the physician should tell the patient what he or she is doing at all times. **A nursing assistant or chaperone should be present during the examination.**

FEMALE SEXUAL DYSFUNCTION

Sexual dysfunction is categorized by the Sexual Function Health Council of the American Foundation of Urologic Disease (AFUD) by failure of one or more of the phases of the sexual response cycle involving desire, arousal, or orgasm. Sexual dysfunction also includes pain disorders (Box 28-2).

Female sexual dysfunction (FSD) is a common condition affecting 30% to 65% of American women. Prevalence often increases with age. Sexual dysfunction can be subdivided into three different categories, depending on whether it is **primary** (realistic sexual expectations have never been met under any circumstances), **secondary** (all phases have functioned in the past, but one or more no longer does), **or situational** (the response cycle functions under some circumstances, but not others). When a patient complains of hypoactive sexual desire, it is important to determine what her preferences are in contrast to those of her partner. A woman who desires intercourse twice a week may be perfectly normal but not func-

Box 28-2. American foundation of urologic disease (AFUD) consensus classification of female sexual dysfunction

I.   **Sexual Desire Disorders***
   A. Hypoactive sexual desire disorder
   B. Sexual aversion disorder
II. **Sexual Arousal Disorders***
III. **Orgasmic Disorder***
IV. **Sexual Pain Disorders***
   A. Dyspareunia
   B. Vaginismus
   C. Other sexual pain disorders

*Each disorder can be subtyped as lifelong versus acquired, generalized versus situational and by origin (organic, psychogenic, mixed, or unknown).

tioning well in a relationship in which her partner desires coitus daily. Sexual dysfunction can occur in homosexual or heterosexual relationships, or even in masturbatory situations.

SEXUAL FUNCTION DISORDERS
DESIRE PHASE DISORDERS

Sexual desire appears to be an appetite similar to hunger, controlled by a dopamine-sensitive excitatory center, in balance with a serotonin (5-hydroxytryptamine)-sensitive inhibitory center. **In both males and females, testosterone appears to be the hormone responsible for initially programming these centers during gestation and for maintaining their threshold of response.** Stimulation and ablation experiments in cats and other mammalian species have located these centers within the limbic system, with significant nuclei in the hypothalamic and preoptic regions. For a woman, desire results from a complex of biologic inputs, as well as psychologic inputs, including her feelings about her partner.

Disorders of sexual desire include hypoactive sexual desire disorder and sexual aversion disorder. Lack of desire involves a decrease or absence of fantasy. **Sexual aversion disorder** may result from prior sex-associated trauma and personal aversion. Often in established relationships, decreased desire may result from sexual activity becoming too routine. Also, lack of privacy or external stresses, especially stress in the relationship, may initiate this disorder. Another important category of causes of hypoactive desire arises in the context of unrelated disease.

Women may fear sex with a partner who has had a heart attack or may have decreased desire themselves following a mastectomy or hysterectomy.

AROUSAL PHASE DISORDERS

Sexual arousal disorder is defined as the inability to attain or maintain sufficient sexual excitement, expressed as a lack of subjective excitement or somatic response such as genital lubrication. Estrogen is the hormone responsible for maintaining the vaginal epithelium and allowing transudation and lubrication to occur. Its deficiency (with breastfeeding or after menopause) is by far the most common cause of excitement phase dysfunction in women. Extragenital changes during the excitement phase include an increase in heart rate and blood pressure; enhanced muscle tension throughout the body; an increase in breast size, nipple erection, and engorgement of the surrounding areolae; and a sex flush. The latter is an erythematous morbilliform skin change over the chest, neck, and face that occurs to a noticeable degree in 75% of women. Some women do not recognize these symptoms as excitement and may experience difficulty and even failure on that basis.

ORGASMIC PHASE DISORDERS

During the orgasmic phase, a series of reflex clonic contractions of the levator sling and related genital musculature occur, mediated primarily via the sympathetic nervous system and occurring at the same 0.8 to 1 second intervals as seen in male ejaculation. Extragenital reactions during orgasm include contraction of muscle groups throughout the body (including the uterus), maximal intensity of the sex flush, and maximal elevations of heart rate, blood pressure, and respiratory rate.

Orgasmic disorder is characterized by difficulty with or absence of attaining orgasm following sufficient sexual stimulation and arousal. Many times anorgasmia is situational. Many women experience orgasm only with manual or oral clitoral stimulation but not with penile thrusting alone. If they are willing to increase direct clitoral stimulation before, during, or after penile penetration, they may achieve a wholly satisfactory sexual adaptation. Women who have been orgasmic in the past but have lost that capacity should be carefully screened for organic or pharmacologic causes, and changes in their relationship or relationships should be carefully explored.

Most women with primary anorgasmia have usually had minimal or no effective stimulation from self or partner. These patients should be encouraged to learn how to achieve orgasm through self-stimulation and then to share this new information with their partners. Increasing the intensity of stimulation should increase the intensity of response.

SEXUAL PAIN DISORDERS

Dyspareunia is genital pain associated with sexual intercourse. It is helpful to categorize dyspareunia into three groups for easier diagnosis and treatment: (1) **pain with intromission** (often due to vestibulitis, vaginismus, fissures, or other vulvar lesions), (2) **mid-vaginal pain** (often due to lack of lubrication, surgical scars, or urethral diverticulosis) and (3) **deep thrust dyspareunia** (often due to endometriosis, interstitial cystitis, pelvic adhesions, or neoplasms).

Vaginismus is defined as severe pain and/or involuntary spasm of the distal vaginal and pelvic floor muscles during attempted penetration. Examination reveals no organic pathologic condition, but the pubococcygeal muscles are tight, and vaginal penetration by speculum or examining finger is painful and difficult, if not impossible Often affected women harbor fantasies about the inadequacy of their vaginas to accommodate a speculum or penis and fear that penetration will damage them. These women respond remarkably well to education and reassurance. Others may have been traumatized by early sexual or other abuse and require more intensive psychologic therapy. One important issue is whether they are able and motivated to participate with their partners in a stepwise desensitization program. This involves the slow, gentle vaginal insertion of dilators of gradually increasing size under the patient's own control. Once sufficient progress has been made, the partner's fingers and, ultimately, his penis may be substituted for the dilators. Alleviation of the problem is usually accomplished in 3 to 6 months.

ETIOLOGY OF SEXUAL DYSFUNCTION

As a general rule, primary problems are predominantly psychogenic and tend to be of longer duration. Secondary problems are often associated with the onset of a disease process or the use of a pharmacologic agent. If such an association cannot be established, deterioration in the patient's relationship or some other chronologically related change in the patient's life experience should be sought. It is important to consider psychologic causes, such as depression or anxiety; organic causes, such as atherosclerosis, diabetes, or genital infections; and pharmacologic causes (Box 28-3). Factors initiating a problem may be different from those maintaining it. For example, drugs may precipitate a problem, but if anxiety and fear of failure sustain the difficulty, discontinuation of the drug may not rectify the problem.

MANAGEMENT OF SEXUAL DYSFUNCTION

Hormone therapy is valuable in a limited number of situations. Estrogen (oral or vaginal application) may improve desire, arousal, and orgasm by decreasing dyspareunia due to vaginal atrophy. **Testosterone improves desire and arousal, but should be used only in hypoandrogenic women, especially those after surgical menopause.** Sildenafil (Viagra), used mostly in men with erectile dysfunction, inhibits cyclic guanosine monophosphate (cGMP) breakdown (cGMP functions as a messenger in the nitric oxide mediated–relaxation of genital smooth muscle), therefore increasing clitoral and vaginal smooth muscle relaxation as well as improving lubrication. **The use of sildenafil in women has not,** however, **been as effective as in men.** Other agents under investigation are L-arginine, phentolamine, and prostaglandin E1.

A clitoral vacuum device (the EROS-CTD) has been approved by the FDA and is said to improve clitoral blood flow and engorgement. **Fantasy therapy is helpful for hypoactive desire** and **sensate focusing therapy is helpful for excitement phase defects.**

Box 28-3. Some drugs that can diminish sexual function in women
Antihypertensive agents: Reserpine, propranolol, methyldopa, atenolol, spironolactone Antidepressant medications: Tricyclics or selective serotonin reuptake inhibitors (SSRIs) Hypnotic agents: Alcohol, barbiturates, tranquilizers or diazepam Narcotics: Heroin or methadone Antipsychotic agents: Fluphenazine or chlorpromazine Stimulants: Cocaine or amphetamines Hallucinogens: Lysergic acid (LSD) or mescaline Diuretics: Acetazolamide

TREATMENT SUCCESS

As a group, orgasmic difficulties seem to respond to treatment most readily. For example, primary orgasmic difficulties may be resolved by means of guided masturbatory training and cognitive behavioral sex therapy. Secondary anorgasmia is more often associated with emotional or psychiatric disorders and relationship issues, so the treatment response may be less positive. **Excitement phase dysfunctions do not have such positive outcomes, although problems with lubrication can nearly always be resolved satisfactorily. Lack of desire is the most resistant to treatment.** Persons with little desire often have little internal motivation to seek more frequent sexual activity or to pursue help. Fewer than 50% of such patients show definite improvement. When the relationship is poor, behavioral approaches directed toward the sexual problem are rarely successful. In contrast to erectile disorder and premature ejaculation, studies using medical and pharmacologic interventions for female arousal or orgasmic disorders are still ongoing but show some promise.

Suggested Reading

Berman JR, Goldstein I: Female sexual dysfunction. Urol Clin North Am 28:405–416, 2001.

Copland LJ, Jarrell JF: Textbook of Gynecology. Philadelphia, WB Saunders, 2000.

Holmes KK, Sparling PF: Sexually Transmitted Diseases. New York, McGraw-Hill, 1999.

Masters WH, Johnson VE: Human Sexual Response. Boston, Little, Brown & Company, 1986.

Yadav J, Gennarelli LA, Ratakonda U: Female sexuality and common sexual dysfunctions: Evaluation and management in a primary care setting. Prim Care Update Ob Gyn 8:5–11, 2001.

29 Domestic Violence and Sexual Assault

Catherine Marin DeUgarte

DOMESTIC VIOLENCE

Domestic violence is defined as an intentional violent or controlling behavior by a person who is in an intimate or close relationship with the victim. Domestic violence can include verbal abuse, intimidation, social isolation, and physical assault, such as a punch, a kick, a threat, a severe beating, an act of sexual assault, or even murder. It occurs in every age group, in all ethnic groups, in every occupation, and in every socioeconomic group. While most often perpetrated by a man against a woman, domestic violence also occurs in the context of family violence, which can include elder abuse and child abuse. Partner violence can also occur between same-sex partners.

The prevalence of domestic violence is not known, but it is considerable. In one study of women seeking care in an emergency room (ER), 54% of study participants said they had been threatened or injured at some time in their lives by a partner, and 24% said they had been injured by a current partner. One in three women presenting to an ER with injuries has symptoms related to domestic violence. More than 20% of violent crimes against women and 30% of female murders are committed by intimate partners. It is estimated that nearly 500,000 elderly persons in domestic settings in the United States are abused or neglected. Seventy percent of such elder abuse is perpetrated by a family member.

The abuser often provides for and is in love with the victim, making it difficult for the victim to seek help. Other obstacles to leaving the abuser include: (1) fear, (2) economic support, (3) social isolation, (4) feelings of failure, (5) promises of change, and (6) previously unanswered calls for help. It is important to understand the cycle of violence that exists in these relationships and how that might affect a woman's ability to leave her situation (Figure 29-1).

Domestic violence should be suspected if any of the following occurs: injury to torso, face, or genitals; defensive injuries (abdomen or breasts for pregnant women); injuries that are bilateral, multiple, unexplained or inconsistent with the history; delay between injury and arrival to hospital; multiple ER visits; chronic pain, especially chronic headaches, abdominal pain, or back pain; sleep or appetite complaints; psychologic distress (e.g., depression); rape/sexual assault; or a partner in the room who is reluctant to leave or answers all the questions for the patient.

ASSESSING THE LIKELIHOOD OF DOMESTIC VIOLENCE

It may be difficult for health care providers to bring up the topic of possible domestic violence. Because of the alarming frequency of this problem, however, it is important to ask all women, when alone with them, if they feel safe in their own home. Depending on the circumstances and if there is any suspicion of physical abuse, they should be asked directly if a partner has hit, kicked, hurt, or ever threatened them. If a positive response is obtained, it is important to document any physical findings. Pictures and drawings should be used.

It is important to tell the victim that she is not alone, that help is available to her, and that her partner's behavior is unacceptable. In addition to the need to comply with any reporting requirements (some states mandate reporting to appropriate

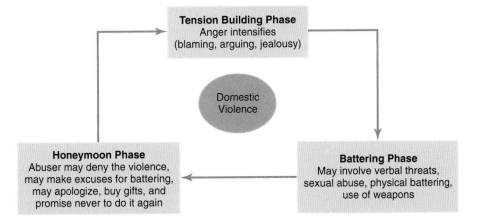

Figure 29-1. Cycle of violence. *From American College of Obstetricians and Gynecologists (ACOG): Domestic violence. Educational Bulletin No. 257. Washington, DC, ACOG, December 1999.*

authorities if there are acute injuries), social workers and other professionals should be consulted. The patient should be provided with hotline information (see Box 29-1) that she may wish to keep in a safe place such as in her shoes. In addition, health care providers should be prepared to provide a referral for her partner to seek help as a "batterer" or perpetrator of domestic violence.

SEXUAL ASSAULT AND RAPE

Sexual assault and rape have different technical or legal definitions depending on the state or country involved. However, any sexual act performed on a person without his/her consent is classified as sexual assault. Sexual assault includes any unwanted genital, anal, or oral penetration by a part of the attacker's body or by any object. Rape, on the other hand, is generally a violent attack that may or may not stem from the perpetrator's sexual desire. Very often, the perpetrator uses sex as a means to control another person. Whatever the rapist's intent, rape is definitely not a welcomed sexual experience for the victim. During any act of rape, the victim's predominant feeling is one of fear for her life or fear of mutilation.

Women of all ages, ethnicities, and socioeconomic groups can be victims of sexual assault, although the very young, the mentally and physically disabled and the elderly are more vulnerable. **Nearly 75% of assaults are perpetrated by someone known to the victim,** such as husbands (marital rape), boyfriends (date rape), fathers (incest), mothers' boyfriends, other relatives, or work associates. The American Medical Association (AMA) reports that 20% of women under 21 years of age have been sexually assaulted. Other estimates are that 41% of women (of all ages) have been victims of actual or attempted sexual assault and 50% of these have been victims more than once. **Death occurs in about 1% of sexual assaults (including rapes), and serious injury occurs in 4%.**

MEDICAL CARE FOR SEXUAL ASSAULT

The medical consultation should proceed only after a supportive, caring relationship has been established. The adult or adolescent woman should be actively involved in the consultation so that she may regain a feeling of control over what has and is happening to her. **The purposes of the consultation are to provide her acute medical care, to gather evidence, and to transition her into the long-term care she will need for psychologic recovery.** These objectives should be explained to her, and she should be allowed to dictate the pace of the questioning and the order of the examination.

During the interview and examination phases, a chaperone and/or patient advocate should be present. Careful attention must be paid to the rules governing the chain of evidence to maintain the legal integrity and utility of all the specimens, photos, and other materials collected. The woman should be asked about the detailed specifics of her assault in order to direct the collection of needed evidence and to address any risk of injury or infection. Information about her recent menstrual history, use of medications, recent immunizations, contraceptive use, and past medical and surgical history is important.

A thorough physical examination is needed to evaluate possible injuries **because 40% of all women who are sexually assaulted sustain injuries.** If possible, photographs or sketches should be obtained of the injured areas. The Centers for Disease Control (CDC) recommend routine testing for gonorrhea and chlamydia from specimens collected from any site of penetration or attempted penetration. Wet mount and culture for trichomonas are routine, and a microscopic evaluation for bacterial vaginosis and candidiasis is prudent in a woman with a vaginal discharge. Serum tests for human immunodeficiency virus (HIV), hepatitis B, and syphilis are needed for baseline evaluation.

Prophylaxis is suggested as preventive therapy. This includes hepatitis B vaccination (if previously unvaccinated) and appropriate antibiotics for sexually transmitted disease (see Chapter 23). **It is critical to provide any woman at risk for pregnancy with emergency contraception** (see Chapter 27). If prophylaxis for HIV is considered necessary, consultation with an HIV specialist is recommended. Tetanus toxoid should be administered to an unprotected, injured woman.

PSYCHOLOGIC SEQUELAE OF SEXUAL ASSAULT

Sexual assault is almost always associated with both immediate and long-term effects on victims. These effects have been termed the *rape trauma syndrome* and involve the following two phases:

1. **Acute/disorganization phase:** This phase lasts from days to weeks. **Immediately after the experience, victims frequently appear calm, although preoccupied and inattentive.** They are anxious, have difficulty sleeping, and commonly express shock, disbelief, fear, guilt, and shame. The psychologic problems that may result are varied and can mimic those seen in the aftermath of other kinds of traumatic experiences. **Among those expected in the acute phase of adjustment are irritability, tension, anxiety, depression, fatigue, and persistent ruminations.** Somatic symptoms of a general nature may occur, such as headaches or irritable bowel syndrome, or symptoms may be more specific to the reproductive system, such as vaginal irritation or discharge. Behavioral problems, such as overeating and alcohol or substance abuse may also surface, particularly when such problems have been evident in the past The long-term sequelae include changes in lifestyle, the occurrence of disturbing dreams and nightmares, and the persistence of phobic reactions. **Fear persists as the predominant feeling.** These reactions often make it difficult for the victim to concentrate effectively on everyday activities and relationships.

2. **Integration and resolution phase**: During this phase, victims begin to accept the assault, but problems at work or with relationships may persist.

The management of the sexual assault victim in the acute phase influences long-term adjustment. Many rape victims may manifest **posttraumatic stress disorder.** The likelihood of this disorder developing is high, owing to the abrupt nature of the crime, its violence, the passivity and helplessness imposed on the victim, and the high probability of receiving physical as well as psychologic trauma. **The lifetime prevalence of posttraumatic stress disorder in rape victims is approximately 50%.**

In addition to attending to immediate physical and emotional needs, the initial evaluation provides an opportunity to prepare the victim for the long-term psychologic impact of the experience. This preparation is intended to diminish the long-term consequences and to enable the woman to recognize the common psychosocial sequelae when they occur, thus enabling her to seek professional help at an early stage.

Longer-term reactions involve nightmares, phobic reactions, and sexual fears. Stimuli associated with the rape, such as a similar-looking man or similar surroundings, may be associated with flashbacks. Flashbacks may also occur during pelvic examinations Reactions to the sexual assault may result in problems with sexual behavior and functioning. **Loss of libido is a common response to stressful or traumatic circumstances of any kind. Other complaints include vaginismus, impaired vaginal lubrication, and loss of orgasmic capacity.** These problems may be even more likely if the assault occurred at home while the woman was asleep. Preparing the woman for these eventualities can be extremely helpful in preventing sexual dysfunction from developing or persisting. Giving permission for a lower-than-usual sexual drive during the period following the assault may remove some performance anxiety. Explaining how anxiety and stress can inhibit

> **Box 29-1. Key phone numbers for medical professionals and victims**
>
> **National Domestic Violence Hotline:** 1-800-799-SAFE (7233 or 7234) TTY 1-800-787-3224 (hearing impaired)
> **RAINN (Rape, Abuse, Incest National Network) Hotline:** 1-800-656-HOPE
> **National Child Abuse Hotline:** 1-800-4-A-CHILD (1-800-422-4453)
> **Elderly Abuse Hotline:** 1-800-922-2275
> **Disabled Person Abuse Hotline:** 1-800-426-9009

sexual responsiveness and providing ways in which this can be overcome are also important.

AFTERCARE PLANNING

Careful follow-up must be arranged. If the patient used the prophylactic therapies, a return visit is needed in one week to review the initial laboratory results and to monitor her progress. Repeat testing is needed only if the woman is symptomatic. If she did not receive prophylaxis, repeat testing for gonorrhea, chlamydia and trichomonas should be performed in 2 weeks and

for syphilis in 6 weeks. Repeat serum tests for HIV should be performed at 6, 12, and 24 weeks after the assault regardless of whether or nor prophylactic measures were taken.

Before discharging the patient, it is important to ensure that she has a safe place to go and a suitable means of transportation. She should also be given (in writing) the names, addresses, and phone numbers of resources available in the community to meet her medical, legal, and psychosocial needs related to the assault (Box 29-1).

Suggested Readings

American College of Obstetricians and Gynecologists: Sexual assault. Educational Bulletin No. 257. Washington, DC, ACOG, December 1999.

American College of Obstetricians and Gynecologists: Domestic violence. Educational Bulletin No. 257. Washington, DC, ACOG, December 1999.

Centers for Disease Control and Prevention: Sexually transmitted diseases guidelines 2002. MMWR 51(No. RR-6):1–80, 2002.

Guidelines for Treatment of Victims of Sexual Assault. Sacramento, State of California Department of Health Services, 1976.

Martin CA, Warfield MC, Braen ER: Physician's management of the psychological aspects of rape. JAMA 249:501–503, 1983.

30

Breast Disease: A Gynecologic Perspective

Neville F. Hacker

It is important that gynecologists be expert in breast examination, diligent about screening asymptomatic women for breast cancer, familiar with common benign and malignant disorders of the breast, and conversant with the various therapeutic options.

SCREENING OF THE BREAST IN ASYMPTOMATIC WOMEN
SELF-EXAMINATION

Many breast cancers are detected by women themselves, and monthly breast self examination should be promoted. Written information should be supplemented by practical training. There is no solid evidence that breast self examination reduces breast cancer mortality, but it is reasonable to assume that a woman's increased awareness of her own breasts may lead to an earlier diagnosis.

Breast Self-Examination Technique

The patient may be invited to perform the examination after each menstrual period. She should commence the technique in the upright position, carefully inspecting the breasts initially with her arms by her sides and then with her arms raised above her head. She should palpate the supraclavicular and axillary regions for the presence of nodes. The patient should then lie down and systematically palpate each quadrant of the breast against the chest wall, using the flat of her fingers. Finally, she should palpate the areolar areas and then compress the nipples for evidence of secretion.

Breast Examination by Physician

A complete breast examination should be performed by a physician at least annually. The breasts are first inspected with the patient in an upright position. The contour and symmetry are observed, and any skin changes or nipple retraction is noted. **Skin retraction because of tethering to an underlying malignancy may be highlighted by having the patient extend her arms over her head.**

Palpation of the breast, areola, and nipple is performed with the flat of the hand. If any mass is palpated, its fixation to deep tissues should be determined by asking the patient to place her hands over her hips and contract her pectoral muscles. Each axilla is then carefully examined while the patient's arm is supported. The supraclavicular fossae are also palpated for lymphadenopathy. **Following palpation in the upright position, the examination is repeated in the supine position.**

MAMMOGRAPHY

Radiologic examination of the breast is an important component of the screening process carried out in asymptomatic women and should be performed in conjunction with a thorough physical examination. **Densities and fine calcifications constitute suspicious findings, and clinically inapparent malignancies of less than 1 cm in diameter may be detected.**

Mammograms of high quality can be made with about 0.3 cGy or less of radiation, so there is little, if any, risk of this technique causing breast cancer.

In the Breast Cancer Detection Demonstration Project carried out by the American Cancer Society and the National Cancer Institute, **89% of 3557 cancers were correctly identified by mammography, 41.6% of which were not clinically detectable.**

The American Cancer Society recommends annual mammograms starting at age 40 years.

ULTRASONOGRAPHY

Ultrasonography can differentiate cystic from solid masses and may demonstrate solid tissue that is potentially malignant within or adjacent to a cyst. It is also useful for imaging palpable focal masses in women younger than 30 years, reducing the need for x-ray studies in this population.

MAGNETIC RESONANCE IMAGING

Magnetic resonance imaging (MRI) may be a useful adjunct in breast imaging. Reported advantages include improved staging and treatment planning, enhanced evaluation of the augmented breast, better detection of recurrences, and possibly improved screening of high-risk women.

DIAGNOSIS OF BREAST LESIONS

Physiologic nodularity and cyclic tenderness caused by the changing hormonal milieu must be distinguished from benign or malignant pathologic changes. **Definitive diagnosis of breast neoplasms may be made by open biopsy or by fine-needle (22-gauge) aspiration cytology.**

FINE-NEEDLE BIOPSY

Fine-needle aspiration biopsy of the palpably suspicious lump in the breast can be performed in the outpatient clinic. Smears are prepared from the aspirate to allow cytologic evaluation. In experienced hands, the test is both sensitive and specific. **A negative result should never be accepted as definitive when there are clinical or mammographic indications that the lesion may be malignant.** In the presence of a palpable lump, fine-needle aspiration cytology should make it possible to diagnose breast cancer without formal excisional biopsy in about 90% of cases, allowing the subsequent management of the patient to be discussed before operation.

OPEN BREAST BIOPSY

Small masses may undergo **excisional biopsy,** whereas large masses should undergo **incisional biopsy,** or occasionally core-cutting needle biopsy. Absolute indications for open breast biopsy are listed in Box 30-1. Relative indications for breast biopsy include those women with a clinically benign mass but a positive family or personal history of breast cancer, a history of atypical hyperplasia, or an equivocal finding on mammography or cytology.

Open breast biopsy may be performed as an outpatient procedure under local anesthesia or as an inpatient procedure under general anesthesia. Women with large breasts who have small, deeply situated lesions are not good candidates for outpatient biopsies nor are those who have a nonpalpable lesion detected by mammography.

COMMON BENIGN BREAST DISORDERS
FIBROCYSTIC CHANGES

The earlier term *fibrocystic disease* **has little clinical value, and the term was abandoned by the College of American Pathologists in 1985.** Lesions formerly grouped together under the designation of fibrocystic disease represent a pathologically heterogeneous group of diseases that can be divided into three separate histologic categories: nonproliferative lesions, proliferative lesions (hyperplasia) without atypia, and atypical hyperplasias.

HYPERPLASIA

Hyperplasia is the most common benign breast disorder and is present in about 50% of women. Histologically, the hyperplastic changes may involve any or all of the breast tissues (lobular epithelium,

---

Box 30-1. Absolute indications for open breast biopsy

Clinically suspicious (dominant) mass that persists through a menstrual cycle, regardless of mammographic findings; if fine-needle aspiration cytology is unequivocally positive, most surgeons proceed directly to definitive treatment.

Cystic mass that does not completely collapse on aspiration (residual solid component) or that contains bloody fluid.

Spontaneous serous or serosanguineous nipple discharge; in the absence of a mass, a "trigger point" should be demonstrable.

ductal epithelium, and connective tissue). **When the hyperplastic changes are associated with cellular atypia, there is an increased risk for subsequent malignant transformation.**

It is postulated that the hyperplastic changes are caused by a relative or absolute decrease in production of progesterone or an increase in the amount of estrogen. Estrogen promotes the growth of mammary ducts and the periductal stroma, whereas progesterone is responsible for the development of lobular and alveolar structures. Patients with hyperplasia improve dramatically during pregnancy and lactation because of the large amount of progesterone produced by the corpus luteum and placenta and the increased production of estriol, which blocks the hyperplastic changes produced by estradiol and estrone.

The disorder usually occurs in the premenopausal years. Clinically, the lesions are usually multiple and bilateral and are characterized by pain and tenderness, particularly premenstrually.

Treatment depends on the age of the patient, the severity of the symptoms, and the relative risk of the development of breast cancer. Women older than 25 years should undergo baseline mammography to exclude carcinoma. **Cysts may be aspirated to relieve pain** (Figure 30-1). If the fluid is clear and the lump disappears, careful follow-up only is indicated. **Open biopsy is required if the fluid is bloody or if there is any residual mass following aspiration.**

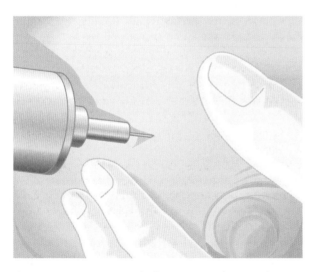

Figure 30-1. Aspiration of a breast cyst. Ultrasound may be used to differentiate a solid from a cystic breast mass.

FIBROADENOMA

Composed of both fibrous and glandular tissue, the fibroadenoma is the most common benign tumor found in the female breast. Clinically these tumors are sharply circumscribed, freely mobile nodules that may occur at any age but are common before the age of 30 years. They usually are solitary and generally are removed when they reach 2 to 4 cm in diameter, although **giant forms up to 15 cm in diameter occasionally occur and have malignant potential.** Pregnancy may stimulate their growth, and regression and calcification usually eventuate post-menopausally. These larger tumors require surgical excision for definitive diagnosis and cure.

INTRADUCTAL PAPILLOMA

Papillary neoplastic growths may develop within the ducts of the breast, most commonly just before or during menopause. They are rarely palpable and are usually diagnosed because of a bloody, serous, or turbid discharge from the nipple. **Mammography and cytologic examination of the fluid are helpful in investigating nipple discharge. Excisional biopsy of the lesion and involved duct is the treatment of choice.**

Histologically there is a spectrum of lesions ranging from those that are clearly benign to those that are anaplastic and give evidence of invasive tendencies.

GALACTOCELE

A galactocele is a cystic dilatation of a duct that is filled with thick, inspissated, milky fluid. It presents during or shortly after lactation and implies some cause for ductal obstruction, such as inflammation, hyperplasia, or neoplasia. Often multiple cysts are present. **Secondary infection may produce areas of acute mastitis or abscess formation.** Needle aspiration is usually curative. If the fluid is bloody or the mass does not disappear completely, excisional biopsy is required.

BREAST CANCER

Breast cancer is the most common female malignancy, accounting for 30% of malignancies in women. It is second only to lung cancer as the leading cause of cancer deaths in women. Over 214,000 new cases are diagnosed annually in the United States, and nearly

40,000 of these women will die from the disease. **In the US, there is a 1 in 8 to 9 chance that a woman will develop breast cancer during her lifetime, if she lives to 90 years of age.**

ETIOLOGY

Established risk factors for breast cancer are shown in Table 30-1, but 75% of women develop the disease despite having no apparently increased susceptibility.

The incidence and mortality rates for breast cancer are approximately five times higher in North America and northern Europe than they are in many Asian and African countries. Migrants to the US from Asia (principally Chinese and Japanese) do not experience a substantial increase in risk, but their first-generation and second-generation descendants have rates approaching those of the white population in the US. The difference may be related to dietary customs.

Menopausal hormone replacement therapy appears to produce a small increased risk of breast cancer, and the estrogen—progestin regimen increases the risk beyond that associated with estrogen alone.

About 5% to 10% of breast cancer cases are hereditary, resulting from mutations in the *BRCA1* or *BRCA2* gene. Hereditary breast cancer is particularly common in premenopausal women. Women with a mutated *BRCA1* or *BRCA2* gene have up to a 70% risk of developing breast cancer by age 65 years.

TUMOR TYPES

The mammary epithelium gives rise to a wide variety of histologic tumor types. **About 80% of all breast cancers are nonspecific infiltrating ductal carcinomas.** These tumors usually induce a significant fibrotic response and are stony hard to clinical palpation. **Less common types include lobular, medullary, mucinous, tubular, and papillary.** In many tumors, several patterns coexist.

Paget's disease of the breast occurs in about 3% of breast cancer patients. It represents a specialized form of intraductal carcinoma that arises in the main excretory ducts of the breasts and extends to involve the skin of the nipple and areola, producing an eczematoid appearance. **The underlying carcinoma, although invariably present, can be palpated clinically in only about two-thirds of patients.**

Inflammatory breast cancer represents 1% to 4% of cases and is often seen in pregnancy. It is characterized clinically by warmth and redness of the overlying skin and induration of the surrounding breast tissues. Biopsies of the erythematous areas reveal malignant cells in subdermal lymphatics, causing an obstructive lymphangitis. Inflammatory cells are rarely present. **Most patients have signs of advanced cancer at the time of diagnosis, including palpable regional lymph nodes and distant metastases.**

TUMOR SPREAD

Breast cancer spreads by local infiltration as well as by lymphatic or hematogenous routes. Locally, the tumor infiltrates directly into the breast parenchyma, eventually involving the overlying skin or the deep pectoral fascia.

Lymphatic spread is mainly to the axillary nodes, and 40% to 50% of patients have involvement of these nodes at the time of diagnosis. The second major area for lymph node metastases is the internal mammary node chain. These nodes are most likely to be involved when the primary lesion is medially or centrally situated. **The supraclavicular nodes are usually involved only after axillary node involvement.**

Hematogenous spread occurs mainly to the lungs and liver, but other common sites of involvement include bone, pleura, adrenals, ovaries, and brain.

Table 30-1. Established risk factors for breast cancer

Risk Factor	Relative Risk
Age (≥50 vs. <50 yr)	6.5
Family history of breast cancer	
First-degree relative	1.4–13.6
Second-degree relative	1.5–1.8
Age at menarche (<12 vs. ≥14 yr)	1.2–1.5
Age at menopause (≥55 vs. <55 yr)	1.5–2.0
Age at first live birth (>30 vs. <20 yr)	1.3–2.2
Benign breast disease	
Breast biopsy (any histologic finding)	1.5–1.8
Atypical hyperplasia	4.0–4.4
Hormone replacement therapy	1.0–1.5

Data from Armstrong K et al: N Engl J Med 342(8):564–571, 2000.

STAGING

Several systems of staging for cancer of the breast have been recommended. The one recommended by the American Joint Committee on Cancer is shown in Box 30-2.

CLINICAL FEATURES

Carcinoma of the breast is usually painless and may be freely mobile. A serous or bloody nipple discharge may be present. With progressive growth, the tumor may become fixed to the deep fascia. **Extension to the**

Box 30-2. Staging of breast cancer*

PRIMARY TUMOR (T)
- TX: Primary tumor cannot be assessed
- T0: No evidence of primary tumor
- Tis: Carcinoma in situ; intraductal carcinoma, lobular carcinoma in situ, or Paget's disease of the nipple with no associated tumor
- T1: Tumor 2.0 cm or less in greatest dimension
  - T1mic: Microinvasion 0.1 cm or less in greatest dimension
  - T1a: Tumor more than 0.1 but not more than 0.5 cm in greatest dimension
  - T1b: Tumor more than 0.5 cm but not more than 1.0 cm in greatest dimension
  - T1c: Tumor more than 1.0 cm but not more than 2.0 cm in greatest dimension
- T2: Tumor more than 2.0 cm but not more than 5.0 cm in greatest dimension
- T3: Tumor more than 5.0 cm in greatest dimension
- T4: Tumor of any size with direct extension to (a) chest wall or (b) skin.
  - T4a: Extension to chest wall
  - T4b: Edema (including peau d'orange) or ulceration of the skin of the breast or satellite skin nodules confined to the same breast
  - T4c: Both of the above (T4a and T4b)
  - T4d: Inflammatory carcinoma.

REGIONAL LYMPH NODES (N)
- NX: Regional lymph nodes cannot be assessed (e.g., previously removed)
- N0: No regional lymph node metastasis
- N1: Metastasis to movable ipsilateral axillary lymph node(s)
- N2: Metastasis to ipsilateral axillary lymph node(s) fixed to each other or to other structures
- N3: Metastasis to ipsilateral internal mammary lymph node(s)
- pN1biv: Metastasis to a lymph node 2.0 cm or more in greatest dimension
- pN2: Metastasis to ipsilateral axillary lymph node(s) fixed to each other or to other structures

- pN3: Metastasis to ipsilateral internal mammary lymph node(s)

DISTANT METASTASIS (M)
- MX: Presence of distant metastasis cannot be assessed
- M0: No distant metastasis
- M1: Distant metastasis present (includes metastasis to ipsilateral supraclavicular lymph nodes)

AMERICAN JOINT COMMISSION ON CANCER STAGE GROUPINGS

Stage 0
- Tis, N0, M0

Stage I
- T1, N0, M0

Stage IIA
- T0, N1, M0
- T1, N1, M0
- T2, N0, M0

Stage IIB
- T2, N1, M0
- T3, N0, M0

Stage IIIA
- T0, N2, M0
- T1, N2, M0
- T2, N2, M0
- T3, N1, M0
- T3, N2, M0

Stage IIIB
- T4, Any N, M0
- Any T, N3, M0

Stage IV
- Any T, Any N, M1

skin may cause retraction and dimpling, whereas ductal involvement may cause nipple retraction. Blockage of skin lymphatics may cause lymphedema and thickening of the skin, a change referred to as *peau d'orange* (Figure 30-2).

TREATMENT

With increasing awareness of the likelihood of early hematogenous spread and an increasing number of early lesions being diagnosed, the present trend is toward a more conservative surgical approach to breast cancer in conjunction with adjuvant radiation and, if necessary, chemotherapy or hormonal therapy.

Surgery

Radical mastectomy, as first described in 1894 by Halsted and Meyer, was for many years the standard operation for operable breast cancer. The procedure consists of an en bloc dissection of the entire breast, together with the pectoralis major and minor muscles and the contents of the axilla. At present, breast-conserving surgery is increasingly practiced. **Survival rates after conservative surgery are equal to those after radical mastectomy.** Although the size of the primary carcinoma is not a limiting factor for breast conservation, if the breast is small, breast conservation is unsatisfactory even for small tumors and is impractical for large tumors.

Routine axillary lymph node dissection has progressively been replaced by lymphatic mapping and sentinel lymph node resection as a less morbid means of determining the tumor status in the axilla. Routine examination of the sentinel node should include serial sectioning, immunohistochemical staining for cytokeratin, and hematoxylin and eosin staining. If the sentinel node is negative, the remaining nodes will be negative with an accuracy of about 95%, so axillary dissection may be avoided. If the node is positive, axillary dissection should be performed.

Breast reconstruction after mastectomy is an integral part of the treatment of breast cancer. It should be available to any woman who desires it, provided that her general condition allows for operation and her expectations for reconstruction are realistic. The procedure may be performed at the time of the mastectomy or may be delayed for at least 3 months.

Radiation Therapy

Conservative surgery is almost always performed in conjunction with external radiation to the breast. This approach gives equivalent outcomes to radical mastectomy, and functional and cosmetic results are improved. External beam therapy is used, with 4500 to 5000 cGy delivered to the entire breast. **The ipsilateral supraclavicular and internal mammary nodes may be treated if there are multiple positive axillary nodes. The axilla is not routinely irradiated following an axillary node dissection because of the high incidence of lymphedema.**

ADJUVANT THERAPY

Adjuvant systemic therapy is used for most patients with early breast cancer, regardless of lymph node status. Overall, adjuvant therapy reducers the risk of relapse by about one third, and reduces the risk of death by 25%.

Current recommendations for adjuvant chemotherapy and hormonal therapy are as follows:

- Premenopausal patients with estrogen-receptor (ER)-negative tumors should receive adjuvant chemotherapy.

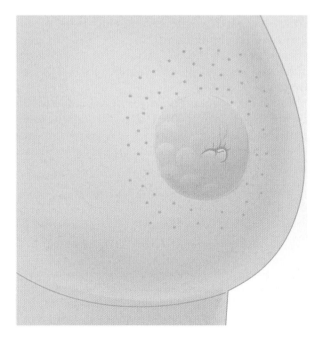

Figure 30-2. Carcinoma of the breast. Note the nipple retraction and the *peau d'orange* appearance.

- Premenopausal patients with ER-positive tumors should be considered for hormonal therapy in addition to chemotherapy.
- Postmenopausal patients with ER-positive tumors who have negative nodes should be treated with adjuvant tamoxifen or both chemotherapy and tamoxifen, and those with positive nodes should receive both tamoxifen and chemotherapy.
- Postmenopausal patients with ER-negative tumors should receive adjuvant chemotherapy.

Tamoxifen should be continued for 5 years. An added bonus of Tamoxifen is a 50% reduction in the risk of cancer in the contralateral breast. More recently, aromatase inhibitors such as anastrazole have been shown to be possibly superior to Tamoxifen.

Chemotherapy usually consists of anthracycline-based regimens (e.g., 4 cycles of Adriamycin and cyclophosphamide; six cycles of 5-fluorouracil, Adriamycin, and cyclophosphamide; or six cycles of 5-fluorouracil, epirubicin, and cyclophosphamide), but current protocols are investigating the role of taxanes in conjunction with anthracyclines. **Preliminary evidence indicates that the addition of taxanes can further improve outcomes.**

In patients with established metastases, symptoms may be palliated with combination chemotherapy. Partial responses are obtained in 50% to 75% of patients, and complete clinical responses are obtained in 5% to 25%. The median duration of response is about 12 months.

Trastuzumab (Herceptin), a humanized monoclonal antibody directed against HER2/neu (human epidermal growth factor receptor 2, also referred to as c-erbB-2), has been approved by the US Food and Drug Administration (FDA) for the treatment of patients with metastatic breast cancer. Its efficiency is predicted by either HER2/neu protein overexpression or gene amplification.

High-dose chemotherapy with autologous bone marrow or peripheral stem cell support in women at high risk of relapse, such as those with multiple lymph node metastases, is experimental. It should be carried out only in clinical trials.

PROGNOSIS

Although prognosis is related to the stage of the disease and the age of the patient (older patients have a better prognosis), **the status of the axillary lymph nodes is the single-most important prognosticator.** ER status is also of independent prognostic significance; patients with ER-negative tumors have a poorer prognosis.

In the National Surgical Adjuvant Breast Project, patients with negative lymph nodes had an actuarial 5-year survival of 83%, compared with 73% for patients with one to three positive nodes, 45% for those with four or more positive nodes, and 28% for those with more than 13 positive nodes.

BREAST CANCER IN PREGNANCY

About 3% of breast cancers occur during pregnancy, complicating approximately 1 in every 3000 pregnancies. Diagnosis is usually delayed because small masses are more difficult to palpate in hypertrophied breasts. Needle aspiration or open biopsy, however, should be performed promptly on any suspicious mass.

The treatment is essentially the same as for the nonpregnant patient except that lumpectomy and removal of axillary nodes followed by postoperative irradiation would not be appropriate with a continuing pregnancy. **For patients with nodal metastases, abortion is advisable in the 1st trimester of pregnancy because of the teratogenic risks of the adjuvant chemotherapy.** In the 3rd trimester, chemotherapy should be delayed until after delivery, although surgery should occur promptly after diagnosis.

Stage for stage, prognosis for pregnant patients is not much worse than that for nonpregnant patients. There is no indication to advise against subsequent pregnancy for breast cancer patients who have no evidence of recurrence.

Suggested Reading

Adjuvant therapy for breast cancer: NIH Consensus Statement 17(4):1–35, 2000.

ATAC Trialists' Group: Arimidex, tamoxifen alone or in combination: Anastrozole alone or in combination with tamoxifen versus tamoxifen alone for adjuvant treatment of postmenopausal women with early breast cancer: first results of the ATAC randomised trial. Lancet 359(9324):2131–2139, 2002.

Early Breast Cancer Trialists' Collaborative Group: Tamoxifen for early breast cancer: An overview of the randomised trials. Lancet 351(9114):1451–1467, 1998.

Robson M, Gilewski T, Haas B, et al: BRCA-associated breast cancer in young women. J Clin Oncol 16(5):1642–1649, 1998.

Schairer C, Lubin J, Troisi R, et al: Menopausal estrogen and estrogen-progestin replacement therapy and breast cancer risk. JAMA 283:485–491, 2003.

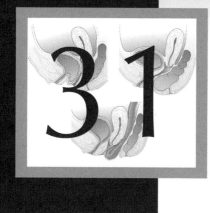

Gynecologic Procedures

Michael S. Broder and Joseph C. Gambone

Advances in surgical instrumentation and technique have resulted in more effective and efficient reproductive health care for women. The gynecologic surgeon should have a high level of training during residency followed by an ongoing commitment to retraining and retooling as effective procedures are added or substituted for outdated ones. All facilities should have an active quality assessment program to continuously evaluate the appropriateness of gynecologic care (including surgery) and to endeavor to improve its performance.

It is not the purpose of this chapter to qualify the reader as a gynecologic surgeon. It is, however, essential that students and residents become familiar with the basic principles of common gynecologic surgical procedures so that they can properly assist in the operating room and carry out perioperative care.

APPROPRIATENESS OF GYNECOLOGIC PROCEDURES

Before any procedure or surgery begins, the most appropriate option (when more than one exists) for an individual patient must be selected, with optimal patient involvement in the decision-making process preceding informed consent.

At least 80% of gynecologic surgical procedures are considered to be elective; that is, there are other alternative treatments to be considered. The appropriateness of performing these procedures should be evaluated by physician and patient on an individual basis (Table 31-1).

CREDENTIALING AND TRAINING

The rapid introduction of new technology can present a challenge to the surgeon, who will need to keep up with the most advanced procedures, and to the institution, which is required to be certain that those who are granted surgical privileges have been properly trained and are currently qualified.

A useful classification for credentialing purposes stratifies procedures into the following levels: Level 1, procedures not requiring additional training after residency (e.g., dilatation and curettage [D&C], cervical conization, adnexal excision, and abdominal or vaginal hysterectomy); Level 2, procedures requiring additional training (e.g., laparoscopic myomectomy); and Level 3, procedures requiring advanced training and special skills generally acquired during subspecialty training (e.g., radical hysterectomy, tubal anastomosis, or oocyte harvesting).

As new procedures are incorporated into basic residency training, they can be reclassified.

INFORMED CONSENT AND GENERAL RISKS ASSOCIATED WITH PROCEDURES

The patient should be thoroughly counseled about surgical risks as part of the process of informed consent (see Chapter 1). In general, risks fall into three categories: risks of anesthesia, intraoperative risks, and postoperative complications. Risks of anesthesia depend on the type of anesthesia used (awake sedation, regional anesthesia, or inhalation agents). Regional anesthesia carries the risk of infection, postprocedure spinal headaches, and failure (the need for an inhalation agent in addition to the regional anesthesia). Inhalation agents may be associated with the risk of aspiration pneumonia, allergic reaction to the agent, and damage to teeth or airways if intubation is necessary. Stroke, myocardial infarction, and death can result. The intraoperative risks include excessive

Table 31-1. The PREPARED checklist

P is the procedure
R is the reason or indication
E is the expectation
P is the preference that the patient may have (e.g., to avoid surgery, or the side effects of medication)
A is the alternative or alternatives
R is the risk or risks
E is the expense (hospital costs and surgeon's fees)
D is the decision to perform or not to perform the procedure

PREPARED is a useful mnemonic checklist to preoperatively assess the appropriateness of a health care procedure, including elective gynecologic surgery. An analysis of each gynecologic or other health care procedure can be carried out and the patient completely and efficiently counseled using this format.

bleeding and unintended damage to organs or tissue. Postoperative risks include infection, persistent bleeding, and thrombosis, all of which can lead to significant morbidity or even mortality. The specific risks of each procedure are listed below.

ENDOMETRIAL SAMPLING PROCEDURES

One of the most common minor gynecologic surgical procedures is dilatation of the cervix and curettage of the endometrium (D&C). Recent advances in office-based instrumentation for diagnosis (hysteroscopy, endometrial biopsy [Figure 31-1], and ultrasonic evaluation of endometrial thickness) have resulted in an

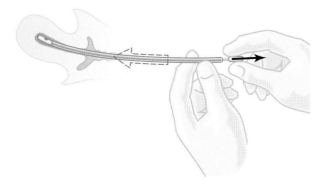

Figure 31-1. Endometrial sampling using the pipelle instrument. A flexible hollow plastic tube is inserted and held in the uterine cavity as the stylet is withdrawn creating a vacuum and resulting in aspiration of tissue.

appropriate decrease in the use of D&C. **However, if cancer of the cervix or endometrium is suspected, a thorough fractional curettage may be the best procedure to confirm its presence**.

INDICATIONS

D&C may be a diagnostic or a therapeutic procedure. A diagnostic D&C is performed for irregular menstrual bleeding, heavy menstrual bleeding, or postmenopausal bleeding, unless an endometrial biopsy has already revealed a diagnosis of malignancy. Irregularities in the contour of the endometrial cavity, either congenital (e.g., uterine septum) or acquired (e.g., submucous myomata), are sometimes determined during the operation. The finding of a thin endometrium on a transvaginal ultrasound (generally <5 mm) may eliminate the need for biopsy or D&C in some women. In patients under 40 years of age with irregular bleeding, hormonal manipulation preceded by office endometrial sampling frequently obviates the need for curettage.

The D&C may have a therapeutic effect in patients with heavy or irregular bleeding from endometrial hyperplasia, endometrial polyps, or small, pedunculated submucous myomas. Unwanted 1st-trimester pregnancies are usually evacuated by dilatation and suction curettage, although nonsurgical techniques are now available.

TECHNIQUE

The operation is performed with the patient in the dorsal lithotomy position. Most D&Cs are now performed on an outpatient basis. Paracervical blocks and local anesthesia are frequently employed.

A pelvic examination is done under anesthesia, and after sterile preparation, a weighted speculum is placed in the posterior vagina. The cervix is grasped with a single-toothed or double-toothed tenaculum. A Kevorkian curette is used for curettage of the endocervical canal. The depth of the uterine cavity is determined with a uterine sound, and the cervix is then dilated with a set of graduated dilators. A small polyp or ovum forceps is introduced through the dilated cervix and gently rotated to remove any endometrial polyps. A thorough curettage is done with a sharp curette, proceeding with each stroke in either a clockwise or a counterclockwise manner to ensure that the entire uterine cavity has been covered.

COMPLICATIONS

The most common surgical complications of D&C are hemorrhage, infection, perforation of the uterus, and laceration of the cervix. **Perforation of the uterus, even in experienced hands, is a not uncommon complication and occurs particularly with a retroverted uterus, during pregnancy, or in postmenopausal patients with endometrial cancer.** As long as no bowel or large blood vessels are injured, careful observation and antibiotics may be all the therapy that is required.

Except in an acute emergency, such as an infected incomplete abortion, D&C should be done reluctantly in the presence of infection.

CERVICAL PROCEDURES

Conization of the cervix is a procedure in which a cone-shaped portion of the cervix is removed for diagnostic or occasionally for therapeutic purposes. The section of the tissue surrounding the external os represents the base of the removed specimen. The apex is either close to the internal os (Figure 31-2A) or close to the external os (Figure 31-2B). Conization may also be performed in an office setting using loop electrosurgical excision (Figure 31-2C) or large loop excision of the transformation zone of the cervix. **Loop excision should not be used before identification of a cervical intraepithelial lesion that requires treatment.**

The technique of cryoablation is commonly used to treat condylomas of the cervix, vagina, and vulva. These procedures almost always are office-based, and little if any anesthesia is required.

The letters in the acronym *laser* stand for light amplification by the stimulated emission of radiation. **Laser instruments are sources of intense beams of light energy.** When used in surgery, this radiant energy is converted inside the cell to thermal or acoustic energy, resulting in controlled vaporization or coagulation of tissue. Lasers come in longer wavelengths (carbon dioxide [CO_2]) or newer and shorter wavelengths (neodymium–yttrium-aluminum-garnet [Nd:YAG], potassium-titanyl-phosphate [KTP], and argon) that can be propagated along flexible optical fibers. This allows delivery of energy for cutting, vaporization, and coagulation to tissues in locations unreachable by a CO_2 laser.

Because of the additional expense of laser equipment and the lack of evidence for improvements in outcome, **the routine use of this technology has been questioned.** Nevertheless, laser technology has

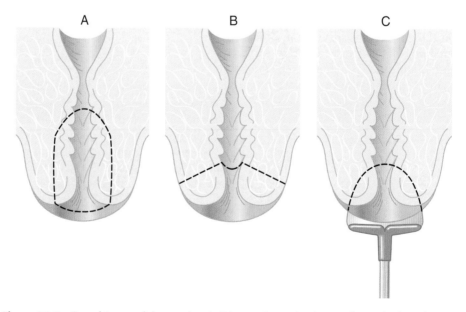

Figure 31-2. Cone biopsy of the cervix. *A,* Diagnostic conization performed when the squamocolumnar junction is not fully visualized colposcopically. *B,* Therapeutic conization performed for disease involving the ectocervix and distal endocervical canal. *C,* Loop electrosurgical excision procedure (LEEP). The goal of the procedure is to remove the cervical tissue to just above the squamocolumnar junction, including any visible lesions.

been applied to conization of the cervix, removal of leiomyomas (myomectomy), and destruction of the ectopic endometrial implants of endometriosis.

PELVIC ENDOSCOPY

Gynecologic endoscopy (laparoscopy and hysteroscopy) is widely used for the diagnosis and treatment of reproductive organ disease and dysfunction. Laparoscopy and hysteroscopy have largely moved from the hospital operating room to the freestanding surgical outpatient unit, and with smaller instruments (needle-scopes) and more refined fiberoptic technology, even into the office setting. **Because of the expense involved, the value of these techniques must be considered in terms of outcome, particularly the long-term health and functional status of the patient.**

LAPAROSCOPY

The laparoscope is an instrument for viewing the peritoneal cavity (Figure 31-3). Both pelvic and upper abdominal structures can be inspected.

The indications for laparoscopy are both diagnostic and therapeutic (Table 31-2). **Laser technology can be applied to operative laparoscopic procedures both to excise and to vaporize areas of pathology.**

Absolute contraindications to laparoscopy include bowel obstruction and large hemoperitoneum with hypovolemic shock. In patients who have had multiple previous laparotomies, a history of peritonitis, previous bowel surgery, or a lower midline abdominal incision, open laparoscopy is preferable. In these conditions, the peritoneal cavity is opened through a small subumbilical incision under

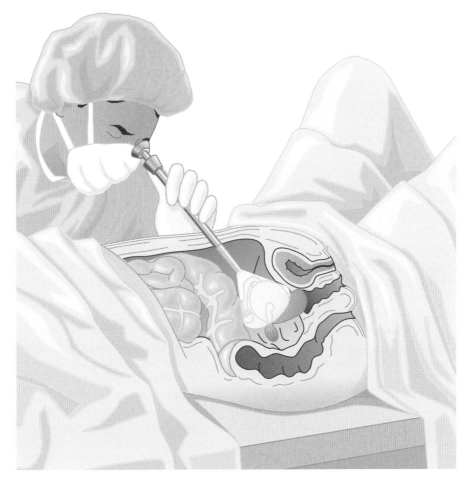

Figure 31-3. Diagnostic laparoscopy.

Table 31-2. Diagnostic and therapeutic indications for laparoscopy: An illustrative evaluation

Indication/Procedure	Diagnostic Value*	Therapeutic Value*
Sterilization	N/A	++++
Ectopic gestation	+++	+++
Infertility	++	+++
Pelvic pain	++	++
Endometriosis	+++	+++
Cancer		
Cervical	+	+
Endometrial	+	+
Ovarian	+++	++
Ovarian surgery	++	+++
Myomectomy	N/A	+
Urogynecology	N/A	++
Laparoscopic hysterectomy	N/A	+
Laparoscopically assisted vaginal hysterectomy	N/A	+++

+, Questionable value; ++, possible value; +++, probable value; ++++, documented value (cost-effective); N/A, not applicable.

*Value = $\dfrac{\text{Outcomes}}{\text{Resource use}}$, or not what *can* be done, but what *should* be done.

direct vision before introduction of the trocar and sheath.

TECHNIQUE

The procedure is performed with the patient in a modified dorsal lithotomy position (i.e., with knee crutches), usually under general anesthesia. An intrauterine manipulator is inserted to help in the visualization of the pelvic organs. A pneumoperitoneum is created by inserting a spring-loaded needle, such as a Veress needle, into the peritoneal cavity via the subumbilical fold, and insufflation with either CO_2 or nitrous oxide is begun. The trocar and surrounding sheath are then inserted through a small subumbilical incision.

The lighted telescope is inserted into the sheath and advanced slowly. With the patient in the Trendelenburg position (upper body lower than the pelvis), visualization of pelvic organs confirms that the peritoneal cavity has been entered. Gas may be added intermittently and automatically to maintain a sufficient pneumoperitoneum. To perform a second punc-

ture, which is sometimes necessary, especially in laparoscopic surgical procedures, the abdominal wall is transilluminated to identify the position of the inferior epigastric vessels, and a 4- to 6-mm trocar and sheath are inserted under laparoscopic guidance through a small incision at the pubic hairline. A probe or other surgical instrument (e.g., surgical scissors) is passed through the second sheath.

On completion of the procedure, hemostasis is checked, the gas is released from the peritoneal cavity, and the instruments are withdrawn. The small skin incisions are closed with a clip or single subcuticular suture.

INDICATIONS

The following are indications for laparoscopy:
1. **Tubal sterilization.** The most common indication for the use of the laparoscope in gynecology is sterilization.
2. **Ectopic pregnancy.** The laparoscope is commonly used for the removal of tubal pregnancies that do not meet the criteria for medical therapy.
3. **Pelvic infection.** Although it is not routinely used for diagnosis of pelvic inflammatory disease (PID), the laparoscope can provide confirmation of a diagnosis when there is a diagnostic dilemma.
4. **Infertility.** Routine laparoscopic evaluation of the infertile woman is widely recommended but controversial because of a lack of controlled evidence of improved outcome. Advanced assisted reproductive techniques, such as in vitro fertilization (IVF) and gamete intrafallopian transfer (GIFT), may involve laparoscopic procedures. Recently, however, the aspiration of oocytes for IVF has been more commonly performed transvaginally using ultrasonic guidance (see Chapter 35).
5. **Pelvic pain.** Acute and chronic pelvic pain can be investigated using the laparoscope.
6. **Endometriosis.** The laparoscope has become a widely used intervention for the diagnosis, staging, and treatment of ectopic endometrial tissue in both overtly symptomatic (pelvic pain) and silently symptomatic (infertility) patients. Laser coagulation, thermal vaporization, excision of endometriosis, and aspiration of endometriomas results in consistent, but sometimes temporary, improvement of pain

and moderate improvement in fertility potential. Repeated procedures and the need for medical adjuvant treatment are common.

7. **Ovarian neoplasms.** Because of the need to rule out pelvic malignancies, the laparoscope can be used as a less invasive procedure to evaluate a persistent small adnexal mass. Laparoscopic ovarian cystectomy or salpingo-oophorectomy allows a tissue diagnosis to be made. **Laparoscopic aspiration of cysts can be dangerous and may result in dissemination of an unsuspected ovarian cancer. Ovarian biopsy is seldom indicated, and in premenopausal patients with simple cystic enlargement, a trial of hormonal suppression or observation is indicated instead of immediate surgical intervention.** Most such lesions will be functional cysts that will spontaneously regress. The laparoscope in expert hands has been advocated for staging and "second-look" procedures in patients with ovarian cancer. These procedures have become feasible since the advent of laparoscopic lymphadenectomy, but incision-site recurrences are a potential problem.

8. **Myomectomy.** Laparoscopic myomectomy remains controversial because of the possibility that smaller leiomyomas will be removed because they *can* be rather than because they *should* be. **Advocates of the procedure recommend that fibroids larger than 6 cm not be removed using the laparoscope.**

9. **Urogynecologic procedures.** Urethropexy can be performed laparoscopically with reported success rates comparable to procedures performed percutaneously (see Chapter 24).

10. **Hysterectomy.** The laparoscope has been used recently to replace an abdominal procedure (laparoscopic hysterectomy), to assist in a vaginal hysterectomy (LAVH), and to convert an abdominal hysterectomy to a vaginal hysterectomy.

COMPLICATIONS

Insufflation of the abdominal wall may occur from failure to enter the peritoneal cavity with the Veress needle. Perforation of a viscus, especially adherent bowel, may occur at the time of insertion of the trocar and sheath. Once the instruments have been successfully introduced into the peritoneal cavity, lack of adequate hemostasis or coagulation burns of a viscus may occur. A poor pneumoperitoneum increases the risk of these complications.

Bowel burns during fulguration are the most serious complication of laparoscopy, although the most common complications are related to the anesthesia. Bowel burns result either from direct contact with the bowel or from a unipolar spark and are usually not detected at the time of the procedure. Several days later, bowel perforation with peritonitis may become evident. **The increased use of bipolar instruments has diminished the occurrence of this serious complication.** There is an increased risk of anesthetic complications in a patient with a pneumoperitoneum.

HYSTEROSCOPY
INDICATIONS AND USES

During the last 100 years, the hysteroscope has seen a progressive improvement in light sources, optical systems, distending media, and electronic equipment, and the instrument now has a wide variety of indications and benefits in clinical gynecology. Hysteroscopy has substantially improved accuracy when compared with x-ray hysterography, and in some cases it may be more effective than diagnostic D&C in detecting intrauterine pathology such as endometrial polyps or submucous myomata.

HYSTEROSCOPIC INSTRUMENTATION

The hysteroscope (Figure 31-4) consists of a telescope and a sheath through which the telescope is inserted. For pure diagnostic use, the telescope is inserted alone, whereas for operative capabilities it is inserted in conjunction with other instruments.

Two different types of telescopes are used today: rigid and fiberoptic. Rigid telescopes are most commonly 4 mm in diameter, but they are available in sizes as small as 2.9 mm. They are unbending telescopes, housing a system of ground lenses of varying thickness separated by columns of air of varying height.

Operating instruments such as rigid or flexible scissors, graspers, biopsy forceps, or even laser fibers are inserted through operating channels, which may be part of the outer sheath itself, or through separate devices interposed between the telescope and the outer sheath, which are called bridges. In addition to the standard operating instruments, some bridges have attachable electrodes and finger-controlled

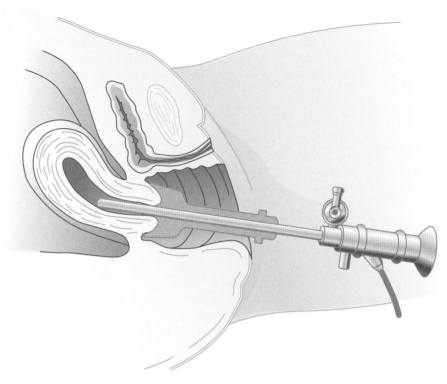

Figure 31-4. Diagnostic hysteroscopy.

mechanisms to allow the performance of precision intrauterine surgery.

OFFICE VS. HOSPITAL-BASED HYSTEROSCOPY

As telescopes have become progressively narrower, they now can be safely inserted into the cervical canal with minimal pain. Several manufacturers now have small office-based telescopes that use physiologic low-viscosity distention fluids such as saline or Ringer's lactate. These allow the performance of hysteroscopy with little more than a paracervical block in patients who are bleeding, and they do not cause the shoulder pain and uterine spasm that often accompany use of carbon dioxide as a distention medium. **At present, a significant number of hysteroscopies are being performed as office procedures.**

OPERATIVE PROCEDURES
Infertility

When abnormalities such as intrauterine synechiae or septa are found, hysteroscopic correction is associated with a high rate of success. Synechiae, almost always the result of trauma such as curettage or other uterine surgery, may vary from mild to severe, obliterating only a small part or almost all of the endometrial cavity. **A third of patients with intrauterine synechiae have no apparent menstrual abnormalities.** The majority of reports of treatment of these adhesions cite the use of hysteroscopic scissors for incision, although lasers or electrical knife electrodes also have been reported to be useful. **In infertile patients, conception rates up to 60% and a reduction of pregnancy wastage by 50% have been reported after incision of synechiae (uncontrolled studies).**

Probably the most rewarding of all hystero-scopic procedures is the excision of an intrauter-ine septum, a congenital anomaly that occurs in up to 1% of women. Usually performed as an out-patient procedure, excision of the septum is a relatively short procedure, with minimal bleeding and minimal risks. It is best performed with mechanical scissors as opposed to electrical or laser devices so as to limit the spread of thermal injury to adjacent healthy myometrium.

In most cases it is necessary to monitor the depth of incision by concomitant laparoscopy or ultrasonography to reduce the risk of uterine perforation.

Abnormal Uterine Bleeding

The hysteroscopic evaluation of the patient with abnormal uterine bleeding frequently uncovers the presence of submucous myomas or endometrial polyps.

Small endometrial polyps can be removed very easily using hysteroscopic scissors or grasping forceps inserted through an accessory channel of the operating hysteroscope, or they can be removed blindly with a polyp forceps followed by reinspection hysteroscopically to ensure complete removal. Because the endocervical canal is rarely dilated larger than 10 mm to accommodate the operating instruments, polyps or myomas that are significantly larger than this must be morcellated before removal. The use of mechanical methods for morcellation (scissors) is almost impossible, owing to their delicate construction and their small size. Morcellation with a laser fiber has been reported, but the procedure is slow and tedious. **The urologic resectoscope has been used to morcellate or vaporize all or part of such lesions.** Electrodes composed of thin wires, rollerballs, roller cylinders, and grooved vaporization tips, coupled with continuous (cutting) electrical waveforms, allow simple removal of such lesions.

Endometrial Ablation

Endometrial ablation is the destruction of the uterine lining for the treatment of chronic menorrhagia. It is performed when more conservative treatments, such as hormone therapy and curettage, are unsuccessful and when the more radical alternative of hysterectomy is undesirable or contraindicated.

Two general methods of endometrial ablation have emerged. The first type requires hysteroscopic visualization and employs electrical or laser energy to shave, vaporize, or coagulate the endometrial surface.

Following a preoperative drug regimen to suppress the endometrial thickness (danazol or leuprolide), hysteroscopic laser surgery can be performed on an outpatient basis under general or regional anesthesia in about 1 hour. A hysteroscope is introduced into the uterus and a fiberoptic delivery system is passed through the operating channel. Resectoscopic endometrial ablation has become a more popular technique than laser ablation, and it appears to be at least as effective; its advantages are a significantly shorter operating time and much less expensive equipment.

Amenorrhea occurs in up to 68% of patients after resectoscopic ablation, whereas hypomenorrhea occurs in more than 90% of cases. Continued excessive bleeding is believed to be more likely when multiple myomas or severe adenomyosis exists.

A more recent method of endometrial ablation does not require hysteroscopic visualization. These techniques use either a reservoir for the delivery of heat to the endometrial surface or microwave energy directed at the endometrium to render it unresponsive to hormonal stimulaton. Because they are narrower than operative hysteroscopes and their attachments and can be inserted blindly into the uterine cavity, these methods are intended for office use and for use by surgeons who may not have the experience or skills needed for laser or resectoscopic surgery.

COMPLICATIONS OF OPERATIVE HYSTEROSCOPY

Operative hysteroscopy generally comprises procedures that are relatively simple and safe, resulting in few complications. The overall complication rate for almost 14,000 hysteroscopic procedures was reported as being 2%, with major complications (perforation, hemorrhage, fluid overload, bowel or urinary tract injury) occurring in less than 1% of procedures. **The most significant risks of operative hysteroscopy are perforation of the uterus, excessive bleeding, and distention medium hazards (e.g., gas embolism, fluid overload, anaphylactic shock).** Much less frequent and less serious complications include infections (e.g., endometritis, pelvic inflammatory disease), traumatic cervical lacerations, and postoperative cervical stenosis.

HYSTERECTOMY

Hysterectomy is the most commonly performed major gynecologic operation and among the top five most commonly performed major surgical procedures in the United States. It can be performed either abdominally or vaginally. Although some indications for hysterectomy remain controversial, high patient satisfaction levels and increasing safety for the procedure has been reported.

Table 31-3 provides a useful list of indications for abdominal or vaginal hysterectomy.

ABDOMINAL HYSTERECTOMY

A simple total hysterectomy is the most commonly performed procedure for benign uterine disease and involves the "simple" excision of the uterine corpus and cervix. **It may be performed intrafascially,** in which case the surgeon stays safely within the endopelvic fascia that surrounds the cervix and upper vagina, **or extrafascially,** in which case the investing fascia of the cervix and upper vagina is removed with the specimen. **A subtotal hysterectomy excises the**

uterine corpus, usually at the level of the internal cervical os, or the cervical canal may be cored out from above. **A radical hysterectomy involves the wide excision of the parametrial tissue laterally** (Figure 31-5) **along with the uterosacral ligaments posteriorly** after the rectum is dissected free and after each ureter is dissected out of its tunnel beneath the uterine artery.

Indications

The indications for simple **total abdominal hysterectomy** may include such benign conditions as uterine myomas, endometriosis, chronic PID,

---

Table 31-3. Hysterectomy: Indication list with criteria

ACUTE CONDITION
A-1*   Pregnancy catastrophe (e.g., severe hemorrhage)
A-2   Severe infection (e.g., ruptured tubo-ovarian abscess)
A-3*   Operative complication (e.g., uterine perforation)

BENIGN DISEASE
B-1   Leiomyomas
       Symptomatic (e.g., bleeding, pressure)
       Asymptomatic (≥12 wk size, confuses adnexal evaluation)
B-2   Endometriosis (distinct endometriosis, unresponsive to hormoneal suppression or conservative surgery)
B-3   Adenomyosis (with symptomatic menometrorrhagia unresponsive to treatment)
B-4   Chronic infection (e.g., recurrent pelvic inflammatory disease)
B-5   Adnexal mass (e.g., ovarian neoplasm)
B-6   Other (operator-defined, criteria-specified)

CANCER OR SIGNIFICANT PREMALIGNANT DISEASE
C-1   Invasive disease of reproductive organs
C-2   Significant preinvasive disease of the uterus (CIN-3 or adenomatous hyperplasia of the endometrium with cellular atypia)
C-3   Cancer of adjacent or distant organ (gastrointestinal, genitourinary, or breast cancer)

DISCOMFORT (NO CONFIRMING TISSUE PATHOLOGY EXPECTED)
D-1*   Chronic pelvic pain (negative laparoscopy and nonsurgical treatment attempted)
D-2*   Pelvic relaxation (symptomatic)
D-3*   Recurrent uterine bleeding (unresponsive to hormone regulation, curettage, or endometrial ablation—normal-size uterus)
D-4*   Other (operator-defined, criteria specified)

EXTENUATING CIRCUMSTANCES (NOT SPECIFICALLY INDICATED BUT POSSIBLY JUSTIFIED—REQUIRES PREOPERATIVE PEER REVIEW)
E-1*   Sterilization (extenuating circumstances)
E-2*   Cancer prophylaxis (e.g., recurrent CIN after cone biopsy or persistent adenomatous hyperplasia of the endometrium without atypia)
E-3*   Other—listing extenuating circumstances

CIN, Cervical intraepithelial neoplasia.
*Denotes indications for which tissue pathology is not expected to confirm the preoperative diagnosis.
Data from Gambone JC, Lench JB, Slesinski MJ, et al: Validation of hysterectomy indications and the quality assurance process. Obstet Gynecol 73:1045, 1989.

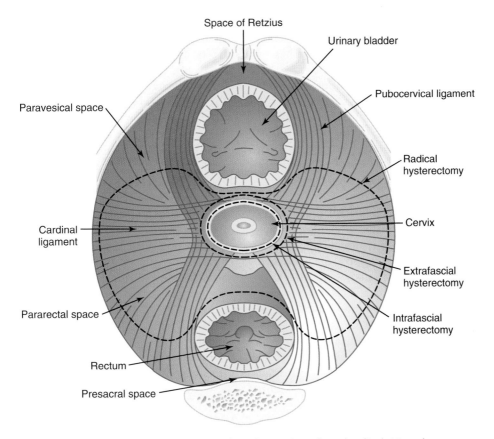

Figure 31-5. Types of hysterectomy: extrafascial, intrafascial, and radical. Note the extensive amount of parametrial tissue that is removed in a radical hysterectomy.

stage I endometrial cancer, and uterine bleeding that is unresponsive to more conservative measures. In some cases, a subtotal hysterectomy may be preferred. In this procedure, the cervix is left in situ, either to provide support for the vagina or because of possible involvement of the cervix in sexual response.

A **radical hysterectomy** is indicated for stage Ib and occasionally stage IIa cervical cancer. Endometrial cancer with gross cervical involvement may also be managed by radical hysterectomy.

In women who undergo hysterectomy at or after menopause, the uterine adnexa (fallopian tubes and ovaries) are usually removed. However, there are few studies weighing the risks and benefits of removing these normal organs. Before menopause, the option of preserving the ovaries at the time of hysterectomy vs. the expense and possible dangers of hormonal replacement therapy must be thoroughly discussed with the patient preoperatively.

In general, the ovaries are preserved at hysterectomy for benign disease before menopause unless there is a strong family history of breast or ovarian cancer. The choice of incidental oophorectomy along with incidental appendectomy awaits a thorough, prospective quality-of-life analysis (economic and medical) to guide gynecologic surgeons and their patients.

TECHNIQUE

Abdominal hysterectomy is carried out with the patient in the supine position, usually under general anesthesia. First, a thorough pelvic and abdominal examination under anesthesia is carried out and recorded. The choice of incision depends on the indication for the procedure. A vertical incision is advisable in patients who have had several prior abdominal operations, are extremely obese, or in whom extensive adhesions or endometriosis is anticipated. In patients with restricted benign disease, incisions along the lines of Langer (transverse in the lower abdomen) achieve a better cosmetic result. The various lower abdominal incisions and their anatomy are discussed in Chapter 3 and depicted in Figure 3-12.

After making the abdominal incision into the peritoneal cavity, the upper abdomen is manually explored with special reference to the liver, gallbladder, stomach, spleen, and paraaortic lymph nodes, and a reference to each must be recorded in the operative note. The intestines are inspected in cases of cancer with careful attention to mesenteric lymph nodes and the vermiform appendix. The patient is then placed in the Trendelenburg position (tilted with upper body lower than the pelvis), and the abdominal viscera are packed out of the pelvis with laparotomy tapes.

Each round ligament is clamped, incised, and ligated. The peritoneum on both sides is incised lateral to the infundibulopelvic ligament. This allows entry to the retroperitoneum between the leaves of the broad ligament exposing the ureter and pelvic vessels. The vesicouterine fold of the peritoneum is incised transversely between the incised round ligaments, and the bladder (adherent to the peritoneum) is reflected inferiorly off the fascia of the lower uterine segment, cervix, and upper vagina.

If the adnexa are to be removed, the ureters are identified and the infundibulopelvic ligaments with the ovarian vessels are clamped, cut, and tied. The medioposterior leaf of the broad ligament is incised toward the uterus, thus exposing the uterine artery and veins as they course superiorly toward the utero-ovarian vascular anastomosis just below the ovarian ligament. If the uterine adnexa are to be preserved, the ovarian ligaments are clamped, incised, and ligated on each side.

The uterine vessels thus exposed are stripped of their adventitial tissue (skeletonized), clamped at the level of the internal cervical os, incised, and securely ligated bilaterally. The ligated uterine vessels are reflected laterally, allowing access to the cardinal ligament (of Mackenrodt). Staying medial to the ligated uterine vessels, the cardinal ligament on either side is clamped, incised, and ligated with a transfixion ligature. It may take several bites to free the cardinal ligaments from the lower cervix and upper vagina.

The peritoneum just below the posterior surface of the cervix is incised transversely between the uterosacral ligaments, and the rectum is reflected from the posterior aspect of the cervix and upper vagina. The uterosacral ligaments are clamped, incised, and ligated, which frees them from the cervix and upper vagina. The total uterus (corpus and cervix) is removed by cutting across the vagina just below the cervix, with care taken to sufficiently reflect the urinary bladder and rectum inferiorly to avoid injury. **The vaginal cuff is normally closed with absorbable sutures,** incorporating the cardinal and uterosacral ligaments into each lateral angle of the vagina to preclude the later development of a vaginal vault prolapse. If the uterosacral ligaments are widely separated, they may be plicated to prevent the formation of an enterocele. **Progressive circular sutures (of Moschowitz) may be placed to obliterate a particularly large pouch of Douglas, which also portends an increased risk of enterocele.**

Three points in the procedures present a particular risk for injury to the ureter: (1) as the infundibulopelvic ligaments are clamped and incised, (2) as the uterine vessels are ligated, and (3) as the cardinal ligaments are clamped if the urinary bladder is not sufficiently reflected inferiorly. **Use of the retroperitoneal approach, with identification of the ureters bilaterally and careful reflection of the bladder inferiorly, prevents ureteric injury.**

VAGINAL HYSTERECTOMY

Vaginal hysterectomy, if feasible, is preferable to the abdominal approach because it avoids a visible scar, is associated with less pain, affords an opportunity to correct pelvic relaxation, and generally requires less postoperative hospitalization and disability.

Indications

Ideally, vaginal hysterectomy is elected for benign disease when the uterus is mobile, is less than 12 gestational weeks in size, is characterized by some pelvic relaxation, and is expected to contain few or no adhesions from endometriosis, PID, or multiple prior lower abdominal operations. The procedure is most commonly performed in association with the correction of uterine prolapse, cystocele, rectocele, or enterocele in postmenopausal women.

The advent of laparoscopically assisted vaginal hysterectomy has greatly expanded the indications for the vaginal approach by freeing up adnexal adhesions, facilitating simultaneous removal of the tubes and ovaries, and identifying conditions that would not safely be managed at the time of vaginal hysterectomy.

Technique

The principles of the operation are similar to those of abdominal hysterectomy except that ligation of the ligaments and vessels proceeds in the reverse order. The patient is placed in the dorsolithotomy position after induction of anesthesia. The bladder is emptied, and a thorough pelvic examination is performed. A weighted vaginal retractor is placed in the vagina, a tenaculum is placed on the cervix, and the uterus is drawn down toward the vaginal introitus and tested for descent and mobility. A transverse incision is made through the vaginal epithelium between the uterosacral ligaments at the posterior junction of the cervix and vagina. The peritoneum of the cul-de-sac is bluntly mobilized and sharply entered. Adhesions of the cul-de-sac and posterior uterine wall are excluded by finger exploration. The uterosacral ligaments are clamped, cut, and ligated, allowing additional descent of the uterus.

At this point, the vaginal epithelial incision is extended circumferentially around the cervix, and the bladder is advanced superiorly along the anterior uterine wall, exposing the anterior uterovesical fold of the peritoneum, which is sharply entered. The pubo-cervical ligaments (bladder pillars) containing the ureters are bluntly displaced laterally and the cardinal ligaments are clamped, cut, and ligated, allowing further descent of the uterus.

An angle retractor (e.g., Heaney, Deaver) is placed into the opening of the anterior vesicouterine fold of the peritoneum, and the urinary bladder is retracted anteriorly. The uterine vessels are clamped, usually with a Heaney clamp, ensuring that the tips of the clamp include the peritoneal edge both anteriorly and posteriorly and that the tips are snug against the lateral uterine wall so as to include all of the uterine vessels. The clamped vessels are cut and securely ligated. Some surgeons prefer to double clamp and ligate this pedicle because the vessels tend to retract superiorly, and if they escape the clamps or ligature, they may be difficult to retrieve.

Downward traction on the uterus should allow full exposure of the round ligament, fallopian tubes, ovarian ligament, and utero-ovarian vascular anastomosis, and these structures are clamped as a group, cut free of the uterus, and securely ligated. Because this pedicle is quite bulky, especially in premenopausal patients, it is wise to double clamp and ligate this pedicle, first with a loop hemostatic ligature and then with a transfixion ligature.

If the adnexa are to be removed, the suspensory ligament of the ovary is addressed instead of the ovarian ligament. With Allis clamps, the fimbriated end of the fallopian tube and ovary are drawn inferiorly into the operative field, which brings the suspensory ligament of the ovary into full view, allowing it to be clamped, cut, and ligated while taking special care to avoid the adjacent ureter. To visualize the ureter more clearly, the round ligament may be initially and separately clamped and ligated, which opens up the lateral extraperitoneal space. This phase of the procedure may be quite difficult in a premenopausal primigravida with good pelvic support, and it should be attempted only by the experienced gynecologic surgeon.

The peritoneum is then closed with a pursestring suture or one or more transverse U-sutures, leaving the pedicles in an extraperitoneal position. As with an abdominal hysterectomy, the uterosacral ligaments may be plicated with one or more sutures to avoid an enterocele. The ovarian and/or round ligaments may be sutured together in the midline, but this is optional, as they add little to no pelvic support. The cardinal ligaments, however, should each be sutured to the lateral aspect of the vaginal cuff to provide vaginal support, to increase vaginal depth, and to prevent the later development of a vaginal vault prolapse. The cardinal ligaments should not be sutured together across the midline, as that might shorten the vagina. The vaginal epithelium is then closed with interrupted absorbable sutures. To allow drainage of the operative site, the vaginal wound may be left open after ensuring hemostasis with a running locked suture or careful electrocautery of the vaginal cuff. If the bladder pillars are plicated to correct a cystocele or if a urethropexy is employed to correct stress incontinence, catheter drainage of the bladder may be employed for 24 to 48 hours postoperatively.

COMPLICATIONS OF HYSTERECTOMY

Complications associated with any abdominal or pelvic surgery include anesthesia complications, hemorrhage, atelectasis, wound infection, urinary tract infection, thrombophlebitis, and pulmonary embolism. **Atelectasis occurs most commonly in the first 24 to 48 hours** and can be prevented and treated with aggressive pulmonary toilet. **Wound infection usually occurs about 5 days postoperatively** and is associated with redness, tenderness, swelling, and increased warmth around the wound.

Treatment may require systemic antibiotics, opening the incision, draining the discharge, local debridement, and wound care. **Urinary tract infection can occur at any time in the postoperative period,** and urine for microscopy and culture should be obtained from any patient with a postoperative fever. **Thrombophlebitis (with possible subsequent pulmonary embolism) is manifested by fever and leg swelling or pain; it usually occurs 7 to 12 days postoperatively.** Pulmonary embolism may occur even in the absence of signs of thrombophlebitis. **Wound disruption after abdominal hysterectomy with evisceration of intestines is generally heralded by a profuse serous discharge from the wound (peritoneal fluid) 4 to 8 days postoperatively.** When evisceration is suspected, the wound should be explored in the operating room.

The most common intraoperative complication of abdominal or vaginal hysterectomy is bleeding from the infundibulopelvic or utero-ovarian pedicle, the uterine vascular pedicle, or the vaginal cuff. When postoperative hemorrhage occurs, bleeding from the vaginal cuff can sometimes be identified and controlled vaginally. **If bleeding is sufficient to cause hypotension, laparotomy may be required to tie off the bleeding vascular pedicle.**

Infection is common to both procedures and is manifested by fever and lower abdominal pain. Examination often reveals tenderness and induration of the vaginal cuff, which indicative of pelvic cellulitis. This can usually be treated with antibiotic therapy. **Administration of prophylactic cephalosporin perioperatively has proven beneficial in controlling infection in vaginal hysterectomies performed in premenopausal patients.**

Injury to the ureter is the most serious complication of hysterectomy and usually occurs during the abdominal procedure, particularly during a difficult dissection for PID, endometriosis, or pelvic cancer. Ureteral injury can also occur during a vaginal hysterectomy. If not detected intraoperatively, fever and flank pain can develop postoperatively, and a ureterovaginal fistula or urinoma may become apparent 5 to 21 days after surgery. **If noted intraoperatively, a ureteral injury can be repaired by implanting the proximal cut end of the ureter into the bladder or by anastomosing the proximal and distal ends of the transected ureter over a ureteric stent.**

Intraoperative injury to the rectum or bladder, if recognized, should be repaired immediately. If a bladder repair is necessary, an indwelling catheter (suprapubic or transurethral) should be left on free drainage for 5 to 7 days. On rare occasions it may be necessary to back up an extensive rectal injury repair with a colostomy.

Suggested Reading

Berek JS: Surgical techniques. *In* Berek JS, Hacker NF (eds): Practical Gynecologic Oncology, 2nd ed. Baltimore, MD, Williams & Wilkins, 1994, pp 519–560.

Gambone JC, Reiter RC, Lench JB: Short-term outcome of incidental hysterectomy at the time of adnexectomy for benign disease. J Womens Health 1:197–200, 1992.

Gimpelson RJ: Office hysteroscopy. Clin Obstet Gynecol 35:270–281, 1992.

Hatch KD, Berek JS: Intraepithelial disease of the cervix, vagina, and vulva. *In* Berek JS (ed): Novak's Gynecology, 13th ed. Philadelphia, Lippincott, William & Wilkins, 2002, p 489.

Kovac SR: Guidelines to determine the route of hysterectomy. Obstet Gynecol 85:18–23, 1995.

PART FOUR

Reproductive Endocrinology and Infertility

Larry R. Laufer

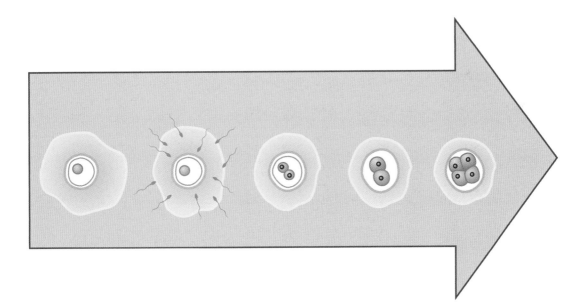

Puberty and Disorders of Pubertal Development

Catherine Marin DeUgarte, Richard P. Buyalos, Jr, and Larry R. Laufer

Puberty encompasses the development of secondary sexual characteristics and the acquisition of reproductive capability. During this transition, usually between 10 and 16 years of age, a variety of physical, endocrinologic, and psychologic changes accompany the increasing levels of sex steroids.

The onset of pubertal changes is determined primarily by genetic factors, but it is also influenced by: **geographic location** (girls in metropolitan areas, at altitudes near sea level, or at latitudes close to the equator tend to begin puberty at an earlier age), **nutritional status** (obese children have an earlier onset of puberty, and those who are malnourished or who have chronic illnesses associated with weight loss have a later onset of menses. Excessive exercise relative to the caloric intake can also delay the onset of puberty. It has been proposed that an "invariant mean weight" of **48 kg (106 lb)** is essential for the initiation of menarche in healthy girls), and **psychological factors** (severe neurotic or psychotic disorders as well as chronic isolation may interfere with the normal onset of puberty through a mechanism similar to adult hypothalamic amenorrhea).

In the United States and Western Europe, a decrease in the age of menarche (age at first menses) was noted between 1840 and 1970. This trend has leveled off in the last 25 years (Figure 32-1). **At present, the mean age of menarche is approximately 12.4 years in the United States.**

ENDOCRINOLOGIC CHANGES OF PUBERTY
FETAL AND NEWBORN PERIOD

The fetal hypothalamic-pituitary-gonadal axis is capable of producing adult levels of gonadotropins and sex steroids. By 20 weeks' gestation, levels of gonadotropins—follicle-stimulating hormone (FSH) and luteinizing hormone (LH)—rise dramatically in both male and female fetuses (Figure 32-2). **The female fetus acquires the lifetime peak number of oocytes by mid-gestation,** and she experiences a brief period of follicular maturation and sex steroid production in response to elevated gonadotropin levels in utero. This transient increase in serum estradiol (a sex steroid) acts on the fetal hypothalamic-pituitary unit, resulting in a reduction of gonadotropin secretion (negative feedback effect), which in turn reduces estradiol production. This indicates that the inhibitory effect of sex steroids on gonadotropin release is operative before birth.

In both male and female fetuses, serum estradiol is primarily of maternal and placental origin. With birth and the acute loss of maternal and placental sex steroids, the negative feedback action on the hypothalamic-pituitary axis is lost, and gonadotropins are once again released from the pituitary gland, reaching adult or near adult concentrations in the early neonatal period. **In the female infant, peak levels of gonadotropins are generally seen by 3 months of age and then slowly decrease until a nadir is reached by the age of 4 years.** In contrast to gonadotropin levels, sex steroid concentrations decrease rapidly to prepubertal values within 1 week after birth and remain low until the onset of puberty.

CHILDHOOD

The hypothalamic-pituitary-gonadal axis in the young child is suppressed between the ages of 4 and 10 years. The hypothalamic-pituitary system

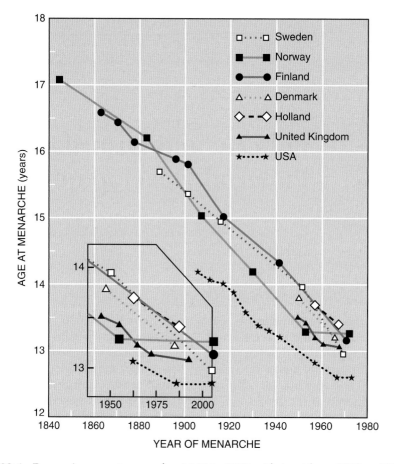

Figure 32-1. Decreasing age at menarche, 1840 to 1978 with inset from 1950 to 2000, indicating a leveling off (about 12.4 years in the USA) since 1975. *Adapted from Styne DM, Grumbach MM: Disorders of puberty in the male and female. In Yen SSC, Jaffe RB, Barbieri RL (eds): Reproductive Endocrinology: Physiology, Pathophysiology and Clinical Management, 4th ed. Philadelphia, WB Saunders, 1999.*

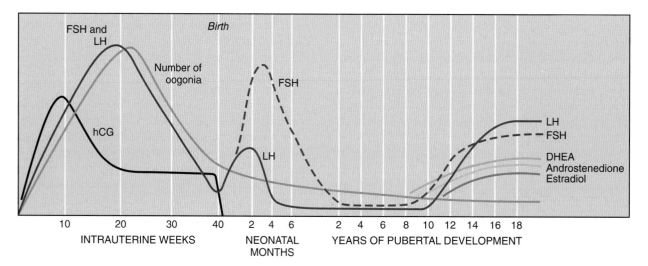

Figure 32-2. Changes in the concentration of gonadotropins (LH and FSH), sex steroids (DHEA, androsteinedionne, and estradiol), and the number of oogonia throughout fetal life and pubertal development. hCG, human chorionic gonadotropin; LH, luteinizing hormone; FSH, follicle-stimulating hormone; DHEA, dehydroepiandrosterone. *Adapted from Speroff L, Glass RH, Kase NG: Neuroendocrinology. In Speroff L (ed): Clinical Gynecologic Endocrinology and Infertility, 6th ed. Baltimore, MD, Williams & Wilkins, 1999.*

regulating gonadotropin release has been termed the **gonadostat. Low levels of gonadotropins and sex steroids during this prepubertal period are a function of two mechanisms: maximal sensitivity of the gonadostat to the negative feedback effect of the low, circulating levels of estradiol** present in prepubertal children, and **intrinsic central nervous system inhibition of hypothalamic gonadotropin-releasing hormone (GnRH) secretion.** These mechanisms occur independent of the presence of functional gonadal tissue. This is clearly demonstrated in children with gonadal dysgenesis. Agonadal children display elevated gonadotropin concentrations during the first 2 to 4 years of life, followed by a decline in circulating FSH and LH levels by 6 to 8 years of age. By 10 to 12 years of age, gonadotropin concentrations spontaneously rise once again, eventually achieving castration levels. This pattern of gonadotropin secretion in early childhood is similar to that of children with normal gonadal function. **This indicates that an intrinsic central nervous system regulator of GnRH release is the principal inhibitor of gonadotropin secretion from 4 years of age until the peripubertal period.**

LATE PREPUBERTAL PERIOD

In general, androgen production and differentiation by the zona reticularis of the adrenal cortex are the initial endocrine changes associated with puberty. Serum concentrations of dehydroepiandrosterone (DHEA), dehydroepiandrosterone sulfate (DHEA-S), and androstenedione rise between the ages of 8 and 11 years. **This rise in adrenal androgens induces the growth of both axillary and pubic hair and is known as** *adrenarche* **or** *pubarche.* This increase in adrenal androgen production occurs independent of gonadotropin secretion or gonadal steroid levels and the mechanism of its initiation is not understood at this time. Recent studies indicate that girls who undergo premature pubarche are more likely to develop polycystic ovarian syndrome (PCOS) as adults.

PUBERTAL ONSET

By approximately the eleventh year of life, there is a gradual loss of sensitivity by the gonadostat to the negative feedback of sex steroids (Figure 32-3). As a consequence of this reduced negative feedback effect, GnRH pulses (with their mirroring pulses of FSH and LH) increase in amplitude and frequency.

The factor (or factors) that reduce the sensitivity of the gonadostat are not completely understood. Some studies indicate that a rise in the concentration of leptin, a hormone produced by adipocytes (fat cells) that mediates appetite satiety, precedes and is necessary for this change. This, in turn, supports the connection between minimum weight or total body fat and the onset of puberty. **A further decrease in sensitivity of the gonadostat combined with the loss of intrinsic central nervous system inhibition of hypothalamic GnRH release is heralded by prominent sleep-associated increases in GnRH secretion.** This nocturnal-dominant pattern gradually shifts into an adult-type secretory pattern, with GnRH pulses occurring every 90 to 120 minutes throughout the 24-hour day.

The increase in gonadotropin release promotes ovarian follicular maturation and sex steroid production, which induces the development of secondary sexual characteristics. By mid- to late puberty, maturation of the positive-feedback mechanism of estradiol on LH release from the anterior pituitary gland is complete, and ovulatory cycles are established.

SOMATIC CHANGES OF PUBERTY

Physical changes of puberty involve the development of secondary sexual characteristics and the acceleration of linear growth (gain in height). The classification of breast and pubic hair development by Marshall and Tanner is employed for descriptive and diagnostic purposes (Figures 32-4 and 32-5).

STAGES OF PUBERTAL DEVELOPMENT

The first physical sign of puberty is usually breast budding (thelarche), followed by the appearance of pubic or axillary hair (pubarche or adrenarche). Unilateral breast development is not uncommon in early puberty and may last up to 6 months before the development of the contralateral breast. **Maximal growth or peak height velocity is usually the next stage, followed by menarche (the onset of menstrual periods).** The final somatic changes are the appearance of adult pubic hair distribution and adult-type breasts. In approximately 15% of normal girls, however, the development of pubic hair occurs prior to breast development. The sequence of pubertal changes generally occurs over a period of 4.5 years, with a normal range of 1.5 to 6 years (Figure 32-6).

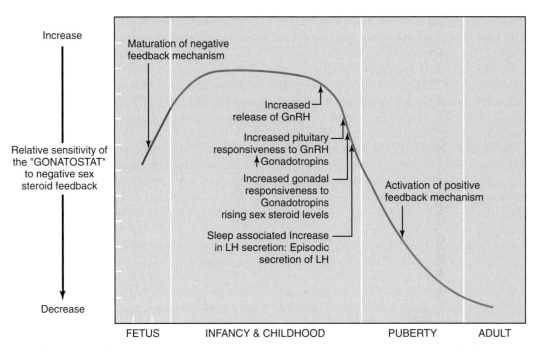

Figure 32-3. Changes in setpoint of the hypothalamic-pituitary unit (gonadostat) (*solid lines*) and the maturation of the negative and positive feedback mechanisms from fetal life to adulthood in relation to the normal changes of puberty. This figure does not illustrate the change in the sex steroid--independent intrinsic central nervous system inhibitory mechanism that is observed from late infancy to puberty. GnRH, gonadotropin-releasing hormone; LH, luteinizing hormone. *Adapted from Styne DM, Grumbach MM: Disorders of puberty in the male and female.* In *Yen SSC, Jaffe RB (eds): Reproductive Endocrinology: Physiology, Pathophysiology and Clinical Management, 2nd ed. Philadelphia, WB Saunders, 1991.*

ADOLESCENT GROWTH SPURT

In general, the pubertal girl's growth spurt is seen 2 years earlier than that of the boy. Growth hormone, estradiol, and insulin-like growth factor I (somatomedin-C) are involved in the adolescent growth spurt. Peak height velocity occurs approximately 1 year before the onset of menarche. There is limited linear growth after menarche, as gonadal steroid production accelerates fusion of the long bone epiphyses.

BODY COMPOSITION AND BONE AGE

There are no significant differences in skeletal mass, lean body mass, or percentage of body fat between prepubertal boys and prepubertal girls. On attaining sexual maturity, girls generally have less skeletal and lean body mass and a greater percentage of body fat than boys.

Bone age correlates well with the onset of secondary sexual characteristics and menarche. Bone age is determined by using radiographs of the left (or nondominant) hand and wrist, elbow, or knee and comparing them with an index population. Osseous maturation is particularly useful in the evaluation of adolescents with delayed onset of puberty. Bone maturation, chronological age, and height can also be used to predict the final adult stature from standardized nomograms (see PDA for growth calculators).

PRECOCIOUS PUBERTY

Precocious puberty refers to the development of any sign of secondary sexual maturation at an age earlier than 2.5 standard deviations (SD) less than the expected age of pubertal onset. In North America, these ages are 8 years for girls and 9 years for boys. The incidence of precocious puberty is 1 in 10,000 children in North America, and it is

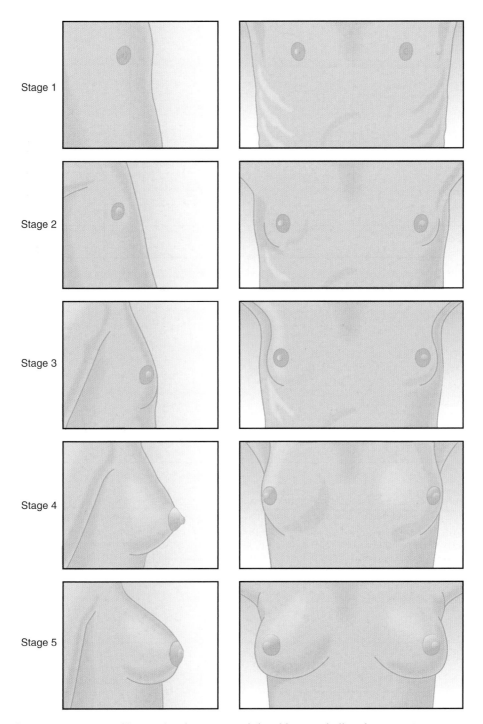

Figure 32-4. Stages of breast development as defined by Marshall and Tanner. *Stage 1,* Preadolescent; elevation of papilla only. *Stage 2,* Breast bud stage; elevation of breast and papilla as a small mound with enlargement of the areolar region. *Stage 3,* Further enlargement of breast and areola without separation of their contours. *Stage 4,* Projection of areola and papilla to form a secondary mound above the level of the breast. *Stage 5,* Mature stage; projection of papilla only, resulting from recession of the areola to the general contour of the breast. *Adapted from Marshall WA, Tanner JM: Variations in pattern of pubertal changes in girls. Arch Dis Child 44:291, 1969.*

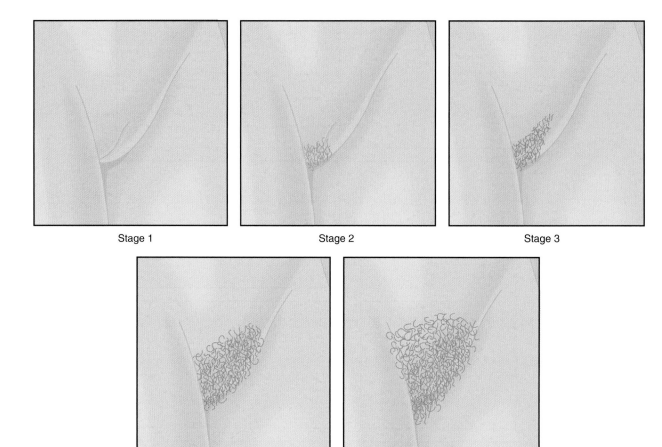

Stage 1   Stage 2   Stage 3

Stage 4   Stage 5

Figure 32-5. Stage of female pubic hair development according to Marshall and Tanner. *Stage 1,* Preadolescent; absence of pubic hair. *Stage 2,* Sparse hair along the labia; hair downy with slight pigment. *Stage 3,* Hair spreads sparsely over the junction of the pubes; hair is darker and coarser. *Stage 4,* Adult-type hair; there is no spread to the medial surface of the thighs. *Stage 5,* Adult-type hair with spread to the medial thighs assuming an inverted triangle (∇) pattern.

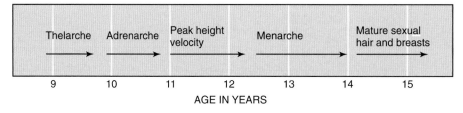

Figure 32-6. Sequence of physical changes during pubertal development.

approximately five times more common in girls. **In 75% of cases of precocious puberty in girls, the cause is idiopathic.** A thorough evaluation to eliminate a serious disease process, and to arrest potential premature osseous maturation that may affect the normal growth pattern, is mandatory.

The early development of secondary sexual characteristics may promote psychosocial problems for the child and should be carefully addressed. **Typically, these girls are taller than their peers as children but ultimately are shorter as adults owing to the premature fusion of the long-bone epiphyses.** A classification system for female precocious puberty is shown in Box 32-1.

Precocious puberty may be divided into two major subgroups: **heterosexual precocious puberty** **(development of secondary sexual characteristics opposite those of the anticipated phenotypic sex) and isosexual precocious puberty (premature sexual maturation that is appropriate for the phenotype of the affected individual).**

Investigations for females with precocious puberty are shown in Box 32-2.

HETEROSEXUAL PRECOCITY

In females, heterosexual precocity results from virilizing neoplasms, congenital adrenal hyperplasia, or exposure to exogenous androgens.

Androgen-secreting neoplasms in females are either ovarian (most commonly an arrhenoblastoma) or adrenal in origin and are exceedingly rare in childhood. They are diagnosed by abdominal physical and radiological examinations and are treated by surgical removal.

Congenital adrenal hyperplasia most commonly results from a defect of the adrenal enzyme 21-hydroxylase leading to excessive androgen production. More severe forms of this defect cause the birth of a

---

Box 32-1. Classification of female precocious puberty

HETEROSEXUAL PRECOCIOUS PUBERTY
Virilizing neoplasm
  Ovarian
  Adrenal
Congenital adrenal hyperplasia (adrenogenital syndrome)
Exogenous androgen exposure

ISOSEXUAL PRECOCIOUS PUBERTY
Incomplete isosexual precocious puberty
  Premature thelarche
  Premature adrenarche
  Premature pubarche
Complete isosexual precocious puberty
  True isosexual precocious puberty
    Constitutional (idiopathic)
    Organic brain disease
      Central nervous system tumors
      Head trauma
      Hydrocephalus
      CNS infection (abscess, encephalitis, meningitis)
  Pseudoisosexual precocious puberty
    Ovarian neoplasm
    Adrenal neoplasm
    Exogenous estrogen exposure
    Advanced hypothyroidism
    McCune-Albright syndrome
    Peutz-Jeghers syndrome

Adapted from Brenner PF: Precocious puberty in the female. *In* Mishell DR Jr, Davajan V (eds): Infertility, Contraception and Reproductive Endocrinology, 3rd ed. Cambridge, MA, Blackwell Scientific Publications, 1991, p 349.

Box 32-2. Laboratory tests used selectively to evaluate female precocious puberty

RADIOLOGIC
Serial bone age (isosexual precocity)
Magnetic resonance imaging (MRI) or computed tomography (CT) of the brain with optimal visualization of hypothalamic region and sella turcica (true isosexual precocity)
MRI, CT, or ultrasonography of abdomen, pelvis, or adrenal gland (heterosexual precocity, pseudoisosexual precocity)

LABORATORY
Luteinizing hormone (LH) and follicle-stimulating hormone (FSH)
Dehydroepiandrosterone sulfate (DHEA-S), testosterone (heterosexual precocity)
17-OH progesterone, 11-deoxycortisol (suspected congenital adrenal hyperplasia [CAH] causing heterosexual precocity)
Thyroid function tests [TSH, free T_4] (isosexual precocious puberty)
GnRH stimulation test: LH measurement after 100 mcg of GnRH given intravenously (to differentiate gonadotropin-dependent from gonadotropin-independent isosexual precocity).

female with ambiguous genitalia. If untreated, progressive virilization during childhood and short adult stature will result. A less severe form of this defect, referred to as late onset adrenal hyperplasia, can cause premature pubarche and an adult disorder resembling polycystic ovary syndrome. The treatment of this disorder includes replacement of cortisol with a related glucocorticoid and surgical correction of any anatomic abnormalities in the first few years of life.

ISOSEXUAL PRECOCIOUS PUBERTY

Complete isosexual precocious puberty results in the development of the full complement of secondary sexual characteristics and increased levels of sex steroids. It may arise from premature activation of the normal process of pubertal development involving the hypothalamic-pituitary-gonadal axis, which is called **true isosexual precocity.** Exposure to estrogen, independent of the hypothalamic-pituitary axis (such as from an estrogen-producing tumor), is called **pseudoisosexual precocity.**

True Isosexual Precocity

In females, 90% of cases are constitutional or are associated with a central nervous system hamartoma. It may be diagnosed by the administration of exogenous GnRH with a resultant rise in LH levels equivalent to that seen in older girls who are undergoing normal puberty. **In approximately 10% of girls with the true form of precocious puberty, a central nervous system disorder is the underlying cause.** This includes tumors, obstructive lesions (hydrocephalus), granulomatous diseases (sarcoidosis, tuberculosis), infective processes (meningitis, encephalitis, or brain abscess), neurofibromatosis, and head trauma. It is postulated that these conditions interfere with the normal inhibition of hypothalamic GnRH release. **Children with precocious puberty secondary to organic brain disease often exhibit neurologic symptoms before the appearance of premature sexual maturation.** Evaluation of true isosexual precocity should include magnetic resonance imaging scanning of the head for lesions.

Pseudoisosexual Precocity

Pseudoisosexual precocity occurs when estrogen levels are elevated and cause sexual characteristic maturation without activation of the hypothalamic-pituitary axis. In these girls, the GnRH stimulation test does not induce pubertal levels of gonadotropins. Causes include ovarian tumors and cysts, exogenous estrogenic compound use, McCune-Albright syndrome, severe prolonged hypothyroidism, and Peutz-Jeghers syndrome. Curiously, when the initial cause of pseudoisosexual precocity is eliminated, some girls go on to develop true isosexual precocity.

Some ovarian tumors can be felt on abdominal examination and are usually unilateral. Other lesions may require radiological imaging for diagnosis. Treatment of these lesions is surgical.

The McCune-Albright syndrome (polyostotic fibrous dysplasia) **represents 5% of cases of female precocious puberty** and consists of sexual precocity, multiple cystic bone defects that fracture easily, and *cafe au lait* spots with irregular borders most frequently on the face, neck, shoulders, and back, and adrenal hypercortisolism. Hyperthyroidism may also occur in this syndrome. The pathophysiology involves a somatic mutation in affected post-zygotic tissues, which causes them to function independent of their normal stimulating hormones.

Prolonged severe hypothyroidism has been hypothesized to cause pituitary gonadotropin release in response to the persistently elevated secretion of thyroid-releasing hormone (TRH). Concomitant elevated prolactin levels may also occur with the development of galactorrhea. Ovarian cysts may occasionally develop, and bone age may be retarded. This is the only form of precocious puberty associated with delayed bone age. Treatment is with thyroid replacement therapy.

The Peutz-Jeghers syndrome has been associated with a rare sex cord tumor with annular tubules, which may be estrogen secreting. Because this syndrome of gastrointestinal tract polyposis and mucocutaneous pigmentation has also been reported in association with a granulosa-theca cell tumor, children with this disorder should be screened for the development of gonadal neoplasms.

Incomplete isosexual precocity is the early appearance of a single secondary sexual characteristic. These conditions include: **premature thelarche,** the isolated appearance of breast development before the age of 4 years (unilateral or bilateral) that resolves spontaneously within months and that is probably secondary to transient estradiol secretion, **premature adrenarche,** the isolated appearance of axillary hair before the age of 7 years that is the result of premature androgen secretion by the adrenal gland; and **premature pubarche,** the isolated appearance of pubic hair in girls before 8 years of age.

In general, premature thelarche and premature adrenarche are of little clinical significance and are associated with appropriate sexual maturation. Therapy for these conditions is not required. Both conditions are more common in girls than in boys. **Premature pubarche may be associated with late-onset adrenal hyperplasia.** It is not possible to diagnose an incomplete form of sexual precocity on a single evaluation, and interval examinations of bone age are necessary to rule out true precocious puberty.

TREATMENT OF TRUE ISOSEXUAL PRECOCIOUS PUBERTY

Approximately 75% of cases of precocious puberty in girls prove to have a constitutional or idiopathic cause, and these patients are candidates for GnRH agonist (e.g., Luprelide) therapy. These girls require treatment to prevent further sex steroid release and accelerated epiphyseal fusion. **If the condition is left untreated, fewer than 50% of girls with idiopathic precocity will attain an adult height of 5 feet.**

GnRH agonists are the most effective therapy for idiopathic precocity. Long-term GnRH agonist treatment suppresses pituitary release of LH and FSH, resulting in the decline of gonadotropin levels to prepubertal concentrations and arrest of gonadal steroid secretion. Clinically, normal gonadotropin release, sex steroid production, and pubertal maturation will resume 3 to 12 months after discontinuation of GnRH agonist therapy.

The final adult stature of girls with GnRH-dependent causes of precocious puberty is strongly influenced by their chronologic age at diagnosis and initiation of treatment. When GnRH agonist treatment is initiated before the chronologic age of 6 years, the final adult height is increased by 2% to 4% (Figure 32-7). In contrast, the final adult height is usually not affected when the chronologic age at diagnosis and treatment is greater than 6 years of age.

The majority of children with sexual precocity have few significant behavioral problems, but emotional support is important in these children. **Behavioral expectations by family members and teachers should be based on the child's chronologic age, which determines psychosocial development, and not on the presence of secondary sexual characteristics.**

DELAYED PUBERTY

Although there is wide variation in normal pubertal development, the vast majority of girls in the United States begin pubertal maturation by the age of 13 years. **Failure to undergo thelarche by age 14 years requires evaluation.** A physiologic delay in the onset of puberty occurs in only 10% of girls with delayed puberty, and exclusion of other diagnoses is necessary. **Physiologic delays in puberty tend to be familial.** A careful history must be taken, with special attention to the patient's past general health, height, dietary habits, and exercise patterns. Details about the pubertal development of the patient's siblings and parents should be obtained. Box 32-3 lists tests that are performed to evaluate girls with delayed puberty.

In general, the causes of delayed onset of puberty can be subdivided into two categories: **hypogonadotropic hypogonadism and hypergonadotropic hypogonadism.** Disorders resulting in hypogonadotropic hypogonadism that may cause primary or secondary amenorrhea are discussed in Chapter 33. Chromosomal abnormalities or injury to the ovaries by surgery, chemotherapy, or radiation may cause hypergonadotropic hypogonadism. When the patient's abnormal karyotype includes the presence of a Y chromosome, gonadectomy must be performed to prevent malignant neoplastic transformation.

A growing list of single gene disorders resulting in delayed or absent female puberty is being documented in the literature.

Kallmann syndrome presents with hypogonadotropic hypogonadism and anosmia/hyposmia. It may result from a mutation of the KAL gene on the

---

Box 32-3. Radiologic and laboratory tests used to evaluate female delayed puberty

RADIOLOGIC
Magnetic resonance imaging or computed tomography of the brain with optimal visualization of hypothalamic region and sella turcica (hypogonadotropic hypogonadism)

LABORATORY
Follicle-stimulating hormone (FSH)
Karyotype (delayed puberty, ambiguous genitalia)
Progesterone (delayed puberty secondary to 17-hydroxylase [P450c17] deficiency)
Prolactin (hypogonadotropic hypogonadism)

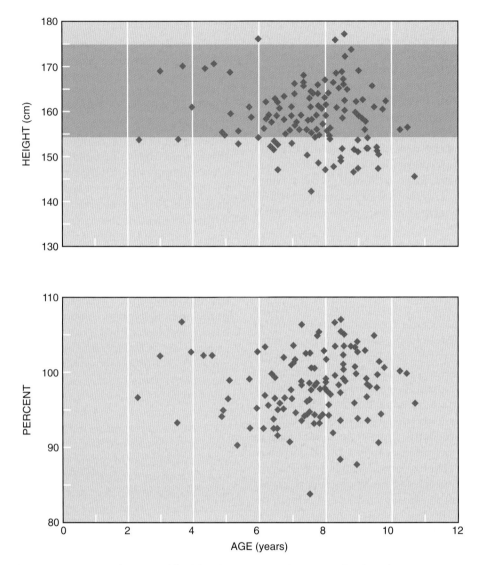

Figure 32-7. Scatter diagram of final height vs. age at diagnosis of girls with GnRH-dependent precocious puberty who were treated with GnRH agonist therapy (*top*). The *shaded area* represents the range of normal adult height for North American women. *Bottom*, Percentage target height (final target height/target height × 100) vs. the age at diagnosis. *Modified from Kletter GD, Kelch RP: Effects of gonadotropin-releasing hormone analogue therapy on adult stature in precocious puberty. J Clin Endocrinol Metab 79:333, 1994.*

X chromosome or from autosomal mutations that prevent the embryologic migration of GnRH neurons into the hypothalamus. These individuals may have other anomalies of midline structures of the head. One in 50,000 females is affected.

Mutations of the GnRH receptor gene in females have resulted in low gonadotropin levels with primary amenorrhea or delayed puberty.

FSH β-subunit gene mutations and **FSH receptor gene mutations** have been associated with primary amenorrhea and varying degrees of incomplete development of secondary sexual characteristics.

Females with **aromatase deficiency** present at puberty with progressive virilization, absence of thelarche, and primary amenorrhea.

17-Hydroxylase (P450c17) deficiency interferes with production of the androgenic and estrogenic steroids, resulting in deficient or absent pubertal development. The accumulation of progesterone prior to the block leads to excessive synthesis of the mineralocorticoid, 11-deoxycorticosterone, that generally causes hypertension and hyokalemia.

Adolescents who present with permanent hypoestrogenism require estrogen therapy as described in Chapter 33, to complete the development of secondary sexual characteristics. Hormone therapy with estrogen plus a progestin or with a low-dose oral contraceptive after establishment of secondary sexual characteristics is required to avoid menopausal symptoms and to prevent osteoporosis. To further maximize bone mineral accretion, 1500 mg of elemental calcium and 400 mg of vitamin D daily are recommended. This should be combined with regular weight-bearing exercise.

Suggested Reading

Speroff L, Glass RH, Kase NG: Abnormal puberty and growth problems. *In* Speroff L (ed): Clinical Gynecologic Endocrinology and Infertility, 6th ed. Baltimore, MD, Williams & Wilkins, 1999.

Styne DM, Grumbach MM: Puberty in the male and female: Its physiology and disorders. *In* Yen SSC, Jaffe RB, Barbieri RL (eds): Reproductive Endocrinology: Physiology, Pathophysiology and Clinical Management, 4th ed. Philadelphia, WB Saunders, 1999.

Amenorrhea, Oligomenorrhea, and Hyperandrogenic Disorders

Larry R. Laufer and Ketan S. Patel

Amenorrhea, or the absence of menses, is a common symptom of several pathophysiologic states. This condition traditionally has been divided into primary amenorrhea, in which menarche (the first menses) has not occurred, and secondary amenorrhea, where menses has been absent for 6 months or more. A more functional or clinical division of menstrual disorders based on initial history and physical examination would be: primary amenorrhea with sexual infantilism, primary amenorrhea with breast development and müllerian anomalies, and amenorrhea/oligomenorrhea with breast development and normal müllerian structures. The last group includes disorders causing primary as well as secondary amenorrhea, oligomenorrhea, and the hyperandrogenic states (Box 33-1).

PRIMARY AMENORRHEA

The diagnosis of primary amenorrhea is made when no spontaneous uterine bleeding has occurred by the age of 16 years. The work-up should be initiated sooner if there is no evidence of breast development (thelarche) by age 14 years or if the patient has failed to menstruate spontaneously within 2 years of thelarche. The presence of normal breast development confirms gonadal secretion of estrogen, and the presence of pubic and axillary hair confirms gonadal secretion of androgens as well as the presence of functional androgen receptors.

PRIMARY AMENORRHEA WITH SEXUAL INFANTILISM

Patients with primary amenorrhea and no secondary sexual characteristics (sexual infantilism) display the absence of gonadal hormone secretion. The differential diagnosis is based on whether the defect is the result of a lack of gonadotropin secretion (**hypogonadotropic hypogonadism**) or of an inability of the ovaries to respond to gonadotropin (**gonadal agenesis/dysgenesis**). The distinction can be made by the measurement of serum follicle-stimulating hormone (FSH). **Patients with hypogonadotropic hypogonadism have low FSH levels, whereas patients with gonadal dysgenesis have elevated FSH levels in the menopausal range (>40 IU/L).** The measurement of serum luteinizing hormone (LH) is of no additional diagnostic value. The absence of breast development is indicative of inadequate secretion of estrogen, and measurement of estradiol adds little to the differential diagnosis.

Hypogonadotropic hypogonadism may be caused by lesions of the hypothalamus or pituitary gland or by functional disorders, which result in inadequate gonadotropin-releasing hormone (GnRH) synthesis and release. It may also represent constitutionally delayed puberty, which is a diagnosis of exclusion. **Patients with primary amenorrhea caused by hypogonadotropic hypogonadism may have a craniopharyngioma or other central nervous system tumor, and therefore, magnetic resonance imaging (MRI) of the hypothalamic-pituitary area is recommended** (this applies to patients with secondary amenorrhea and hypogonadotropic hypogonadism as well).

Hypogonadotropic hypogonadism may be the result of a general process of pituitary failure. These patients should be screened for other pituitary hormone deficiencies by testing for thyroid stimulating hormone (TSH), growth hormone (GH), and adrenocorticotropic hormone (ACTH).

Box 33-1. Clinical classification of menstrual disorders

PRIMARY AMENORRHEA WITH SEXUAL INFANTILISM
Hypergonadotropic hypogonadism
Gonadal agenesis/dysgenesis
17-Hydroxylase (P450c17) deficiency

PRIMARY AMENORRHEA WITH BREAST DEVELOPMENT AND MÜLLERIAN ANOMALIES
Complete androgen insensitivity syndrome (46 XY)
Normal karyotype (46 XX)
  Imperforate hymen
  Transverse vaginal septum
  Cervical agenesis
  Meyer-Rokitansky-Kuster-Hauser syndrome

AMENORRHEA/OLIGOMENORRHEA WITH BREAST DEVELOPMENT AND NORMAL MÜLLERIAN STRUCTURES
Pregnancy
Uterine defects (e.g., Asherman's syndrome)
Hypoestrogenism
  hypothalamic-pituitary dysfunction (e.g., anorexia nervosa)
  Premature ovarian failure
Hyperprolactinemia
Mild hypothalamic dysfunction (normoestrogenic)
Hyperandrogenism

The latter is done by measuring a fasting morning cortisol level.

Patients with gonadal agenesis/dysgenesis have elevated FSH levels. These patients should have karyotype determinations. The differential diagnosis includes patients with 45 XO (Turner syndrome), a structurally abnormal X chromosome, mosaicism with or without a Y chromosome, and pure gonadal dysgenesis (46 XX and 46 XY), as well as conditions with normal karyotypes resulting in the failure of a normal gonad to develop (such as galactosemia). Although most affected patients show no signs of secondary sexual characteristics, occasionally an individual with mosaicism or Turner syndrome has sufficient follicular activity and secretes enough estrogen to cause breast development, menstruation, ovulation, and rarely, pregnancy.

A second gonadal cause of sexual infantilism is 17-hydroxylase (P450c17) deficiency, which pre-vents the synthesis of sex steroids (see Figure 33-1). These individuals have hypertension and hypokalemia caused by mineralocorticoid excess.

Patients with sexual infantilism may be induced to undergo thelarche by very gradually increasing estrogen doses, for example, starting with 0.3 mg conjugated estrogens every other day and slowly increasing over 1 to 3 month intervals (guided by the presence or absence of mastalgia). Those individuals with persistent hypogonadotropic hypogonadism who seek fertility will need therapy with either human menopausal gonadotropin (hMG) injections or pulsatile GnRH given by a continuously worn pump. Patients with gonadal dysgenesis and 17-hydroxylase deficiency can achieve pregnancy only by in vitro fertilization (IVF), using donated oocytes.

PRIMARY AMENORRHEA WITH BREAST DEVELOPMENT AND MÜLLERIAN ANOMALIES

Patients with primary amenorrhea, breast development, and Müllerian anomalies all fail to demonstrate a visible or palpable uterine cervix on physical examination. They fall into two categories: those with complete androgen insensitivity syndrome (46 XY) and those with a karyotype of 46 XX. The distinction can be made by the serum testosterone level. Patients with complete androgen insensitivity syndrome have male levels of testosterone.

The karyotype in patients with androgen insensitivity syndrome is 46 XY, and they have testes that are often intraabdominal. Breast development (with smaller nipples and areolae than normal) is caused by an enzymatic conversion of male levels of androgen to estrogen. The testes in these patients secrete normal male amounts of Müllerian-inhibiting substance; hence, patients have only a vaginal dimple and no uterus or tubes. Treatment should consist of gonadal resection to avoid malignant neoplasia once puberty is complete and the creation of a neovagina when the patient is prepared to be sexually active. Psychological counseling is also an important component in the care of these patients.

Patients with primary amenorrhea, breast development, and a karyotype of 46 XX with anatomical anomalies have levels of testosterone appropriate for females. One should suspect an imperforate hymen in adolescents who report monthly dysmenorrhea in the absence of menstrual flow. On examination, these patients often present with a vaginal bulge and a midline cystic mass on rectal examination. Ultrasonography confirms the presence of a normal uterus and ovaries with hematocolpos. These patients can be successfully treated by hymenectomy.

Alternatively, women may present with similar symptoms but no lower vaginal bulge. When ultrasonography confirms a normal uterus and ovaries, one should suspect the possibility of **a transverse, obstructing vaginal septum or cervical agenesis.** MRI is the diagnostic method of choice in these patients. If the MRI scan confirms a transverse septum, surgical correction is indicated. These procedures can be extremely difficult, and the surgeon must be prepared to use tissue expanders, split-thickness skin grafts, or other techniques to effect a functional vagina. Surgical construction of a functional cervix is extremely unlikely. In general, it is recommended that these women undergo hysterectomy.

Finally, **rectal examination and ultrasonography may show the absence of a uterus indicating Meyer-Rokitansky-Küster-Hauser syndrome.** This syndrome is characterized by a failure of the Müllerian ducts to fuse distally and to form the upper genital tract. These patients usually have bilateral rudimentary uterine tissues (anlagen), fallopian tubes, and ovaries. It is uncommon to have functional endometrial tissue within the anlagen. On occasion, the ovaries are not visible on ultrasonography because they have not descended into the pelvis. In these cases, computed tomography (CT) or MRI may identify them well above the pelvic brim.

Creation of a neovagina can be accomplished by using one of two general approaches. The Frank method of vaginal dilatation uses dilatation of the vaginal pouch with vaginal forms (usually thermoplastic acrylic resin [Lucite] dilators) over the course of weeks to months. Alternatively, a McIndoe vaginoplasty, which involves the surgical creation of a neovaginal space using a split-thickness skin graft, may be performed. Both of these methods should be initiated in proximity to the time when the patient anticipates having vaginal intercourse.

Congenital anatomic abnormalities of the uterus or vagina, or both, are often associated with renal abnormalities such as a unilateral solitary kidney or a double collecting system, among others.

These patients should have an intravenous pyelogram or other diagnostic study to confirm the normalcy of the urinary system.

AMENORRHEA/OLIGOMENORRHEA WITH BREAST DEVELOPMENT AND NORMAL MÜLLERIAN STRUCTURES

All other menstrual disorders in which the patient has breast development and a demonstrable cervix and uterine fundus on physical examination may cause primary as well as secondary amenorrhea (absence of menses for 6 months or more). **All patients with menstrual bleeding disorders should be tested for pregnancy.**

Once pregnancy has been excluded, these patients can be characterized as shown in Box 33-1. Initial history-taking should include questions about the timing of the menstrual disorder (present since puberty or new), significant weight change, strenuous exercise activities, increased facial hair, and the presence or absence of hot flashes. A comprehensive list of all medications should be compiled.

Investigations should include a serum prolactin level (preferably fasting), and if the patient is amenorrheic, a FSH level and a progestin challenge test. Failure of the patient to have withdrawal bleeding after taking a progestational agent indicates pregnancy, severe hypoestrogenism, or a uterine defect. The latter condition can be ruled out by the presence of withdrawal bleeding following sequential estrogen and progestin therapy.

UTERINE DEFECTS

Women who do not have withdrawal bleeding after hormonal challenge testing and who have a history of uterine instrumentation, particularly a dilation and curettage (D&C) following vaginal delivery or pregnancy termination may have Asherman's syndrome, with characteristic intrauterine synechiae. Because there is no ovarian or hormonal abnormality, these patients may have normal ovulatory cycles with cyclic premenstrual symptoms. Patients with Asherman's syndrome may be evaluated by hysterosalpingography (HSG) and transvaginal ultrasonography. Hysteroscopic treatment with excision of synechiae is the treatment of choice. The results are often disappointing in terms of subsequent fertility.

SECONDARY AMENORRHEA ASSOCIATED WITH HYPOESTROGENISM

The differential diagnosis for patients with amenorrhea associated with hypoestrogenism is

hypothalamic-pituitary dysfunction, premature ovarian failure, or hyperprolactinemia. The first group of women has low FSH and prolactin levels, the second group have high FSH and normal prolactin levels, and the third group has high prolactin and low FSH levels.

The hypothalamic-pituitary dysfunction group includes: patients with severe weight loss or excessive exercise resulting in a low percentage body fat, psychiatric stress, (e.g., anorexia nervosa), wasting from severe systemic diseases such as disseminated malignancies, pituitary or central nervous system lesions, and pituitary failure.

As with hypogonadotropic hypogonadism and sexual infantilism, these patients should be evaluated for the status of the other pituitary hormones and by MRI of the hypothalamus and pituitary gland. When this condition cannot be resolved by identifying an underlying cause (e.g., excessive exercise), estrogen and progestin therapy, usually in the form of a combined oral contraceptive pill, is given to reduce the risk of osteoporosis caused by chronic hypoestrogenism. In the case of anorexia nervosa, ovarian hormone therapy without weight gain will not totally prevent osteoporosis. Fertility restoration will require human menopausal gonadotropin (hMG) injections or continuous pulsatile GnRH (see Chapter 35).

Premature ovarian failure is defined as ovarian failure before the age of 40 (see Chapter 36). In patients younger than 30 years of age when they present, failure may be caused by a chromosomal disorder. A karyotype is done to check for mosaicism (some cells bearing a Y chromosome). If cells with a Y chromosome are present, gonadectomy to prevent malignant transformation is indicated.

Other causes of premature ovarian failure include ovarian injury from surgery, radiation or chemotherapy, galactosemia, and autoimmunity. When premature ovarian failure is secondary to autoimmunity, other endocrine organs may be affected as well. There are no specific laboratory tests available for autoimmune ovarian failure. Therefore, patients with unexplained ovarian failure should be screened for diabetes (fasting glucose), hypothyroidism (TSH and free T4), hypoparathyroidism (serum calcium), and hypocortisolism (fasting morning cortisol). It is not unusual for patients with premature ovarian failure to have episodes of normal ovarian and menstrual function. Patients with premature ovarian failure require hormone therapy (estrogen and a progestin) to reduce the risk of osteoporosis.

AMENORRHEA WITH HYPERPROLACTINEMIA

Hyperprolactinemia that is severe or that is associated with menstrual disturbance or galactorrhea should be confirmed by a second test, preferably in the fasting state, as food ingestion may cause transient hyperprolactinemia. At the same time that the repeat prolactin level is drawn, a TSH level should be obtained to test for hypothyroidism. A biologically inactive complex of prolactin and immunoglobulin, called big prolactin, can give a physiologically insignificant elevation. Hence, the presence of a clinical abnormality should initiate the decision to test for hyperprolactinemia. **If clinically significant hyperprolactinemia is not explained by hypothyroidism or drug use, a CT or MRI scan of the sella turcica should be performed.**

Galactorrhea is the most frequently observed abnormality associated with hyperprolactinemia. The secretion may occur spontaneously or only after breast manipulation. Both breasts should be examined gently by palpating the gland moving from the periphery to the nipple. To confirm galactorrhea, a smear may be prepared and examined microscopically for the presence of multiple fat droplets (indicating milk). **Besides galactorrhea, hyperprolactinemia frequently causes oligomenorrhea or amenorrhea.**

PHARMACOLOGIC AGENTS AFFECTING THE SECRETION OF PROLACTIN

Drugs may cause hyperprolactinemia and nonphysiologic galactorrhea. **Responsible agents include tranquilizers, antidepressants, antihypertensive agents, narcotics, metaclopramide, and estrogen.** The mechanism of drug-induced hyperprolactinemia is secondary to reduced hypothalamic secretion of dopamine, depriving the pituitary of a natural inhibitor of prolactin release.

When clinically indicated, patients with hyperprolactinemia caused by medications should be encouraged to discontinue the medication for at least 1 month. If hyperprolactinemia persists, or if the patient cannot interrupt the medication, a complete evaluation is indicated.

PATHOLOGIC FACTORS AFFECTING SECRETION OF PROLACTIN

In about 3% to 5% of patients with galactorrhea and hyperprolactinemia, the underlying cause is **primary hypothyroidism.** These patients have a low serum free thyroxine (T_4) level; as a consequence, they lack negative feedback on the hypothalamic-pituitary axis, resulting in increased secretion of thyrotropin-releasing hormone (TRH). TRH, in turn, stimulates elevated levels of TSH and prolactin. **Patients with primary hypothyroidism should be given T_4 replacement therapy.** Further evaluation is often unnecessary.

Pituitary adenomas may cause hyperprolactinemia. Their etiology is unknown. About 50% of patients with hyperprolactinemia have radiographic changes in the sella turcica compatible with an adenoma. Most patients have normal or somewhat low baseline levels of FSH. **Hypothalamic tumors** may cause hyperprolactinemia by damaging the hypothalamus or by compression of the pituitary stalk interfering with the production or transport of dopamine. Craniopharyngiomas are the most common of these lesions.

The empty sella syndrome is characterized by herniation of the subarachnoid membrane into the pituitary sella turcica through a defective or incompetent sella diaphragm and may coexist with prolactin-secreting pituitary adenomas.

Patients with **acute or chronic renal failure** may have hyperprolactinemia because of delayed clearance of the hormone. These patients rarely require treatment other than for their renal failure.

Patients with scars from previous chest surgery, including breast implants, may have galactorrhea caused by **peripheral nerve stimulation.** Herpes zoster of the area including the breasts, as well as other forms of breast stimulation, can produce galactorrhea and sometimes hyperprolactinemia by the same mechanism.

TREATMENT OF GALACTORRHEA AND HYPERPROLACTINEMIA

The objectives of therapy for patients with galactorrhea or hyperprolactinemia include the elimination of lactation, the establishment of normal estrogen secretion, and the induction of ovulation when fertility is desired. The recommended forms of management are periodic observation, drug therapy, and surgery.

Observation

Periodic observation is indicated in menstruating women with galactorrhea who have either normal serum prolactin levels or idiopathic elevations of prolactin. **As long as the galactorrhea is not socially embarrassing and the patient has regular menses (confirming normal estrogen levels), there is no need to institute treatment.** Patients with oligomenorrhea who do not desire fertility should be treated with progestins to induce regular uterine bleeding. Failure to induce withdrawal bleeding with progestins is suggestive of hypoestrogenism and, if verified by low serum levels of estradiol (<30 pg/mL) and a negative pregnancy test, hormone therapy (estrogen and a progestin) should be initiated. Long-term treatment with bromocriptine (for hyperprolactinemia) in women with normal estrogen levels is not indicated.

Observation can be extended to some women with radiologic evidence of a pituitary microadenoma (<1 cm in diameter). **Because the growth rate of microadenomas is slow, an annual measurement of serum prolactin is appropriate in patients with normal estrogen levels.** The size of the tumor increases in only a small percentage of women with microadenomas who do not receive any treatment.

Pharmaceutical Therapy

Patients with hyperprolactinemia may suffer from galactorrhea and anovulation with resulting infertility. In more severe cases they may be hypoestrogenic, which places them at risk for developing osteoporosis. **Anovulatory patients without demonstrable tumors by MRI, for whom the only issues are prevention of osteoporosis and cycle regulation, may be treated with combination oral contraceptives.**

The ergot compounds, bromocriptine and cabergoline, act as dopamine agonists to reduce prolactin secretion and allow for the restoration of cyclic, physiologic estrogen secretion. Bromocriptine has a high initial incidence of side effects such as headache, nausea, and orthostatic hypotension. As a consequence, it should be started at a dose of 1.25 to 2.5 mg at bedtime and slowly increased in divided doses to tolerance and restoration of normal prolactin levels. Some patients tolerate bromocriptine better when it is given vaginally. Cabergoline is taken in twice-weekly doses beginning at 0.25 mg and increasing the dose up to a maximum of 1 mg twice weekly. It is better tolerated and more convenient to take than bromocriptine, but is also more expensive.

Ninety-five percent of women without radiographic evidence of an adenoma require 5 mg/day of bromocriptine, whereas about 50% of patients with adenomas require higher doses of bromocriptine to resume regular menses. Usually, menses resume and galactorrhea resolves after about 6 weeks of bromocriptine therapy in women without adenomas. If an adenoma is present, it takes another 3 or 4 weeks for bromocriptine to become effective. Return of ovulation requires an average of 10 weeks without a tumor and 16 weeks with a microadenoma. Restoration of normal menstrual cycles and pregnancy may occur without complete normalization of the serum prolactin level. Discontinuation of therapy usually results in the return of hyperprolactinemia, leading to galactorrhea and amenorrhea. Up to 25% of patients without demonstrable tumors will have prolonged euprolactinemia without treatment after more than 6 months of therapy.

Patients with macroadenomas (>1 cm diameter) should have visual field testing and screening of the other pituitary hormones. A repeat MRI is done 6 months after the full therapeutic dose of bromocriptine is reached. As long as shrinkage of the adenoma is demonstrated, bromocriptine therapy is continued. **Surgery should be performed for patients with significant visual field defects or symptoms that cannot be relieved by medical therapy.**

Bromocriptine therapy is usually discontinued as soon as a pregnancy is confirmed. The patients with macroadenomas should have visual fields carefully examined in each trimester of pregnancy. If abnormalities in the visual fields develop, bromocriptine treatment should be instituted or increased and maintained for the rest of the pregnancy. There is no increase in fetal malformations as a result of bromocriptine treatment, and the drug can be discontinued after the completion of pregnancy to allow for breast-feeding.

Surgery

If surgery is required, the trans-sphenoidal route for the microsurgical exploration of the sella turcica permits the removal of the pituitary adenoma while preserving the functional capacity of the remaining gland.

Cure rates of 50% to 80% have been reported for patients with microadenomas and rates of 10% to 30% have been reported for patients with macroadenomas. Potential morbidity includes transient or persistent diabetes insipidus, hemorrhage, meningitis, cerebrospinal fluid leak, and panhypopituitarism. Fifty percent of patients followed for 5 to 10 years after successful resection of the adenoma have recurrence of hyperprolactinemia without radiologic evidence of tumor.

SECONDARY AMENORRHEA/ OLIGOMENORRHEA DUE TO MILD HYPOTHALAMIC DYSFUNCTION

Patients who are diagnosed as consistently having adequate levels of estrogen but who are anovulatory may have a mild form of hypothalamic anovulation caused by nutrition/exercise mismatch, psychological stress, previous use of Depo-Provera, recent pregnancy, or lactation. If contraception is not required and fertility is not desired, periodic progestin withdrawal to confirm a normal estrogen levels and observation may be appropriate. If hypoestrogenism is demonstrated, the previously outlined evaluation and management plans apply. For patients with normal estrogen levels who desire fertility, clomiphene citrate is the initial therapy.

HYPERANDROGENIC DISORDERS, HIRSUTISM, AND VIRILISM

Hirsutism (more apparent facial and chest hair caused by conversion to the dark, thick terminal hair form) and virilism (severe hirsutism with temporal balding, deepening of the voice or clitoromegaly) are clinical manifestations of abnormal androgen effect. Androgens in women are normally produced in the ovaries and the adrenal glands (see Figure 33-1). Hyperandrogenic disorders may be divided into functional and neoplastic disorders of the adrenal or ovary (Box 33-2).

Box 33-2. Hyperandrogenic disorders

ADRENAL DISORDERS
Congenital adrenal hyperplasia (CAH)
Cushing's syndrome
Adrenal adenomas and carcinomas

OVARIAN DISORDERS
Polycystic ovarian syndrome (PCOS)
Hyperthecosis
Hilus cell hyperplasia
Ovarian neoplasms
    Sertoli-Leydig cell tumors
    Hilus cell tumors
    Lipoid cell tumors

NORMAL ANDROGEN METABOLISM

The formation of androgens results from the metabolism of cholesterol via the Δ^5 or Δ^4 pathway (Figure 33-1). The stimulus for ovarian androgen production is LH. The control of adrenal androgen production is currently unclear, although the presence of ACTH is required.

Approximately one half of serum testosterone and androstenedione originates in the ovary, whereas the other half arises from the adrenal gland. Dehydroepiandrosterone (DHEA) and its sulfate, DHEA-S are primarily products of adrenal androgen production and serve as markers for this tissue. **After secretion by the ovaries or adrenal glands, most androgens are bound in the circulation to specific proteins, especially sex hormone–binding globulin (SHBG). In the bound form, androgens are biologically inactive.** For example, in normal women, approximately 99% of serum testosterone is protein-bound and therefore largely inactive. The active nonprotein-bound or free fraction represents only about 1% of the total circulating testosterone.

When androgens reach the target tissue, they are further metabolized, which may result in more potent intracellular hormones. **Testosterone is converted within the cell to dihydrotestosterone (DHT), which possesses greater biologic potency than its precursor.** The skin is capable of this conversion. The pilosebaceous unit in the skin consists of the sebaceous gland and the hair follicle, both of which are sensitive to androgenic regulation. Frequently, hirsutism is accompanied by oily skin and acne. Some women with hyperandrogenic states, such as East Asian women with polycystic ovarian syndrome (PCOS), do not have hirsutism because of reduced skin sensitivity to androgens.

HYPERANDROGENIC DISORDERS
ADRENAL DISORDERS
Congenital Adrenal Hyperplasia

Congenital adrenal hyperplasia (CAH) is a general term used to describe an assortment of clinical entities that arise from inborn glandular enzyme deficiencies associated with overproduction of steroids.

The most common condition is 21-hydroxylase deficiency. In 20% of cases, the defect is complete, whereas in 80% it is incomplete or partial. **The most severe form of CAH usually occurs in the newborn and is manifested by ambiguous genitalia in female**

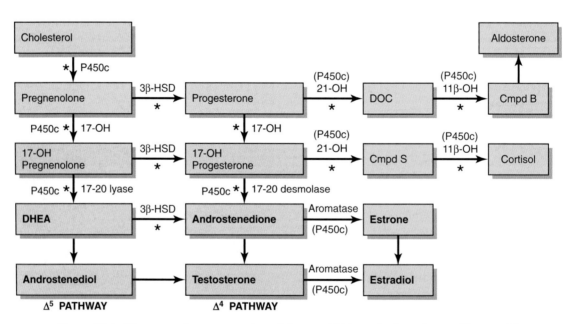

Figure 33-1. Diagrammatic representation of the steroid biosynthetic pathways. The *asterisk* refers to specific enzyme defects that result in congenital adrenal hyperplasia (CAH). OH, hydroxylase; HSD, hydroxysteroid dehydrogenase; P450c, cytochrome P450; DOC, desoxycorticosterone; cmpd B, corticosterone; cmpd S, II-desoxycortisol.

newborns. A very mild form of this disorder has been recognized in young women soon after puberty (late-onset 21-hydroxylase deficiency). The diagnosis is suggested by an adolescent onset of hirsutism with or without regular menstrual function.

Because 21-hydroxylase is responsible for the conversion of 17-hydroxyprogesterone to 11-deoxycortisol (compound S), a deficiency of 21-hydroxylase results in an accumulation of 17-hydroxyprogesterone, which is detectable in the circulation. As a result, this specific enzyme disorder is marked by an elevated serum 17-hydroxyprogesterone level as well as increases in its Δ^4 metabolites androstenedione and testosterone (Figure 33-1). **This disease is inherited as an autosomal recessive trait.**

Cushing's Syndrome

The second major adrenal disease leading to excess androgen production is Cushing's syndrome or persistent hypercortisolism. Characteristic manifestations include truncal obesity, moonlike faces with plethora, hypertension, impaired glucose tolerance, muscle wasting, osteoporosis, abdominal striae, and supraclavicular and cervical spinal fat pads. Other symptoms include hirsutism, acne, and irregular menstrual function. Emotional lability is common in patients with Cushing's syndrome. This disorder may arise from a cortisol-producing tumor of the adrenal gland or from excessive pituitary ACTH production.

Adrenal Neoplasms

Adrenal tumors resulting in androgenization without symptoms and signs of glucocorticoid excess are rare. Adenomas, which produce androgens only, generally secrete large amounts of DHEA-S. Adrenal carcinomas may produce large amounts of both glucocorticoids and androgens.

OVARIAN DISORDERS
Polycystic Ovarian Syndrome

In general, 4% to 6% of women of reproductive age suffer from some form of PCOS. Polycystic ovarian syndrome is a chronic condition that has been defined as chronic anovulation or oligoovulation with clinical or laboratory evidence of hyperandrogenism, both of which occur in the absence of any other underlying condition. Its onset generally occurs at the time of puberty.

Clinically, the most common symptoms of PCOS are hirsutism (90%), menstrual irregularity (90%), and infertility (75%). In most patients, the ovaries contain multiple follicular cysts that are inactive and arrested in the midantral stage of development. The cysts are located peripherally in the cortex of the ovary (Figure 33-2). The ovarian stroma is hyperplastic and may contain nests of luteinized theca cells that produce androgens. Approximately 20% of hormonally normal women may also have polycystic-appearing ovaries.

In PCOS, hyperandrogenism results from an overproduction of androgen by the ovary and often the adrenal gland. It is unclear what the ultimate underlying pathophysiology of this condition is or whether it is a single clinical entity. **Patients with PCOS exhibit increased LH pulse frequency, resulting in higher circulating levels of LH.** It is likely that these patients exhibit increased LH levels because of either increased GnRH secretion from the arcuate nucleus of the hypothalamus or increased pituitary sensitivity to GnRH. **The increased LH level promotes androgen secretion from ovarian theca cells, leading to elevated levels of intraovarian-derived androgens.** This then leads to atresia of developing follicles and interferes with the normal development of a dominant ovarian follicle. The normal secretory pattern of estrogen is disrupted and the midcycle LH surge does not occur, resulting in

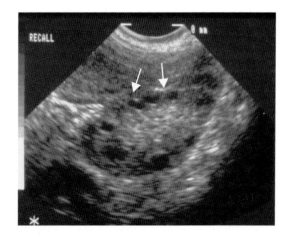

Figure 33-2. Transvaginal ultrasonography in a woman with polycystic ovarian disease. The multiple subcapsular cysts, with their "string of pearls" appearance (arrows), are common in this syndrome.

anovulation and lack of progesterone production. **The excessive amounts of androgen are peripherally converted to estrogen. The unopposed estrogens may cause adenomatous hyperplasia of the endometrium or rarely endometrial carcinoma.** Other important effects of the increased estrogen levels are the stimulation of pituitary LH release and the inhibition of FSH release, which further interferes with normal folliculogenesis.

Some PCOS patients have excessive androgen production from the adrenal glands as well as the ovaries. The mechanism of excess adrenal androgen production in this disorder is unknown.

An association exists between abnormal androgen production and insulin resistance with hyperinsulinism. In PCOS, insulin sensitivity is decreased, leading to insulin hypersecretion compared with height- and weight-matched control women. Receptor studies performed in these patients have indicated normal receptor numbers and binding. Most likely, insulin resistance in PCOS is caused by a postreceptor phosphorylation defect.

Hyperinsulinemia is related to excessive production of ovarian androgens. Basal insulin concentrations and insulin responses to a glucose load have shown a positive linear relationship to serum testosterone and androstenedione levels. Moreover, in vitro studies of ovarian stroma from hyperandrogenic women have revealed that testosterone and androstenedione responses to insulin and LH are significantly amplified compared with those of normal tissue. In addition, animal studies have demonstrated that insulin increases LH release from cultured pituitary cells.

Increased androgens as well as insulin generally reduce hepatic production and secretion of SHBG. When SHBG production is suppressed, the amount of free testosterone may be dramatically increased even though the overall increase in total testosterone is moderate or small. Thus, the physical manifestations of hyperandrogenism may seem dramatic in relation to the level of total testosterone.

Hyperthecosis and Hilus Cell Hyperplasia

Hyperthecosis and hilus cell hyperplasia are functional hyperandrogenic conditions that are marked by higher androgen levels than are seen in PCOS. **In hyperthecosis, nests of luteinized stroma cells are seen.** The appearance of the remainder of the ovary is similar to that seen in PCOS.

Hilus cell hyperplasia is seen most often when estrogen feedback from ovarian follicles is minimal or absent as a result of gonadal dysgenesis or menopause. The resulting elevation of gonadotropin levels leads to hilus cell hyperplasia. Why this condition develops in *only* a minority of patients with low estrogen states is unknown.

Ovarian Neoplasms

Androgen-producing ovarian tumors are extremely uncommon and include Sertoli-Leydig cell tumors, hilus cell tumors, lipoid cell tumors, and virilizing conditions associated with hyperplasia of the stroma surrounding non-hormone producing neoplasms. These tumors include cystic teratomas, Brenner tumors, serous cystadenomas, and Krukenberg's tumors (see Chapter 21).

IDIOPATHIC HIRSUTISM

Some patients exhibit mild to moderate hirsutism without an elevation in circulating levels of androgens with regular ovulation. This condition has been referred to as *familial, constitutional,* or *idiopathic* hirsutism. This form of hirsutism may occur as a result of increased tissue conversion of testosterone to DHT.

EVALUATION
HISTORY

Functional disorders often first appear during puberty and tend to progress slowly, with the signs of androgen excess developing over several years. In contrast, **neoplastic disorders can occur at any time.** They most often arise many years after puberty, and their manifestations appear abruptly. Progression is rapid, and these patients frequently present with the recent onset of virilism. There is some overlap with functional disorders in that 15% of patients with PCOS can also exhibit signs of virilization, particularly temporal balding and clitoromegaly.

EVALUATION OF A TUMOR
Physical Examination

A bimanual pelvic examination may identify ovarian enlargement. Asymmetrical ovarian enlargement associated with the rapid onset of virilizing signs usually indicates an androgen-producing tumor.

Laboratory Evaluation

The laboratory evaluation of patients with virilism or hirsutism, or both, is aimed primarily at identification of a neoplastic disorder. The most appropriate screening tests are measurements of **serum total testosterone** and **DHEA-S**. DHEA-S serves as a marker of adrenal androgen production and is extremely useful in the detection of an adrenal neoplasm. **Values of DHEA-S in excess of 8000 ng/mL should be viewed as highly suspicious for an adrenal tumor.**

Marked elevations of testosterone may indicate the presence of an ovarian or adrenal androgen-producing tumor. About 80% of patients with an androgen-producing ovarian tumor have peripheral testosterone concentrations greater than 200 ng/dL. It is uncommon for patients with functional disorders to have testosterone levels greater than 200 ng/dL, and such a finding indicates that a neoplasm must be ruled out.

Almost 20% of patients with androgen-producing tumors have testosterone levels less than 200 ng/dL. In this group of patients, clinical features, such as the sudden onset and rapid progression of signs, are important in raising sufficient suspicion to go on to more definitive evaluation. **Virilization is present in 98% of patients with tumors, regardless of the peripheral level of testosterone.**

A pelvic ultrasound should be obtained whenever any high-risk features are present. Androgen-secreting tumors of the adrenal gland can be detected by CT or MRI.

If any of these clinical or laboratory findings indicates the presence of an androgen-secreting tumor, and it cannot be located by imaging studies, selective venous catheterization may be carried out and androgens measured in the venous blood from each adrenal gland and ovary.

EVALUATION OF A FUNCTIONAL DISORDER

Once an androgen-producing tumor has been excluded, attention may then be focused on possible functional disorders. The presence of hirsutism and oligomenorrhea indicates PCOS in most cases.

Physical Examination

Approximately half of patients with hyperandrogenic disorders are obese, and many exhibit evidence of acne and hirsutism. At the time of physical examination, the ovaries are usually cystic and enlarged bilaterally (4 to 6 cm), although in some women ovarian enlargement does not occur. The diagnosis is based primarily on the history and physical examination, with laboratory findings helpful but inconsistent.

Laboratory Evaluation

Dehydroepiandrosterone sulfate (DHEAS). In approximately half of PCOS patients, an adrenal component of the hyperandrogenic state may be demonstrated by an elevation in the serum of the weak androgen, DHEAS.

Prolactin. Up to 20% of patients who present with chronic anovulation have hyperprolactinemia associated with elevated estrogen levels and chronic anovulation.

Serum 17-hydroxyprogesterone. In the presence of regular menstrual cycles, congenital adrenal hyperplasia caused by 21-hydroxylase deficiency should be considered. The appropriate screening test for this condition is a **serum 17-hydroxyprogesterone** level obtained at 8:00 AM. The time of day is important because of the normal diurnal adrenal secretion pattern. With concentrations greater than 3 ng/mL, ACTH stimulation testing is the definitive method of diagnosis. When Cushing's syndrome is suspected, an overnight dexamethasone suppression test should be performed. Dexamethasone 1 mg is given orally at bedtime, and serum cortisol is measured in an 8:00 AM fasting specimen. Normal is <5 µg/dL.

Treatment

Treatment of hirsutism or virilism is guided by the nature of the underlying disease, the severity of clinical symptoms and signs, and the ultimate desires of the patient. **If an ovarian or adrenal neoplasm exists, surgical removal of the tumor is indicated.** In premenopausal women, unilateral salpingo-oophorectomy is usually sufficient for an ovarian tumor and preserves future childbearing potential. In postmenopausal women, the treatment is usually a total abdominal hysterectomy and bilateral salpingo-oophorectomy.

PCOS is by far the most common functional ovarian disorder causing hirsutism, but the management of PCOS depends on the patient's presentation. **The therapy for the hirsutism in PCOS patients is ovarian suppression, which is usually achieved by**

administration of an estrogen-progestin contraceptive. Estrogen-progestin treatment suppresses gonadotropins, which allows regression of the overproduction of testosterone and androstenedione by the ovary. Estrogen also stimulates SHBG production, which decreases free testosterone levels.

All patients with PCOS and chronic anovulation are at risk for the development of endometrial hyperplasia and endometrial cancer. Hence, management in patients not taking combined oral contraceptives should always include progestin-induced maturation of the endometrium to reduce this risk. This may be accomplished with 10 mg oral medroxyprogesterone acetate given daily for 10 to 12 days every other month.

The problems of insulin resistance and hyperandrogenism may have a significant effect on cardiovascular morbidity. Women with PCOS and hyperandrogenism have increased levels of low-density lipoprotein cholesterol (LDL cholesterol) and reduced levels of high-density lipoprotein cholesterol (HDL cholesterol). They are also at increased risk for developing hypertension and diabetes mellitus. Thus, patients with PCOS and chronic anovulation should be counseled regarding nutrition, exercise, and other cardiovascular risk factors.

Patients with functional adrenal hyperandrogenism are treated by the administration of glucocorticoid (0.5 mg dexamethasone every other day), which replaces deficient cortisol and provides sufficient negative pituitary feedback to restore normal ACTH secretion.

In patients with Cushing's syndrome, treatment is surgical removal of the source of excess cortisol or ACTH (adrenal or pituitary tumor).

ANTIANDROGENIC AGENTS

Antiandrogenic agents have been advocated for the treatment of hirsutism, particularly when ovarian or adrenal suppression has failed or is contraindicated. **The most commonly used drug for hirsutism in women in the US is spironolactone.** This aldosterone antagonist competes for testosterone-binding sites, thereby exerting a direct antiandrogenic effect at the target organ. In addition, spironolactone interferes with steroid enzymes and decreases testosterone production. Because this medication opposes the action of aldosterone, serum potassium levels may rise and should be monitored.

COSMETIC TREATMENT

Suppression of abnormal androgen production generally suppresses future hair growth but does not immediately cause the existing hirsutism to disappear. Improvement of the existing hirsutism may not be observed for up to 1 year, when most older hairs have degenerated and fallen out. To obtain good cosmetic results, some local hair removal is usually required in addition to the biochemical manipulation. Local methods include shaving, depilatory creams, and electrolysis.

Plucking of individual hairs should be discouraged because growth of surrounding hair follicles may be stimulated by this technique.

Suggested Reading

American College of Obstetricians and Gynecologists: Evaluation and Treatment of Hirsute Women, ACOG technical bulletin No. 203. Washington, DC, ACOG, March 1995.

Franks S: Polycystic ovary syndrome. N Engl J Med 333:853, 1995.

Kletzky OA, Davajan V, Nakamura RM, et al: Clinical categorization of patients with secondary amenorrhea using progesterone-induced uterine bleeding and measurement of serum gonadotropin levels. Am J Obstet Gynecol 121:695, 1975.

Kletzky OA, Marrs RP, Davajan V: Management of patients with hyperprolactinemia and normal or abnormal tomograms. Am J Obstet Gynecol 147:528, 1983.

Martin TL, Kim M, Malarky WB: The natural history of idiopathic hyperprolactinemia. J Clin Endocrinol Metab 60:855, 1985.

34 Dysfunctional Uterine Bleeding

J. George Moore and Joseph C. Gambone

Dysfunctional uterine bleeding (DUB) is defined as abnormal uterine bleeding (AUB) in women between menarche and menopause that cannot be attributed to medications, blood dyscrasias, systemic diseases, trauma, uterine neoplasms, or pregnancy. This form of AUB is almost always caused by aberrations in the hypothalamic-pituitary-ovarian hormonal axis resulting in anovulation. Usually, a diagnosis of DUB is made by excluding other treatable causes of AUB. The bleeding is generally from a proliferative, or discordant (mixed), endometrium. In most cases, it is associated with anovulatory or oligo-ovulatory ovarian cycles (e.g., polycystic ovarian syndrome [PCOS]), and estrogen levels are frequently unopposed by progesterone. On occasion, it occurs with apparently normal ovulatory cycles. It is one of the most common problems dealt with in the gynecologic clinic or private office.

The bleeding patterns of DUB are defined in Box 34-1. Taken together, the abnormal patterns of bleeding are sometimes designated as menometrorrhagia.

Most DUB occurs during the years around the menarche (11 to 14 years of age) or menopause (45 to 50 years of age). During the perimenopausal years, the anovulatory bleeding is mainly caused by the declining functional capacity of the ovary. In adolescence, the anovulatory bleeding may be caused by a failure of the hypothalamic-pituitary system to respond to the positive feedback effect of estrogen.

Abnormalities of menstrual bleeding are felt to be associated with alterations in endometrial vascular homeostasis. A normal efficient menstrual cycle is discussed in detail in Chapter 4, and the usual normal events are briefly summarized as follows:

First, gradually increasing estrogen levels support and maintain the growth of endometrium during the proliferative phase of the menstrual cycle. The proliferative phase is variable in length, but it generally lasts 13 days from the onset of menses to the luteinizing hormone surge. The increasing level of estrogen supports growth, prevents breakthrough bleeding, and stimulates an increase in endometrial progesterone receptors.

Second, about 24 hours after the luteinizing hormone (LH) surge, ovulation occurs and the corpus luteum forms. It produces estrogen and progesterone in increasing amounts and lasts for about 14 days unless an intervening pregnancy prolongs it by secretion of human chorionic gonadotropin. With the demise of the corpus luteum, the levels of estrogen and progesterone fall precipitously and the decidual portion of the endometrium desquamates.

Third, during the luteal phase of the endometrial cycle, there is a marked increase in tissue levels of prostaglandin $F_{2\alpha}$ which is a powerful vasoconstrictor, and this eventually leads to endometrial ischemia. The process allows for a complete sloughing of the outer two-thirds of the endometrium and avoids prolonged menstruation. During anovulatory cycles, the resulting nonsecretory endometrium contains less prostaglandin and is less apt to initiate an efficient menstrual period of short duration. The unopposed estrogenic effect is likely to result in cycles of irregular duration and prolonged menses. With repeated cycles of unopposed estrogen, endometrial hyperplasia or even cancer may develop.

DIAGNOSIS

The diagnosis of DUB is usually made by excluding other causes of abnormal uterine bleeding. A possible

<table>
<tr><td>

Box 34-1. Patterns of dysfunctional uterine bleeding (DUB)

POLYMENORRHEA
Abnormally frequent menses at intervals <24 days

MENORRHAGIA (HYPERMENORRHEA)
Excessive and/or prolonged menses (>80 mL and >7 days) occurring at normal intervals

METRORRHAGIA
Irregular episodes of uterine bleeding

MENOMETRORRHAGIA
Heavy and irregular uterine bleeding

KLEINE REGNUNG (LITTLE SHOWER)
Scant bleeding at ovulation for 1 or 2 days

</td><td>

Box 34-2. Nondysfunctional causes of abnormal uterine bleeding (AUB)

IATROGENIC
Exogenous estrogen (e.g., oral contraceptives)
Aspirin
Heparin/coumadin
Tamoxifen
Intrauterine device

DYSCRASIAS
Thrombocytopenia
Increased fibrinolysins
Autoimmune disease
Leukemia
Von Willebrand's disease

SYSTEMIC DISORDERS
Hepatic disease (impaired metabolism of estrogens)
Renal disease (hyperprolactinemia)
Thyroid disease

TRAUMA
Laceration
Abrasion
Foreign body

ORGANIC CONDITIONS
Complications of pregnancy
Uterine leiomyomas
Malignancies of cervix or corpus
Endometrial polyp
Adenomyosis
Endometritis
Endometrial hyperplasia

</td></tr>
</table>

unexpected pregnancy should always be ruled out initially. Box 34-2 lists possible causes of abdominal uterine bleeding to be considered. A **pelvic examination** must be performed to verify that the source of bleeding is uterine and not the result of a cervical, rectal, vaginal, vulvar, or urethral lesion. **Iatrogenic causes** such as oral contraceptive-induced breakthrough bleeding or bleeding associated with an intrauterine device should be considered. **Dyscrasias of the blood** such as von Willebrand's disease should be ruled out. **Systemic diseases** such as liver, renal, or thyroid conditions may represent treatable causes of AUB. **Trauma,** although unusual, is an occasional cause of vaginal and even uterine bleeding and should be considered at the time of the pelvic examination. Organic causes of AUB include tumors, infections, and complications of pregnancy. **Benign tumors and growths** include endocervical and endometrial polyps, leiomyomata (uterine fibroids), adenomyosis, and endometrial hyperplasia. **Malignant neoplastic conditions** include cervical and uterine cancers. **Infections** that may cause AUB include cervicitis, endometritis, and pelvic inflammatory disease.

Two investigations are most useful for confirming DUB: a pelvic ultrasound and an endometrial biopsy. If they are both normal and show nothing more than a nonsecretory endometrium, a presumptive diagnosis of DUB is highly likely. Other tests and procedures that may be indicated to exclude other causes of AUB are listed in Box 34-3.

MANAGEMENT

The management of DUB becomes relatively clear once other more serious causes of bleeding have been excluded, particularly endometrial or cervical cancer. For less significant bleeding, observation and expectant management may be reasonable. Box 34-4 lists the appropriate hormonal management of significant DUB.

Heavy endometrial hemorrhage from menarche through the perimenopause may require high-dose estrogens (sometimes given intravenously) to support the endometrium and diminish bleeding. If the bleeding substantially abates, lower-dose oral estrogen followed by, or in combination with, a progestin can then

---

Box 34-3. Evaluation of dysfunctional uterine bleeding (DUB)

LABORATORY EVALUATION*

Complete blood count
Platelet count
Serum iron and iron-binding globulin
Coagulation studies (prothrombin time and partial thromboplastin time)
Bleeding time
Urinary hCG assay
Thyroid function studies
Serum progesterone
Liver function studies
Prolactin levels
Serum FSH levels

DIAGNOSTIC PROCEDURES*

Cervical cytology (Papanicolaou smear)
Endometrial biopsy
    Pipelle (flexible syringe suction curette)
    Office curette (Novak, Randall type)
    Vacuum (Vabra) curette
Pelvic ultrasonic imaging
Hysteroscopy, hysterosonogram, and/or D&C

*Used selectively based on history and physical examination.

Box 34-4. Hormonal management of dysfunctional uterine bleeding (DUB)

MASSIVE INTRACTABLE BLEEDING
25 mg IV of conjugated estrogens

CONTINUED MANAGEMENT AFTER MASSIVE BLEEDING HAS ABATED
Conjugated estrogens 2.5 mg orally daily for 25 days*
May double the dose if bleeding recurs or increases
Add 10 mg of medroxyprogesterone acetate (MPA)† for last 10 days of treatment
Allow 5–7 days for withdrawal bleeding

MANAGEMENT OF MODERATE MENOMETRORRHAGIA ESTROGEN-PROGESTIN COMBINATION
Conjugated estrogen,* 1.25 mg orally each day for 25 days with 10 mg MPA† orally for the last 10 days of the estrogen treatment
Oral contraceptive (e.g., Triphasil)‡ for 21 days with a 7-day withdrawal
CYCLIC PROGESTIN—MPA†, 10 mg orally each day for 10–15 days each month, usually for a 3 month trial; a 5–7 day period of menstrual withdrawal should follow cessation of the MPA each month

*May substitute other oral estrogen (e.g., ethinyl estradiol .02).
†May substitute other progestin (e.g., Megace, 5 mg).
‡May substitute other combined oral contraceptives.

---

be initiated. If the bleeding is unremitting, dilatation and curettage may be necessary.

The more common and less urgent type of DUB is best managed by cyclic estrogens with a progestin added in the latter 10 to 15 days of the 25-day estrogen cycle (see Box 34-4). A 5- to 7-day withdrawal bleed is expected each month as the medications are withdrawn on the 21st or 25th day. The cycle is repeated each month for 3 to 6 months, after which a normal pattern may be spontaneously established. Oral contraceptives should not be used for women in their 40s who are smokers, because of the high content of estrogens and their association with thrombophlebitis and myocardial infarction. **Cyclic progestins alone may be used for younger patients who are likely to have sufficient endogenous estrogens to prime the endometrial progesterone receptors.** These drugs are unlikely to be effective after prolonged bleeding. Only when these measures are ineffective, should a dilation and curettage or hysteroscopy and biopsy be performed.

For older patients who do not respond to medical therapy and who do not anticipate later pregnancies, more radical and potentially permanent therapeutic measures may be considered. **Endometrial ablation** at the time of hysteroscopy provides an amenorrhea rate of up to 75% and relief of excessive bleeding in most of the remainder. However, about 10% continue to have bleeding problems. **Vaginal hysterectomy** may be appropriate for women who have associated problems such as pelvic relaxation or severe dysmenorrhea or for patients who are refractory to endometrial ablation.

Although DUB is annoying or even distressing, it is seldom life-threatening. Conservative treatment, after a thorough evaluation, is generally successful, although it may extend over several months and the problem may recur.

The important issue is to rule out unsuspected pregnancies and genital tract cancers, reserving hysterectomy for those patients with significant precancerous lesions or refractory problems.

Suggested Reading

American College of Obstetricians and Gynecologists: Dysfunctional uterine bleeding, ACOG Technical Bulletin Number 134. Washington, DC, ACOG, 1989.

Association of Professors of Gynecology and Obstetrics: Clinical Management of Abnormal Uterine Bleeding, Educational Series on Women's Health Issues. Boston, Jespersen and Associates, 2002.

35

Infertility and Assisted Reproductive Technologies

David R. Meldrum

A couple is considered infertile after unsuccessfully attempting to achieve pregnancy for 1 year. Infertility is termed *primary* when it occurs without any prior pregnancy and *secondary* when it follows a previous conception. Some conditions, such as azoospermia, endometriosis, and tubal occlusion, are more common in women with primary infertility, but virtually all conditions occur in both settings, making the distinction of little clinical significance.

Conception requires the juxtaposition of the male and female gametes at the optimal stage of maturation, followed by transportation of the conceptus to the uterine cavity at a time when the endometrium is supportive of its continued development and implantation (see Chapter 4). For these events to occur, the male and female reproductive systems must be both anatomically and physiologically intact, and coitus must occur with sufficient frequency for the semen to be deposited in close temporal relationship to the release of the oocyte from the follicle. **Even when fertilization occurs, it is estimated that more than 70% of resulting embryos are abnormal and fail to develop or become nonviable shortly after implantation.** Therefore, it is not surprising that 10% to 15% of couples experience infertility.

Considering the vast complexity of the reproductive process, it is remarkable that **80% of couples achieve conception within 1 year.** More precisely, 25% conceive within the first month, 60% within 6 months, 75% by 9 months, and 90% by 18 months. The steadily decreasing rate of monthly conception demonstrated by these figures most likely reflects a spectrum of fertility extending from highly fertile couples to those with relative infertility. After 18 months of unprotected sexual intercourse, the remaining couples have a low monthly conception rate without treatment, and many may have absolute defects preventing fertility (sterility).

GENERAL PRINCIPLES OF EVALUATION

Conception requires adequate function of multiple physiologic systems in both partners. Infertility may result from either one major deficiency (e.g., tubal occlusion) or multiple minor deficiencies. Failure to realize this important dictum may lead the inexperienced practitioner to overlook additional factors that might be more amenable to treatment than the one that has been identified. **Infertility in about 40% of infertile couples has multiple causes.** Therefore, with rare exceptions, a complete infertility evaluation should be performed on each couple.

Age substantially decreases the rate of conception because of decreased coital frequency and reduced embryo quality. From a large study of donor insemination, the strictly age-related reduction appears to be about one-third for women aged 35 to 45 years. It is reasonable to begin the basic evaluation at 6 months in older patients and to consider starting treatment for unexplained infertility earlier in women past 35 years of age.

BASIC EVALUATIONS

Evaluation and therapy may be started earlier when obvious defects are identified, or they may be delayed, for instance, when a correctable factor, such as infrequent intercourse, is identified.

In general, the first 6 to 8 months of evaluation involve relatively simple and noninvasive tests and

the performance of a radiologic evaluation of tubal patency (hysterosalpingogram), which can sometimes have a therapeutic effect. Operative evaluation by laparoscopy is thus reserved for the small proportion of couples who have not conceived after 18 to 24 months or who have specific abnormalities or indications of a probable pelvic factor.

To keep the status of the evaluation in mind, it is helpful to arrange the workup under a series of five categories that can be mentally reviewed at each visit. Table 35-1 shows the approximate incidence and the tests involved in the evaluation of each category. In 5% to 10% of couples, no explanation can be found (idiopathic infertility).

ETIOLOGIC FACTORS
MALE COITAL FACTOR
History

The history from the male partner should cover any pregnancies previously sired; any history of genital tract infections, such as prostatitis or mumps orchitis; surgery or trauma to the male genitalia or inguinal region (e.g., hernia repair); and any exposure to lead, cadmium, radiation, or chemotherapeutic agents. Excessive consumption of alcohol or cigarettes or unusual exposure to environmental heat should be elicited. Some medications such as furantoins and calcium channel blockers reduce sperm quality or function.

Physical Examination

The normal location of the urethral meatus should be ensured. Testicular size should be estimated by comparison with a set of standard ovoids. The presence of a varicocele should be elicited by asking the patient to perform Valsalva's maneuver in the standing position. Rectal massage of the prostate and seminal vesicles should bring forth sufficient secretions at the urethral meatus to allow microscopic examination for white blood cells.

Investigations

A semen analysis should be performed following a 2- to 4-day period of abstinence. The entire ejaculate should be collected in a clean, nontoxic container. Until relatively recently, the full range of normal variation was not appreciated. Characteristics of a normal semen analysis are shown in Table 35-2.

An excessive number of leukocytes (more than 10 per high-power field) may indicate infection, but special stains are required to differentiate polymorphonuclear leukocytes from immature germ cells. Semen quality varies greatly with repeated samples. An accurate appraisal of abnormal semen requires at least three analyses. Periodic reassessment is necessary. A few weeks should pass between each sample to reflect fluctuations in spermatogenesis.

Endocrine evaluation of the male with subnormal semen quality may uncover a specific cause. Hypothyroidism can cause infertility, but there is no place for the empirical use of thyroxine. Low levels of gonadotropins and testosterone may indicate hypothalamic-pituitary failure. An elevated prolactin concentration may indicate the presence of a prolactin-producing pituitary tumor. An elevated level of follicle-stimulating hormone (FSH) generally indicates substantial parenchymal damage to the testes, as inhibin, produced by the Sertoli cells of the seminiferous tubules, provides the principal feedback control of FSH secretion. A response to any

Table 35-1. Common infertility factors

Factor	Incidence (%)	Basic Investigations
Male-coital	40	Semen analysis Postcoital test
Ovulatory	15–20	Urinary luteinizing hormone self-test* Serum progesterone* Endometrial biopsy*
Cervical	5	Postcoital test
Uterine-tubal	30	Hysterosalpingogram Laparoscopy
Peritoneal	40	Laparoscopy

*Investigations only when menses are regular (every 22 to 35 days); oligoamenorrhea requires additional testing.

Table 35-2. Characteristics of normal semen analysis

Characteristics	Quantity
Semen volume	2–5 mL
Sperm count	Greater than 20 million/mL
Sperm motility	Greater than 50%
Normal forms	Greater than 30%
White blood cells	Fewer than 10 per high-power field or 1×10^6/mL

treatment is unlikely in the presence of an elevated level of FSH. However, the level of FSH is not helpful in predicting whether sperm will be recovered with testicular sperm extraction.

Treatment

The couple should be advised to have intercourse approximately every 1 to 2 days during the periovulatory period (e.g., days 10 through 18 and particularly days 12 through 16 of a 28-day cycle). **Because infrequent coitus is a common contributing factor, firm advice in this regard can be beneficial.** This "scheduled intercourse" can be disruptive and stressful, however, and insemination using husband/partner sperm may relieve considerable pressure on a couple whose biologic drives do not match the physiologic necessity.

Lubricants and postcoital douching should be avoided, and the woman should be advised to lie on her back for at least 15 minutes after coitus to prevent rapid loss of semen from the vagina.

Smoking should be reduced or stopped, as should intake of alcohol. The use of saunas, hot tubs, or tight underwear should be discouraged, as should exposure to other environments that raise scrotal temperature, because these factors may affect spermatogenesis.

Low semen volume may provide insufficient contact with the cervical mucus for adequate sperm migration to occur. This may be remedied by insemination with the male partner's semen. When a high semen volume coexists with a low count, infertility may result because a lower density of sperm contacts the cervical mucus. **At present, these abnormalities of volume are most commonly treated with sperm washing and intrauterine insemination (IUI).**

If low sperm density (oligospermia) or low motility (asthenospermia) is caused by hypothalamic-pituitary failure, injections of human menopausal gonadotropins (hMGs) may be effective. The suppressive effects of **hyperprolactinemia** on hypothalamic function **can be reversed by the administration of bromocriptine,** a dopamine agonist. When low semen quality coexists with a varicocele (dilatation and incompetence of the spermatic veins), improved semen quality, particularly motility, may occur with ligation of this venous plexus. Various medications (clomiphene, human chorionic gonadotropin [hCG], testosterone, and hMG) have been tried when no cause is apparent (idiopathic

oligoasthenospermia), but none has proved effective. Recent placebo-controlled studies of clomiphene have shown no significant benefit. Because approximately 3 months is required for spermatogenesis and sperm transport to occur, more frequent semen checks during treatment are unnecessary and serve only to discourage the patient.

If semen quality cannot be improved, IUI with close timing of the insemination to the precise point of ovulation is effective. By washing and concentrating the sperm into a small volume by centrifugation, large numbers of sperm can be placed into the uterus. Without washing, IUI must be limited to small amounts of semen, owing to marked cramping. Accurate timing may be accomplished either by measurement of daily luteinizing hormone (LH) concentrations or by controlled stimulation of the cycle with clomiphene or hMG, followed by administration of hCG when follicular diameter as seen by ultrasonography indicates maturity. Insemination may then be carried out within a few hours of ovulation, which occurs 36 to 44 hours following the LH surge or hCG injection. When urinary LH testing is used, there is a delay of several hours between the onset of the surge and the positive urine test. It is advisable to test in the afternoon or evening, with insemination the following morning.

In-vitro fertilization (IVF) is an effective treatment for the male factor because a relatively small number of sperm are required to inseminate each oocyte. With intracytoplasmic sperm injection (ICSI), only one viable sperm for each egg is necessary. Finally, insemination with donor sperm is effective when the male factor is refractory to treatment.

OVULATORY FACTOR
History

Most women with regular cycles (every 22 to 35 days) are ovulating, particularly if they have premenstrual molimina (e.g., breast changes, bloating, and mood change). Recent studies indicate reduced fecundity associated with very irregular cycles.

Investigations

The simplest screening tests to confirm reasonably normal ovulation are serial measurement of urinary LH, which assesses the duration of luteal

function, and the midluteal level of serum progesterone, which assesses the level of luteal function. The interval from the urinary LH surge to the onset of menses should be at least 12 days. An older test of ovulation, the basal body temperature, is now seldom used because of its inaccuracy in showing anovulation and in indicating the timing of ovulation. A progesterone level of greater than 5 ng/mL indicates ovulatory activity, but midluteal concentrations usually exceed 10 ng/mL in cycles in which conception can take place. Because of the marked pulsatile secretion of progesterone, a level between 5 and 10 ng/mL should be found in the normal luteal phase.

In spite of ovulation, an inadequate luteal phase may be responsible for infertility. If there are indications that a luteal phase defect may be present (e.g., history of spontaneous abortion), an endometrial biopsy should be taken from the upper anterior aspect of the uterine fundus, and histologic development should be carefully dated. If the day of the biopsy, timed to 11 or 12 days following the LH surge, lags by more than 2 days in at least two cycles, a luteal phase defect is present. It has been shown that prospective timing from the LH surge rather than retrospectively from the onset of menses helps to reduce false-positive results.

Treatment

Correction of a luteal phase defect is generally possible by the use of vaginal progesterone suppositories, 25 mg twice daily, beginning on the second or third day after ovulation, or by the use of clomiphene citrate, or hMG. The latter two treatments are accompanied by an increased risk of multiple pregnancy, however, and clomiphene citrate may itself cause a luteal phase defect.

In women whose menses are less frequent than every 35 days (oligomenorrhea), it is helpful to induce more frequent ovulation, thus increasing the opportunity for pregnancy and improving the ability to time coitus. Ovulation induction should always be preceded by a thorough workup, as discussed in Chapter 33, because conditions causing anovulation may be worsened by pregnancy or may complicate it. In addition, ovarian failure seldom responds to attempts to induce ovulation.

The choice of the most appropriate technique for ovulation induction is determined by the patient's specific diagnosis. With this approach, regular ovulation can be restored in more than 90% of anovulatory women. Provided that these patients persevere with treatment for an adequate period of time, and no other infertility factors are present, their fertility should approximate that of normal women.

Pituitary insufficiency requires the injection of hMG (FSH and LH). Hypothalamic amenorrhea is caused by infrequent or absent pulsatile release of gonadotropin-releasing hormone (GnRH). GnRH is highly effective when administered in small pulses subcutaneously or intravenously in these patients every 90 to 120 minutes by a small portable infusion pump. If this treatment is not available, hMG is quite effective, but with a much higher risk of multiple pregnancy. Hyperprolactinemia and its suppressive effect on the hypothalamus are specifically treated by use of the dopamine agonists bromocriptine (Parlodel) or carbergoline (Dostinex).

Most of the remaining patients with anovulation have some form of polycystic ovarian syndrome (PCOS) and generally respond to clomiphene, an orally active antiestrogen. Anovulation occurs in patients with polycystic ovaries because of chronic, mild suppression of FSH release and the antagonistic effect of androgens on the response of the follicle to FSH. These women often have both increased ovarian and increased adrenal androgen production. Clomiphene, by inhibiting the negative feedback effect of endogenous estrogen, causes a rise of FSH and stimulation of follicular maturation. One of the principal causes of excessive ovarian androgen production is higher circulating insulin concentrations because of insulin resistance. Metformin, which reduces glucose mobilization and increases insulin sensitivity, is currently being used together with clomiphene or gonadotropins to improve response as well as to reduce an excessive response to ovulation induction. Metformin can also be used alone and may result in ovulation and pregnancy.

Two other treatments have been used to decrease the inhibitory effect of androgens. First, surgical excision of androgen-producing ovarian stroma (wedge resection) induces ovulation, but it is not as effective as clomiphene treatment and may cause infertility by inducing periadnexal adhesions. Laparoscopic procedures to create multiple craters in the ovary with cautery or laser have been used to achieve similar effects. Second, dexamethasone, which suppresses adrenal androgens, may be helpful in cases of PCOS with elevated dehydroepiandrosterone sulfate (DHEA-S) levels to make clomiphene treatment more effective in inducing ovulation and pregnancy at lower dosages.

If ovulation does not occur with clomiphene, follicular development may be occurring, but the normal LH surge may fail to occur. This results in lack of follicular rupture. **Assessment by serial pelvic ultrasonography and carefully timed hCG administration may lead to normal ovulation. If follicular maturation is not occurring, ovulation induction will require low-dose FSH or hMG.**

The main complications of ovulation induction are related to excessive stimulation of the ovaries. Substantial enlargement of the ovary with clomiphene citrate can generally be avoided by examining the ovaries before each treatment course and by using the lowest effective dose. Cystic ovarian enlargement is not an uncommon complication of hMG treatment. **The hyperstimulation syndrome can be a critical illness associated with marked ovarian enlargement and exudation of fluid and protein into the peritoneal cavity.** The use of serum estradiol measurements, transvaginal ultrasonic scanning, and low-dose gonadotropin have greatly reduced the incidence of hyperstimulation syndrome. By starting at 1 ampule (75 U) and increasing the dose by half an ampule every 7 days if follicular maturation is not detected, there is a marked reduction in the incidence of multifollicular development, hyperstimulation, and multiple pregnancy. **Multiple pregnancy occurs in 6% to 8% of clomiphene citrate conceptions, with less than 1% of cases exceeding two babies.** Multiple gestation occurs in 20% to 30% of hMG conceptions, and 5% of these conceptions are multiple births of more than two. Ultrasonic monitoring appears to reduce this risk if the hCG is withheld in the presence of an excessive number of mature follicles. **Current use of a low-dose regimen of hMG or pure FSH reduces the overall risk of multiple pregnancy to about 5%.**

CERVICAL FACTOR

During the few days before ovulation, the cervix produces profuse watery mucus (Spinnbarkeit) that exudes out of the cervix to contact the seminal ejaculate. To assess its quality, the patient must be seen during the immediate preovulatory phase (days 12 to 14 of a 28-day cycle). Spuriously abnormal results can be reduced by timing the test to the morning after the urinary LH surge.

Investigations

The amount and clarity of the mucus is recorded. **The spinnbarkeit may be tested by touching the mucus with a piece of pH paper and lifting vertically. The mucus should extend in a thread to at least 6 cm. The pH should be 6.5 or greater. A postcoital (Sims-Huhner) test is performed 2 to 12 hours after intercourse to assess the number and motility of spermatozoa that have entered the cervical canal.** The number of sperm, however, does not correlate well with semen quality, recovery of sperm from the cul-de-sac, or subsequent fertility. Consequently, the predictive value of this test for fertility is low.

Treatment

Any cervical infection is treated by prescribing a 10-day course of doxycycline, 100 mg twice daily, for both partners. Persistent chronic cervicitis may be treated with cryotherapy if antibiotic treatment fails. Poor mucus quality can be treated with a small dose of estrogen from day 7 until ovulation, but **intrauterine insemination of washed sperm appears to be more effective.**

UTERINE-TUBAL FACTOR

Abnormalities of the uterine cavity are seldom the cause of infertility. Large submucosal myomas or endometrial polyps may be associated with infertility and 1st-trimester spontaneous abortions. The role of intramural myomas is not clear, although myomectomy has been associated with conception in 40% to 50% of couples in uncontrolled series and some studies with IVF have shown reduced conception with intramural myomas. Subserous fibroids do not affect fecundity.

Tubal occlusion may occur at three locations: the fimbrial end, the midsegment, or the isthmus-cornu. Fimbrial occlusion is by far the most common. Prior salpingitis is a common cause of tubal occlusion, although about one-half of cases are unassociated with any such history. Isthmic-cornual occlusion can be congenital or caused by mucus plugs, endometriosis, tubal adenomyosis, or prior infection.

Investigations

Tubal abnormalities may be diagnosed by hysterosalpingography (HSG) or laparoscopy. To perform a hysterosalpingogram, an occlusive cannula is placed in the cervix, and the instillation of a radiopaque dye is followed with image intensification under fluoroscopy. Selected radiographs are taken for permanent documentation (Figure 35-1). Anesthesia generally is not required. A water-soluble dye is used initially to confirm tubal patency because of the adverse effects of sequestration of an oil-based dye within the lumen of an occluded tube. If patency is confirmed, an oil-based dye is then instilled because of its prominent therapeutic effect in women with unexplained infertility. If only one tube fills with dye, the hysterosalpingogram should be considered normal, as this finding is usually, although not invariably, caused by the dye following the path of least resistance.

Serious infections can result from hysterosalpingography. A normal pelvic examination, negative cervical cultures, and prophylactic doxycycline should reduce this risk to a minimum.

Treatment

In most circumstances, microsurgical tuboplasty is more effective than conventional surgical techniques for reversal of tubal occlusion. About 60% to 80% of patients achieve pregnancy after reversal of sterilization using microsurgical techniques. Most recently tubal reanastomosis has been carried out laparoscopically, with good results in highly experienced hands.

Neosalpingostomy, which is required following fimbriectomy, is associated with a success rate of about 40% to 50%. When performed for fimbrial

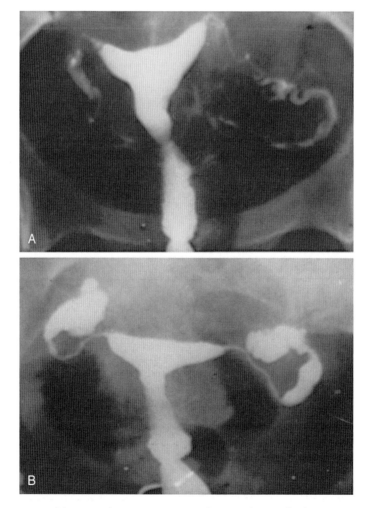

Figure 35-1. Normal hysterosalpingogram (HSG) showing free spill of contrast material (*A*) and bilateral hydrosalpinges (*B*).

occlusion, neosalpingostomy is associated with a success rate of 20% to 30%, although it has reached 40% with long-term follow-up. Most often this is done by laparoscopy. Because a hydrosalpinx reduces the success rate of IVF by about 50%, any hydrosalpinx not repaired should be removed, or its communication with the uterus interrupted by cautery.

For an isthmic-cornual occlusion caused by disease, clearing the obstruction with oral danazol has been reported when the occlusion coexists with peritoneal endometriosis. Selective catheterization has restored patency in the majority of proximal occlusions and should be the first line of therapy. Microsurgical resection and reanastomosis is associated with a 50% to 60% pregnancy rate. **If the intramural portion of the tube is occluded, reimplantation is required, with a new opening being made into the endometrial cavity.** A substantially lower rate of success is achieved in this circumstance, a laparotomy is required, and similar success can be achieved with a single cycle of IVF.

At least 10% of conceptions after repair of diseased tubes are ectopic pregnancies. Anastomosis of healthy tubes carries a risk of ectopic pregnancy of about 3% to 5%. This possibility must always be considered in the management of an early pregnancy following tuboplasty.

PERITONEAL FACTOR

Laparoscopy identifies previously unsuspected pathologic conditions in 30% to 50% of women with unexplained infertility. Endometriosis is the most common finding. Periadnexal adhesions may be found and may hold the fimbriae away from the ovarian surface or entrap the released oocyte.

Endometriosis may interfere with tubal motility, cause tubal obstruction, or cause adhesions that directly disturb the pick-up of the oocyte by the fimbriae. Other mechanisms of endometriosis-associated infertility must exist as well because even minimal endometriosis has some negative effect. In a randomized study of laparoscopic cautery versus no treatment for minimal endometriosis, treatment resulted in one out of eight affected women conceiving. These same women, however, may conceive with other treatments used for unexplained infertility. **There is a strong trend toward omitting laparoscopy in women who have no symptoms indicating pelvic disease and who have a normal pelvic examination, a normal HSG, and a normal pelvic ultrasound.** A serum titer for antichlamydia antibodies may be helpful if this approach is taken, to avoid overlooking occult pelvic adhesions.

Treatment of endometriosis depends on its extent and is discussed fully in Chapter 26. **If substantial adhesions or endometriomas are present, laparoscopic surgery is preferable because** these conditions generally do not respond to medical management. Intermediate and mild disease may respond similarly to stimulation with hMG plus IUI or surgical therapy (the latter being slightly more effective), with the choice depending largely on the preferences of the patient for one or the other treatment. **With more advanced operative laparoscopic techniques, most endometriosis can be removed or ablated** without laparotomy by using advanced instrumentation, lasers, or fulguration.

Danazol, gonadotropin-releasing hormone agonists, or oral medroxyprogesterone acetate are effective treatments for symptomatic disease, with continuous oral contraception therapy being generally inferior. If minimal disease with scattered implants is found, simple cautery at the time of laparoscopy should suffice.

Periadnexal adhesions may be lysed by operative laparoscopy or may require laparotomy. Microsurgical techniques diminish adhesions. The most effective adjunct in preventing recurrent scarring is the placement of an artificial tissue barrier, separating the raw surfaces during the early period of healing.

UNEXPLAINED INFERTILITY

No cause is found for infertility in 5% to 10% of patients who have documented ovulation, normal semen analyses, and a normal HSG. The problem may be primarily one of sperm transport because IUI with washed sperm appears to increase the rate of conception.

In other cases, a defect in the ability of the sperm to fertilize the egg may be present because a lower rate of fertilization is noted in couples with unexplained infertility who undergo IVF compared with couples in whom there is a tubal cause for infertility. **Another male problem that may not be detected by routine evaluation is the presence of antisperm antibodies.**

Other possible mechanisms of unexplained infertility include minimal endometriosis and mildly reduced ovarian reserve (reduced number of normal oocytes without hormonal abnormalities such as elevated FSH levels).

Intrauterine insemination, usually with superovulation induction (stimulation of multiple folliculogenesis with hMG) and hCG timing, is employed next. The final therapy is IVF.

ASSISTED REPRODUCTIVE TECHNOLOGIES

The last resort for infertile couples with any of the aforementioned factors and failure of lesser treatments is the procedure of IVF and embryo transfer (Figure 35-2). In most cases of tubal occlusion in which the rate of success with tubal repair is low (less than 30%), IVF is preferable to surgery because of the more rapid conception rate and the lower ectopic pregnancy rate. **Even severe male factors can be effectively treated with IVF by using ICSI, with fertilization rates of 60% to 70% of injected oocytes and pregnancy rates similar to those of non-male factor IVF (30 to 35%).**

TECHNIQUE

A gonadotropin-releasing hormone agonist (GnRH-a) is given to prevent premature LH release. It is commonly started in the midluteal phase or overlapped with an oral contraceptive. After ovarian suppression (with GnRH-a), **the ovaries are stimulated with FSH or hMG, or both,** on the second or third day of the next cycle. Follicle size is assessed by transvaginal ultrasonic scanning.

An injection of hCG (usually 10,000 U) is given by injection based on follicle size and estradiol levels to induce the resumption of meiosis and completion of oocyte maturation. Thirty-five hours after the hCG injection, multiple oocytes are aspirated under transvaginal ultrasonic guidance. After a further period of in vitro maturation, washed sperm are added or a single sperm is injected (ICSI) into each oocyte. Fertilization may be identified 14 to 18 hours after insemination by the visualization of two pronuclei. The conceptus is then transferred to the uterine cavity 2 to 5 days after oocyte retrieval by means of a tiny catheter. In some cases, the hatching process is aided by making an artificial opening in the zona pellucida ("assisted hatching"). Surplus embryos not transferred at the time of the IVF treatment can be frozen, stored, and transferred in a later menstrual cycle in the event of failure or for additional pregnancies.

OUTCOME

The pregnancy rate with IVF has been highly variable from center to center, owing to the complexity of the techniques required, whereas the pregnancy rate with Gamete Intrafallopian Transfer (GIFT), a technique where oocytes and washed sperm are mixed and placed into the fallopian tube or tubes, has been more consistent. **The mean live delivery rate per retrieval with IVF in 1998 was 29%, with 2% of clinical pregnancies being ectopic.** Most studies have not shown any increase of fetal abnormalities.

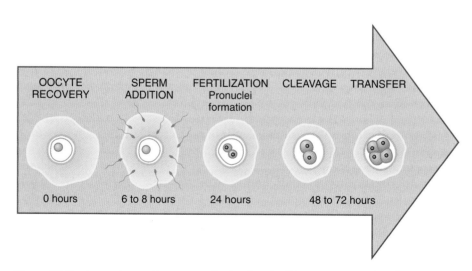

Figure 35-2. Approximate time course for in vitro fertilization (IVF) and embryo transfer.

EGG DONATION

It is possible to achieve pregnancy with IVF and embryo transfer using donor eggs, with a higher success rate than in regular IVF (41% per retrieval in 1998). The eggs generally come from young fertile women (known or anonymous volunteers). The recipient can be programmed for optimal uterine receptivity by replacement doses of estradiol and progesterone. Estradiol and progesterone must be continued until the placenta takes over in the late 1st trimester. **The excellent success of egg donation mandates the conservation of the uterus whenever future fertility is desired, even if the ovaries must be removed.**

OVERALL SUCCESS OF INFERTILITY THERAPY

Conventional therapies result in conception in 50% to 60% of infertile couples. The application of the newer treatments described here should enable even more couples who are willing to exhaust all measures to reach their goal.

Suggested Reading

Dodson WC, Haney AF: Controlled ovarian hyperstimulation and intrauterine insemination for treatment of infertility. Fertil Steril 55:457, 1991.

Federation CECOS, Schwartz D, Mayaux MG: Female fecundity as a function of age: Results of artificial insemination in 2193 multiparous women with azoospermic husbands. N Engl J Med 1:404, 1982.

Investigation of the infertile couple. Birmingham, AL, American Fertility Society, 1991.

Meldrum DR: In vitro fertilization and embryo transfer. *In* Droegemueller W, Sciarra J (eds): Gynecology and Obstetrics. Philadelphia, JB Lippincott, 1996.

Meldrum DR: Low dose follicle-stimulating hormone therapy for polycystic ovarian disease. Fertil Steril 55:1039, 1991.

Watson A, Vandekerckhove P, Lilford R, et al: A meta-analysis of the therapeutic role of oil soluble contrast media at hysterosalpingography: A surprising result? Fertil Steril 61:470, 1994.

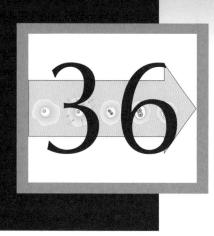

36

Climacteric

Larry R. Laufer and Joseph C. Gambone

The "climacteric" refers to the phase in a woman's reproductive life when a gradual decline in ovarian function results in decreased sex steroid production, and its sequelae. Because this phase is a normal consequence of the aging process, it should not be considered an endocrinopathy. Menopause literally refers to the last menstrual period. The exact time of menopause is usually made in retrospect; that is, 1 year without menses. **In most women, menopause occurs between the ages of 50 and 55 years, with an average age of 51.5 years,** but some have their menopause before the age of 40 (premature menopause), whereas a few may menstruate until they are in their 60s.

Women are born with about 1.5 million oocytes (primary ovarian follicles) and reach menarche (first menstruation) with about 400,000 potentially responsive eggs. Most women ovulate about 400 times between menarche and menopause, but during this time nearly all oocytes are lost. When all the oocytes either have ovulated or become atretic, the ovary is no longer capable of responding to pituitary gonadotropins, and the production of estrogen, progesterone, and other ovarian follicular hormones is reduced. These lower levels of hormones often result in unpleasant and even harmful physical, psychological, and sexual changes in postmenopausal women. **The climacteric phase and postmenopause is now recognized as a time of decreased hormonal production with associated problems that may reduce the quality and even the quantity of life for many women.**

HORMONAL CHANGES

Menopause rarely occurs as a sudden loss of ovarian function. **For some years before menopause, the** ovary begins to show signs of impending failure. Anovulation becomes common with resulting unopposed estrogen production and irregular menstrual cycles (see Chapter 34). On occasion, heavy menses, endometrial hyperplasia, and increasing mood and emotional changes may occur. In some women, hot flashes (or flushes) and night-sweats begin well before menopause is reached. These **perimenopausal symptoms may last 3 to 5 years before there is complete loss of menses and postmenopausal levels of hormones are reached.**

Some women may suffer a more dramatic loss of estrogen. This usually occurs following a surgical intervention that removes or damages the ovaries or their blood supply. On occasion, women have an early ("artificial") menopause following chemotherapy or radiotherapy for cancer. **Women who reach menopause before the age of 40 years are said to have premature menopause or premature ovarian failure.** Other causes of premature ovarian failure include karyotype abnormalities involving the X chromosome, galactosemia, and autoimmune disorders that may cause failure of various endocrine organs.

Some women continue to produce estrogen in substantial amounts for many years after menopause. **Androstenedione from the ovary and the adrenal gland is converted in peripheral fat tissues to estrone, which is then capable of maintaining the vagina, skin, and bone in reasonable cellular tone and reducing the incidence of flashes.** Although this unopposed estrogen may be beneficial to women, it may also be responsible for the increased incidence of endometrial or breast cancer among obese women. For this reason, it is important that obese postmenopausal women, in particular those who may have no signs or symptoms of estrogen deficiency, have regular examinations to monitor the endometrial and breast tissues.

OVARIAN SENESCENCE

The ovary produces a sequence of hormones during a normal menstrual cycle, each sequence being induced by gonadotropic hormones from the pituitary. Under the influence of luteinizing hormone (LH), cholesterol from the liver is converted in theca cells of the ovarian follicle to pregnenolone (Figure 36-1). The pregnenolone then becomes the substrate for all further ovarian sex steroid production, and under the influence of enzymes within the theca, granulosa and luteal cells, androgen, estrogen, and progesterone are produced. The induction of these sex hormones depends on the presence of viable oocytes and normal ovarian stroma and the production of follicle-stimulating hormone (FSH) and LH in adequate amounts. When the ovary becomes depleted of oocytes, the ability to produce sex hormones is diminished.

ESTROGEN

Following menopause, ovarian estradiol (E2) values decline (only 10 to 50 pg/mL of E2 may be found), **but estrone levels may be higher.** Estrone

(E1) can be produced by peripheral conversion of androstenedione from the ovary and the adrenal gland. In some women, the amount of postmenopausal estrogen may be considerable.

ANDROGENS

Women normally produce significant quantities of androgens during the metabolic conversion of cholesterol to estradiol. In this process, both androstenedione and testosterone are formed, and although the major portion is aromatized to estradiol, some androgens circulate. After menopause, there is a decrease in the level of circulating androgens, with androstenedione falling to less than half that found in normal menstruating young women, whereas testosterone gradually diminishes over about 3 to 4 years. Even though postmenopausal women produce less androgens, they tend to be more sensitive to them because of the lost opposition of estrogen. This sometimes results in unwelcome signs such as excessive facial hair growth and decreased breast size.

PROGESTERONE

With anovulation before and ovarian failure during menopause, the production of proges-

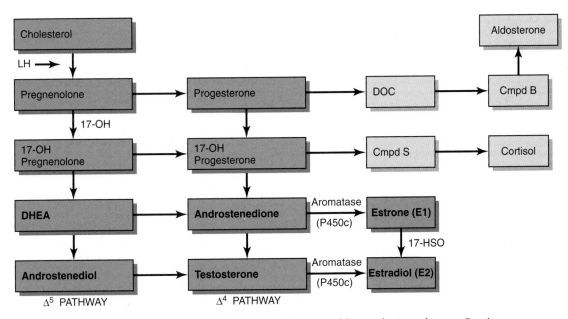

Figure 36-1. Diagrammatic representation of the steroid biosynthetic pathways. Ovarian sex steroid pathways are in red. P450c, cytochrome P450; LH, luteinizing hormone; DH, hydroxylase; DHEA, dehydroepiandrosterone; DOC, desoxycorticosterone; cmpd B, corticosterone; cmpd S, II-desoxycortisol.

terone declines to low levels that are insufficient to induce the cytoplasmic enzymes (estradiol dehydrogenase and estrone sulfuryltransferase) that convert estradiol to the less potent estrone sulfate. There is not only insufficient progesterone to prevent the mitotic activity of estrogen, but also insufficient progesterone to induce secretory activity in the endometrium. As a consequence, perimenopause is often associated with irregular vaginal bleeding, endometrial hyperplasia and cellular atypia, and an increased incidence of endometrial cancer.

GONADOTROPINS

The two gonadotropins, LH and FSH, are produced in the anterior pituitary gland. **When levels of estrogen are low, the arcuate nucleus and paraventricular nucleus in the hypothalamus are induced to secrete increasing amounts of gonadotropin-releasing hormone (GnRH) into the pituitary portal circulation.** This, in turn, stimulates an increased release of LH and FSH into the circulation. The mechanism responsible for the pulsatile release of GnRH (and subsequent LH release) is also thought to be responsible for inducing the hot flash, which so characterizes menopause. Typical levels of FSH in postmenopausal women are greater than 40 IU/L.

CLINICAL MANIFESTATIONS

Loss of estrogen is associated with an increased risk of well-documented adverse effects such as urogenital atrophy and osteoporosis (Table 36-1). Although postmenopausal women have a higher incidence of heart disease and of cancer, the relationship between these

Table 36-1. Consequence of estrogen loss

Symptoms (early)	Hot flushes (flashes) Insomnia Irritability Mood disturbances
Physical changes (intermediate)	Urogenital atrophy Stress (urinary) incontinence Skin collagen loss
Diseases (late)	Osteoporosis Dementia of the Alzheimer's type (possible) Cardiovascular disease (unclear relationship) Cancers, for example, colon (unclear relationship)

adverse events and ovarian function and hormonal therapy remain unclear and controversial.

GENERAL SYMPTOMS

About 85% of women experience hot flashes as they pass through the climacteric, but about half of these women are not seriously disturbed by them. For about 40% of affected women, the hot flash is a most distressing experience. Flashes may occur as frequently as every 30 to 40 minutes, but more often they occur about 8 to 15 times daily. There may be associated sweating, dizziness, and palpitations. Often, the hot flash is preceded by an aura, which may awaken the woman and disturb her sleep. **As a consequence of frequent flashes at night, insomnia, tiredness, and irritability are common.** Women are often given sedatives, hypnotics, or psychotropic drugs in an attempt to relieve these symptoms caused by estrogen deficiency. Some complain of confusion, loss of memory, lethargy, and inability to cope, as well as mild depression. Some studies indicate that the hypoestrogenic state may be associated with a loss of the sense of balance, possibly resulting in an increased risk of falling. It is uncertain whether these symptoms result directly from estrogen deficiency affecting the neurotransmission processes or whether they are secondary to the loss of sleep and the disturbing vasomotor symptoms. Whatever the cause, women may improve considerably when appropriate hormonal therapy (estrogen and a progestagen or estrogen alone) is initiated. **Severe or even sustained moderate depression should never be attributed solely to climacteric hormonal changes.**

UROGENITAL SYMPTOMS

The vagina is very sensitive to estrogen, and it responds to this hormone by producing a thick moist epithelium with an acidic secretion (pH of about 4.0). The absence of estrogen results in a thin, dry epithelium with an alkaline secretion (pH >7.0). The postmenopausal vagina shrinks in diameter and splits and tears easily, and these changes may result in severe dyspareunia. **The bladder and vagina are derived from the same embryologic tissue, so it is not surprising that some postmenopausal women also complain of urinary frequency and dysuria.** The elastic capacity of the bladder is decreased even though the urinary output remains constant. As a result, frequency, urgency, and nocturia occur. Although some urinary incontinence is inevitable with age, some women may experience significant loss of urine in part because of hormonal decline during the climacteric and after menopause. Hormone therapy may help this condition, but surgical intervention may be necessary to correct incontinence (see Chapter 24).

OSTEOPOROSIS

Remodeling of bone continues throughout life, but with estrogen deprivation, the osteoclastic activity far exceeds the osteoblasts' ability to lay down bone. Under these conditions, osteopenia and finally osteoporosis occur. An early clinical sign of osteoporosis is a loss of height greater than 1.5 inches because of vertebral compression fracture, which may be accompanied by acute and chronic back pain. Other important osteoporotic events include wrist and hip fractures. **Ten to 15 years after menopause has occurred, women begin to fracture their bones at a rate exceeding that of men by a factor of three-fold to fivefold.** About 200,000 women break a hip each year in the United States, and the annual cost of osteoporotic fractures and their complications has been estimated to be in excess of $14 billion. The earlier women are deprived of estrogen in their lives, the earlier osteoporotic bone loss begins. **Most calcium is lost from trabecular bone, and as a consequence, the spinal column and femoral neck are the bones most commonly fractured.**

Risk factors for osteoporosis include a family history of osteoporosis, slender body composition, Caucasian and Asian ethnic origin, sedentary lifestyle, alcohol consumption, cigarette smoking, thyroid excess, or use of corticosteroid or anticonvulsant medications. The North American Menopause Society recommends bone mineral density screening for osteoporosis in women with risk factors who are 50 years of age or older and in women without risk factors who are 65 years or older. The preferred screening modality is dual-energy x-ray absorptiometry measurements of the total hip and spine. The results of these studies are expressed in T scores, which are standard deviations (SDs) from the peak bone mineral density of normal young adults. Osteoporosis is defined as a T score of less than –2.5 SD. Drug therapy is recommended in postmenopausal women with a T score of less than –2.5 SD or a T score of –2.0 to –2.5 SD plus an additional risk factor for fracture. If bone mineral density measurements are used to monitor the effects of drug therapy, they should be repeated after at least 2 years of treatment.

Reducing the risk of osteoporotic fracture entails several changes of diet and lifestyle. **Postmenopausal women should consume 1200 to 1500 mg of calcium and 400 to 600 U of vitamin D daily, which are contained in two to three portions of dairy products.** Those who cannot or will not include dairy products in their meals should be encouraged to use calcium and vitamin D supplements. Excess supplementation should be discouraged to avoid renal complications. **Walking and weight-bearing exercise both help to increase bone mineral mass and reduce the risk of fracture-causing falls.** The risk of falling can be reduced further by elimination of throw rugs in the home, placement of handrails in the bathroom, and minimizing the use of alcoholic beverages. **Smoking should be discouraged** for many other health reasons in addition to osteoporosis prevention. Patients receiving replacement therapy for hypothyroidism should be tested to ensure that they are not receiving an excessive (and potentially bone density—depleting) dose.

Pharmacologic treatments for osteoporosis include estrogen (with or without a progestin), selective estrogen receptor modulators (SERMs), biphosphonates, calcitonin, and parathyroid hormone. Recently released data from the Women's Health Initiative study demonstrated that combined estrogen/progestin therapy reduced postmenopausal total fractures by 24% compared to controls, with a 34% reduction of hip fractures. This translates to a reduction of the hip fracture rate from 15 to 10 cases per 10,000 postmenopausal women per year. **SERMs, such as raloxifene, have been found to be beneficial for the prevention of vertebral fractures,** but data are lacking regarding the prevention of hip fracture. **Biphosphonates, such as alendronate, are effective in both preventing and, at higher doses, treating osteoporosis** without requiring long-term, continued usage. In general, biphosphonates have few adverse side effects. However, they must be taken properly (empty stomach, upright position, and with a large glass of water) to minimize the risk of esophagitis and esophageal ulcers. Both calcitonin and parathyroid hormone are second-line adjunctive treatments for osteoporosis.

OVARIAN HORMONE THERAPY

For four decades, ovarian hormone therapy has been advocated for an expanding set of prophylactic indications. Initially, hormone therapy was provided for the treatment of hot flashes and symptoms of genitouri-

Table 36-2. Some of the inherent biases in observational studies	
Selection bias	Hormone therapy users may be different from non-users in terms of behaviors and disease risk
Prescribing bias	Only well women are given hormone therapy
Prevention bias	Monitoring and treatment are more intensive in women on hormone therapy
Compliance bias	Women with greater adherence (even to placebo) have better outcomes
Recall bias	Women who develop a disease have a better recollection of treatments taken
Prevalence-incidence bias	Early adverse effects of hormone therapy not observed if user dies before becoming part of cohort

nary atrophy. Later, increasing evidence revealed that prevention of osteoporosis was a specific benefit of ovarian hormone therapy. More recently, ovarian hormone therapy has been advocated for the prevention or delay of arteriosclerotic heart disease and Alzheimer's disease through a number of diverse mechanisms. These latter two proposed benefits were suggested by the results of observational cohort and case–control studies. Other observational studies have raised concerns about ovarian hormone therapy and the risks of thrombotic disease and breast cancer. Although observational studies provide useful information, they are subject to several sources of bias. Table 36-2 lists some of the biases that may occur during observational studies.

Randomized controlled trials tend to minimize the biases of observational studies. However, they are difficult and time-consuming to do when the conditions being observed are relatively uncommon. The WHI study* is attempting to sort out the risks and benefits of ovarian hormone therapy. Over 16,000 women were entered into one arm of the study comparing a combined preparation of conjugated estrogens and medroxyprogesterone acetate with placebo. After 5 years of follow-up, this combined ovarian hormone arm was halted in July of 2002. **The previously reported protection from osteoporotic fracture**

*Women's Health Initiative (WHI) study, sponsored by the US National Institutes of Health.

was confirmed by the WHI study. In addition, a 37% reduction in the rate of colorectal cancer was found. This would result in six fewer cases of colorectal cancer (10 vs. 16) per 10,000 women per year. **Combined ovarian hormone use, however, was found to increase the risks for coronary artery disease events (by 29%), stroke (by 41%), thromboses (by 100%), and breast cancer (by 26%).** Although most of the risks increased after 1 to 2 years of use, increased risk of breast cancer became apparent only after 4 years of use. There was no significant increase in death rates between treatment and placebo groups (Figure 36-2). No data concerning Alzheimer's disease was reported from this study as of the end of 2003.

Although definite limitations of the WHI study have been identified, **the findings have had a significant effect on clinical practice, and the routine use of hormone therapy after the menopause is now viewed with caution.** On the basis of the WHI study, **a consensus is developing that combined ovarian hormone therapy is indicated primarily for the relief of significant menopausal symptoms such as frequent hot flashes, genitourinary discomfort, and other quality-of-life issues.** The length of treatment should be minimized depending on the individual patient's clinical course and preference, after informed consent. Whether this more restrictive approach applies to younger hypoestrogenic women such as those who undergo premature menopause or bilateral oophorectomy is unclear. The need for prevention and treatment of osteoporosis may be determined by bone densitometry studies rather than ovarian status, *per se*, with biphosphonates or raloxifene as the first line of treatment in the absence of concomitant significant menopausal symptoms.

MANAGEMENT OF OVARIAN HORMONAL THERAPY

Women who still have a uterus and elect to use unopposed estrogen for the treatment of menopausal symptoms are at significant risk of developing endometrial hyperplasia and endometrial adenocarcinoma. Concurrent progestin is protective for endometrial disease and may be given for 12 days per month or for 14 days per quarter with predictable uterine bleeding on withdrawal. **Patients who seek complete amenorrhea may use continuous combined estrogen/progestin** (e.g., conjugated estrogens, 0.625 mg, and medroxyprogesterone

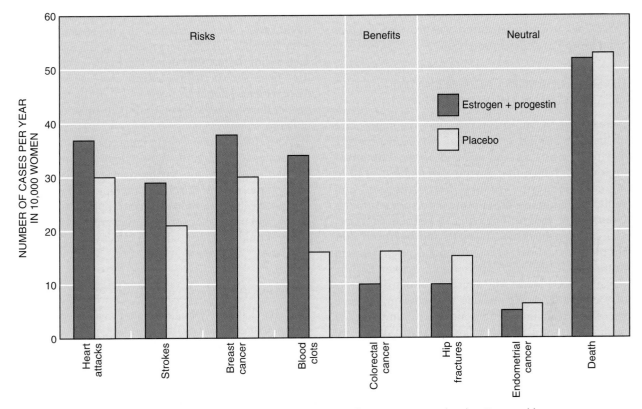

Figure 36-2. Disease rates for women on estrogen plus progestin or placebo. Reported by the Women's Health Initiative (WHI) Study Group, 2002.

acetate, 2.5 mg daily). This latter regimen is characterized by unpredictable breakthrough bleeding, with a majority of patients achieving amenorrhea within a year.

Severe continuous bleeding or intermittent bleeding for more than 6 months of hormonal therapy should prompt a search for uterine pathology. Optimization of menopausal symptom control while reducing adverse side effects of therapy may be accomplished by using the lowest effective dose and by substituting continuous transdermal estrogen for oral estrogen preparations when symptoms are not adequately controlled. When the patient's main concerns are with genitourinary symptoms, vaginal estrogen cream, tablets, or rings may be used on an "as needed" basis without necessarily adding a progestin.

SELECTIVE ESTROGEN RECEPTOR MODULATORS

The biologic effect of estrogenic substances is mediated by the translocation of a ligand-estrogen receptor complex into the nucleus where various estrogen-responsive genes are activated or repressed. At least two estrogen receptors, α and β, are presently known to exist. They exert different biologic effects and exist in different proportions in different tissues. In addition, different ligands bound in complex with the same receptor manifest different biologic activity. The use of SERMs attempts to take advantage of these facts to produce some but not all of the biologic effects of native estradiol. SERMs in use today include clomiphene, tamoxifen, and raloxifene. Unlike estradiol and other SERMs in current use, **raloxifene does not stimulate endometrial or breast duct epithelial proliferation.** However, **raloxifene does seem to reduce osteoclast activity and prevent osteoporosis (at least in the spine).** Hence, raloxifene has the bone-sparing effect of estradiol without the risk of endometrial hyperplasia/carcinoma, and in fact, it may prove to be protective of breast cancer in the same way as tamoxifen. However, **raloxifene appears to worsen rather than**

ameliorate vasomotor symptoms. Perhaps new SERMs discovered in the future will provide symptom relief as well as skeletal protection.

LIFESTYLE CHANGES AND ALTERNATIVE TREATMENTS FOR THE CLIMACTERIC

Increasingly, an emphasis is placed on the importance of lifestyle changes as a strategy for decreasing the inevitable effects of the aging process. **The most important change that anyone can make overall to increase longevity, reduce heart disease, and reduce calcium loss from bone is to stop smoking. Controlling weight, engaging in regular exercise, and eating a healthier, low-fat, and balanced diet should be strongly recommended,** especially in women with diabetes, hypertension, or significantly elevated blood lipids. All counseling about the effects of menopause should include a discussion of these issues and recommendations along with any possible medical therapies. In particular, **the statin drugs are especially important for postmenopausal women with unfavorable lipid profiles, as they significantly reduce the risk of cardiovascular disease and serendipitously protect against osteoporosis.**

Recently, phytoestrogens (plant products that are functionally or structurally similar to estrogen) and herbal substances have been marketed to consumers as the "natural" alternative to traditional hormone therapy for the symptoms of perimenopause and menopause. Women should be made aware that even placebos may decrease some of the symptoms, such as hot flashes, and that some herbal preparations have been shown to be ineffective or even harmful. Also, patients should be made aware of the less rigorous evaluation and regulation that these products undergo.

With proper counseling, appropriate screening, and professional care, the signs, symptoms, and sequelae of the climacteric can be managed successfully. Short-term use of hormonal therapy for symptom control, healthy lifestyle changes, appropriate monitoring, and medical or surgical intervention when necessary should provide a safe and effective level of care.

Suggested Reading

American College of Obstetricians and Gynecologists: Risk of breast cancer with estrogen-progestin replacement therapy. Committee Opinion No. 262. Washington, DC, ACOG, 2001.

American College of Obstetricians and Gynecologists: Use of botanicals for management of menopausal symptoms. Practice Bulletin No. 28. Washington, DC, ACOG, 2001.

Management of Postmenopausal Osteoporosis Position Statement of the North American Menopause Society. Menopause, 9(2): 84–101, 2002.

Menstrual Cycle–Influenced Disorders

Larry R. Laufer and Joseph C. Gambone

The human menstrual cycle is unique as a physiologic process in that it involves mechanisms that change on a daily basis rather than remaining stable to maintain homeostasis. This process of change is carried out through the many intricate hormonal interactions between the hypothalamic region of the brain, the pituitary gland, the ovaries, and to some extent, the adrenal glands and the pancreatic islets of Langerhans (see Chapter 4). To a large degree, the subject matter of reproductive endocrinology deals with disturbances of this inter-glandular hormonal communication that may result in irregular or absent menstrual cycles.

There is a second group of menstrual cycle–associated disorders, the hallmark of which is regular ovulatory cycles that cause dysfunction of other organ systems. In these menstrual-influenced disorders, the causative factors are not abnormal concentrations of the hormones of the hypothalamic-pituitary-ovarian (HPO) axis, but rather the factors are atypical end-organ responses to normal levels of gonadotropins and sex steroids. A common feature of these disorders is the inability to distinguish between affected women and normal controls by measurement of the traditional HPO hormones. Interestingly, in many cases, relief from the symptoms of these disorders can be obtained by intentionally disrupting or abolishing regular menstrual function. The quintessential menstrual influenced disorder is premenstrual syndrome, or PMS.

PREMENSTRUAL SYNDROME AND PREMENSTRUAL DYSPHORIC DISORDER

The acronyms PMS for premenstrual syndrome and PMDD for premenstrual dysphoric disorder refer to the same pathologic process at opposite ends of the symptom spectrum (Figure 37-1). In both PMS and PMDD, patients experience adverse physical, psychologic, and behavioral symptoms during the luteal phase of the menstrual cycle. There is a crescendo of symptom intensity up to the time that menses begins with quick resolution thereafter. Some patients have a brief surge of symptomatology at the time of ovulation in mid-cycle.

As many as 80% of regularly ovulating women experience some degree of physical and psychologic premenstrual symptomatology. Those who have mild to moderate symptoms are said to have PMS. In 5% or less of women, these symptoms are so severe that they seriously interfere with usual daily functioning or personal relationships. These women are characterized as having PMDD.

Common symptoms reported by patients include depressed mood, anxiety, affective lability and irritability, decreased interest in regular activity, difficulty concentrating, fatigue, change of appetite, sleep disturbance, and feelings of being overwhelmed. Physical symptoms include breast swelling and tenderness, bloating (a sense of abdominal swelling), weight gain, edema, and headache. The diagnosis of these disorders is confirmed by the predominant occurrence of symptoms in the luteal phase as documented on a menstrual calendar of two consecutive cycles.

A formal set of diagnostic criteria has been proposed in the fourth edition of **The Diagnostic and Statistical Manual (DSM-IV) of the American Psychiatric Association for PMDD** (Table 37-1). Although the DSM-IV definition of PMDD specifies that this is not just an exacerbation of another disorder, the dividing line between PMDD and other

Spectrum Of Premenstrual Syndromes

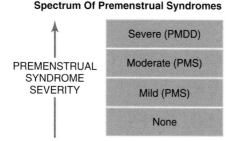

Figure 37-1. Spectrum of premenstrual syndromes.

neuropsychiatric disorders is not so clear cut. For example, **46% of PMDD patients have a history of a prior major depressive episode.** Moreover, patients with PMDD and clinical depression share similar sleep electroencephalogram (EEG) alterations, and they are both responsive to the selective serotonin reuptake inhibitor (SSRI) antidepressants.

Although PMS/PMDD patients and controls do not differ in their average cyclic levels of sex steroids, gonadotropins, prolactin, or cortisol, **there exists a strong basis to believe that these disorders have a hormonal rather than purely psychologic basis.** First, abolition of the menstrual cycle with gonadotropic-releasing hormone (GnRH) agonists, pregnancy, menopause, or spontaneous anovulation, provides symptomatic relief, whereas sequential ovarian hormone therapy in hypogonadal patients can induce PMS/PMDD symptoms. Second, cycles with higher luteal phase levels of estradiol are associated with more severe symptoms.

The physiologic mechanism that results in the occurrence of PMS/PMDD is not well understood. Evidence exists that the phenomenon arises, in part, from atypical metabolism of progesterone to the steroid, allopregnanolone, within the central nervous system. In turn, allopregnanolone interacts with the γ-aminobutyric acid (GABA) and serotonin neurons to influence the regions of the brain responsible for emotion and subjective perception. In addition, the GABA and serotoninergic neurons may be inherently dysfunctional in PMS/PMDD patients, especially in those with severe depressive symptoms—hence the overlap between PMDD and clinical depression. Major depressive disorder (MDD) persists, however, on a daily basis for weeks without a relationship to the menstrual cycle. **MDD may be exacerbated during the luteal phase of the menstrual cycle and can even coexist with PMDD in some women.** In such cases both PMDD and MDD need to be treated (Table 37-2).

Table 37-1. Criteria for premenstrual dysphoric disorder (PMDD)

- Symptoms seriously interfere with usual functioning/relationships.
- Premenstrual timing confirmed by menstrual calendar in two consecutive cycles.
- Symptoms resolve after the onset of menses.
- Symptoms are not an exacerbation of another disorder.
- At least 5 premenstrual symptoms:
  1. At least one of the following:
     Depressed mood
     Marked anxiety
     Marked affective lability
     Marked irritability
  2. Other possible symptoms:
     Decreased interest in regular activities
     Difficulty in concentrating
     Lethargy/fatigue
     Appetite change/food cravings
     Sleep disturbance
     Feelings of being overwhelmed
     Physical symptoms (breast swelling and tenderness, bloating, weight gain, edema, or headache)

Table 37-2. Distinguishing premenstrual dysphoric disorder (PMDD) from premenstrual syndrome (PMS) and major depressive disorder (MDD)

	Predominant Mood Symptoms	Premenstrual Physical Symptoms	Marked Social Impairment	Monthly Cyclicity
Premenstrual syndrome (PMS)	−/+	+	−	Yes
Premenstrual dysphoric disorder (PMDD)	+	+	+	Yes
Major depressive disorder (MDD)	+	−	+	No

Research performed to determine the best therapy for this disorder is problematic, because of the subjective nature of the condition, as well as the wide variation in the severity of the symptoms from one cycle to the next. In addition, external influences at work and at home may affect the severity of the symptoms. Finally, placebo interventions produce significant initial benefits in most PMS/PMDD studies. All of these considerations necessitate prolonged studies, which are expensive and infrequently performed.

TREATMENT

The majority of women who could be characterized as having PMS should be treated individually and conservatively, with **reassurance and mild diuretics** for symptoms such as bloating. The mild anxiety that frequently occurs with PMS may be treated with agents such as **buspirone**. At present, the most effective therapy studied for women with PMDD is the SSRI class of antidepressants. **Fluoxetine taken at dosages of 20 to 60 mg per day during the luteal phase of the cycle** provides significant symptom improvement in 50% to 60% of patients. **Sertraline at 50 to 150 mg per day** is equally effective. Side effects of the SSRIs are usually self-limited and include insomnia and sexual dysfunction.

Other preparations have been effective in at least one randomized controlled trial. They include **calcium carbonate at 1200 mg per day**, for control of mood and behavioral symptoms; **spironolactone at 100 mg per day**, for mood and bloating; and **buspirone at 25 to 60 mg per day** for premenstrual anxiety. **Danocrine and bromocriptine** are effective for the treatment of cyclic mastalgia. Pyridoxine (vitamin B6) at 50 to 100 mg a day has demonstrated mixed results in clinical trials.

GnRH agonists used with estrogen and progesterone "add back" are effective in eliminating PMS/PMDD symptoms. However, this is an expensive therapeutic approach. The trial use of this regimen might be considered in extreme cases in which other therapies are ineffective and the patient is contemplating possible oophorectomy.

Treatments that have been **demonstrated to be ineffective** in randomized controlled trials include oral or vaginal progesterone and conventional use of combined oral contraceptives. With the latter, patients have PMS-like symptoms during the placebo week. **Some individuals may derive relief from continuous oral contraceptives.**

MENSTRUAL MIGRAINE HEADACHES

Migraine headaches, which are believed to result from sequential intracranial vasoconstriction and vasodilation, are known to be influenced by menstrual cycling. They are two to three times more common in women than in men. They improve in approximately 80% of patients during pregnancy but recur postpartum. Usually, migraines resolve following the onset of the menopause. **Sixty percent of women who suffer migraine link the occurrence of their attacks to the menstrual cycle,** and 7% exclusively have migraines on the 2 days before or after the onset of menstruation.

The link between migraine headaches and the hormonal changes of the menstrual cycle is believed to be the phenomenon of estrogen withdrawal. Evidence for this derives from several observations: first, a small proportion of women with menstrual migraine have an upsurge in headache frequency following the preovulatory estradiol surge; second, exogenous estrogen reduces the incidence of migraines; and third, exogenous progesterone may delay the onset of menstruation without preventing the migraine attacks.

Several mechanisms have been proposed to explain why estrogen withdrawal produces migraine headaches. They include abnormal platelet aggregation, central nervous system endogenous opioid dysregulation, and stimulation of increased synthesis of prostaglandin in the central nervous system.

Standard treatment of migraine headaches includes ergotamine, nonsteroidal anti-inflammatory drugs, and antiemetics. In addition, sublingual estradiol taken with the onset of an aura may abort progression to the headache. **Drugs used for the prophylaxis of migraines include nonsteroidal inflammatory drugs, beta-blockers, calcium channel blockers, and antidepressants.** Monitoring of the menstrual cycle by basal body temperature charting or the use of a luteinizing hormone surge detector kit permits the initiation of increased dosage of these agents for more effective headache prevention.

Several hormonal protocols may also be effective in preventing menstrual migraines. They include transdermal or oral estrogen begun 48 hours before anticipated menses and continued for 3 to 6 days, continuous oral contraceptive pills for 2 to 4 months with symptomatic treatment during withdrawal intervals, and GnRH agonists with "add back" ovarian hormone replacement. **The ultimate and most radical "hormonal treatment" is hysterectomy with bilateral salpingo-oophorectomy and estrogen-only hormonal therapy.**

CATAMENIAL EPILEPSY

Seventy percent of women epileptics report an increased incidence of seizures premenstrually. Fourteen percent of women epileptics have catamenial epilepsy in which seizures only occur in the perimenstrual phase of the cycle. **This includes all varieties of epilepsy.** In these women, the onset of epilepsy is usually at the time of, or shortly after, menarche. Eight-four percent of catamenial epileptics have significant premenstrual syndrome symptoms in contrast to a 22% incidence of PMS in epileptics whose seizures do not correlate with the menstrual cycle.

Two mechanisms are felt to underlie the phenomenon of catamenial epilepsy, the first being a direct effect of the sex steroids on the neurons of the brain. In vitro, estradiol lowers the seizure threshold of many varieties of neurons whereas progesterone raises the threshold, making a seizure more likely. As a consequence, catamenial epilepsy reflects the effect of a reduced progesterone concentration or progesterone/estradiol ratio during the late luteal phase of the menstrual cycle. This correlates well with several clinical observations: first, some patients with catamenial epilepsy also suffer exacerbations during the preovulatory estradiol surge; second, seizure activity is prone to increase in anovulatory cycles; and third, seizure activity is reduced in incidence during menopause.

A second mechanism explaining this disorder is a reduction in serum level of anticonvulsants during the late luteal phase. This is believed to be mediated by increased hepatic mono-oxygenase activity resulting directly from reduced sex steroid levels. This is the rationale for the treatment option of closely tracking the menstrual cycle and determining anticonvulsant concentrations in the late luteal phase, so that drug dosage may be altered when necessary.

The anticonvulsant effect of progesterone is the basis of using Depo-Provera, progestin-only oral contraceptive pills, or premenstrual progesterone suppositories (50 to 400 mg BID) to reduce seizure activity. GnRH agonist therapy has been helpful for intractable cases. Combined oral contraceptives have inconsistent effects, with some patients suffering exacerbations during the placebo week. Moreover, pill efficacy is reduced by anticonvulsants, resulting in a 6% contraceptive failure rate with low-dose preparations.

OTHER MENSTRUAL INFLUENCED DISORDERS
PREMENSTRUAL ASTHMA

Thirty percent to 40% of female asthmatics report increased symptoms or decreased peak expiratory flow rates in the premenstrual phase of their cycles. Both estradiol and progesterone have bronchodilatory effects. In addition, the sex steroids are postulated to have immune system modulatory effects that may be responsible for this phenomenon. As with other cycle-influenced disorders, monitoring of the cycle to modify glucocorticoid or other inflammatory drug dosage may be helpful.

DIABETES MELLITUS

Seventy percent of female type 1 diabetics report changes in glycemic control premenstrually. Possible mechanisms for this effect include PMS-induced dietary binges and reduction of physical activity. The suggested management is intensified adherence to diet control, exercise, and glucose measurement.

PREMENSTRUAL ACNE

Although acne is worsened by the increased sebum production associated with androgen excess in conditions such as polycystic ovarian syndrome, regularly cycling women have little cyclic variation in androgen levels. The mechanism of premenstrual acne is unclear, but it may be secondary to altered immune function or hormone-related constriction of the pilosebaceous ductal orifice in the late luteal phase.

OTHER CONDITIONS

In some individuals, the following conditions may be influenced by the menstrual cycle: rheumatoid arthritis, irritable bowel syndrome, hereditary angioedema, aphthous ulcers, Behçet's syndrome, acute intermittent porphyria, paroxysmal supraventricular tachycardia, multiple sclerosis, glaucoma, urticaria, erythema multiforme, and myasthenia gravis. Interestingly, in the case of the last named condition, 25% to 50% of female patients improve premenstrually.

Suggested Reading

American College of Obstetricians and Gynecologists: Practice Bulletin on Premenstrual Syndrome, No. 15. Washington, DC, ACOG, 2000.

Case AM, Reid RL: Menstrual cycle effects on common medical conditions. Comp Therapeutics 27:65–71, 2000.

Kessel B: Premenstrual syndrome: Advances in diagnosis and treatment. Obstet Gynecol Clin North Am 27:625–631, 2000.

Rapkin A, Mikacich J: Premenstrual syndrome: Gynaecology or psychiatry? Reprod Med Rev 9(3):223–239, 2001.

PART FIVE | Gynecologic Oncology

Neville F. Hacker

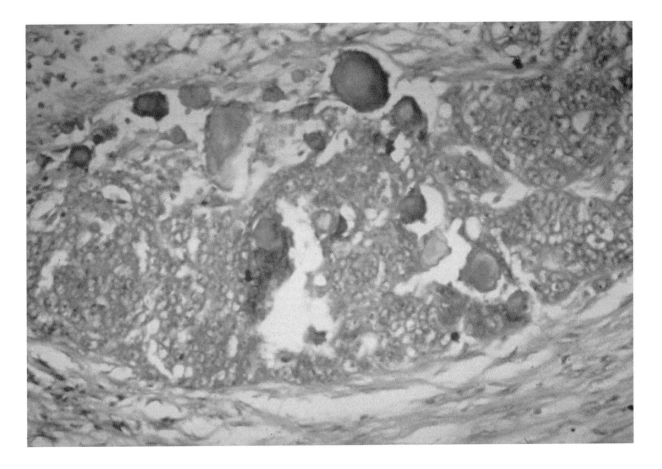

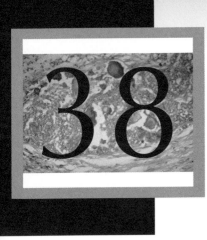

Principles of Cancer Therapy

Neville F. Hacker

The standard modalities for the management of gynecologic cancer are surgery, chemotherapy, radiation therapy, and hormonal therapy. In this chapter, the principles of chemotherapy, radiation therapy, and hormonal manipulation are discussed, together with the principles of pain management and end-of-life issues. Immunotherapy, biologic response modifiers, and hyperthermia are at present experimental modalities and are not included.

CELLULAR BIOLOGY

The characteristic feature of malignant tumor growth is its uncontrolled cellular proliferation, which requires replication of DNA. There are two distinct phases in the life cycle of all cells: **mitosis** (M phase), during which cellular division occurs, and **interphase,** the interval between successive mitoses.

Interphase is subdivided into three separate phases (Figure 38-1). Immediately following mitosis is the G_1 **phase,** which is of variable duration and is characterized by a diploid content of DNA. DNA synthesis is absent, but RNA and protein synthesis occur. During the shorter **S phase,** the entire DNA content is duplicated. This is followed by the G_2 **phase,** which is characterized by a tetraploid DNA content and by continuing RNA and protein synthesis in preparation for cell division. When mitosis occurs, a duplicate set of chromosomal DNA is inherited by each daughter cell, thus restoring the diploid DNA content. Following mitosis, some cells leave the cycle temporarily or permanently and enter the G_0 **or resting phase.**

The growth fraction of the tumor is the proportion of actively dividing cells. The higher the growth fraction, the fewer the number of cells in the G_0 phase and the faster the tumor-doubling time.

Chemotherapeutic agents and radiation kill cells by first-order kinetics, which means that a constant proportion of cells is killed for a given dosage, regardless of the number of cells present. Both therapeutic modalities are most effective against actively dividing cells because cells in the resting (G_0) phase are better able to repair sublethal damage. Unfortunately, both therapeutic modalities also suppress rapidly dividing normal cells, such as those in the gastrointestinal mucosa, bone marrow, and hair follicles.

CHEMOTHERAPY

One of the major advances in medicine since the 1950s has been the successful treatment of certain disseminated malignancies, including choriocarcinoma and germ cell ovarian tumors, with chemotherapy.

CLASSIFICATION OF CHEMOTHERAPEUTIC AGENTS

Chemotherapeutic agents act primarily by disrupting nuclear DNA, and thus inhibiting cellular division. They may be subdivided into two categories according to their mode of action relative to the cell cycle:

1. **Cell cycle–nonspecific agents,** such as alkylating agents, cisplatin, and paclitaxel, exert their damage at any phase of the cell cycle. They may damage resting as well as cycling cells, but the latter are much more sensitive.
2. **Cell cycle–specific agents** exert their lethal effects exclusively or primarily during one phase of the cell cycle. Examples include hydroxyurea and methotrexate, which act primarily during the S phase; bleomycin, which acts in the G_2

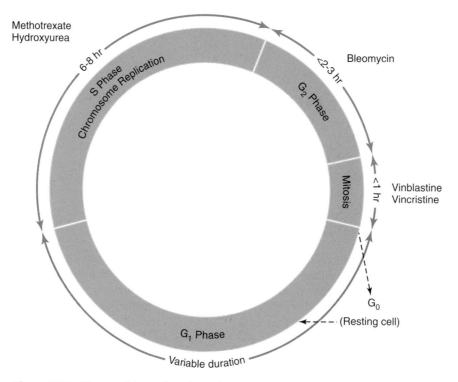

Methotrexate
Hydroxyurea

6-8 hr

S Phase
Chromosome Replication

Bleomycin

<2-3 hr

G₂ Phase

Mitosis

<1 hr

Vinblastine
Vincristine

G₀

(Resting cell)

G₁ Phase

Variable duration

Figure 38-1. Phases of the cell cycle and sites of action of cell cycle–specific drugs.

phase; and the vinca alkaloids, which act in the M phase.

PRINCIPLES OF CHEMOTHERAPY

Chemotherapeutic agents are selected on the basis of previous experience with particular agents for a given tumor. The drugs are usually given systemically so that the tumor can be treated regardless of its anatomic location. To increase the local concentration, certain drugs may occasionally be administered topically, by intraarterial infusion, or by intrathecal or intracavitary instillation (e.g., intraperitoneal therapy for ovarian cancer).

Chemotherapy is generally not administered if the white cell count is less than 3000/mm³ or if the platelet count is less than 100,000/mm³. Nadir blood counts are obtained 7 to 14 days after treatment, and subsequent doses may need to be reduced, depending on the degree of myelosuppression. Dosage reduction may also be necessary because of toxicity to other organs, such as the gastrointestinal tract, liver, or kidneys.

Resistance to chemotherapeutic agents may be temporary or permanent. Temporary resistance is mainly related to the poor vascularity of bulky tumors, which results in poor tissue concentrations of the drugs and an increasing proportion of cells in the relatively resistant G₀ phase of the cell cycle. Permanent resistance mainly results from spontaneous mutation to phenotypic resistance and occurs most commonly in bulky tumors. Permanent resistance may also be acquired by frequent exposure to chemotherapeutic agents.

CHEMOTHERAPEUTIC AGENTS

The common agents used in the management of gynecologic malignancies may be classified as shown in Table 38-1, along with a summary of the main indications and side effects of these drugs.

Alkylating Agents

The cytotoxicity of alkylating agents results from their ability to cause alkylation to DNA, resulting in cross-linkage between DNA strands and prevention of DNA replication. There is cross-resistance among the various alkylating agents.

Table 38-1. Indications, side effects, and precautions for commonly used chemotherapeutic agents

Drug	Main Indications	Side Effects	Precautions
ALKYLATING AGENTS			
Chlorambucil	Ovarian carcinoma	Bone marrow depression	
Melphalan	Ovarian and tubal carcinoma	Bone marrow depression, leukemia	Avoid prolonged courses (more than 12 cycles) to avoid leukemia
Cyclophosphamide	Ovarian carcinoma, germ cell tumors, squamous carcinomas, sarcomas	Bone marrow depression, nausea and vomiting, alopecia, hemorrhagic cystitis, sterility	Maintain adequate fluid intake to avoid cystitis
ANTIMETABOLITES			
Methotrexate	Gestational trophoblastic disease	Bone marrow depression, nausea and vomiting, stomatitis, alopecia, liver and renal failure, dermatitis	Ensure normal kidney and liver function
5-fluorouracil	Vaginal and vulvar intraepithelial neoplasia (topical application)	Pain and ulceration	
Gemcitibine	Ovarian carcinoma	Bone marrow depression, flu-like illness, skin rash	IV infusion
ANTIBIOTICS			
Actinomycin-D	Gestational trophoblastic disease	Bone marrow depression, nausea and vomiting, diarrhea, stomatitis, alopecia, dermatitis, local tissue necrosis	Administer through running intravenous infusion to avoid extravasation
Doxorubicin	Ovarian carcinoma, recurrent endometrial carcinoma, sarcoma	Bone marrow depression, nausea and vomiting, cardiomyopathy, cardiac arrhythmias, alopecia, local tissue necrosis	Administer through running intravenous infusion; do not exceed total dose of 550 mg/m^2 to avoid cardiac toxicity; avoid if significant heart disease is present
Liposomal doxorubicin	Ovarian cancer	Hand-foot syndrome; less cardiotoxic than doxorubicin	IV infusion
Bleomycin	Germ cell tumors, squamous carcinomas	Pneumonitis and pulmonary fibrosis, alopecia, stomatitis, cutaneous reactions	Do not exceed total dose of 400 U; monitor pulmonary function with carbon monoxide diffusion capacity
PLANT ALKALOIDS			
Vinblastine	Germ cell tumors, sarcomas	Bone marrow depression, nausea and vomiting, stomatitis, diarrhea, local tissue necrosis	Administer through running intravenous infusion
Vincristine	Germ cell tumors, sarcomas	Neurotoxicity, constipation, alopecia, local tissue necrosis; bone marrow depression less marked	Administer through running IV infusion; prophylactic cathartics may be helpful
Etoposide	Germ cell tumors	Bone marrow depression; nausea and vomiting	Administer slowly intravenously

Table 38-1. Indications, side effects, and precautions for commonly used chemotherapeutic agents— cont'd

Drug	Main Indications	Side Effects	Precautions
Paclitaxel	Ovarian carcinoma, breast carcinoma	Myelosuppression, alopecia, allergic reactions, cardiac arrhythmias	Intravenously as a 3–24 hour infusion
Docetaxel	Ovarian and breast cancer	Myelosuppression, alopecia, dermatologic reactions	Intravenous infusion, IV dexamethasone to reduce fluid retention
OTHER DRUGS			
Cisplatin	Ovarian carcinoma, germ cell tumors, squamous carcinomas	Renal toxicity, ototoxicity, neurotoxicity, severe nausea and vomiting, bone marrow depression less marked, hypokalemia, hypomagnesemia	Administer intravenous fluids to maintain urinary output of 100 mL/hr during infusion; discontinue if creatinine clearance <35 mL/hr
Carboplatin	Ovarian carcinoma, germ cell tumors	Bone marrow depression, less gastrointestinal toxicity, less renal toxicity, less neurotoxicity	Suitable for outpatient therapy because no need for high urinary output
Hexamethylmelamine	Ovarian carcinoma	Bone marrow depression, nausea and vomiting, neurotoxicity, depression	Given orally
Topotecan	Ovarian cancer	Bone marrow depression	IV for 5 days every 3 weeks

Antimetabolites

Antimetabolites are compounds that closely resemble normal intermediaries, for which they may substitute in biochemical reactions, and thereby produce a metabolic block; for example, **methotrexate** competitively inhibits the enzyme dihydrofolate reductase, thus preventing the conversion of dihydrofolate to tetrahydrofolate. The latter is required for the methylation reaction necessary for the synthesis of purine and pyrimidine subunits of nucleic acid.

Antibiotics

Antibiotics are naturally occurring antitumor agents elaborated by certain species of *Streptomyces*. They have no single, clearly defined mechanism of action, but many agents in this group intercalate between strands of the DNA double helix, thereby inhibiting both DNA and RNA synthesis and causing oxygen-dependent strand breaks.

Plant Alkaloids

The most common plant alkaloids are the **vinca alkaloids,** which are derived from the periwinkle plant. These include vincristine and vinblastine. They are spindle toxins that interfere with cellular microtubules and cause metaphase arrest.

Other plant alkaloids include the **epipodophyllotoxins** such as etoposide (VP16), which are extracts from the mandrake plant, and **paclitaxel** (Taxol), an extract from the bark of the Pacific yew tree. **Docetaxel (Taxotere)** is the first semisynthetic analogue of paclitaxel. Etoposide appears to act by causing single-strand DNA breaks. Paclitaxel binds preferentially to microtubules, and results in their polymerization and stabilization.

Other Drugs

Cisplatin, one of the more important drugs in gynecologic oncology, causes inhibition of DNA synthesis by forming interstrand and intrastrand linkages. Carboplatin is an analogue of cisplatin with a similar mechanism of action and efficacy, but with less gastrointestinal and renal toxicity.

RADIATION THERAPY

Radiation may be defined as the propagation of energy through space or matter.

TYPES OF RADIATION

There are two main types of radiation: electromagnetic and particulate.

Electromagnetic Radiation

Examples of electromagnetic radiation include the following:
- Visible light
- Infrared light
- Ultraviolet light
- X-rays (photons)
- Gamma rays (photons)

X-rays and gamma rays are identical electromagnetic radiations, differing only in their mode of production. X-rays are produced by bombardment of an anode by a high-speed electron beam; gamma rays result from the decay of radioactive isotopes, such as cobalt 60 (^{60}Co).

X-rays and gamma rays (photons) are differentiated from electromagnetic radiation of longer wavelength by their greater energy, which allows them to penetrate tissues and cause ionization.

Particulate Radiation

Particulate radiation consists of moving particles of matter. Their energy consists of the kinetic energy of the moving particles.

$$\text{Energy} = 0.5 \text{ mass} \times \text{velocity}^2$$

The particles vary greatly in size and include the following:
- Neutrons (no charge)
- Protons (positive charge)
- Electrons (negative charge)

The most commonly used particles are electrons. They may be derived from a linear accelerator, the beam of electrons being directed into the patient without first striking a metal target and producing x-rays. Alternatively, high-energy electrons (called beta particles) may be derived from the radiodecay of an unstable isotope, such as phosphorus 32 (^{32}P). Particulate radiation penetrates tissues less than photons but also produces ionization.

UNIT OF RADIATION MEASUREMENT

The Gray (Gy) is equivalent to an absorbed energy of 1 joule per kilogram of absorbing material.

INVERSE SQUARE LAW

The intensity of electromagnetic radiation is inversely proportional to the square of the distance from the source. Thus, the dose of radiation 2 cm from a point source will be 25% of the dose at 1 cm.

BIOLOGIC CONSIDERATIONS
Ionization of Molecules

Radiation damage is caused by the ionization of molecules in the cell, with the production of free radicals. Because approximately 80% of a mammalian cell is water, most of the cellular radiation damage is mediated by ionization of water and the production of the free radicals H (hydrogen) and OH (hydroxide). Free radicals may cause irreversible damage to DNA, making it impossible for the cell to continue replication. Minor or sublethal damage to DNA, which the cell is capable of repairing, may also occur. RNA, protein, and other molecules in the cell are also damaged, but these molecules can be more readily repaired or replaced.

Oxygen Effect

In the absence of oxygen, cells show a twofold to threefold increase in their capacity to survive radiation exposure. This means that hypoxic cells are less radiosensitive than are fully oxygenated cells. The enhancement of the lethal effects of radiation by oxygen is presumed to occur because the oxygen will combine with the free radicals split from cell targets by the radiation. This prevents the recombination of the free radicals with the targets, which would restore the integrity of the targets.

The effect of oxygen has important clinical implications. First, anemic patients should undergo transfusion before radiation therapy. Second, bulky tumors are usually poorly vascularized and, therefore, are often hypoxic, particularly in the center. Such areas are likely to be relatively resistant to radiation so that viable tumor cells may remain in spite of marked shrinkage of the tumor.

Pharmacologic Modification of the Effects of Radiation

A variety of chemical compounds are capable of enhancing the lethal effects of radiation. Recently, a series of randomized clinical trials has demonstrated a significant survival advantage, particularly in terms of local disease control, when cisplatin-containing chemotherapy is given concurrently with radiation for locoregionally advanced cervical cancer. Some of the regimens tested have included 5-fluorouracil in combination with cisplatin. This is called chemoradiation.

Time-Dose Fractionation of Radiation

Successful radiation therapy requires a delicate balance between dosage to the tumor and that to the surrounding normal tissues. A dose of radiation that is too high sterilizes the tumor but results in an unacceptably high complication rate because of the destruction of normal tissues.

Most normal tissues, such as gastrointestinal mucosa and bone marrow, have a remarkable capacity to recover from radiation damage by the division of stem cells as well as by repair of sublethal radiation damage. Tumors, in general, have less ability to repair and repopulate. This difference can be exploited by administering the radiation in multiple fractions, thereby allowing some recovery, particularly of normal cells, between fractions.

If the interval between each fraction increases, the total dose must increase to produce the same biologic effect because of the amount of recovery that will occur in the interval. **Cells that survive the acute effects of radiation usually repair sublethal damage within 24 hours;** therefore, conventionally fractioned radiation is usually given in daily increments.

When treating the pelvis with external radiation, each fraction is usually 180 to 200 cGy. In treating the whole abdomen, fractions are decreased to 100 to 120 cGy because the tolerance of normal tissues decreases as the volume irradiated increases. The major factors influencing the outcome of radiation therapy are summarized in Box 38-1.

Box 38-1. Major factors influencing the outcome of radiation therapy

Normal tissue tolerance
Malignant cell type
Total volume irradiated
Total dose delivered
Total duration of therapy
Number of fractions
Type of equipment used
Tissue oxygen concentration

Box 38-2. Modalities of radiation therapy

EXTERNAL BEAMS
Kilovoltage ("orthovoltage") (125–400 kV)
Cobalt 60 machine (1.25 MeV)
Linear accelerator (4–35 MeV)
Betatrons (20–42 MeV)
Particle accelerators (e.g., electrons, protons, neutrons)

INTRACAVITARY (CESIUM OR IRIDIUM)
Afterloading applicators (e.g., Fletcher-Suit)
Intraperitoneal (e.g., ^{32}P)

INTERSTITIAL
Permanent
    Seeds (e.g., ^{198}Au, ^{125}I)
Removable
    Ribbons (e.g., ^{192}Ir)
    Needles (e.g., ^{226}Ra, ^{137}Cs)

MODALITIES OF RADIATION THERAPY

The modalities used to deliver radiation therapy are listed in Box 38-2. In general, there are two radiation techniques: teletherapy and brachytherapy. **In teletherapy, a device quite removed from the patient is used, as with external beam techniques. Figure 38-2 is a linear accelerator used to deliver external beam pelvic radiation. In brachytherapy, the radiation source is placed either within or close to the target tissue, as with intracavitary and interstitial techniques.** In contrast to external beam therapy, intracavitary and interstitial techniques allow a high dose of radiation to be delivered to the tumor, whereas dosages to surrounding normal tissues are considerably lower and are determined by the inverse square law.

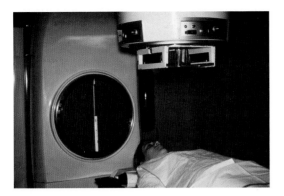

Figure 38-2. Linear accelerator used to deliver external beam pelvic radiation.

Box 38-3. Advantages of megavoltage therapy

Skin sparing
Greater dose at deeper depth in tissues
Shorter treatment times
No differential bone absorption (therefore no bone necrosis)
Can treat larger fields easily (e.g., whole abdomen)

External Beam Therapy

As the energy of the electromagnetic radiation increases, the penetration of the tissues increases, resulting in a relative sparing of the skin and an increased dosage to deeper tissues. At megavoltage energies (1 million electron volts or greater), there is no differential absorption of energy by bone.

Orthovoltage machines are no longer used except to treat skin cancers. Cobalt machines, developed in the early 1950s, have also been largely replaced by linear accelerators, which have a higher range of energies. The advantages of megavoltage therapy over the earlier orthovoltage machines are listed in Box 38-3.

External radiation allows a uniform dose to be delivered to a given field. The tolerance of the normal tissues (e.g., bowel, bladder, liver, kidneys) limits the total dosage that can be delivered. External radiation is usually used to shrink a large tumor mass before brachytherapy. When used alone, it is generally useful only when there is small residual macroscopic or microscopic disease following surgery. With highly radiosensitive tumors (e.g., dysgerminoma), external radiation alone may sterilize even bulky disease.

Intracavitary Radiation

Intracavitary therapy is used particularly in the treatment of cervical and vaginal cancer. **All applicators now in use should be "afterloaded,"** which means that they are placed in the patient and their position checked by radiography before the radioactive substance is loaded into the applicator. The Fletcher-Suit is an example of one afterloading device. Remote afterloading devices, such as the Selectron, allow the radioactive sources to be removed from the applicators when medical or nursing personnel enter the room, thereby significantly limiting staff exposure to radiation.

Radioactive colloids, such as chromic phosphate (^{32}P), may be instilled directly into the peritoneal cavity to treat minimal residual disease, particularly in patients with ovarian cancer. To be effective, these agents must achieve a uniform distribution throughout the cavity, which is difficult to achieve, so such agents are rarely used at present. ^{32}P **is a pure beta (electron) emitter.**

Interstitial Radiation

Interstitial therapy (in which the radioactive source is placed directly in the tumor) may be delivered by removable or permanent implants. **Permanent implants are used for inaccessible tumors. They use radioisotopes such as radon 222 (^{222}Rn) or iodine 125 (^{125}I) seeds** and are usually placed in an unresectable tumor nodule at the time of laparotomy.

Removable implants are placed in tumors that are accessible (e.g., cervical or vaginal tumors). Interstitial therapy has the theoretical advantage of better dose distribution within the tumor but the disadvantage that it is easier to overdose normal tissues, thereby increasing the complication rate. As with intracavitary devices, afterloading devices are now available for interstitial therapy. **The radioisotope of choice for afterloading interstitial implants is iridium 192 (^{192}Ir).**

COMPLICATIONS ASSOCIATED WITH RADIATION

The success of radiation therapy depends on an exploitable gradient of susceptibility to injury in favor of normal tissue. Unfortunately, most malignant tumors are only marginally more sensitive to radiation than are normal tissues, so the total dose that can be delivered, and therefore the radiocurability, is limited by the associated complications.

Acute Complications

Acute reactions to radiation include the following pathologic changes: rapid cessation of mitotic activity, cellular swelling, tissue edema, and tissue necrosis.

In the management of gynecologic tumors, these acute reactions may produce the following effects: **acute cystitis,** manifested by hematuria, urgency, and frequency; **proctosigmoiditis,** manifested by tenesmus, diarrhea, and passage of blood and mucus in the stool; **enteritis,** manifested by nausea, vomiting, diarrhea, and colicky abdominal pain; and **bone marrow depression,** which is uncommon with pelvic radiation but common with whole-abdominal radiation, particularly if the patient has had previous cytotoxic chemotherapy.

Chronic Complications

Chronic complications occur 6 months or more after completion of radiation and are characterized pathologically by the following changes: internal thickening and obliteration of small blood vessels (endarteritis), fibrosis, and permanent reduction in the epithelial and parenchymal cell populations.

Significant chronic complications occur in 5% to 10% of patients receiving 5000 cGy or more of radiation, and they may be slowly progressive over several years.

Common chronic complications of radiation follow.

Radiation Enteropathy

Previous surgery, with resultant loops of adherent small bowel fixed in the pelvis, predisposes the patient to radiation enteritis, particularly when intracavitary or interstitial radiation is used in addition to teletherapy.

Large bowel injuries, which are best diagnosed by sigmoidoscopy or colonoscopy, may include: **proctosigmoiditis,** manifested by pelvic pain, tenesmus, diarrhea, and rectal bleeding; **ulceration,** manifested by rectal bleeding and tenesmus; **rectovaginal fistula,** manifested by passage of stool through the vagina; and **rectal or sigmoid stenosis,** manifested by progressive large bowel obstruction (Figure 38-3 shows a radiation induced stricture of the sigmoid colon).

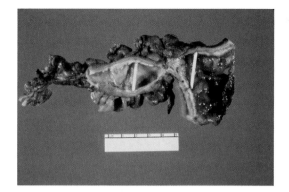

Figure 38-3. Radiation-induced stricture of the sigmoid colon. Note the tight fibrotic constriction, necessitating partial sigmoid colectomy for large bowel obstruction.

Small bowel injuries usually present with cramping abdominal pain and vomiting, or with alternating diarrhea and constipation.

Vaginal Vault Necrosis

This is associated with severe pain and tenderness of the vaginal vault and a profuse discharge.

Urologic Injuries

The following are included in this category: **hemorrhagic cystitis,** which may necessitate frequent blood transfusions and, occasionally, urinary diversion; **vesicovaginal fistula,** manifested by the constant leakage of urine and demonstrable by cystoscopy; **ureterovaginal fistula,** which is also manifested by constant leakage of urine and is demonstrable with an intravenous pyelogram; **ureteric stenosis,** which is manifested by progressive hydronephrosis.

HORMONAL THERAPY

The estrogen receptor (ER) status of primary and metastatic breast cancer has been shown to be of therapeutic and prognostic significance. The ER and progesterone receptor (PR) status of endometrial cancer also have prognostic and therapeutic significance.

MECHANISM OF ACTION OF HORMONAL RECEPTORS

Most steroid hormones influence their target tissues by the following series of steps: passive diffusion of the hormone through the cell membrane, specific binding in the cytoplasm with the hormone receptor, translocation of the receptor-hormone complex to the nucleus, binding of the receptor-hormone complex to an "acceptor" site on the chromatin, and transcription of DNA in a manner characteristic of the specific hormone–target cell interaction, eventually resulting in either an increase or a decrease in specific protein synthesis.

Tamoxifen binds with the ER and is translocated to the nucleus, where it binds to chromatin. It does not influence gene transcription, so functionally, tamoxifen acts as an antiestrogen.

Estrogen exposure increases the production of both ER and PR, whereas progesterone inhibits production of both ER and PR.

CLINICAL APPLICATIONS

Because tumor growth in patients whose tumors contain ER and PR is likely to be stimulated by estrogen exposure, tumor regression should occur if endogenous estrogen production is abolished or if the patient is exposed to a progestin or antiestrogen. **In breast cancer, patients whose tumors contain ER and PR have an 80% response rate to hormonal manipulation,** whereas fewer than 10% of receptor-poor tumors respond.

An objective response to progestin therapy occurs in about one-third of patients with recurrent or metastatic endometrial carcinoma. Progestin therapy is more likely to be effective in well-differentiated endometrial adenocarcinomas than in more poorly differentiated tumors because well-differentiated tumors are the ones that are most likely to contain ER and PR.

ER and PR have been demonstrated in some ovarian adenocarcinomas, particularly endometrioid carcinomas, but the therapeutic implications of these findings await further investigation.

PAIN MANAGEMENT

More than 70% of patients with cancer will develop significant pain at some point in their disease. Proper pain management requires an understanding of pain physiology, pain mechanisms, and the pharmacology of analgesics.

Pain in gynecologic cancer may be the result of soft tissue infiltration, bone involvement, neural involvement, muscle spasm (e.g., psoas spasm), infection within or near tumor masses, or bowel colic.

Therapeutic approaches will vary according to the pain mechanism involved. Consideration must be given to the specific therapeutic measure that may be appropriate in the individual case, such as radiation therapy, chemotherapy, antibiotics, regional nerve block, or surgery.

Peripherally acting drugs such as acetaminophen (paracetamol) should rarely be omitted from analgesic regimens, and rectal suppositories are useful if oral intake is not appropriate. When pain is caused by bone metastases, nonsteroidal anti-inflammatory drugs or bisphosphonates are helpful. Muscle spasm requires muscle relaxants such as diazepam, whereas bowel colic requires anticholinergics such as busulphan.

Opioid use will be necessary for severe pain, although nerve pain and muscle spasm are not well relieved by opioids. A variety of opioids is available, and in general, a low-potency opioid such as codeine or a high-potency opioid such as morphine is combined with a peripherally acting drug such as acetaminophen or aspirin.

Immediate release morphine, which is best given orally or subcutaneously, should be given at regular 4-hour intervals. **Controlled-release morphine tablets are a significant advance in convenience of administration, as they need to be given only every 12 to 24 hours,** once the total 24-hour requirement has been determined from the use of an immediate release preparation. Constipation is a real problem with opioids, and prophylactic laxatives should be prescribed.

Alternative opioids (with equivalency to morphine 5 mg) include oxycodone (5 mg), hydromorphone (1 mg), pentazocine (45 mg), and meperidine (75 mg). **When pain is neurogenic in origin, an opioid and a peripherally acting drug should usually be supplemented by a tricyclic antidepressant, an anticonvulsant, or a corticosteroid.**

END-OF-LIFE ISSUES

When it becomes clear that the patient is dying, the goals are to control symptoms, maintain dignity, and allow time and privacy for communication with loved ones.

Medications should usually be given subcutaneously or rectally, any unnecessary tubes or equipment should be removed to facilitate contact with loved ones, and nursing care should particularly focus on pressure areas, mouth care, and "grooming." Sedation, for example, with sublingual lorazepam 0.5 to 2.5 mg every 4 to 6 hours, may be helpful if the patient is agitated.

Important issues from a patient's perspective are receiving adequate pain and symptom management, avoiding inappropriate prolongation of dying, achieving a sense of control, relieving the burden on caregivers, and strengthening relationships with loved ones.

Suggested Reading

Eifel PJ: Radiation therapy. *In* Berek JS, Hacker NF (eds): Practical Gynecologic Oncology, 3rd ed. Philadelphia, Lippincott Williams & Wilkins, 2000, pp 117–158.

Hortobagyi GN, Theriault RL, Lipton A, Porter L, Blayney D, Sinoff C, et al.: Long-term prevention of skeletal complications of metastatic breast cancer with pamidronate. J Clin Oncol 16:2038–2044, 1998.

Lickiss JN, Philip JAM.: Palliative care and pain management. *In* Berek JS, Hacker NF (eds): Practical Gynecologic Oncology, 3rd ed. Philadelphia, Lippincott Williams & Wilkins, 2000, pp 863–886.

Singer PA, Martin DK, Kelner M: Quality end-of-life care: Patient's perspectives. JAMA 281:163–168, 1999.

Young RC, Markman M: Chemotherapy. *In* Berek JS, Hacker NF (eds): Practical Gynecologic Oncology, 3rd ed. Philadelphia, Lippincott Williams & Wilkins, 2000, pp 83–116.

39 Cervical Dysplasia and Cancer

Neville F. Hacker

Worldwide, cervical cancer is the most common cause of death from cancer in women, with 80% of cases occurring in developing countries. In developed countries, regular screening with Papanicolaou smears has markedly decreased the incidence of the disease, and most cases now occur in women who have not had regular smears. In the US, cervical cancer now ranks only eleventh among cancers in women, with 10,520 new cases expected in 2004, and 3900 deaths.

ETIOLOGY AND EPIDEMIOLOGY

Cervical cancer and its precursors have been associated with several epidemiologic variables (Box 39-1). It is relatively rare before 20 years of age; the average age at onset is 47 years of age.

It is now believed that almost all cases of cervical cancer are caused by exposure to a high-risk human papilloma virus (HPV), such as type 16, 18, 31, 33, or 35. Types 6 and 11 have been associated with cervical condylomas and low-grade cervical intraepithelial neoplasia (CIN). In the future, it is hoped that a vaccine will be developed that can be given to teenage girls and virtually eliminate cervical cancer as a public health problem.

The adolescent cervix is believed to be more susceptible to carcinogenic stimuli because of the active process of squamous metaplasia, which occurs within the transformation zone during periods of endocrine change. This squamous metaplasia is normally a physiologic process, but under the influence of the HPV, cellular alterations occur that result in an atypical transformation zone. These atypical changes initiate a process called CIN, which is the preinvasive phase of cervical cancer.

CIN represents a spectrum of disease, ranging from CIN I (mild dysplasia) to CIN III (severe dysplasia and carcinoma in situ). At least 35% of patients with CIN III will develop invasive cancer within 10 years, whereas lower grades of CIN may spontaneously regress.

SCREENING OF ASYMPTOMATIC WOMEN

The American College of Obstetricians and Gynecologists (ACOG) has recommended that all women, once they have become sexually active, should undergo an annual physical examination, including a Papanicolaou smear. Less rigorous screening, such as every 2 to 5 years following two or three normal Papanicolaou smears, has been proposed by some as being more cost-effective for low-risk women. Because having a sexual partner with multiple partners is a major risk factor, relatively few women belong to the low-risk group and it is better to regard any woman who has ever been sexually active as being "at risk." Recently, ACOG stated that less frequent screening is appropriate at the discretion of the treating physician. **Both the endocervical canal and the ectocervix should be sampled when taking the Papanicolaou smear.**

The false-negative rate for conventional pap smears for high-grade intraepithelial lesions is generally reported to be about 20%, but it is higher for glandular lesions and for invasive cancers.

New technologies have been developed to decrease the false negative rate. Thin Prep (Cytyc Corporation) and AutoCyte PREP (TriPath Imaging) are automated liquid-based slide-preparation systems. With liquid-based cytology, the spatula or brush taking the smear is

Box 39-1. Risk factors for cervical cancer

- Young age at first coitus (<20 yr)
- Multiple sexual partners
- Sexual partner with multiple sexual partners
- Young age at first pregnancy
- High parity
- Lower socioeconomic status
- Smoking

placed into a fixative solution, instead of smearing the cells directly onto a glass slide. Blood, mucus, and inflammatory cells are eliminated and a monolayer smear is then automatically prepared by a machine. **Auto Pap Guided Screening System (Tripath Imaging) is a semiautomated computerized image-processor** that selects slides requiring reading by a cytotechnician, thereby eliminating many normal smears from manual reading.

CERVICAL TOPOGRAPHY

During early embryonic development, the cervix and upper vagina are covered with columnar epithelium. During intrauterine development, the columnar epithelium of the vagina is progressively replaced by squamous epithelium. At birth, the vagina is usually covered with squamous epithelium, and the columnar epithelium is limited to the endocervix and the central portion of the ectocervix. **In about 4% of normal female infants and about 30% of those exposed to diethylstilbestrol in utero, the columnar epithelium extends onto the vaginal fornices.** Macroscopically, the columnar epithelium has a red appearance because it is only a single cell layer thick, allowing blood vessels in the underlying stroma to show through it.

The embryologic squamous and columnar epithelia are designated the original or native squamous and columnar epithelia, respectively. The junction between them at or near the external cervical os is called the original squamocolumnar junction.

Throughout life, but particularly during adolescence and a woman's first pregnancy, metaplastic squamous epithelium covers the columnar epithelium so that a new squamocolumnar junction is formed more proximally. This junction moves progressively closer to the external os and then up the endocervical canal. **The transformation zone is the area of metaplas-

tic squamous epithelium located between the original squamocolumnar junction and the new squamocolumnar junction** (Figure 39-1).

CLASSIFICATION OF AN ABNORMAL PAPANICOLAOU SMEAR

In 1988, a consensus meeting was convened by the Division of Cancer Control of the National Cancer Institute to review existing terminology and to recommend effective methods of cytologic reporting. As a result of this meeting, **the Bethesda system** was devised and **(1) requires a statement regarding the adequacy of the specimen** for diagnosis, **(2) diagnostic categorization** (normal or other), and **(3) a descriptive diagnosis.** A revised Bethesda system was developed in 2001 and is shown in Box 39-2.

CERVICAL INTRAEPITHELIAL NEOPLASIA

With CIN, there is abnormal epithelial proliferation and maturation above the basement membrane. Involvement of the inner one-third of the epithelium represents CIN I, involvement of the inner one-half to two-thirds represents CIN II, and full-thickness involvement represents CIN III (Fig. 39-2). The disease is asymptomatic.

COLPOSCOPY

The colposcope is a stereoscopic binocular microscope of low magnification, usually 10× to 40×.

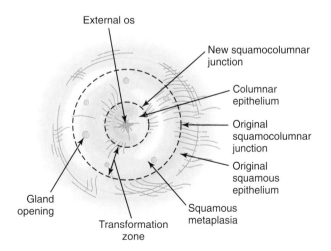

Figure 39-1. Schematic representation of the transformation zone.

Box 39-2. The 2001 Bethesda classification of cytologic abnormalities (abridged)

SPECIMEN ADEQUACY
Satisfactory for evaluation (note presence/absence of endocervical/transformation zone component)
Unsatisfactory for evaluation . . . (specify reason)
Specimen rejected/not processed . . . (specify reason)
Specimen processed and examined, but unsatisfactory for evaluation of epithelial abnormality because of (specify reason)

GENERAL CATEGORIZATION (OPTIONAL)
Negative for intraepithelial lesion or malignancy
Epithelial cell abnormality
Other

INTERPRETATION/RESULT
Negative for Intraepithelial Lesion or Malignancy
Organisms (e.g., *Trichomonas vaginalis*)
Reactive cellular changes associated with inflammation (includes typical repair), radiation, intrauterine contraceptive device
Atrophy

EPITHELIAL CELL ABNORMALITIES
Squamous Cell
Atypical squamous cells of undetermined significance (ASCUS) cannot exclude HSIL (ASC-H)
Low-grade squamous intraepithelial lesion (LSIL) encompassing: human papillomavirus/mild dysplasia/cervical intraepithelial neoplasia (CIN I)
High-grade squamous intraepithelial lesion (HSIL) encompassing: moderate and severe dysplasia, carcinoma in situ; CIN 2 and CIN 3
Squamous cell carcinoma

Glandular Cell
Atypical glandular cells (AGC) (specify endocervical, endometrial, or not otherwise specified)
Atypical glandular cells, favor neoplastic (specify endocervical or not otherwise specified)
Endocervical adenocarcinoma in situ (AIS)
Adenocarcinoma

Other (e.g., endometrial cells in a woman ≥40 years of age)

Illumination is centered, and the focal length is between 12 and 15 cm.

To perform a colposcopic examination, an appropriately-sized speculum is inserted to expose the cervix, which is cleansed with a cotton pledget soaked in 3% acetic acid to remove adherent mucus and cellular debris. A green filter can be employed to accentuate the vascular changes that frequently accompany pathologic alterations of the cervix.

At colposcopy, the original or native squamous epithelium appears gray and homogeneous. The columnar epithelium appears red and grapelike. **The transformation zone can be identified by the presence of gland openings that are not covered by the squamous metaplasia and by the paler color of the metaplastic epithelium compared with the original squamous epithelium. Nabothian follicles may also be seen in the transformation zone. Normal blood vessels branch like a tree.**

EVALUATION OF A PATIENT WITH AN ABNORMAL PAPANICOLAOU SMEAR

An algorithm for the evaluation of patients with abnormal Papanicolaou smears is presented in Figure 39-3.

Any patient with a grossly abnormal cervix should have a punch biopsy performed, regardless of the results of the Papanicolaou smear.

Patients with atypical squamous cells of undetermined significance (ASCUS) found on their smear may have a repeat smear in 6 months. Alternatively, HPV testing, such as with the Hybrid Capture assay (Digene Diagnostics, Silver Spring, MD) may be used to triage such patients. About 6% to 10% of patients with an ASCUS smear will have high-grade CIN on colposcopy, and 90% of these can be detected by HPV testing for high-risk viral types.

The colposcopic hallmark of cervical intraepithelial neoplasia is an area of sharply delineated acetowhite epithelium—that is, epithelium that appears white after the application of acetic acid. It is thought that the acetic acid dehydrates the cells and that there is increased light reflex from areas of increased nuclear density. **Within the acetowhite areas, there may or may not be abnormal vascular patterns.**

There are two basic changes in the vascular architecture in patients with CIN: punctation and mosaicism. Punctation is caused by single-looped capillaries lying within the subepithelial papillae, seen end-on as a "dot" as they course toward the surface of the epithelium. Mosaicism is caused by a fine network of capillaries disposed parallel to the surface in a mosaic pattern. Punctate and mosaic patterns may be

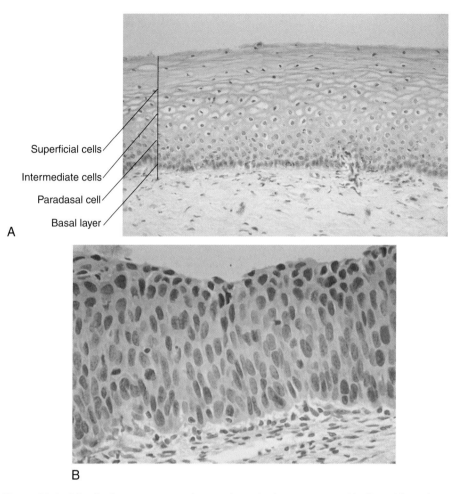

Superficial cells
Intermediate cells
Paradasal cell
Basal layer

A

B

Figure 39-2. Histologic appearance of normal cervical squamous epithelium (*A*) and carcinoma in situ (*B*) of the cervix. In the normal epithelium, note the orderly maturation from the basal layer to the parabasal cells, glycogenated intermediate cells, and flattened superficial cells. In the carcinoma in situ, the entire thickness of the epithelium is replaced by immature cells that are variable in size and shape and have irregular nuclei. Mitotic figures are seen in the lower two-thirds of the epithelium.

seen together within the same area of the cervix. The more dilatated and irregular the punctate and mosaic capillaries and the greater the intercapillary distance, the more atypical is the tissue on histologic examination. Similarly, the whiter the lesion, the more severe the dysplasia.

With microinvasive carcinoma, extremely irregular punctate and mosaic patterns are found, as are small atypical vessels. **The irregularity in size, shape, and arrangement of the terminal vessels becomes even more striking in frankly invasive carcinoma, with exaggerated distortions of the vascular architecture producing comma-shaped,** **corkscrew-shaped, and dilated, blind-ended vessels.**

BIOPSY AND ENDOCERVICAL CURETTAGE

If the colposcopic examination is satisfactory, which implies that the entire transformation zone has been visualized, a punch biopsy specimen is taken from the worst area or areas, together with an endocervical curettage specimen. The endocervical curettage is not performed in patients who are pregnant.

A diagnostic cone biopsy of the cervix is indicated if:

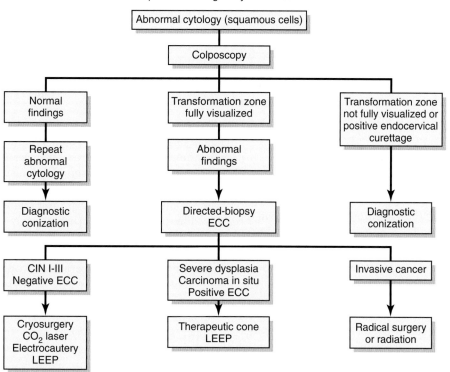

Figure 39-3. Algorithm for evaluation of patients with an abnormal Papanicolaou smear and a grossly normal-appearing cervix. ECC, endocervical curettage; LEEP, loop electrodiathermy excision procedure.

Colposcopic examination is unsatisfactory.

Endocervical curettings show a high-grade lesion.

Papanicolaou smear shows a high-grade lesion that is not confirmed on punch biopsy.

Papanicolaou smear indicates adenocarcinoma in situ.

Microinvasion is present on the punch biopsy.

TREATMENT OF INTRAEPITHELIAL NEOPLASIA

Superficial ablative techniques, such as loop electrodiathermy excision procedure (LEEP), cryosurgery, carbon dioxide laser, or electrocoagulation, are appropriate if the entire transformation zone is visible.

LOOP EXCISION OF THE TRANSFORMATION ZONE

Loop excision of the transformation zone (LLETZ) has gained popularity because **the equipment is relatively cheap, it can be performed on an outpatient basis under local anesthesia, and tissue is obtained for histologic evaluation.** Hence, occult invasive lesions should be more readily diagnosed. In unskilled hands, diathermy artifact may make histologic interpretation impossible.

LASER

Destruction of the transformation zone by carbon dioxide laser (*l*ight *a*mplification by *s*timulated *e*mission of *r*adiation) ablation can be performed as an outpatient procedure, but requires local anesthesia. Bleeding may sometimes occur, but scarring is minimal and large lesions may be destroyed with low failure rates (in the order of 5% to 10%). The equipment is expensive, so laser has lost favor in most centers.

CRYOSURGERY

The **cryosurgery** technique is a relatively painless outpatient procedure that can be performed without anesthesia. There is no bleeding, and the equipment is cheap. However, **there is a high failure rate for large lesions and for lesions extending down glandular crypts.** It is mainly useful for CIN I or CIN II involving 1 or 2 quadrants. The major side effect is a rather copious vaginal discharge that persists for several weeks.

ELECTROCOAGULATION

Success rates of up to 97% have been reported for electrocoagulation. It causes more discomfort than the other techniques, and it **requires general anesthesia.** Cervical stenosis may occasionally occur.

CERVICAL CONIZATION

Cervical conization is mainly a diagnostic technique, but it may be used for treatment. Provided that the margins of resection are clear, cure rates are as high as those with hysterectomy for intraepithelial lesions. **Bleeding, infection, cervical stenosis, and cervical incompetence are the major complications. Laser conization decreases the risk of cervical stenosis compared with cold knife conization.**

Hysterectomy is rarely necessary for the treatment of CIN. It may be applicable when sterilization is desired for other reasons in a patient with CIN III or when there is concomitant uterine or adnexal disease.

Persistence and recurrence rates combined are approximately 2% to 3% after hysterectomy. This number should be significantly reduced by using colposcopy and Schiller's staining (Lugol's iodine) preoperatively to exclude intraepithelial neoplasia in the upper vagina.

INVASIVE CANCER
SYMPTOMS

Invasive cancer usually presents with postcoital, intermenstrual, or postmenopausal vaginal bleeding. In patients who are not sexually active, bleeding from cervical cancer usually does not occur until the disease is quite advanced (unlike patients with endometrial cancer, who almost always bleed early).

Persistent vaginal discharge, pelvic pain, leg swelling, and urinary frequency are usually seen with advanced disease. In developing countries, it is not uncommon for patients to present with loss of urine or stool from the vagina, because of fistula formation.

PHYSICAL FINDINGS

Patients with cervical cancer usually have a normal general physical examination. Weight loss occurs late in the disease. With advanced disease, there may be enlarged inguinal or supraclavicular lymph nodes, edema of the legs, ascites, pleural effusion, or hepatomegaly, but these are not commonly seen.

The pelvic examination in early cervical cancer may reveal a cervix that appears normal, especially if the lesion is endocervical. Visible disease may take several forms: ulcerative, exophytic, granular, or necrotic. The cervix may be friable and bleed on palpation. There is often an associated serous, purulent, or bloody discharge. The lesion may involve the upper portion of the vagina and extend toward the introitus. The cervix may be distorted or completely replaced by tumor (Figure 39-4).

The rectovaginal examination is essential to determine the extent of involvement. **The degree of cervical expansion and spread to the parametria are much more easily detected with a finger in the rectum, as is extension into the uterosacral ligaments.** On occasion, a palpable mass on the pelvic wall representing an enlarged node can be felt.

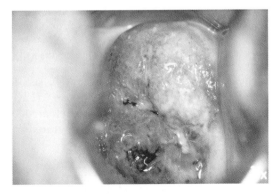

Figure 39-4. Invasive squamous cell carcinoma of the cervix. Note the irregular, ulcerated surface of the ectocervix. A biopsy of such a lesion is mandatory.

PATHOLOGIC FEATURES

Most uterine cervical cancers are squamous in origin. Adenocarcinomas and adenosquamous carcinomas are increasing in incidence and account for about 20% to 25% of cases. Melanomas and sarcomas occur rarely.

PATTERNS OF SPREAD

Invasive cervical cancer spreads by direct invasion of cervical stroma, corpus, vagina, and parametrium; lymphatic spread to pelvic and then paraaortic lymph nodes (Figure 39-5); and hematogenous spread, particularly to the lungs, liver, and bone.

PREOPERATIVE INVESTIGATIONS
CLINICAL STAGING

The official International Federation of Gynaecology and Obstetrics staging for cervical cancer is a clinical staging method based on physical examination and noninvasive testing (Table 39-1). **Studies allowed include biopsies, cystoscopy, sigmoidoscopy, chest and skeletal radiographs, intravenous pyelography, and liver function tests.** Lung metastases are seen in about 5% of patients with advanced disease and almost never in early disease.

For patients with advanced disease, an abdominal and pelvic computed tomographic scan is helpful in planning management, but the results do not influence the FIGO stage.

Laboratory studies may reveal abnormalities with advanced disease, the most common being anemia from bleeding, elevated blood urea nitrogen and creatinine levels if the ureters are obstructed, and abnormal liver function tests if there are liver metastases. **Ureteric obstruction occurs in about 30% of patients with stage III disease and in 50% of patients with stage IV disease.** Hypercalcemia may denote bone metastases.

SURGICAL STAGING

Because of the lack of sensitivity and specificity of computed tomography (CT) scanning, surgical staging was introduced in many centers in the 1970s for patients with advanced disease, to better determine the extent of disease before radiation therapy. Particularly relevant was the status of the para-aortic lymph nodes. **The incidence of para-aortic lymph node metastases is approximately 20% in stage II disease and 30% in stage III, and the status of the para-aortic nodes is the single most important prognostic factor.**

Most centers discontinued surgical staging because the improvement in survival was relatively low, particularly with the use of prophylactic extended field radiation. In the 1990s, some centers introduced laparoscopic surgical staging, but it is likely that in the future, position-emission tomographic (PET) scanning will prove to be a suitable noninvasive technique for the identification of patients with para-aortic lymph node metastases in advanced cervical cancer.

TREATMENT OF INVASIVE CANCER
STAGE IA (MICROINVASIVE CARCINOMA)

A preoperative diagnosis of microinvasive carcinoma can be made only on the basis of a cone biopsy of the cervix, which allows multiple-step sections to be taken at 2-mm intervals. With a punch biopsy, the sampling of the cervix is too limited, and a more frankly invasive focus may be missed. The concept of microinvasive carcinoma has only been applied to squamous lesions in the past, but recent evidence indicates that it may also apply to glandular lesions, although an occasional adenocarcinoma will have a skip lesion higher in the endocervical canal.

When the depth of invasion on cone biopsy is 3 mm or less, horizontal dimension is 7 mm or less (stage Ia1), and there is no lymphatic or vascular space involvement, an extra-fascial abdominal or vaginal hysterectomy is appropriate treatment. Cervical conization alone may suffice if the patient

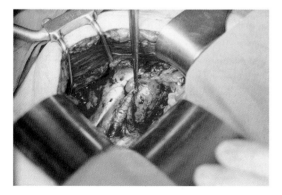

Figure 39-5. Grossly enlarged lymph node at the bifurcation of the common iliac artery in a patient with stage Ib2 carcinoma of the cervix. Large nodes such as this can cause ureteric obstruction.

Table 39-1. The International Federation of Gynecology and Obstetrics (FIGO) staging of cervical carcinoma

Stage	
PREINVASIVE CARCINOMA	
Stage 0	Carcinoma in situ, intraepithelial carcinoma (cases of stage 0 should not be included in any therapeutic statistics).
INVASIVE CARCINOMA	
• Stage I	The carcinoma is strictly confined to the cervix.
Stage Ia	Invasive cancer is identified only microscopically. All gross lesions even with superficial invasion are Ib cancers. Invasion is limited to a measured stromal invasion, with a maximal depth of 5 mm and a horizontal extension of not more than 7 mm.
Stage Ia1	Measured invasion of stroma not greater than 3 mm in depth and 7 mm in width.
Stage Ia2	Measured invasion of stroma greater than 3 mm and not greater than 5 mm and width not greater than 7 mm.
Stage Ib	Clinical lesions confined to the cervix or preclinical lesions greater than stage Ia.
Stage Ib1	Clinical lesions not greater than 4 cm in size.
Stage Ib2	Clinical lesions greater than 4 cm in size.
• Stage II	The carcinoma extends beyond the cervix but has not extended to the pelvic wall or to the lower third of the vagina.
Stage IIa	No obvious parametrial involvement.
Stage IIb	Obvious parametrial involvement.
• Stage III	The carcinoma has extended to the pelvic wall. On rectal examination there is no cancer-free space between the tumor and the pelvic wall. The tumor involves the lower third of the vagina. All cases with hydronephrosis or nonfunctioning kidney should be included, unless they are known to be due to another cause.
Stage IIIa	Tumor involves lower third of the vagina with no extension to the pelvic wall.
Stage IIIb	Extension onto the pelvic wall and/or hydronephrosis or nonfunctioning kidney.
• Stage IV	The carcinoma has extended beyond the true pelvis or has clinically involved the mucosa of the bladder or rectum. A bullous edema, as such, does not permit a case to be allotted to stage IV.
Stage IVa	Spread of the growth to adjacent organs.
Stage IVb	Spread to distant organs.

desires to maintain her fertility, as long as the cone margins are free of disease and the endocervical curettings (taken after the conization) are negative. **For stage Ia2 disease, or if there is lymphatic or vascular space involvement, most gynecologic oncologists recommend modified radical hysterectomy and pelvic lymph node dissection.** If childbearing is desired, large-cone biopsy or radical trachelectomy combined with pelvic lymphadenectomy may be offered.

STAGE Ib

Stage Ib disease may be treated by either radical hysterectomy and bilateral pelvic lymphadenectomy or radiation therapy. The advantage of surgery is that the ovaries may be spared in younger women, surgical staging may be carried out, and chronic radiation complications may be avoided, particularly vaginal stenosis, radiation proctitis, and radiation cystitis.

The results of treatment by either method are similar when both the surgeon and the radiotherapist are knowledgeable and skilled. Chemoradiation is often chosen for Stage Ib2 lesions, but primary surgery followed by tailored external beam therapy is a valid alternative approach. Patients with deep stromal penetration and extensive vascular space invasion but negative lymph nodes may receive a "small field" of pelvic radiation, whereas patients with positive common iliac or para-aortic nodes may receive extended field radiation, often combined with cisplatin.

Radical Hysterectomy

In this procedure, the uterus is removed along with adjacent portions of the vagina, cardinal ligaments, uterosacral ligaments, and bladder pillars.

The most common complication of radical hysterectomy is bladder dysfunction, which occurs as a result of interruption of the autonomic nerves traversing the cardinal and uterosacral ligaments. Normal bladder function is usually restored within 1 to 3 weeks, but 1% to 2% of patients have permanent dysfunction necessitating lifelong self-catheterization.

The most serious complication of radical hysterectomy is ureteric fistula or stricture, which occurs in 1% to 2% of cases. A less common but life-threatening complication is deep venous thrombosis, with or without pulmonary embolism. The incidence of pulmonary embolism can be reduced with the use of early ambulation, together with prophylactic low-dose subcutaneous heparin and external pneumatic calf compression at the time of surgery and before adequate postoperative mobilization. Some degree of lymphedema occurs in 15% to 20% of patients having a pelvic lymphadenectomy.

Radiation Therapy

For patients with stage Ib2 disease, most centers use primary chemoradiation, using weekly cisplatin as the radiation sensitizer. **Therapy usually begins with external radiation in an attempt to shrink the central tumor and improve the dosimetry of the subsequent intracavitary therapy.**

External radiation may also be used postoperatively for patients with lymph node metastases or inadequate surgical margins. The addition of weekly cisplatin (40 mg/m^2, intravenously) during external beam therapy has been shown to improve survival.

STAGE IIa

In patients with minimal involvement of the vaginal fornix, radical surgery or chemoradiation therapy may be employed. With more extensive involvement of the upper vagina, chemoradiation therapy alone is the treatment of choice.

STAGE IIb

Most patients with stage IIb lesions are treated with a combination of external beam chemoradiation and intracavitary brachytherapy. **If positive para-aortic or high common iliac lymph nodes are detected by surgical staging, or preoperative scanning, extended-field radiation may be employed** to treat all of the para-aortic lymph nodes up to the diaphragm.

STAGES IIIa AND IIIb

Patients with stage IIIa and stage IIIb disease are treated with chemoradiation therapy, usually external beam followed by intracavitary brachytherapy. In patients with locally advanced disease, distortion of the cervix and vagina may make brachytherapy difficult to apply. Therefore, a higher dose of external therapy, up to 6000 to 7000 cGy, may be necessary. Alternatively, interstitial radiation may be given to get a better dose distribution than would be possible with intracavitary therapy.

STAGE IVa

Pelvic chemoradiation therapy is used in most patients with stage IVa lesions. If radiation therapy results in only partial tumor regression, a "salvage" pelvic exenteration may be performed. **Primary pelvic exenteration is performed only rarely,** usually when the patient presents with a rectovaginal or vesicovaginal fistula.

STAGE IVb

Patients with stage IVb disease may receive some pelvic radiation therapy to palliate bleeding from the vagina, bladder, or rectum. Because distant metastases are present, however, chemotherapy is often employed but is only palliative.

RECURRENT OR METASTATIC DISEASE
Chemotherapy

The effectiveness of chemotherapy is limited for metastatic cervical cancer.

Several drugs have been tested and found to be active in up to 35% of cases. Most responses are partial, and the patients usually progress within 12 months. **The most active agents are cisplatin, bleomycin, mitomycin C, methotrexate, and cyclophosphamide.**

Pelvic Exenteration

Pelvic exenteration is generally reserved for patients who have a central recurrence following pelvic irradiation. **Total exenteration involves removal of the pelvic viscera, including the uterus, tubes, vagina, ovaries, bladder, and rectum** (Figure 39-6). Depending on the site and extent of the disease, the operation may be limited to an anterior exenteration, which spares the rectum, or a posterior exenteration, which spares the bladder.

Following the extirpative surgery, pelvic reconstruction is necessary. If the bladder is removed, the ureters must be implanted into a portion of the small or large bowel that has been isolated from the remainder of the gastrointestinal tract to form a conduit. A continent conduit may be created, particularly in younger patients. When the disease is confined to the upper vagina and rectovaginal septum, the lower rectum and anal canal may be preserved and reanastomosed to the sigmoid colon. A temporary colostomy is often required to protect the reanastomosis because

of the prior irradiation. **Vaginal reconstruction can be performed using a split-thickness skin graft, bilateral gracilis myocutaneous grafts, a rectus abdominus myocutaneous flap, or a segment of large intestine.**

Relatively few patients with recurrent cancer of the cervix are suitable to undergo pelvic exenteration because of metastases outside the pelvis or fixation of the tumor to structures that cannot be removed, such as the pelvic side wall. If an extensive metastatic workup is negative for cancer, patients undergo exploratory laparotomy with a view to pelvic exenteration. If the tumor is discovered to have spread to pelvic or para-aortic lymph nodes or to intraabdominal viscera, the procedure is abandoned.

In selecting patients who may be suitable for pelvic exenteration, the triad of unilateral leg edema,

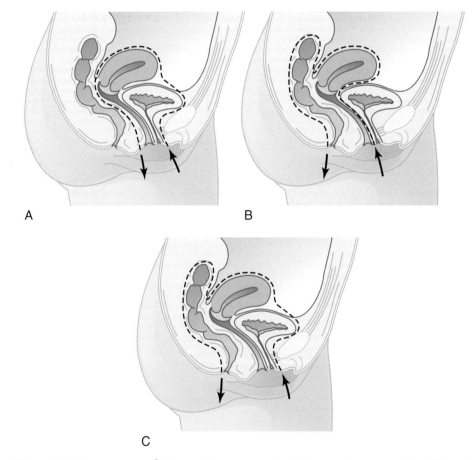

A

B

C

Figure 39-6. Organs removed in anterior exenteration *(A)*, posterior exenteration *(B)*, and total pelvic exenteration *(C)*.

sciatic pain, and ureteral obstruction is ominous and indicates unresectable disease in the pelvis.

CERVICAL CARCINOMA IN PREGNANCY

Carcinoma of the cervix associated with pregnancy usually implies diagnosis during pregnancy or within 12 months postpartum. It is relatively uncommon, invasive carcinoma occurring in approximately 1 in 2200 pregnancies. The proportion of patients with invasive cancer who are pregnant or within 12 months postpartum is about 1 in 34 cases, and the average age at occurrence is about 34 years.

SYMPTOMS

The symptoms are similar to those in nonpregnant patients, with painless vaginal bleeding being the most common. During pregnancy, this symptom can readily be attributed to conditions such as threatened abortion or placenta previa, so there is often an unnecessary delay in diagnosis.

DIAGNOSIS

Screening cervical cytologic studies lead to the diagnosis in most cases. The pregnant cervix lends itself to colposcopic evaluation because the columnar eversion or gaping of the cervical os that occurs during pregnancy facilitates adequate visualization of the transformation zone. **Pregnancy tends to exaggerate the colposcopic features of CIN so that overdiagnosis is more likely than the reverse.** Endocervical curettage should not be performed during pregnancy because of the risk of rupturing the membranes. **Cone biopsy, if required, is best performed during the 2nd trimester to avoid the possibility of induced abortion in the 1st trimester and severe hemorrhage and premature labor in the 3rd trimester.** Unfortunately, about half of the patients are not diagnosed until the postpartum period. The later the diagnosis is made, the more likely the cancer is to be in an advanced stage.

MANAGEMENT

CIN III diagnosed during pregnancy should be managed conservatively, with the pregnancy allowed to proceed to term, vaginal delivery anticipated, and appropriate therapy carried out 6 to 8 weeks postpartum.

Microinvasive carcinoma of the cervix diagnosed by conization of the cervix during pregnancy may also be managed conservatively, the pregnancy being allowed to continue to term with colposcopic surveillance of the cervix at 28 weeks. At term, either cesarean hysterectomy or vaginal delivery followed by postpartum extrafascial hysterectomy is appropriate, unless further childbearing is desired.

Frankly invasive cancer requires relatively urgent treatment. After 22 to 26 weeks, it is reasonable to continue the pregnancy until fetal viability (about 32 weeks) if the patient desires. The general principles of treatment are essentially the same as those in the nonpregnant patient. For early lesions, radical hysterectomy may be performed. Before 20 weeks' gestation, this is performed with the fetus in situ. After that time, hysterotomy through a high incision in the uterine fundus is performed to remove the fetus, followed by radical hysterectomy and bilateral pelvic lymphadenectomy.

For some patients with early disease and for all patients with advanced disease, the alternative to radical surgery is radiation therapy. For patients with disease diagnosed in the 1st trimester, external irradiation is initiated to shrink the tumor. Abortion usually occurs spontaneously during the course of external therapy; if it does not, uterine curettage should be performed before brachytherapy. After the 1st trimester, it is preferable to perform a hysterotomy through a high incision in the corpus before instituting radiotherapy.

If a decision is made to await fetal viability, it is important to be certain by ultrasonography that the fetus is apparently healthy and to obtain a mature lecithin-to-sphingomyelin ratio to ensure fetal lung maturity before delivery. Neoadjuvant chemotherapy using cisplatin and etoposide has been used to try to "contain" the disease. Because of the increased risk of hemorrhage and infection likely to be associated with delivery through a cervix containing gross cancer, classic cesarean section is the preferred method of delivery. **For patients in whom inadvertent vaginal delivery has occurred, there is no evidence to indicate that the prognosis is altered.**

Prognosis for Cervical Cancer

Prognosis is related directly to clinical stage (Table 39-2). With higher stage disease, the frequency of nodal

Table 39-2. Carcinoma of the cervix: survival by FIGO stage

Stage	Patients	5-Year Survival (%)
Ia1	787	94.6
Ia2	313	92.6
Ib1	986	90.4
Ib2	440	79.8
IIa	993	76.0
IIb	2775	73.3
IIIa	131	50.5
IIIb	2271	46.4
IVa	258	29.6
IVb	196	22.0

Data from the Annual Report on the Results of Treatment in Gynaecological Cancer. Patients treated 1993–1995. J Epidemiol Biostat 24:5–44, 2001.

metastasis escalates, and the 5-year survival rate diminishes. Adenocarcinomas and adenosquamous carcinomas have a somewhat lower 5-year survival rate than do squamous carcinomas, stage for stage.

Matched, controlled studies have demonstrated identical survivals for pregnant and nonpregnant patients.

Suggested Reading

Hacker NF: Cervical cancer. *In* Berek JS, Hacker NF (eds): Practical Gynecologic Oncology, 3rd ed. Philadelphia, Lippincott Williams & Wilkins, 2000, pp 345–405.

Ho GY, Bierman R, Beardsley L, Chang CJ, Burk RD: Natural history of cervicovaginal papillomavirus infection in young women. N Engl J Med 338:423–428, 1998.

Landoni F, Maneo A, Colombo A, Placa F, Milani R, Perego P, et al: Randomized study of radical surgery versus radiotherapy for stage IB-IIA cervical cancer. Lancet 359:535–540, 1997.

Ostor A, Rome R, Quinn M: Microinvasive adenocarcinoma of the cervix: A clinicopathologic study of 77 women. Obstet Gynecol 89:88–93, 1997.

Rose PG, Bundy B, Watkins EB, et al: Concurrent cisplatin-based radiotherapy and chemotherapy for locally advanced cervical cancer. N Engl J Med 340:1144–1153, 1999.

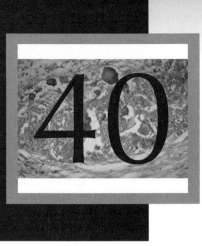

40 Ovarian Cancer

Jonathan S. Berek

Ovarian cancer is the fifth most common cancer among females in the United States, accounting for one-fourth of all gynecologic cancers. It is the leading cause of death from gynecologic cancer because it is difficult to detect before it disseminates. In 2004, 25,800 new cases and more than 15,000 deaths are expected from this disease. Most women with ovarian cancer are in the fifth or sixth decade of life.

ETIOLOGY AND EPIDEMIOLOGY

The cause of ovarian cancer is unknown. The patient characteristics found to be associated with an increased risk for epithelial ovarian cancer include white race, late age at menopause, family history of cancer of the ovary or breast, and prolonged intervals of ovulation uninterrupted by pregnancy. There is an increased prevalence of ovarian cancer in nulliparous women and those who have been infertile.

The incidence of ovarian cancer varies in different geographic locations. Western countries, including the United States, have rates that are three to seven times greater than those in Japan. Second-generation Japanese immigrants to the United States have an incidence of ovarian cancer similar to that of American women. White Americans experience ovarian cancer about 1.5 times more frequently than do black Americans.

It has been estimated that between 5% and 10% of epithelial ovarian cancers occur in women with a hereditary predisposition. In women with hereditary cancers, two or more first-degree relatives on either the paternal or maternal side typically have had the disease. **The pattern of inheritance is autosomal dominant and is associated with breast and ovarian cancers that tend to occur in younger women (median age approximately 50 years).** These germline mutations are found on the autosomes—BRCA1 is on chromosome 17 and BRCA 2 on Chromosome 13. **The Lynch II syndrome, nonpolyposis colorectal cancer syndrome, is associated with mutations in the mismatch repair genes.** Adenocarcinomas of the ovary, breast, colon, stomach, pancreas, and endometrium are seen in the families of these individuals.

The use of oral contraceptives has been found to protect against ovarian cancer, possibly because of suppression of ovulation. It has been postulated that **incessant ovulation may predispose to malignant transformation in the ovary.**

Patients with a known germ line mutation (e.g., BRCA1 and BRCA2 mutations) may be offered prophylactic salpingo-oophorectomy once childbearing has been completed, and this operation is highly protective for ovarian and fallopian tube carcinomas. Indeed, the risk of subsequent breast cancer is also significantly reduced in these women. There is still a small risk of peritoneal carcinoma after prophylactic salpingo-oophorectomy.

Some case-control studies have suggested that the use of postmenopausal estrogen replacement therapy may increase the risk of ovarian cancer, but these data are controversial.

It has also been postulated that a causative agent could enter the peritoneal cavity through the lower genital tract. For example, the perineal use of asbestos-contaminated talc has been linked to the development of epithelial ovarian cancer. This possibility remains controversial, although **tubal ligation and hysterectomy are both associated with a decreased risk of the disease.**

SCREENING FOR OVARIAN CANCER

Population screening for ovarian cancer is not feasible because ultrasonography and available tumor markers, for example, CA 125, lack specificity and sensitivity for early-stage disease. CA 125 is more useful in postmenopausal women because false-positive measurements occur commonly in premenopausal women in association with endometriosis, pelvic inflammatory disease, or uterine fibroids. Patients with a strong family history of epithelial ovarian cancer may benefit from surveillance with serial transvaginal ultrasonography and serum CA-125 titers.

CLINICAL FEATURES
SYMPTOMS

Unfortunately, many patients in whom ovarian cancer develops are relatively asymptomatic before dissemination takes place. In early-stage disease, the patient may complain of nonspecific symptoms or irregular menses if she is premenopausal. Symptoms of a mass compressing the bladder or rectum, such as urinary frequency or constipation, may bring the patient to a physician. Sometimes the patient complains of a lower abdominal or pelvic "fullness" or of dyspareunia. Only rarely does a patient present with acute symptoms, such as pain secondary to torsion, rupture, or intracystic hemorrhage.

In advanced-stage disease, patients most often present with abdominal pain or swelling. The latter may be from the tumor itself or from associated ascites. On careful questioning, there has usually been a history of vague abdominal symptoms, such as bloating, constipation, nausea, dyspepsia, anorexia, or early satiety. Premenopausal patients may complain of irregular menses or heavy vaginal bleeding. **Postmenopausal bleeding is occasionally a symptom of ovarian neoplasms, particularly functional stromal tumors.**

SIGNS

The disease is frequently misdiagnosed for several months because patients with nonspecific abdominal symptoms do not receive a vaginal and rectal examination. **A solid, irregular, fixed pelvic mass is suggestive of ovarian cancer, and if combined with an upper abdominal mass, ascites, or both, the diagnosis is almost certain.**

PREOPERATIVE EVALUATION

The diagnosis of ovarian cancer requires a laparotomy or laparoscopy. Routine preoperative hematologic and biochemical studies should be obtained, as should a chest radiograph. A pelvic and abdominal computed tomography (CT) scan will exclude liver metastases, but it is not mandatory.

A Papanicolaou smear should be obtained to evaluate the cervix, but this test is of limited value in detecting ovarian cancer. **Endometrial biopsy and endocervical curettage are necessary in patients with abnormal vaginal bleeding, because concurrent primary tumors occasionally occur in the ovary and endometrium.** In the presence of a pelvic mass, it is preferable not to perform abdominal paracentesis for cytologic evaluation of ascitic fluid, because seeding of the abdominal wall may occur.

An abdominal radiograph may be useful in a younger patient to locate calcifications associated with a benign cystic teratoma (dermoid cyst), which is the most common neoplasm in patients younger than 25 years of age. **In patients with occult blood in the stool or significant intestinal symptoms, a barium enema or lower gastrointestinal endoscopy should be obtained** to rule out a primary colonic cancer with ovarian metastasis.

Similarly, **an upper gastrointestinal barium study or endoscopy is important if there are significant gastric symptoms.** Breast cancer may also metastasize to the ovaries, so **bilateral mammograms should be obtained if there are any suspicious breast masses.**

Pelvic ultrasonography, particularly transvaginal ultrasonography with or without color Doppler studies, **may be useful** for smaller (<8 cm) masses in premenopausal women. Masses that are predominantly solid or multilocular have a high probability of being neoplastic, whereas unilocular cystic masses are generally functional cysts. In postmenopausal women, ultrasonography may also be useful because small, unilocular cysts (<5 cm) that are stable are generally benign.

Several tumor markers have been investigated, but none has been consistently reliable. **The tumor-associated antigen CA 125 is elevated in only about 50% of women with stage I ovarian cancer.** When this assay is elevated, it is useful for monitoring the clinical course of the disease.

DIFFERENTIAL DIAGNOSIS

Ovarian malignancies must be differentiated from benign neoplasms and functional cysts of the ovaries. In addition, a variety of gynecologic conditions can simulate a neoplastic process, including tuboovarian abscess, endometriosis, and a pedunculated uterine leiomyoma. Nongynecologic causes of pelvic tumor must also be excluded, such as an inflammatory or neoplastic disease of the colon or a pelvic kidney.

MODE OF SPREAD

Ovarian cancer typically spreads by exfoliating cells that disseminate and implant throughout the peritoneal cavity. The distribution of intraperitoneal metastases tends to follow the circulatory path of peritoneal fluid, so **metastases are commonly seen on the posterior cul-de-sac, paracolic gutters, right hemidiaphragm, liver capsule, and omentum.** Implants are also common on the bowel serosa and its mesenteries. In general, they grow around the intestines, encasing them with tumor, without invading the bowel lumen. Widespread bowel metastases can lead to a functional obstruction known as carcinomatous ileus.

Lymphatic dissemination to the pelvic and para-aortic nodes is common, particularly with advanced disease. Extensive blockage of the diaphragmatic lymphatics is at least partially responsible for the development of ascites. Hematogenous metastases are not common, and parenchymal metastases to the liver and lungs are seen in only about 2% of patients at initial presentation.

Death from ovarian cancer usually results from progressive encasement of abdominal organs, leading to anorexia, vomiting, and inanition. The bowel obstruction caused by tumor growth is often incomplete and intermittent and may last for several months before the patient's demise.

STAGING

The standard staging system for ovarian cancer is presented in Table 40-1. **Ovarian cancer is surgically staged** according to the International Federation of Gynecology and Obstetrics (FIGO) staging system.

Even though all microscopic disease may appear to be confined to the ovaries at the time of laparotomy, microscopic spread may have already occurred; thus, patients must undergo a thorough "surgical staging." Procedures necessary to stage ovarian cancer are shown in Box 40-1.

Table 40-1.	**International Federation of Gynecology and Obstetrics (FIGO) staging for primary carcinoma of the ovary**
Stage I	Growth limited to the ovaries.
Stage Ia	Growth limited to one ovary; no ascites. No tumor on the external surface; capsule intact.
Stage Ib	Growth limited to both ovaries; no ascites. No tumor on the external surfaces; capsules intact.
Stage Ic	Tumor either stage Ia or Ib but with tumor on the surface of one or both ovaries or with capsule ruptured or with ascites present containing malignant cells or with positive peritoneal washings.
Stage II	Growth involving one or both ovaries with pelvic extension.
Stage IIa	Extension or metastases, or both, to the uterus or tubes, or both.
Stage IIb	Extension to other pelvic tissues.
Stage IIc	Tumor either stage IIa or IIb but with tumor on the surface of one or both ovaries or with capsule or capsules ruptured or with ascites present containing malignant cells or with positive peritoneal washings.
Stage III	Tumor involving one or both ovaries with peritoneal implants outside the pelvis or positive retroperitoneal or inguinal nodes, or both. Superficial liver metastasis equals stage III. Tumor is limited to the true pelvis, but with histologically proven malignant extension to small bowel or omentum.
Stage IIIa	Tumor grossly limited to the true pelvis with negative nodes but with histologically confirmed microscopic seeding of abdominal peritoneal surfaces.
Stage IIIb	Tumor of one or both ovaries with histologically confirmed implants of abdominal peritoneal surfaces, none exceeding 2 cm in diameter. Nodes negative for disease.
Stage IIIc	Abdominal implants >2 cm in diameter or positive retroperitoneal or inguinal nodes, or both.
Stage IV	Growth involving one or both ovaries with distant metastasis. If pleural effusion is present, there must be positive cytologic test results to allot a case to stage IV. Parenchymal liver metastasis equals stage IV.

Box 40-1. Requirements for staging or "second-look" operation

MULTIPLE CYTOLOGIC ASSAYS
Free ascitic fluid, if present
Peritoneal "washings" (50 mL of normal saline)
Pelvic cul-de-sac
Both paracolic gutters
Both hemidiaphragms

MULTIPLE INTRAPERITONEAL BIOPSIES
Pelvis
Cul-de-sac peritoneum
Bladder peritoneum
Pedicles of infundibulopelvic ligaments
Any adhesions

Abdomen
Both paracolic gutters
Bowel serosa and mesenteries
Omentum
Any adhesions

EXTRAPERITONEAL BIOPSIES
Pelvic and para-aortic lymph nodes

*Procedures performed in patients with no visible evidence of metastatic disease.

CLASSIFICATION

The histologic classification of ovarian neoplasms is listed in Table 40-2. These lesions fall into four categories according to their tissue of origin. **Most ovarian neoplasms (80% to 85%) are derived from coelomic epithelium and are called epithelial carcinomas.** Less common tumors are derived from primitive germ cells, specialized gonadal stroma, or nonspecific mesenchyme. In addition, the ovary can be the site of metastatic carcinomas, most often from the gastrointestinal tract or the breast.

EPITHELIAL OVARIAN CARCINOMAS
PATHOLOGIC FEATURES

The main histologic subtypes of epithelial carcinomas are serous (about 40%), mucinous (about 25%), endometrioid (about 20%), and clear cell (about 5%). Malignant Brenner tumors and undifferentiated carcinomas are uncommon.

Serous tumors resemble fallopian tube epithelium histologically (Figure 40-1). About 30% of patients with stage I and stage IIa disease have bilateral involvement. On gross examination, serous carcinomas have an irregular and multilocular appearance (Figure 40-2).

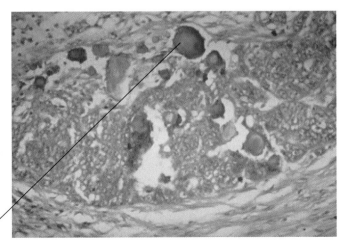

Psammoma bodies

Figure 40-1. Papillary serous cystadenocarcinoma. This tumor frequently contains numerous psammoma bodies, which are shown here. Their origin is uncertain, but it has been suggested that they may reflect an immune reaction against the tumor or, more simply, represent alteration to the secretions from the malignant cells. There is no relationship between the presence of psammoma bodies and the malignancy of the tumor.

Table 40-2. Histogenetic classification of primary ovarian neoplasms

Derivation	Type of Tumor

Coelomic epithelial origin (80%–85%)	"Common" epithelial tumors; benign, borderline, malignant
	  Serous tumor
	  Mucinous tumor
	  Endometrioid tumor
	  Clear cell (mesonephroid) tumor
	  Brenner tumor
	Undifferentiated carcinoma
	Carcinosarcoma or malignant mixed mesodermal tumors

Germ cell origin (10%–15%)	Teratoma
	  Mature teratoma
	  Solid adult teratoma
	  Dermoid cyst
	  Struma ovarii
	  Malignant neoplasms secondarily arising from teratomatous
	    tissues (squamous carcinoma, carcinoid tumor, sarcoma)
	  Immature teratoma
	Dysgerminoma
	Endodermal sinus tumor
	Embryonal carcinoma
	Choriocarcinoma
	Gonadoblastoma*
	Mixed germ cell tumors

Specialized gonadal-stromal origin (3%–5%)	Granulosa-theca cell tumors
	  Granulosa cell tumor
	  Thecoma
	Sertoli-Leydig tumors
	  Arrhenoblastoma
	  Sertoli cell tumor
	Gynandroblastoma
	Lipid cell tumors

Nonspecific mesenchymal origin (fewer than 1%)	Fibroma, hemangioma, leiomyoma, lipoma Lymphoma Sarcoma

Data from Hart WR, Morrow CP: The ovaries. In Romney SL, Gray MJ, Little AO, et al (eds): Gynecology and Obstetrics: The Health Care of Women, 2nd ed. New York, McGraw-Hill, 1981.
*Combined germ cell and specialized gonadal-stromal elements.

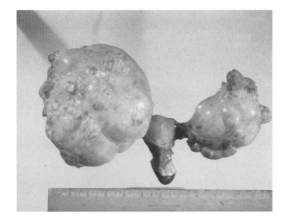

Figure 40-2. Bilateral serous cystadenocarcinomas. A uterus with both ovaries grossly enlarged by multilocular tumors with papillary excrescences on their serosal surfaces.

Mucinous tumors histologically resemble endocervical epithelium and are often large, measuring 20 cm or more in diameter. They are bilateral in 10% to 20% of patients.

Endometrioid tumors closely resemble carcinomas of the endometrium and arise in association with primary endometrial cancer in about 20% of patients. In early-stage disease, they are bilateral in about 10% of cases. Approximately 10% of endometrioid ovarian carcinomas are associated with endometriosis, although malignant transformation of endometriosis occurs in fewer than 1% of patients.

Clear cell carcinomas of the ovary are uncommon. **In about 25% of cases, they occur in association with endometriosis.**

The Brenner tumor represents only 2% to 3% of all ovarian neoplasms, and fewer than 2% of these tumors are malignant. **About 10% of Brenner tumors occur in conjunction with a mucinous cystadenoma or dermoid cyst in the same or opposite ovary.**

Tumors of low malignant potential or borderline histologic appearance exist for each histologic type. **Approximately 5% to 10% of malignant serous tumors are borderline** (Figure 40-3), **whereas 20% of malignant mucinous tumors fall into this category.** The endometrioid, clear cell, and Brenner tumors are only rarely borderline.

MANAGEMENT OF EPITHELIAL OVARIAN CANCER

The initial approach to all patients with ovarian cancer is surgical exploration of the abdomen and pelvis.

Early-Stage Disease

Definitive diagnosis requires an intraoperative frozen section. In patients with no gross evidence of disease beyond the ovary, the standard operation is total abdominal hysterectomy, bilateral salpingo-oophorectomy, infracolic omentectomy, and thorough surgical staging, as shown in Box 40-1. Patients who wish to preserve fertility may have a unilateral salpingo-oophorectomy. **In patients with grade 1 or grade 2 tumors confined to one or both ovaries after surgical staging, no further treatment is necessary.** Patients with poorly differentiated (grade 3) tumors are subsequently treated with systemic chemotherapy.

Advanced-Stage Disease

In patients with advanced disease, cytoreductive surgery ("debulking") is required. The objectives are to remove the primary tumor and all of the metastases, if possible. **If all macroscopic disease cannot be removed, an attempt should be made to reduce individual tumor nodules to 1 cm or less in diameter.** Patients in whom this goal is achieved are said to have had "optimal" cytoreduction, which can be achieved in about 70% of patients. In addition to a total or subtotal abdominal hysterectomy, bilateral salpingo-oophorectomy, omentectomy, and resection of peritoneal metastases, optimal cytoreduction may necessitate bowel resection; therefore, **all patients having surgery for suspected ovarian cancer should have a bowel preparation preoperatively.**

In retrospective studies, patients whose individual residual tumor nodules are 1 cm in diameter or less before the commencement of chemotherapy have been shown to have longer median survivals and more complete responses to therapy. The longest survival is seen in patients in whom all visible tumor has been removed before treatment.

In patients who are medically unfit or have a poor performance status, usually because of a

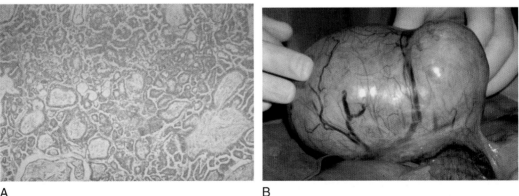

A   B

Figure 40-3. *(A)* Serous tumor—borderline. (Papillary serous cystadenocarcinoma of low malignant potential.) The papillary pattern filling the cyst lumen is very complex, and the epithelium is, in places, more than one cell thick. Mitotic figures are present, although not abundant. *(B)* Large borderline tumor mobilized out of the pelvis. Note the smooth surface and large blood vessels coursing over the surface.

large pleural effusion and massive ascites, it may be prudent to give two or three cycles of neoadjuvant chemotherapy before undertaking radical surgery. If the disease does not respond to chemotherapy, as evidenced by the failure to resolve the malignant effusions, the patient should be offered palliative care only. Usually, the effusions resolve completely, and an "interval" cytoreductive operation can be safely undertaken.

Following primary cytoreductive surgery, combination chemotherapy is given, most commonly carboplatin and paclitaxel. Single-agent therapy with paclitaxel, or carboplatin, is occasionally used for frail or elderly patients. During chemotherapy, the patient's response is monitored with serial CA 125 levels. If the values rise or plateau within 12 months, it is advisable to change to second-line drugs, such as liposomal-encapsulated doxorubicin, topotecan, etoposide, gemcytabine, or experimental chemotherapeutic agents. If the progression-free interval has been greater than 12 months, the patient may respond to further paclitaxel or carboplatin chemotherapy. Response to second-line chemotherapy is in the range of 20% to 50%, but patients are not considered to be curable after their initial relapse. Secondary cytoreduction may be appropriate if the disease-free interval is 24 months or longer.

It is unclear whether patients with "metastatic" borderline tumors benefit from chemotherapy.

The intraperitoneal route for the administration of chemotherapy remains experimental.

Second-Look Laparotomy

In patients who are clinically free of disease after completing a prescribed course of chemotherapy (usually about six cycles), a "second-look" laparotomy may be performed to determine whether the patient has had a complete response to chemotherapy. It is unclear whether the performance of a second-look laparotomy and the administration of further treatment ultimately prolong survival, so the surgery is discretionary and should generally be confined to research settings. If there is no macroscopic or microscopic evidence of disease at second-look laparotomy, essentially the same procedures as are carried out for surgical staging should be performed (see Box 40-1). If gross disease is present, an attempt should be made to resect persistent disease to facilitate a response to subsequent therapy.

PROGNOSIS

Patients with stage I disease have 5-year survival rates of 75% to 95%, depending on the histologic grade.

Almost all patients with carefully staged Ia grade 1 ovarian cancer are cured surgically, whereas the 5-year survival rate for patients with poorly differentiated bilateral lesions is as low as 75%. The 5-year survival rate for patients with stage II disease is about 65%. Despite aggressive primary surgery and combination chemotherapy, the 5-year survival rate for patients with advanced-stage disease is about 20%, although the median survival is between 2 and 3 years. Patients with advanced-stage disease who have negative findings on second-look laparotomy have a 5-year survival rate of about 60%. Patients whose tumors are associated with BRCA1 and BRCA2 mutations may have a somewhat better prognosis, but this issue is unclear.

Patients who have borderline ovarian tumors can be expected to have a prolonged survival. If the disease is confined to the ovary, the vast majority of tumors never recur. Five- and 10-year survival rates are 95% to 100%, but late recurrences may occur, and 20-year survival rates are approximately 85% to 90%. Patients who initially present with metastatic disease are more likely to exhibit subsequent clinical evidence of disease, although the rate of progression is slow; most live at least 5 years.

GERM CELL TUMORS

Germ cell tumors of the ovary account for only about 2% to 3% of all ovarian malignancies. They occur predominantly in young patients and frequently produce either human chorionic gonadotropin (hCG) or α-fetoprotein (AFP), which serve as tumor markers. The most common germ cell tumors are the dysgerminoma and immature teratoma. Endodermal sinus tumors, embryonal tumors, and nongestational choriocarcinomas are less common. Mixed germ cell tumors are not uncommon.

DYSGERMINOMAS

Dysgerminomas occur predominantly in children and young women. About 10% are bilateral. These tumors, of varying malignant virulence, are occasionally seen in patients with gonadal dysgenesis or the testicular feminization syndrome. In such patients, the dysgerminoma may arise in a gonadoblastoma. In about two-thirds of patients, the disease is confined to the ovaries at the time of diagnosis. About 10% of dysgerminomas are associated with other germ cell malignancies. **Pure dysgerminomas do not produce the tumor markers hCG and AFP, but commonly produce lactate dehydrogenase (LDH).**

Treatment

In most patients, the contralateral ovary and the uterus can be preserved. **Surgical staging,** as outlined earlier in this chapter, **is important. Particular attention should be paid to the pelvic and para-aortic lymph nodes** because of the propensity of these tumors for lymphatic dissemination. If disease extends beyond one ovary, the treatment of choice is resection and chemotherapy. **The regimen employed for these patients is usually bleomycin, etoposide, and cisplatin.** Carboplatin and paclitaxel are also being tested in these patients. Dysgerminomas are uniquely radiosensitive, and radiotherapy was previously the treatment of choice. However, it is now best reserved for the management of recurrent, chemoresistant disease.

Prognosis

The 5-year survival rate for patients with stage Ia pure dysgerminoma treated with unilateral oophorectomy is about 95%, whereas it is 80% for stage II and 60% to 70% for stage III disease. Recurrences following conservative surgery have at least an 80% 5-year survival rate.

IMMATURE TERATOMAS

Immature teratomas are the second most common malignant ovarian germ cell tumor. About 75% of malignant teratomas are encountered during the first two decades of life. Bilateral lesions are rare, although the other ovary may contain a benign dermoid cyst in about 5% of cases. Like other germ cell tumors, immature teratomas grow fairly rapidly, cause pain early, and are found confined to the ovary in about two-thirds of cases at the time of diagnosis. **Pure immature teratomas do not produce hCG or AFP.** Histologically, the tumors can be graded from 1 to 3 according to the degree of differentiation, with grade 3 tumors being the least differentiated. Neural elements are most frequently seen, but cartilage and epithelial tissues are also common.

Treatment

The primary tumor should be removed. **In young patients, the uterus and contralateral ovary should be preserved to maintain fertility.** All patients with other than stage Ia grade 1 immature teratomas should receive postoperative chemotherapy using bleomycin, etoposide, and cisplatin. Therapy should be given for three to four cycles. A second-look laparotomy is not considered necessary in patients with stage I disease.

Prognosis

Survival correlates with grade and stage of disease. The 5-year survival rate for patients with grade 1 immature teratomas is about 95%, compared with 80% for grade 2 and 60% to 70% for grade 3 disease.

OTHER GERM CELL TUMORS

The endodermal sinus tumor is a rare malignancy. It is also referred to as a *yolk sac* tumor. **Endodermal sinus tumors produce AFP,** which can serve as a useful serum marker for this neoplasm. **Embryonal carcinomas produce both hCG and AFP, whereas choriocarcinomas produce hCG only.** All occur in children and young women, and all grow rapidly. **Bilateral tumors are rare.**

Therapy for these lesions includes surgical resection of the primary tumor followed by systemic combination chemotherapy with bleomycin, etoposide, and cisplatin. Before the advent of effective chemotherapy, these tumors were usually fatal. The overall 5-year survival rate is now about 60% to 70%.

SPECIALIZED GONADAL-STROMAL TUMORS

A group of relatively uncommon tumors is derived from the specialized ovarian stroma. As such, they are often endocrinologically functional, many of them being capable of synthesizing gonadal or adrenal steroid hormones. Because the ovarian stroma has sexual bipotentiality, hormones that are secreted can be either female or male. **Estrogen and progesterone are typically associated with granulosa-theca cell tumors, whereas testosterone and other androgens may be secreted by many Sertoli-Leydig cell tumors. Rarely, lipid cell tumors,** which are usually virilizing, **produce adrenal corticoids** and a clinical cushingoid syndrome.

PATHOLOGIC FEATURES

Granulosa cell tumors are the most common stromal carcinomas. They have a distinct histologic pattern: **small groups of cells called Call-Exner bodies are the hallmark.** They may secrete large amounts of estrogen and can be associated with endometrial cancer in adults or sexual pseudoprecocity in children.

Thecomas, which are only one-third as common as granulosa cell tumors, are rarely malignant. Mixtures of the two types of tumor exist.

Sertoli-Leydig cell tumors (arrhenoblastomas) contain both Sertoli-type and Leydig-type stromal cells and are classically associated with masculinization. **Only 3% to 5% of these tumors are malignant.**

Lipid cell tumors are often referred to as hilar cell tumors because they are located in the ovarian hilus. **Only a rare lipid tumor, usually larger than 8 cm in diameter, behaves in a malignant fashion.**

TREATMENT

Most stromal tumors occur in postmenopausal women, and are best treated by a total abdominal hysterectomy and bilateral salpingo-oophorectomy. Conservation of the uterus and contralateral ovary is appropriate for carefully staged young patients with stage I disease provided that the possibility of an associated adenocarcinoma of the endometrium has been excluded by dilatation and curettage. The tumors are not very chemosensitive.

PROGNOSIS

Granulosa cell tumors, which tend to grow slowly, are usually confined to one ovary at the time of diagnosis. **The 5-year survival rate is approximately 90% for stage I disease. Recurrences are usually detected late** and may result in death 15 to 20 years after removal of the primary lesion.

METASTATIC CANCERS

About 4% to 8% of ovarian malignancies are metastatic, most commonly from either the gastrointestinal tract or the breast. **The Krukenberg tumor is a specific type of metastatic tumor in which "signet-ring" cells are seen in the ovarian stroma histologically.** Most Krukenberg tumors are bilateral and metastatic from the stomach. Rarely, it has not been possible to locate a primary focus, and removal of the ovarian disease has produced apparent cures.

FALLOPIAN TUBE CARCINOMA

Primary carcinoma of the fallopian tube accounts for only 0.1% to 0.5% of gynecologic cancers and is diagnostically confused with ovarian carcinoma. **Most are adenocarcinomas, but sarcomas and mixed tumors can occur.** There is no official staging system for fallopian tube carcinoma, but in general they are staged like ovarian cancer because the mode of dissemination is similar. Bilateral carcinomas are seen in 10% to 20% of patients.

CLINICAL FEATURES

Clinically, **patients can present with a vaginal discharge that is typically watery in nature,** as well as vaginal bleeding, pelvic pain, or some combination of symptoms. In postmenopausal patients, the vaginal discharge may be yellow, watery, and similar to that seen with a urinary fistula. Physical examination may reveal an adnexal mass, but is often unremarkable. **A fallopian tube cancer should be suspected in a postmenopausal patient whose bleeding or abnormal cytologic findings are not explained by endometrial or endocervical curettage.** In most patients, the diagnosis is not made preoperatively.

TREATMENT

The treatment for fallopian tube carcinoma is total abdominal hysterectomy, bilateral salpingo-oophorectomy, and omentectomy. **Surgical staging should be performed in patients whose disease appears to be confined to the pelvis, and cytoreductive surgery is appropriate in patients with metastatic disease.** Postoperatively, combination chemotherapy, including carboplatin and paclitaxel, is usually used for patients with stages II–IV disease.

PROGNOSIS

The prognosis for fallopian tube carcinoma is similar to that for ovarian cancer.

Suggested Reading

Berek JS: Epithelial ovarian cancer. *In* Berek JS, Hacker NF (eds): Practical Gynecologic Oncology, 3rd ed.

Philadelphia, Lippincott Williams & Wilkins, 2000 pp. 457–522.

Bristow RE, Tomacruz RS, Armstrong DK, et al: Survival effect of maximal cytoreductive surgery for advanced ovarian carcinoma during the platinum era: A meta-analysis. J Clin Oncol 20:1248–1259, 2002.

Frank TS, Manley SA, Olopade OI, Cummings S, Garber JE, Bernhardt B, et al: Sequence analysis of BRCA1 and BRCA2: Correlation of mutations with family history and ovarian cancer risk. J Clin Oncol 16:2417–2425, 1998.

McGuire WP, Hoskins WJ, Brady MF, et al: Cyclophosphamide and cisplatin compared with paclitaxel and cisplatin in patients with stage III and stage IV ovarian cancer. N Engl J Med 334:1, 1996.

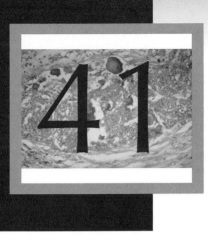

Vulvar and Vaginal Cancer

Neville F. Hacker

VULVAR NEOPLASMS

Malignant tumors of the vulva are uncommon, representing about 4% of malignancies of the female genital tract. Most tumors are squamous cell carcinomas, with melanomas, adenocarcinomas, basal cell carcinomas, and sarcomas occurring much less frequently.

Squamous cell carcinoma of the vulva occurs mainly in postmenopausal women, and the mean age at diagnosis is 65 years. A history of chronic vulvar itching is common.

EPIDEMIOLOGY

Recent studies suggest two different etiologic types of vulvar cancer. **One type is seen mainly in younger patients, is related to human papillomavirus infection and smoking, and is commonly associated with vulvar intraepithelial neoplasia (VIN) of the basaloid or warty type. The more common type is seen mainly in elderly women and is unrelated to smoking or human papillomavirus (HPV) infection; concurrent VIN is uncommon. When VIN is present, it is of the differentiated type.** VIN III appears to carry a significant risk of progression to invasive cancer if left untreated.

About 5% of patients have positive results on serologic testing for syphilis. In the latter group of patients, vulvar cancer occurs at an earlier age and carries a graver prognosis. Although rarely seen in the United States, **vulvar cancer also occurs in association with lymphogranuloma venereum and granuloma inguinale.**

INTRAEPITHELIAL NEOPLASIA

The International Society for the Study of Vulvar Disease recognizes two varieties of intraepithelial neoplasia: squamous cell carcinoma in situ (Bowen's disease) or VIN III, and Paget's disease.

Squamous Cell Carcinoma In Situ: VIN III

During the last 25 years, the incidence of VIN has increased. Younger patients are being affected, and the mean age is approximately 45 years.

Clinical Features

Itching is the most common symptom, although some patients present with palpable or visible abnormalities of the vulva. Approximately half of the patients are asymptomatic. There is no absolutely diagnostic appearance. Most lesions are elevated, but the color may be white, red, pink, gray, or brown (Figure 41-1). **Approximately 20% of the lesions have a "warty" appearance, and the lesions are multicentric in about two thirds of cases.**

Diagnosis

Careful inspection of the vulva in a bright light, with the aid of a magnifying glass if necessary, is the most useful technique for detecting abnormal areas. Colposcopic examination of the entire vulva after the application of 5% acetic acid will sometimes highlight additional acetowhite areas.

Management

The mainstay of treatment is local superficial surgical excision, with primary closure. The microscopic disease seldom extends significantly beyond the colposcopic lesion, so **margins of about 5 mm are**

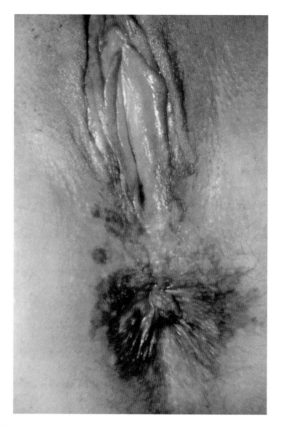

Figure 41-1. VIN III-carcinoma in situ of the vulva. Note the pigmented and multicentric nature of the lesions and the extensive perianal involvement in this patient.

usually adequate. **For extensive lesions involving most of the vulva, a "skinning" vulvectomy,** in which the vulvar skin is removed and replaced by a split-thickness skin graft, **may be used.** Because the subcutaneous tissues are not excised, the cosmetic result is superior to that obtained with vulvectomy.

Laser therapy is also effective, particularly for multiple small lesions, or for lesions involving the clitoris, labia minora, or perianal area. No specimen is available for histologic study after laser ablation, so a liberal number of biopsies must be taken before treatment to exclude invasive cancer.

BOWENOID PAPULOSIS OF THE VULVA

Bowenoid papulosis is a clinical entity that usually affects younger individuals. It is characterized clinically by multiple reddish brown or violaceous papules, and histologically, it is indistinguishable from VIN III. Treatment should be by local excision or laser therapy.

Some lesions may regress spontaneously after pregnancy.

PAGET'S DISEASE

Paget's disease of the vulva predominantly affects postmenopausal white women. Paget's disease also occurs in the nipple areas of the breast.

Clinical Features

Itching and tenderness are common and may be long-standing. **The affected area is usually well demarcated and eczematoid in appearance,** with the presence of white plaquelike lesions. As growth progresses, extension beyond the vulva to the mons pubis, thighs, and buttocks may occur; rarely, it may extend to involve the mucosa of the rectum, vagina, or urinary tract. **In 10% to 20% of cases, Paget's disease is associated with an underlying adenocarcinoma.**

Histologic Features

The disease is an adenocarcinoma in situ and is characterized by large, pale, pathognomonic Paget's cells, which are seen within the epidermis and skin adnexa. **They are rich in mucopolysaccharide, a diastase-resistant substance that stains positive with periodic acid–Schiff.** The intracytoplasmic mucin may also be demonstrated by Mayer's mucicarmine stain. **The Paget's cells are typically located adjacent to the basal layer, both in the epidermis and in the adnexal structures.**

Management

The histologic extent of Paget's disease is frequently far beyond the visible lesion. Local superficial excision with 5- to 10-mm margins is required to clear the gross lesion, exclude underlying invasive cancer, and to relieve symptoms. Recurrences are common and may be treated by further excision or laser therapy. **If an underlying invasive carcinoma is present, the treatment should be the same as for other invasive vulvar cancers.**

INVASIVE VULVAR CANCER
SQUAMOUS CELL CARCINOMA

Squamous cell carcinoma accounts for about 90% of vulvar cancers.

Clinical Features

Patients generally present with a vulvar lump, although long-standing pruritus is common. The lesions may be raised, ulcerated, pigmented, or warty in appearance, and **definitive diagnosis requires biopsy under local anesthesia.** Most lesions occur on the labia majora; the labia minora are the next most common sites. Less commonly, the clitoris or the perineum is involved (Figure 41-2). Approximately 5% of cases are multifocal.

Methods of Spread

Vulvar cancer spreads by direct extension to adjacent structures, such as the vagina, urethra, and anus; **by lymphatic embolization to regional lymph nodes;** and **by hematogenous spread to distant sites,** including the lungs, liver, and bone. In most cases, the initial lymphatic metastases are to the inguinal lymph nodes, located between Camper's

Table 41-1. Incidence of lymph node metastases in relation to lesion size in vulvar cancer			
Lesion Size (cm)	Number	Positive Nodes	Percent
1	40	2	5
1–2	81	13	16
2–4	33	11	33.3
>4	15	8	53.3

Data from Hackër NF, et al.: Vulvar cancer. *In* Haskell CM. (ed) Cancer Treatment, 3rd ed. WB Saunders, Philadelphia, 1990, p 354.

fascia and the fascia lata. From these superficial nodes, spread occurs to the femoral nodes located medial to the femoral vein. Cloquet's node, which is situated beneath the inguinal ligament, is the most cephalad of the femoral node group. **From the inguinofemoral nodes, spread occurs to the pelvic nodes, particularly the external iliac group** (Figure 41-3).

The incidence of lymph node metastases in vulvar cancer is approximately 30%. It is related to the size of the lesion (Table 41-1). **Approximately 5% of patients have metastases to pelvic lymph nodes. Such patients usually have three or more positive unilateral inguinofemoral lymph nodes.** Hematogenous spread usually occurs late in the disease and rarely occurs in the absence of lymphatic metastases.

Staging

In 1989, the International Federation of Gynecology and Obstetrics (FIGO) Cancer Committee introduced a surgical staging system for vulvar cancer. This system was revised in 1994, and the present FIGO staging system is shown in Table 41-2.

Management

In the past, en bloc radical vulvectomy and bilateral inguinofemoral lymphadenectomy, with or without pelvic lymphadenectomy, has been considered the standard treatment for invasive vulvar cancer. **During the past 25 years a more conservative approach has been used for the primary lesion, and the groin dissection has frequently been performed through a separate groin incision.**

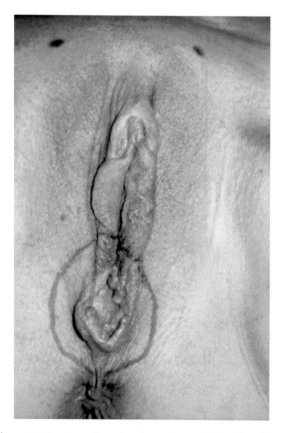

Figure 41-2. A small perineal carcinoma. Note that the remainder of the vulva is normal.

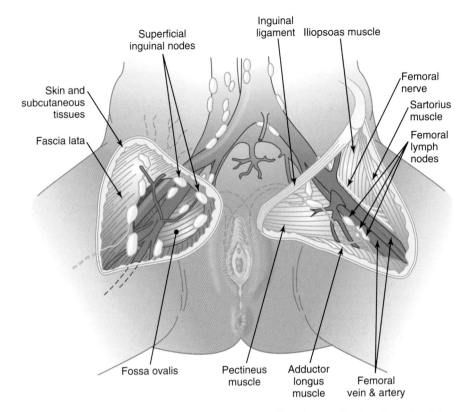

Figure 41-3. Lymphatic drainage of the vulva. Inguinal nodes are displayed on the right side of the groin and femoral nodes are seen on the left side of the groin.

Table 41-2. International Federation of Gynecology and Obstetrics (FIGO) staging of vulvar carcinoma (1994)

Stage	
Stage 0	Carcinoma in situ, intraepithelial carcinoma
Stage I	Tumor confined to the vulva or perineum, or both, and 2 cm or less in greatest dimension; no nodal metastasis
Stage Ia	As above with stromal invasion ≤1 mm
Stage Ib	As above with stromal invasion >1 mm
Stage II	Tumor confined to the vulva or perineum, or both, and more than 2 cm in greatest dimension; no nodal metastasis
Stage III	Tumor of any size with: 1. Adjacent spread to the urethra and/or vagina, and/or the anus. 2. Unilateral regional lymph node metastasis, or a combination
Stage IV	
Stage IVa	Tumor invades any of the following: upper urethra, bladder mucosa, rectal mucosa, pelvic bone or bilateral regional node metastasis, or a combination
Stage IVb	Any distant metastasis including pelvic lymph nodes

Using the separate incision technique, major wound breakdown is significantly reduced, so hospital stays are shorter. **Groin seromas and cellulitis are common acute complications,** while deep venous thrombosis and pulmonary embolism are uncommon. **Chronic complications include lower leg lymphoedema, genital prolapse, and urinary stress incontinence.** Rarely, introital stenosis, pubic osteomyelitis, a femoral hernia, or a rectoperineal fistula may occur.

EARLY VULVAR CANCER

During the past 25 years, much emphasis has been placed on vulvar conservation in an attempt to decrease psychologic morbidity. With respect to the lymphadenectomy, **patients with Stage Ia disease** (i.e., with T1 tumors in whom the depth of penetration is less than 1 mm from the overlying basement membrane) **do not need groin dissection. All other patients require at least an ipsilateral inguinal–femoral lymphadenectomy. For patients with midline lesions invading more than 1 mm, bilateral groin dissection is necessary.** For ipsilateral lesions there is about a 1% risk of involvement of the contralateral nodes if the ipsilateral nodes are negative.

For patients with TI or T2 lesions (i.e., lesions confined to the vulva) a wide and deep local excision (radical local excision) is as effective as radical vulvectomy in preventing local recurrence provided that the remainder of the vulva is normal. For patients with stage I vulvar cancer, there is about a 10% risk of local recurrence, even with radical vulvectomy, and this incidence appears to be no higher with radical local excision. **Surgical margins should be at least 1 cm**.

ADVANCED VULVAR CANCER

The standard management for patients with advanced vulvar cancer involving the proximal urethra, anus, or rectovaginal septum has been pelvic exenteration performed in conjunction with radical vulvectomy and bilateral inguinofemoral lymphadenectomy. Although the 5-year survival rate for such patients approximates 50%, the operative mortality rate is about 10%, and the cure rate is low if there are any involved lymph nodes. **Over the last 20 years, many centers have been using preoperative radiation or chemoradiation to shrink the primary tumor, followed by more conservative surgical excision.** Bilateral groin node dissection, or at least removal of any large, positive nodes is usually performed prior to the radiation therapy. Survival does not seem to be compromised by this approach, and most patients can be spared pelvic exenteration.

MANAGEMENT OF PATIENTS WITH POSITIVE NODES

Patients with more than one nodal micrometastases, (≤5 mm diameter), one macrometastasis

(≥10 mm), or evidence of extra nodal spread should receive postoperative radiation to both groins and to the pelvis.

Prognosis

The overall survival rate for vulvar carcinoma is about 70%. Survival by FIGO stage is shown in Table 41-2. Survival also correlates significantly with lymph node status, since **patients with positive nodes have a 5-year survival rate of about 50%, whereas those with negative nodes have a 5-year survival rate of about 90%.** Patients with one involved node have a good prognosis, regardless of stage, whereas those with three or more involved nodes do poorly, regardless of stage.

MALIGNANT MELANOMA

Malignant melanoma is the second most common type of vulvar cancer. Melanomas may arise de novo or from a preexisting junctional or compound nevus. They occur predominantly in postmenopausal white women and most commonly involve the labia minora or clitoris (Figure 41-4).

Diagnosis and Staging

Any pigmented lesion on the vulva requires excisional biopsy for histologic diagnosis. The FIGO staging of vulvar cancer does not apply well to melanomas, which are usually smaller lesions and tend to metastasize early. **The prognosis correlates more closely with the depth of penetration into the dermis.** Those lesions that penetrate to a depth of 1 mm or less from the granular layer of the epidermis

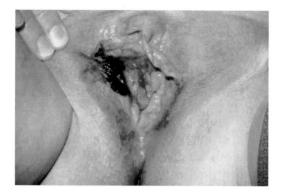

Figure 41-4. Malignant melanoma arising from the right labium minus.

Table 41-3. Survival of vulvar cancer by FIGO Stage (epidermoid invasive cancer only)		
Stage	Patients	5 year Survival
I	193	86.5%
II	247	67.7%
III	201	40.3%
IV	74	21.7%

Data from the Annual Report on the Results of Treatment in Gynecological Cancer. Patients treated 1993–1995. J Epidemiol Biostat 24:153–174, 2001.

rarely metastasize. Clark's levels are not readily applicable to vulvar melanomas.

Management

For the superficial lesions referred to previously, radical local excision alone, with margins of at least 1 cm, is adequate therapy. For lesions with ≥1 mm invasion, **radical local excision of the primary tumor is usually combined with at least ipsilateral inguinal-femoral lymphadenectomy.** Adjuvant therapy with nonspecific immunostimulants or chemotherapeutic agents has been disappointing, although vaccines prepared from the patient's own tumor have shown some promise.

Prognosis

The overall 5-year survival rate for vulvar melanomas is approximately 30%, which is comparable to that for cutaneous melanomas of nongenital origin.

VERRUCOUS CARCINOMA

Verrucous carcinoma is a variant of squamous cell carcinoma and was originally described in the oral cavity. The lesions, which are cauliflower-like in nature, may occur in the cervix, vulva, or vagina. Invasion occurs with a broad "pushing" front, and unless the base of the lesion is submitted for histologic examination, these tumors may be difficult to differentiate from condyloma acuminatum or squamous papilloma. **Metastasis to regional lymph nodes is rare,** but the tumors are locally aggressive and prone to local recurrence unless wide surgical margins are obtained. **Radiation therapy may induce anaplastic transformation and is contraindicated.**

BARTHOLIN'S GLAND CARCINOMA

Adenocarcinomas, squamous cell carcinomas, and rarely, transitional cell carcinomas may arise from the Bartholin's gland and its duct. A history of preceding inflammation of Bartholin's gland is present in about 10% of patients, and malignancies may be mistaken for benign cysts or abscesses. Current management consists of hemivulvectomy and ipsilateral inguinofemoral lymphadenectomy. **Postoperative vulvar irradiation appears to decrease the local recurrence rate for patients with large lesions.**

BASAL CELL CARCINOMA

Basal cell carcinomas of the vulva are rare. They commonly present as a rolled edged "rodent" ulcer, although nodules and macules may occur. They are locally aggressive but nonmetastasizing, so wide local excision is adequate treatment.

Vulvar Sarcoma

Vulvar sarcomas represent 1% to 2% of vulvar malignancies. Many histologic types have been reported, including leiomyosarcomas, fibrosarcomas, neurofibrosarcomas, liposarcomas, rhabdomyosarcomas, angiosarcomas, and epithelioid sarcomas. Leiomyosarcomas are the most common, and recurrences are most likely with lesions larger than 5 cm, with infiltrating margins, and with five or more mitotic figures per 10 high-power fields.

VAGINAL NEOPLASMS
INTRAEPITHELIAL NEOPLASIA

Carcinoma in situ of the vagina (VAIN) is much less common than its counterparts on the cervix or vulva. Most lesions occur in the upper third of the vagina, and the patients are usually asymptomatic.

Etiology

Vaginal intraepithelial neoplasia appears to be related to infection with the wart virus in many cases. Patients with a past history of in situ or invasive carcinoma of the cervix or vulva are at increased risk. Some lesions may occur after irradiation for cervical cancer.

Diagnosis

The diagnosis is usually considered because of an abnormal Papanicolaou smear in a woman who either has had a hysterectomy or has no demonstrable cervical abnormality. Definitive diagnosis requires vaginal biopsy, which should be directed by colposcopy or Lugol's iodine staining. Colposcopic findings are similar to those seen with cervical lesions, although thorough colposcopy of all vaginal walls is technically more difficult. **In postmenopausal patients, a 4-week course of topical estrogen before colposcopy is indicated to enhance the colposcopic features and eliminate those patients with Papanicolaou smear abnormalities due to inflammatory atypia.**

Management

Surgical excision is the mainstay of therapy, and this may require excision of the vaginal apex. At times, extensive disease requires total vaginectomy and creation of a neovagina using a split-thickness skin graft. Laser therapy and topical 5-fluorouracil are alternatives to surgical excision.

SQUAMOUS CELL CARCINOMA OF THE VAGINA

Squamous cell carcinoma of the vagina is uncommon. The mean age of patients at presentation is about 60 years. Up to 30% of patients with primary vaginal cancer have a history of in situ or invasive cervical cancer that was treated at least 5 years earlier. Symptoms consist of abnormal vaginal bleeding, vaginal discharge, and urinary symptoms. On physical examination, ulcerative, exophytic, and infiltrative growth patterns may be seen. About half of the lesions are in the upper third of the vagina, particularly on the posterior wall. Punch biopsy is required to confirm the diagnosis.

Patterns of Spread

Vaginal cancer spreads by direct invasion as well as by lymphatic and hematogenous dissemination. **Direct tumor spread may result in involvement of the bladder, urethra, or rectum, or progressive lateral extension to the pelvic side wall.** The lymphatic drainage from the upper vagina is to the obturator, hypogastric, and external iliac nodes, whereas the lower third of the vagina drains primarily to the inguinofemoral nodes. Hematogenous spread is uncommon until the disease is advanced.

Staging

The FIGO staging for vaginal cancer is clinical, as shown in Table 41-4. All patients should have at least a chest radiograph, intravenous pyelogram, cystoscopy, and sigmoidoscopy. A pelvic and abdominal computed tomographic scan may be useful to detect lymph node enlargement, but a finding of involved nodes does not alter the FIGO stage.

Management

Radiotherapy is the main method of treatment for primary vaginal cancer. Initial treatment usually consists of 4500 to 5000 cGy external irradiation to the pelvis to shrink the primary tumor and treat the pelvic lymph nodes and paravaginal tissues. Brachytherapy is then given, either with intracavitary vaginal applicators, or by interstitial techniques. **When the lower third of the vagina is involved, the groin nodes should either be included in the treatment field or surgically removed.**

Radical surgery has a limited role in the management of vaginal cancer. **Radical hysterectomy, partial vaginectomy, and pelvic lymphadenectomy may be performed for early lesions in the posterior fornix.** Surgery should otherwise be reserved for medically fit patients in whom a central recurrence develops following irradiation. Pelvic exenteration with creation of a neovagina may be appropriate in such patients provided that there are no lymph node metastases at the time of exploratory laparotomy, and adequate surgical margins can be attained.

Table 41-4. International Federation of Gynecology and Obstetrics (FIGO) staging of vaginal cancer	
Stage	**Description**
Stage I	Carcinoma limited to the vaginal wall
Stage II	Carcinoma has involved the subvaginal tissue but has not extended onto the pelvic side wall
Stage III	Carcinoma has extended to the pelvic side wall
Stage IV	Carcinoma has extended beyond the true pelvis or has involved the mucosa of the bladder or rectum
Stage IVa	Spread to bladder or rectum
Stage IVb	Spread to distant organs

Prognosis

The overall 5-year survival for vaginal cancer is about 50%. When corrected for death from inter-current disease, 5-year survival rates should be approximately 85% to 90% for stage I lesions, 55% to 65% for stage II lesions, 30% to 35% for stage III lesions, and 5% to 10% for stage IV lesions.

RARE VAGINAL CANCERS
Adenocarcinoma

Most adenocarcinomas of the vagina are metastatic, usually from the cervix, endometrium, or ovary, but occasionally from more distant sites such as the kidney, breast, or colon. **Most primary vaginal adenocarcinomas are clear cell carcinomas in female offspring of women who ingested diethylstilbestrol (DES) during pregnancy** (see later in this chapter). Primary adenocarcinomas of the vagina not related to DES are rare but may arise in residual glands of müllerian (paramesonephric) origin, Gartner's duct (a remnant of the embryonic wolffian or mesonephric duct), or foci of endometriosis.

Malignant Melanoma

Vaginal melanomas account for fewer than 2% of vaginal malignancies. The mean age at diagnosis is 55 years. The carcinoma usually occurs on the distal anterior wall. **Radical surgery has been the traditional treatment but comparable local control and overall survival maybe obtained with conservative tumor resection and postoperative radiation therapy.** The use of high-dose fractions (greater than 400 cGy) may be beneficial. The prognosis is poor, with an overall 5-year survival rate of 5% to 10%.

Sarcoma

Vaginal sarcomas are rare. In adults, leiomyosarcomas are most common, whereas **in infants and children, sarcoma botryoides predominates.** The latter term comes from the Greek *botrys* (bunch of grapes), which these lesions usually grossly resemble. The mean age at diagnosis of sarcoma botryoides is 2 to 3 years, with a range of 6 months to 16 years. **Histologically the tumor is an embryonal rhabdomyosarcoma.** Treatment consists of **conservative surgical resection** followed by adjuvant chemotherapy, with or without radiation therapy.

DIETHYLSTILBESTROL EXPOSURE IN UTERO

In 1971, an association between in utero exposure to DES and the later development of clear cell adenocarcinoma of the vagina was reported. Since that time, numerous non-neoplastic uterine and vaginal anomalies have been reported in young women exposed in utero to DES. **Vaginal adenosis (vaginal columnar epithelium) is the most common anomaly and is present in about 30% of exposed females.** This tissue behaves similarly to the columnar epithelium of the cervix and is replaced initially by immature metaplastic squamous epithelium. With progressive squamous maturation, complete resolution of this anomaly usually occurs.

Structural changes of the cervix and vagina occur in about 25% of exposed females. Possible changes include a transverse vaginal septum, cervical collar (Figure 41-5), cockscomb (a raised ridge, usually on the anterior cervix), or cervical hypoplasia. Most of these changes tend to disappear as the individual matures. The risk is insignificant if administration was begun after the 22nd week of gestation.

In addition to these changes in the lower genital tract, upper genital tract anomalies occur in at least half of the patients and may be associated with exposure later in pregnancy. **The most common abnormalities are a T-shaped uterus and a small uterine cavity** (less than 2.5 cm in length). Exposed individuals have an increased risk of miscarriage, premature delivery, or ectopic pregnancy, but most are able to deliver a viable infant successfully.

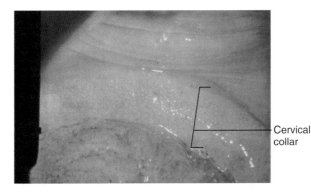

Figure 41-5. A cervical collar in a patient exposed to diethylstilbestrol in utero.

CLEAR CELL ADENOCARCINOMA

The risk of developing a clear cell adenocarcinoma following DES exposure in utero is somewhat less than 1 in 1000. The tumors are rare before age 14 years, and the mean age of patients at diagnosis is about 19 years. Few cases have been reported after 30 years of age, so as DES has not been given during pregnancy for about 30 years, few DES related adenocarcinomas will be seen in the future. Not all patients with vaginal clear cell adenocarcinomas give a history of prior DES exposure in uterus. **For early tumors, radical hysterectomy and vaginectomy (with creation of a neovagina) or radiation therapy is effective. Overall, the 5-year survival rate is about 80%,** which is considerably better than that for squamous cell cancer of the cervix or vagina.

Suggested Reading

Hacker NF: Vulvar cancer. *In* Berek JS, Hacker NF (eds): Practical Gynecologic Oncology, 3rd ed. Philadelphia, Lippincott Williams & Wilkins, 2000, pp 553–596.

Homesley HD, Bundy BN, Sedlis A, et al: Assessment of current International Federation of Gynaecology and Obstetrics staging of vulvar carcinoma relative to prognostic factors for survival (a Gynecologic Oncology Group study). Am J Obstet Gynecol 164:997–1004, 1991.

Hording U, Junge J, Daugaard S, et al: Vulvar squamous carcinoma and papillomaviruses: Indications for two different etiologies. Gynecol Oncol 52:241–246, 1994.

Jones RW, Baranyai J, Stables S: Trends in squamous cell carcinoma of the vulva: The influence of vulvar intraepithelial neoplasia. Obstet Gynecol 90:448–452, 1997.

Kirkbridge P, Fyles R, Rawlings GA, et al: Carcinoma of the vagina—experience at the Princess Margaret Hospital (1974–89). Gynecol Oncol 56:435–443, 1995.

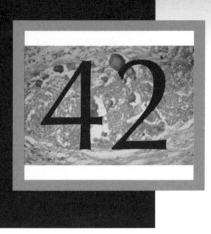

Uterine Corpus Cancer

Neville F. Hacker

Cancer of the endometrium is the most common gynecologic malignancy in the US. For 2004, it is estimated that there will be over 40,000 new cases and 4000 deaths. It is the fourth most common malignancy found in American women after breast, colorectal, and lung cancer, and is predominantly a disease of affluent, obese, postmenopausal women of low parity.

EPIDEMIOLOGY AND ETIOLOGY

The median age for endometrial cancer is about 58 years. The risk factors associated with the development of carcinoma of the endometrium are listed in Box 42-1. **Any factor that increases the exposure to unopposed estrogen increases the risk of endometrial cancer.** If the proliferative effects of estrogen are not counteracted by a progestin, endometrial hyperplasia and possibly adenocarcinoma can result.

Obesity results in an increased extraovarian aromatization of androstenedione to estrone. Androstenedione is secreted by the adrenal glands, whereas the increased peripheral conversion occurs predominantly in fat depots but also in the liver, kidneys, and skeletal muscles. **Granulosa-theca cell tumors of the ovary produce estrogen,** and up to 15% of patients with these tumors have an associated endometrial cancer.

Unopposed estrogenic stimulation from anovulatory cycles occurs in patients who have polycystic ovarian syndrome (Stein-Leventhal syndrome), **and in patients with a late menopause.** In postmenopausal women taking estrogen replacement without a progestin for menopausal symptoms, the risk of cancer developing appears to be both dose-dependent and duration-dependent. This increased risk varies from twofold to 14-fold compared with nonusers. The addition of progestin in a cyclic fashion for 10 to 14 days of the month or in a continuous fashion daily throughout the month eliminates this increased risk. **Women taking tamoxifen for breast cancer have a twofold to threefold increased risk of endometrial cancer.** Young women who use oral contraceptives have been shown to have a lower incidence of subsequent endometrial cancer.

SCREENING OF ASYMPTOMATIC WOMEN

Population screening for endometrial cancer is not feasible, because there is no simple method of cancer detection available. However, screening may be justified for high risk women, including those with a family history of Lynch II Syndrome (hereditary nonpolyposis colorectal cancer syndrome), those with polycystic ovarian disease, any woman with an intact uterus taking unopposed estrogen, and possibly those taking tamoxifen. **Only about 50% of women with endometrial cancer will have malignant cells on a pap smear.**

In the 1990s, transvaginal ultrasonography has been increasingly used for endometrial evaluation. Almost all women with endometrial hyperplasia or carcinoma will have an endometrial thickness of 5 mm or more. **Tamoxifen produces a confusing ultrasonic image, which leads to frequent false positive reports.**

SYMPTOMS

The most common symptom of endometrial cancer is abnormal vaginal bleeding, which is present in 90% of patients. **Postmenopausal bleeding is always abnormal and must be investigated.** The most common

Box 42-1. Risk factors for endometrial cancer

- Obesity
- Nulliparity
- Late menopause
- Diabetes mellitus
- Hypertension
- Breast, colon, or ovarian cancer
- Chronic unopposed estrogen stimulation
- Chronic tamoxifen use

Table 42-1. Etiology of postmenopausal bleeding

Factor	Approximate Percentage
Exogenous estrogens	30
Atrophic endometritis, vaginitis	30
Endometrial cancer	15
Endometrial or cervical polyps	10
Endometrial hyperplasia	5
Miscellaneous (e.g., cervical cancer, uterine sarcoma, urethral caruncle, trauma)	10

conditions associated with postmenopausal bleeding are listed in Table 42-1. In the premenopausal patient, especially after age 35 years, menorrhagia or intermenstrual bleeding may signal an endometrial malignancy.

SIGNS

The general physical examination may reveal obesity, hypertension, and the stigmata of diabetes mellitus. Evidence of metastatic disease is unusual at initial presentation, but the chest should be examined for any effusion and the abdomen carefully palpated and percussed to exclude ascites, hepatomegaly, or evidence of upper abdominal masses.

On pelvic examination, the external genitalia are usually normal. The vagina and cervix are also usually normal but should be carefully inspected and palpated for evidence of involvement. **A patulous cervical os or a firm, expanded cervix may indicate extension of disease from the corpus to the cervix.** The uterus may be of normal size or enlarged, depending on the extent of the disease and the presence or absence of

other uterine conditions, such as adenomyosis or fibroids. The adnexae should be carefully palpated for evidence of extrauterine metastases or an ovarian neoplasm. **A granulosa cell tumor or an endometrioid ovarian carcinoma may occasionally coexist with endometrial cancer.**

DIAGNOSIS

Any woman who presents with postmenopausal bleeding should have a transvaginal ultrasound. If the endometrial thickness is greater than 5 mm, endometrial evaluation is necessary. Outpatient techniques for endometrial sampling include the use of the Kevorkian curette, Vabra aspirator, Gravlee jet washer, and Pipelle cannula. These techniques have a diagnostic accuracy of about 90%. If the endometrial biopsy reveals endometrial cancer, definitive treatment can be arranged. **If the endometrial biopsy is negative for cancer or reveals endometrial hyperplasia, a fractional dilatation and curettage should be performed under general anesthesia.** Specimens from the endometrium and endocervix should be submitted separately for histologic evaluation to determine whether the tumor has extended to the endocervix.

In a premenopausal patient with high-risk factors and abnormal uterine bleeding, the endometrium must be sampled. Failure to respond to medical management or a suspicious transvaginal ultrasound is another indication for endometrial sampling. Hysteroscopy maybe more useful in premenopausal patients A grossly obvious lesion of the cervix or vagina should be biopsied directly.

STAGING

The International Federation of Gynecology and Obstetrics (FIGO) changed from a clinical to a surgical staging system for endometrial cancer in 1988. The new surgical staging, based on pathologic confirmation of the extent of spread, is shown in Table 42-2.

PREOPERATIVE INVESTIGATIONS

In addition to a thorough physical examination, blood studies should include a complete blood count, determinations of hepatic enzymes, serum electrolytes, blood urea nitrogen, serum creatinine, and a coagulation profile. A routine urinalysis should be performed. The only radiologic study necessary is a chest x-ray.

Table 42-2. 1988 FIGO staging of endometrial carcinoma

Stage

Stage Ia	Tumor limited to endometrium
Stage Ib	Invasion through less than one half of the myometrium
Stage Ic	Invasion equal to or more than half of the myometrium
Stage IIa	Endocervical glandular involvement only
Stage IIb	Cervical stroma invasion
Stage IIIa	Tumor invades serosa or adnexa, or both, or positive peritoneal cytologic findings, or both
Stage IIIb	Vaginal metastases
Stage IIIc	Metastases to pelvic or para-aortic lymph nodes, or both
Stage IVa	Tumor invasion of bladder or bowel mucosa, or both
Stage IVb	Distant metastases including intraabdominal or inguinal lymph nodes, or both

Histologic grade does not change the stage

Grade 1	Well differentiated
Grade 2	Moderately differentiated
Grade 3	Poorly differentiated

Additional radiographic procedures, including abdominopelvic computed tomography, intravenous pyelography, bone radiographs, and a barium enema are performed only if indicated.

PATHOLOGIC FEATURES

About 75% of endometrial cancers are pure adenocarcinomas. When squamous elements are present, the tumor is called an adenocarcinoma with squamous differentiation. Such tumors are graded on the glandular component of the lesion. Less often, **clear cell, squamous, or serous carcinomas occur, and all carry a worse prognosis.**

Invasive adenocarcinoma of the endometrium demonstrates proliferative glandular formation with minimal or no intervening stroma. Tumor grade is determined by both the degree of abnormality of the glandular architecture and the degree of nuclear atypia. A lesion that is well differentiated (grade 1) forms a glandular pattern similar to normal endometrial glands (Figure 42-1). A moderately well-differentiated lesion (grade 2) has glandular structures admixed with papillary, and occasionally solid, areas of

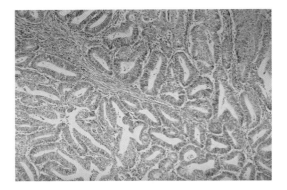

Figure 42-1. Well-differentiated endometrial adenocarcinoma (histologic study). Note the back-to-back glands with minimal intervening stroma and the gland-within-gland pattern.

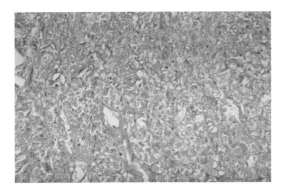

Figure 42-2. Poorly differentiated endometrial adenocarcinoma (histologic study). Note the predominantly solid nature of the tumor with minimal gland formation.

tumor. In a poorly differentiated lesion (grade 3), the glandular structures have become predominantly solid with a relative paucity of identifiable endometrial glands (Figure 42-2).

PATTERN OF SPREAD

Endometrial cancer spreads by (1) direct extension, (2) exfoliation of cells that are shed through the fallopian tubes, (3) lymphatic dissemination, and (4) hematogenous dissemination.

The most common route of spread is direct extension of the tumor to adjacent structures. The tumor may invade through the myometrium and eventually penetrate the serosa. It may also grow downward and involve the cervix. Although uncommon, progressive growth may eventually involve the vagina, parametrium, rectum, or bladder.

Exfoliated cells may pass through the fallopian tubes and implant on the ovaries, the visceral or parietal peritoneum, or the omentum.

Lymphatic spread occurs most commonly in patients with deep myometrial penetration. **Spread mainly occurs to the pelvic lymph nodes and subsequently to the para-aortic lymph nodes, although simultaneous spread to both nodal groups may occur.** In stage I endometrial cancer, the overall incidence of pelvic lymph node metastases is about 12%, and para-aortic metastases occur in about 8% of cases. **In patients with deeply invasive, poorly differentiated stage I adenocarcinomas,** however, **pelvic lymph node metastases occur in up to 40%** of cases. Lymphatic spread is also responsible for vaginal vault recurrences.

Hematogenous dissemination is less common, but it results in parenchymal metastases, particularly in the lungs or liver, or both.

TREATMENT
STAGE I
Surgery

An exploratory laparotomy with total abdominal hysterectomy and bilateral salpingo-oophorectomy is performed on all patients, unless there are absolute medical contraindications (Figure 42-3). On opening the abdomen, peritoneal washings are taken with normal saline for cytologic evaluation. **Approximately 15% of patients with disease confined to the corpus have positive peritoneal cytology.** Retroperitoneal spaces should be opened and evaluated, and any enlarged pelvic or para-aortic lymph nodes should be resected. **Formal surgical staging, including at least pelvic lymphadenectomy, should be performed on high risk patients, including those with serous, clear cell or grade 3 histology; outer half myometrial invasion; or cervical extension.** Laparoscopic surgery, including laparoscopic-assisted vaginal hysterectomy and laparoscopic lymph node dissection, is currently under investigation.

Radiation Therapy

With the advent of surgical staging, less reliance has been placed on adjuvant radiation therapy in the management of patients with endometrial cancer.

Recommendations are as follows (Figure 42-4).
1. Patients with grade 1 or 2 endometrioid carcinomas confined to the inner half of the myometrium may be followed **without adjuvant therapy** (i.e., stage Ia or Ib, grade 1 or 2).
2. Patients with high risk carcinomas with negative pelvic nodes (i.e., any stage Ic cancer; any grade 3, clear cell or serous cancer; or any stage II cancer) may have vault **brachytherapy** (without external beam pelvic radiation).
3. Patients with one positive pelvic node should receive **external pelvic radiation.**
4. Patients with multiple positive pelvic nodes or proven positive paraaortic nodes should receive **extended field radiation** (i.e., pelvic and paraaortic).
5. **Whole abdominal radiation** may be considered for patients with adnexal or omental metastases completely resected.

In patients medically unfit for surgery, radiation therapy alone may be employed. A combination of intracavitary plus external beam radiation is used. The overall 5-year survival rate is about 20% lower than for patients treated with hysterectomy.

STAGE II

If the cervix is grossly normal and involvement is detected only on the histologic evaluation of the endocervical curettage material (occult stage II disease), treatment may be the same as for stage I disease (i.e., total abdominal hysterectomy, bilateral

Figure 42-3. Specimen from a total abdominal hysterectomy and bilateral salpingo-oophorectomy. The uterus has been opened to reveal an exophytic carcinoma on the posterior wall of the corpus.

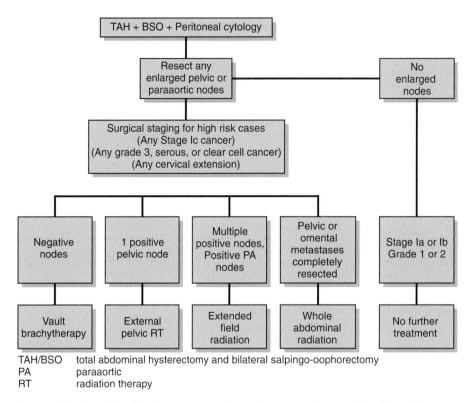

TAH + BSO + Peritoneal cytology

Resect any enlarged pelvic or paraaortic nodes | No enlarged nodes

Surgical staging for high risk cases
(Any Stage Ic cancer)
(Any grade 3, serous, or clear cell cancer)
(Any cervical extension)

Negative nodes | 1 positive pelvic node | Multiple positive nodes, Positive PA nodes | Pelvic or omental metastases completely resected | Stage Ia or Ib Grade 1 or 2

Vault brachytherapy | External pelvic RT | Extended field radiation | Whole abdominal radiation | No further treatment

TAH/BSO   total abdominal hysterectomy and bilateral salpingo-oophorectomy
PA   paraaortic
RT   radiation therapy

Figure 42-4. Algorithm for the treatment of stage I and occult stage II endometrial cancer.

salpingo-oophorectomy, surgical staging, and tailored postoperative radiotherapy).

If the cervix is grossly enlarged, primary radical hysterectomy, bilateral salpingo-oophorectomy, surgical staging, and postoperative external beam therapy for positive lymph nodes is the treatment of choice.

ADVANCED STAGES

For advanced disease, treatment is individualized. The uterus, tubes, and ovaries should be removed, if possible, for palliation of bleeding and other pelvic symptoms. If gross disease is present in the upper abdomen, tumor metastases that are readily removable, such as an omental "cake," should be extirpated in an attempt to improve the patient's quality of life by temporarily decreasing abdominal discomfort and ascites. In addition to preoperative or postoperative radiation, patients with advanced disease also require hormonal therapy, with or without chemotherapy.

RECURRENT DISEASE

Seventy-five percent of recurrences develop within 2 years of treatment. If recurrent disease is detected, the patient should undergo a complete physical examination and metastatic workup. Careful follow-up is particularly important for patients treated without adjuvant therapy. The majority of recurrences in these patients are at the vaginal vault, and 70% to 80% of patients can be salvaged by radiation therapy.

Metastases in other sites, such as the upper abdomen, lungs, or liver, are treated initially with high-dose progestins or antiestrogens. About one-third of recurrent endometrial carcinomas contain estrogen and progesterone receptors, with the more well-differentiated tumors more likely to contain such receptors. As with breast cancer, the likelihood of a patient responding to progestin treatment is increased in patients whose tumor contains estrogen and progesterone receptors. Approximately 80% of such patients respond to progestin therapy, compared with fewer than 10% of patients whose tumor is receptor negative.

Medroxyprogesterone acetate (Provera, 50 mg three times daily; Depo-Provera, 400 mg intramuscularly weekly) or megestrol acetate (Megace), 80 mg twice daily, may be given. **If disease progresses while the patient is receiving progestins, chemotherapy may be offered.** The combination of Carboplatin and paclitaxel (Taxol) gives a response rate of about 50%.

Prognosis

Prognosis is dependent on several variables, including uterine size, histologic type, grade of tumor, depth of myometrial penetration, status of lymph nodes, status of peritoneal cytologic features, and presence or absence of occult adnexal or upper abdominal metastases. **Serous and clear cell endometrial carcinomas have a particularly bad prognosis, and both of these histologic types are prone to early dissemination. Five-year survival rates for these tumor types are less than 50%, even for patients with stage I disease.**

Five-year survival rates for each stage of endometrioid endometrial cancer are presented in Table 42-3.

Follow-Up

Follow-up examinations should be performed every 3 months for 2 years, every 6 months for 3 years, and then annually. It is important to take a vault pap smear on patients who have not had radiation therapy.

Table 42-3. Survival for endometrial cancer by FIGO Stage (N = 5694)

Stage	Patients	5-year Survival (%)
Ia	975	88.9
Ib	2035	90.0
Ic	986	80.7
IIa	342	79.9
IIb	367	72.3
IIIa	457	63.4
IIIb	101	38.8
IIIc	200	51.1
IVa	57	19.9
IVb	174	17.2

Data from the Annual Report on the Results of Treatment in Gynecological Cancer. Patients treated 1993–1995. J Epidemiol Biostat 24:45–86, 2001.

UTERINE SARCOMAS

Uterine sarcomas account for about 3% of uterine cancers. They arise from the stromal components of the uterus, either the endometrial stroma or the mesenchymal and myometrial tissues. As a group, sarcomas tend to be more advanced at the time of diagnosis, are more likely to disseminate hematogenously, and have much lower 2- and 5-year survival rates.

CLASSIFICATION

A classification system for uterine sarcomas is presented in Table 42-4.

Uterine sarcomas can be classified as either *pure*, in which the only malignant tissue is of mesenchymal origin, or mixed, in which malignant mesenchymal and malignant epithelial tissues are present. They may also be classified as homologous, implying that the tissue that is malignant is normally present in the uterus (e.g., endometrial stroma, smooth muscle), **or heterologous,** implying that the tissue that is malignant is not normally present in the uterus (e.g., bone or cartilage). The majority of pure uterine sarcomas are leiomyosarcomas and endometrial stromal sarcomas.

LEIOMYOSARCOMA

Leiomyosarcomas may be associated with a benign leiomyoma of the uterus, but the risk of malignant transformation in a benign fibroid is less than 1%. **The histologic criteria for distinguishing leiomyosarcomas from leiomyomas are the mitotic count (usually greater than 10 per 10 high-power fields), the presence or absence of coagulative necrosis, and the presence or absence of cellular atypia.**

Clinically, the mean age of patients with leiomyosarcoma is about 55 years. Patients with this

Table 42-4. Classification of uterine sarcomas

Type	Homologous	Heterologous
Pure	Leiomyosarcoma	Rhabdomyosarcoma
	Endometrial stromal sarcoma	Chondrosarcoma
		Osteosarcoma
	Endometrial sarcoma	Liposarcoma
Mixed	Carcinosarcoma	Malignant mixed mesodermal tumor

disease may present with pelvic pain, abnormal uterine bleeding, or a pelvic or lower abdominal mass. A sensation of pressure on the bladder or rectum may also be noted.

Most cases are not diagnosed preoperatively but are discovered at the time of exploratory surgery for a probable fibroid. Curettings are usually normal. **If a known fibroid uterus appears to be rapidly enlarging, especially post-menopausally, malignancy should be suspected.**

The treatment of a uterine leiomyosarcoma consists of total abdominal hysterectomy and bilateral salpingo-oophorectomy. Adjuvant pelvic radiation appears to decrease local pelvic recurrence but does not prolong survival because most patients die with distant metastases.

Response rates to chemotherapy are very low.

ENDOMETRIAL STROMAL TUMORS

The three types of stromal tumors are (1) endometrial stromal nodule; (2) endometrial stromal sarcoma, previously known as endolymphatic stromal myosis; and (3) high-grade endometrial sarcoma. The first of these, **the stromal nodule, is a rare benign condition.** There are typically three or fewer mitoses per 10 high-power fields. A hysterectomy is curative.

Endometrial stromal sarcoma is a low-grade lesion. Histologically, there is minimal to no cellular atypia, with usually fewer than five mitoses per 10 high-power fields. There is always evidence of vascular channel invasion. These patients usually present with abnormal vaginal bleeding and often with pelvic pain.

Most patients are cured with total abdominal hysterectomy and bilateral salpingo-oophorectomy. Local and distant recurrences may occur even 10 to 20 years later and require reexploration and resection of disease. Prolonged survival is possible after resection of recurrent disease, and response to progestins is good. Pelvic disease may respond to radiation therapy.

High-grade endometrial sarcoma generally causes abnormal uterine bleeding, and more than half the patients are premenopausal. **The diagnosis can often be made by endometrial biopsy or uterine curettage.** Histologically, there are 10 or more mitoses per 10 high-power fields, and the lesion is composed of very poorly differentiated cells. Aggressive myometrial invasion occurs, and hematogenous spread is common at the time of diagnosis.

The treatment of high grade endometrial sarcoma is total abdominal hysterectomy and bilateral salpingo-oophorectomy. A thorough exploration of the peritoneal cavity and retroperitoneum should be made for evidence of metastases. **Postoperative pelvic irradiation improves local control but does not improve survival.** In patients with metastatic disease, progestogens or chemotherapy may be offered. The best chemotherapeutic agents are cisplatin, doxorubicin, and ifosfamide, but the prognosis is poor.

MIXED MÜLLERIAN SARCOMA

Malignant mixed müllerian tumors account for about 40% of uterine sarcomas. Most patients are postmenopausal and present with vaginal bleeding or discharge. About one-third of patients have tumor growing through the cervix into the vagina as a polypoid mass. **Up to 50% of patients with this lesion have evidence of metastatic disease at the time of diagnosis if surgically staged.**

These tumors aggressively invade the myometrium and disseminate via the lymphatics and the blood stream.

The primary treatment of mixed müllerian sarcoma is the same as that for high-grade endometrial stromal sarcomas. Prophylactic cisplatin and epirubicin may improve survival for patients with stage I or II disease.

Prognosis

The prognosis for uterine sarcomas is poor because of the propensity for hematogenous dissemination. The overall 5-year survival rate is about 35%. Patients with stage I uterine sarcoma have 50% chance of 5-year survival, and patients with disease outside the uterus have a dismal prognosis.

Suggested Reading

Abeler VM, Kjorstad KE, Berle E. Carcinoma of the endometrium in Norway: A histopathological and prognostic survey of a total population. In J Gynecol Cancer 2:9–22, 1992.

Hacker NF: Endometrial cancer. *In* Berek JS, Hacker NF (eds): Practical Gynecologic Oncology, 3rd ed. Philadelphia, Lippincott Williams & Wilkins, 2000, pp 407–448.

Karlsson B, Granberg S, Wikland M, Ylostalo P, Torvid K, Mansal K, et al: Transvaginal ultrasonography of the endometrium in women with postmenopausal bleeding: A Nordic multicenter study. Am J Obstet Gynecol 172:1488–1494, 1995.

Morrow CP, Bundy BN, Kurman RJ, Creasman WT, Heller P, Homesley H, et al: Relationship between surgical-pathological risk factors and outcome in clinical stages I and II carcinoma of the endometrium: A Gynaecologic Oncology Group Study. Gynecol Oncol 40:55–65, 1991.

Parazzini F, La Vecchi C, Bocciolone L, Franceschi S: The epidemiology of endometrial cancer. Gynecol Oncol 41:1–16, 1991.

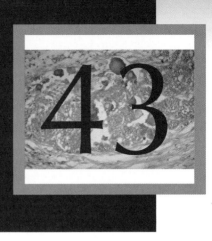

43

Gestational Trophoblastic Neoplasia

Jonathan S. Berek

Gestational trophoblastic neoplasia (GTN) represents a unique spectrum of diseases that includes benign hydatidiform mole; invasive mole (chorioadenoma destruens), which can metastasize; and the frankly malignant variety, choriocarcinoma. About 3000 hydatidiform moles are diagnosed annually in the United States. **The majority of patients (80% to 90%) with GTN follow a benign course, with their disease remitting spontaneously.** Most patients with metastatic disease can be effectively cured with chemotherapy. This diverse group of diseases has a sensitive tumor marker, β-hCG, which is secreted by all of these tumors and allows accurate follow-up and assessment of the disease.

EPIDEMIOLOGY AND ETIOLOGY

The incidence of molar pregnancy is about 1 in every 1500 to 2000 pregnancies among whites in the United States. There is a much higher incidence among Asian women in the United States (1 in 800) and an even higher incidence among women in Asia, for example, Taiwan (1 in every 125 to 200 pregnancies). **The risk of the development of a second molar pregnancy is 1% to 3%,** or as much as 40 times greater than the risk of developing the first molar pregnancy.

Although the cause of GTN is unknown, it is **known to occur more frequently in women younger than 20 years and in those older than 40 years.** It appears that GTN may result from defective fertilization, a process that is more common in both younger and older individuals. Diet may play a causative role. **The incidence of molar pregnancy has been noted to be higher in geographic areas** where people consume less β-carotene (a retinoid) and folic acid.

GENETICS OF GESTATIONAL TROPHOBLASTIC DISEASE

The cytogenetic analysis of tissue obtained from molar pregnancies offers some clue to the genesis of these lesions. Figure 43-1 illustrates the genetic composition of molar pregnancies.

COMPLETE MOLE

The majority of hydatidiform moles are "complete" moles and have a 46 XX karyotype. Specialized studies indicate that both of the X chromosomes are paternally derived. This androgenic origin probably results from fertilization of an "empty egg" (i.e., an egg without chromosomes) by a haploid sperm (23 X), which then duplicates to restore the diploid chromosomal complement (46 XX). Only a small percentage of lesions are 46 XY. **Complete molar pregnancy is only rarely associated with a fetus, and this may represent a form of twinning.**

PARTIAL MOLE

In the "incomplete" or partial mole, the karyotype is usually a triploid, often 69 XXY (80%). The majority of the remaining lesions are 69 XXX or 69 XYY. Occasionally mosaic patterns occur. **These lesions, unlike complete moles, often present with a coexistent fetus.** The fetus usually has a triploid karyotype and is defective.

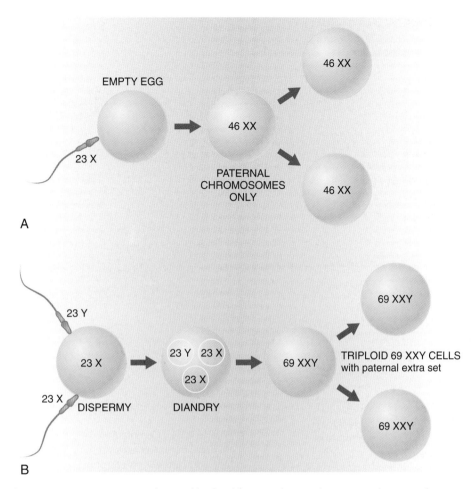

Figure 43-1. Cytogenetic makeup of hydatidiform mole. *A,* Chromosomal origin of a complete mole. A single sperm fertilizes an "empty egg." Reduplication of its 23 X set gives a completely homozygous diploid genome of 46 XX. A similar result follows fertilization of an empty egg by two sperms with two independently drawn sets of 23 X or 23 Y; note that both karyotypes, 46 XX and 46 XY, can ensue. *B,* Chromosomal origin of the triploid, partial mole. A normal egg with a 23 X haploid set is fertilized by two sperms that can carry either sex chromosome to give a total of 69 chromosomes with a sex chromosome configuration of XXY, XXX, or XYY. A similar result can be obtained by fertilization with a sperm carrying the unreduced paternal genome 46 XY (resulting sex complement, XXY only). *Adapted from Szulman AE: Syndromes of hydatidiform moles: Partial vs. complete. J Reprod Med 29:789–790, 1984.*

CHORIOCARCINOMA

Genetic analysis of choriocarcinomas usually reveals aneuploidy or polyploidy, typical for anaplastic carcinomas.

CLASSIFICATION

The term *gestational trophoblastic neoplasia* is of clinical value because often the diagnosis is made and therapy instituted without definitive knowledge of the precise histologic pattern. GTN may be benign or malignant and nonmetastatic or metastatic (Box 43-1).

The benign form of GTN is called hydatidiform mole. Although this entity is usually confined to the uterine cavity, trophoblastic tissue can occasionally embolize to the lungs. **The malignant forms of GTN are invasive mole and choriocarcinoma. Invasive mole is usually a locally invasive lesion,**

Box 43-1. Classification of gestational trophoblastic neoplasia

BENIGN
Hydatidiform mole
- Complete mole
- Incomplete ("partial") mole

MALIGNANT
Invasive mole ("chorioadenoma destruens")
Choriocarcinoma
Malignant GTN may be
- Nonmetastatic
- Metastatic
  - Good prognosis
  - Poor prognosis

GTN, gestational trophoblastic neoplasia.

Box 43-2. Clinical features of metastatic gestational neoplasia with a poor prognosis

- Urinary hCG level greater than 100,000 IU/24 hours or serum hCG level greater than 40,000 IU
- Disease presents more than 4 mo from the antecedent pregnancy
- Metastasis to the brain or liver (regardless of hCG titer or duration of disease)
- Prior failure to respond to single-agent chemotherapy
- Choriocarcinoma after a full-term delivery

hCG, human chorionic gonadotropin.

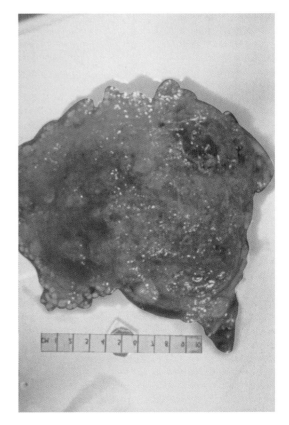

Figure 43-2. Complete hydatidiform mole. Multiple hydropic villi (vesicles), resembling a "bunch of grapes," are admixed with areas of necrosis *(white areas)* and hemorrhage. Note the absence of a fetus.

although it can be associated with metastases. This lesion accounts for the majority of patients who have persistent human chorionic gonadotropin (hCG) titers following molar evacuation. **Choriocarcinoma is the frankly malignant form of GTN.**

Metastatic GTN can be subdivided into "good prognosis" and "poor prognosis" groups, depending on the sites of metastases and other clinical variables (Box 43-2).

PATHOLOGIC FEATURES

Grossly, a hydatidiform mole appears as multiple vesicles that have been classically described as a "bunch of grapes" (Figure 43-2). **The characteristic histopathologic findings associated with a complete molar pregnancy are (1) hydropic villi, (2) absence of fetal blood vessels, and (3) hyperplasia of trophoblastic tissue** (Figure 43-3). Invasive mole differs from hydatidiform mole only in its propensity to invade locally and to metastasize.

A partial mole has some hydropic villi, whereas other villi are essentially normal. Fetal vessels are seen in a partial mole, and the trophoblastic tissue exhibits less striking hyperplasia.

Choriocarcinoma in the uterus appears grossly as a vascular-appearing, irregular, and "beefy" tumor, often growing through the uterine wall. Metastatic lesions appear hemorrhagic and have the consistency of currant jelly. **Histologically, choriocarcinoma consists of sheets of malignant cytotrophoblast and syncytiotrophoblast with no identifiable villi.**

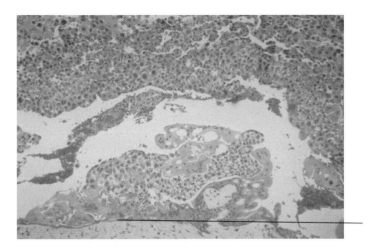

Edge of chorionic villus

Figure 43-3. Histologic appearance of a complete hydatidiform mole. Note the marked trophoblastic proliferation.

HYDATIDIFORM MOLE

SYMPTOMS

Most patients with hydatidiform mole present with irregular or heavy vaginal bleeding during the 1st or early 2nd trimester of pregnancy (Box 43-3). The bleeding is usually painless, although it can be associated with uterine contractions. In addition, **the patient may expel molar "vesicles" from the vagina and occasionally may have excessive nausea, even "hyperemesis gravidarum."** Irritability, dizziness, and photophobia may occur, since **some patients experience preeclampsia. Patients may occasion-ally exhibit symptoms relating to hyperthyroidism,** such as nervousness, anorexia, and tremors.

SIGNS

The patient's vital signs may reveal tachycardia, tachypnea, and hypertension, reflecting the presence of preeclampsia or clinical hyperthyroidism. Fundus-copic examination may show arteriolar spasm. In the rare case of trophoblastic emboli to the pulmonary system, wheezing and rhonchi may be noted on chest examination. Abdominal examination may reveal an enlarged uterus. **Auscultation of the uterus is typically remarkable for the absence of fetal heart sounds.**

On pelvic examination, the grapelike vesicles of the mole may be detected in the vagina. Blood clots may be present. **About half of patients with molar pregnancy present with a uterus that is bigger than expected based on their last menstrual period,** whereas about a fourth has a size compatible with or smaller than gestational age. **Ovarian enlargement by theca-lutein cysts occurs in about one-third of women with molar pregnancies.** This may be difficult to detect until the uterus has been evacuated.

DIAGNOSIS

The β-hCG titers can be high for early pregnancy. This should alert the physician that the patient might have GTN or a multiple gestation. The condition

---

Box 43-3. Diagnosis of hydatidiform mole

CLINICAL DATA
- Bleeding in the first half of pregnancy
- Lower abdominal pain
- Toxemia before 24 wk gestation
- Hyperemesis gravidarum
- Uterus "large for dates" (only 50% of cases)
- Absent fetal heart tones and fetal parts
- Expulsion of vesicles

DIAGNOSTIC STUDIES
- Ultrasonography
- Chest film
- Serum β-hCG higher than normal pregnancy values

β-hCG, beta subunit of human chorionic gonadotropin.

must also be distinguished from a threatened spontaneous abortion or an ectopic pregnancy.

Definitive diagnosis of hydatidiform mole can usually be made ultrasonographically. Ultrasonography is noninvasive and reveals a "snow storm" pattern that is diagnostic.

CLINICAL INVESTIGATIONS

Patients who have the presumptive or definitive diagnosis of hydatidiform mole should have a complete blood count obtained to exclude anemia, which might require a transfusion. They require an assessment of the platelet count, prothrombin time, partial thromboplastin time, and a fibrinogen level, because an occasional patient may experience disseminated intravascular coagulation. Liver and renal function tests should be performed. Blood should be typed and cross-matched in the event that excessive bleeding is encountered at the time of evacuation of the mole. A chest film should be obtained, as should an electrocardiogram if tachycardia is present or if the patient is older than 40 years.

STAGING

The International Federation of Gynecology and Obstetrics (FIGO) staging system for gestational trophoblastic tumors is shown in Table 43-1.

Stage I: Patients with persistently elevated hCG levels and tumor confined to the uterine corpus.

Stage II: Patients with metastases to the vagina or pelvis, or both.

Stage III: Patients with pulmonary metastases with or without uterine, vaginal, or pelvic involvement. The diagnosis is based on a rising hCG level in the presence of pulmonary lesions on chest film.

Stage IV: Patients with advanced disease and involvement of the brain (Figure 43-4), liver, kidneys, or gastrointestinal tract. These

Table 43-1. International Federation of Gynecology and Obstetrics (FIGO) staging of gestational trophoblastic neoplasia

Stage	
Stage I	Disease confined to uterus
Stage Ia	Disease confined to uterus with no risk factors
Stage Ib	Disease confined to uterus with one risk factor
Stage Ic	Disease confined to uterus with two risk factors
Stage II	Gestational trophoblastic tumor extending outside uterus but limited to genital structures (adnexa, vagina, broad ligament)
Stage IIa	Gestational trophoblastic tumor involving genital structures without risk factors
Stage IIb	Gestational trophoblastic tumor extending outside uterus but limited to genital structures with one risk factor
Stage IIc	Gestational trophoblastic tumor extending outside uterus but limited to genital structures with two risk factors
Stage III	Gestational trophoblastic disease extending to lungs with or without known genital tract involvement
Stage IIIa	Gestational trophoblastic tumor extending to lungs with or without genital tract involvement and with no risk factors
Stage IIIb	Gestational trophoblastic tumor extending to lungs with or without genital tract involvement and with one risk factor
Stage IIIc	Gestational trophoblastic tumor extending to lungs with or without genital tract involvement and with two risk factors
Stage IV	All other metastatic sites
Stage IVa	All other metastatic sites without risk factors
Stage IVb	All other metastatic sites with one risk factor
Stage IVc	All other metastatic sites with two risk factors

Risk factors affecting staging include the following: (1) human chorionic gonadotropin greater than 100,000 IU/mL and (2) duration of disease longer than 6 months from termination of antecedent pregnancy.

The following factors should be considered and noted in reporting: (1) prior chemotherapy has been given for known gestational trophoblastic tumor, (2) placental-site tumors should be reported separately, (3) histologic verification of disease is not required.

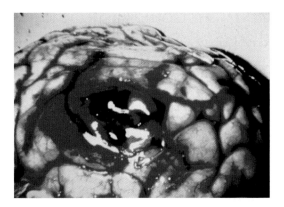

Figure 43-4. Autopsy specimen showing a cerebral metastasis from choriocarcinoma. Brain metastases carry a high mortality.

patients are in the highest risk category, because their disease is most likely to be resistant to chemotherapy. The histologic pattern of choriocarcinoma is usually present, and disease commonly follows a nonmolar pregnancy.

TREATMENT
Evacuation

The standard therapy for hydatidiform mole is suction evacuation followed by sharp curettage of the uterine cavity, regardless of the duration of pregnancy. This should be performed in the operating room with general or regional anesthesia. **Intravenous oxytocin is given simultaneously to help stimulate uterine contractions and reduce blood loss.** This technique is associated with a low incidence of uterine perforation and trophoblastic embolization.

Most patients have an uncomplicated course in the immediate postoperative period. Some require transfusion, however, because of excessive blood loss. Abnormal clotting parameters should be treated with fresh frozen plasma and platelet transfusions, as indicated. Rarely, a patient can experience acute respiratory distress from trophoblastic embolization or fluid overload. Such patients may require respiratory support via a ventilator and careful cardiopulmonary monitoring.

Monitoring Levels of the β Subunit of Human Chorionic Gonadotropin

Following the evacuation of a hydatidiform mole, the patient must be monitored with weekly serum assays of β-hCG. Because the titers drop to a low level, a nonspecific pregnancy test cannot be used because of cross-reactivity with luteinizing hormone. The radioimmunoassay, sensitive to levels of 1 to 5 mIU/mL should be used. Following the evacuation, the β-hCG levels should steadily decline to undetectable levels, usually within 12 to 16 weeks. A normal regression curve for β-hCG levels following evacuation of a molar pregnancy is shown in Figure 43-5.

Chemotherapy

Prophylactic chemotherapy is not indicated in patients with molar pregnancy because 90% of these individuals have spontaneous remissions. If the β-hCG levels plateau or rise at any time, chemotherapy should be initiated. This is discussed later in this chapter.

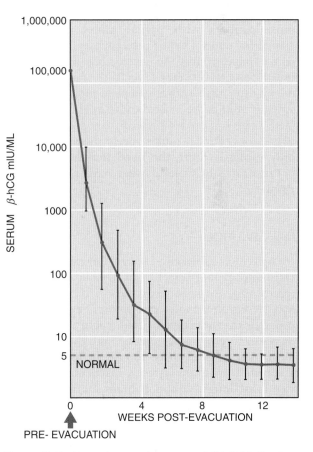

Figure 43-5. Normal regression curve of β-hCG following molar evacuation. *Adapted from Morrow CP, Nakamura R, Schaerth J, et al: Clinical and laboratory correlates of molar pregnancy and trophoblastic disease. Am J Obstet Gynecol 128:428, 1977.*

PARTIAL MOLE

The incomplete or partial mole is usually associated with a developing fetus. **Patients with a partial mole display most of the pathologic and clinical features of patients with a complete mole, although usually in a less severe form.** Partial moles are usually diagnosed later than are complete moles and generally present as a spontaneous or missed abortion.

It is unusual for a partial mole to be detected before the spontaneous termination of a pregnancy. **Ultrasonography performed for other indications may indicate possible "molar degeneration" of the placenta associated with the developing fetus. Under these circumstances, an amniocentesis should be performed to determine whether the karyotype of the coexisting fetus is normal.**

Uterine enlargement is much less common; **most patients with partial moles are** actually **"small for dates."** When preeclampsia occurs with a partial mole, it may be severe, but the condition usually occurs between 17 and 22 weeks, about 1 month later than with a complete mole. The most striking difference between partial and complete moles is related to the malignant potential of the two lesions. **Partial moles rarely metastasize, and only rarely is there the need for chemotherapy because of β-hCG levels that have plateaued or risen.**

INVASIVE MOLE

Invasive mole is usually a locally invasive tumor. It constitutes about 5% to 10% of all molar pregnancies, representing the majority of those with persistent β-hCG levels after molar evacuation. The lesion may penetrate the entire myometrium, rupture through the uterus, and result in hemorrhage into the broad ligament or peritoneal cavity. **Rarely, invasive mole is associated with metastases, particularly to the vagina or lungs, although brain metastases have been documented.**

Histologic confirmation of invasive mole is almost always made at the time of hysterectomy. The latter is usually performed in patients with persistent β-hCG levels following evacuation of a molar pregnancy or in patients with persistent titers despite chemotherapy who have no evidence of metastatic disease. The hysterectomy is usually curative.

PLACENTAL-SITE TROPHOBLASTIC TUMOR

Placental-site trophoblastic tumor is an uncommon but important variant of GTN that consists predominantly of intermediate trophoblast and a few syncytial elements. These tumors produce small amounts of hCG and human placental lactogen relative to their mass, tend to remain confined to the uterus, and metastasize late in their course. In contrast to other trophoblastic tumors, placental-site tumors are relatively insensitive to chemotherapy, so surgical resection of disease is important.

CHORIOCARCINOMA

The frankly malignant form of GTN is choriocarcinoma. **About one half of patients with gestational choriocarcinoma have had a preceding molar pregnancy. In the remaining patients, the disease is preceded by a spontaneous or induced abortion, ectopic pregnancy, or normal pregnancy.** Trophoblastic disease following a normal pregnancy is always choriocarcinoma. The tumor has a tendency to disseminate hematogenously, particularly to the lungs, vagina, brain, liver, kidneys, and gastrointestinal tract.

SYMPTOMS

Most patients with choriocarcinoma present with symptoms of metastatic disease. Vaginal bleeding is a common symptom of uterine choriocarcinoma or vaginal metastasis. Because of the gonadotropin excretion, amenorrhea may develop, simulating early pregnancy. **Hemoptysis, cough, or dyspnea** may occur as a result of lung metastasis. In the presence of central nervous system metastases, the patient may complain of **headaches, dizzy spells, "blacking out,"** or other symptoms referable to a space-occupying lesion in the brain. **Rectal bleeding** or "dark stools" could represent disease that has metastasized to the gastrointestinal tract.

SIGNS

The signs, like the symptoms, are common to many pathologic entities.

Uterine enlargement may be present, with blood coming through the os, as seen on examination with a speculum. A tumor metastatic to the vagina may present with a firm, discolored mass. Occasionally, the patient presents with an **acute abdomen because of**

rupture of the uterus, liver, or theca-lutein cyst. **Neurologic signs,** such as partial weakness or paralysis, dysphasia, aphasia, or unreactive pupils, indicate probable central nervous system involvement.

DIAGNOSIS

Choriocarcinoma is a great imitator of other diseases, so unless it follows a molar pregnancy, it may not be suspected. **In females of reproductive age, a β-hCG measurement to screen for choriocarcinoma should be performed when any unusual symptoms or signs develop.**

INVESTIGATIONS

If the β-hCG level is elevated, the workup of a patient with choriocarcinoma is the same as that for patients with hydatidiform mole, but it should also include a computed tomographic scan of the abdomen, pelvis, and head. In addition, a lumbar puncture should be performed if the computed tomographic scan of the brain is normal because simultaneous evaluation of the β-hCG level in the cerebrospinal fluid and serum may allow detection of early cerebral metastases. **Because the β subunit does not readily cross the blood-brain barrier, a ratio of serum to cerebrospinal fluid β-hCG levels of less than 40:1 suggests central nervous system involvement,** with secretion of the β-hCG directly into the cerebrospinal fluid.

TREATMENT OF GESTATIONAL TROPHOBLASTIC NEOPLASIA

If the β-hCG levels plateau or rise, chemotherapy is required. Because of the sensitivity of this tumor marker, chemotherapy is usually initiated without histologic confirmation of disease. Before initiating chemotherapy, a full metastatic workup must be performed to determine whether there is metastatic disease present and, if so, whether the liver or brain, or both, are involved.

NONMETASTATIC AND METASTATIC GESTATIONAL TROPHOBLASTIC NEOPLASIA WITH A GOOD PROGNOSIS

The chemotherapy most often employed is either methotrexate or actinomycin D (Box 43-4). Methotrexate is usually given as a daily dose for 5 consecutive days or every other day for 8 days,

---

> **Box 43-4. Single-agent chemotherapy for molar pregnancy**
>
> **ACTINOMYCIN D TREATMENT**
> *5-Day Actinomycin D*
> Actinomycin D, 12 µg/kg IV daily for 5 days
> CBC, platelet count, SGOT determination daily
> With response, retreat at the same dose
> Without response, add 2 µg/kg to the initial dose or switch to methotrexate protocol
>
> *Pulse Actinomycin D*
> Actinomycin D, 1.25 mg/m^2 every 2 wk.
>
> **METHOTREXATE TREATMENT**
> *5-Day Methotrexate*
> Methotrexate, 0.4 mg/kg IV or IM daily for 5 days
> CBC, platelet count daily
> With response, retreat at the same dose
> Without response, increase dose to 0.6 mg/kg or switch to actinomycin D protocol
>
> *Pulse Methotrexate*
> Methotrexate 40 mg/m^2 IM weekly
>
> **PROTOCOL FOR METHOTREXATE WITH FOLINIC ACID "RESCUE"**
> Methotrexate 1 mg/kg/day IM or IV on days 1, 3, 5, 7 followed 24 hr later by 0.1 mg/kg/day of folinic acid "rescue" on days 2, 4, 6, 8

IV, intravenously; CBC, complete blood count; SGOT, serum glutamic oxaloacetic transaminase; IM, intramuscularly.

alternating with folinic acid (leucovorin). This folinic acid "rescue" regimen is associated with significantly less bone marrow, gastrointestinal, and liver toxicity. Actinomycin D is given for 5 consecutive days intravenously or every other week as a single dose.

In appropriately selected patients, hysterectomy may be the primary therapy for hydatidiform mole. Women older than 40 years have an increased incidence of choriocarcinoma after molar pregnancy. These patients may decrease their risk of malignant sequelae by undergoing hysterectomy.

METASTATIC GESTATIONAL TROPHOBLASTIC NEOPLASIA WITH A POOR PROGNOSIS

For patients with disease having a poor prognosis, combination chemotherapy is always used. Regimens that have been successfully employed include

methotrexate, actinomycin D, and cyclophosphamide (MAC), or the **modified "Bagshawe" regimen (EMA-CO),** which is a six-drug chemotherapy regimen. The drugs used include etoposide (VP-16), actinomycin D, vincristine, cyclophosphamide, methotrexate, and folinic acid. For patients whose disease fails to improve with these agents, combinations of cisplatin and etoposide or vinblastine, with or without bleomycin, have been used.

In patients with disease metastatic to the brain or liver, radiation is often employed to these areas in conjunction with chemotherapy. The whole brain tolerates an initial dose of 2000 to 3000 cGy, with fractions of approximately 200 cGy per day. Together with systemic chemotherapy, a 50% cure rate can be expected. Liver metastases are usually treated with about 2000 cGy.

FOLLOW-UP STUDIES

Following three normal β-hCG levels, patients with a good prognosis should be followed with monthly levels for 1 year. Patients with a poor prognosis should have monthly titer determinations for 2 years or more. Thereafter, levels should be checked every 3 months until 5 years have elapsed. **Patients should be advised to not become pregnant again within the first 9 to 12 months after molar evacuation and should be given a reliable contraceptive.** If a patient's levels become normal and later are found to be rising, a second metastatic workup must be undertaken before the initiation of secondary therapy.

PROGNOSIS

About 95% to 100% of patients with GTN having a good prognosis are cured of their disease. Patients with poor prognostic features can be expected to be cured in only 50% to 70% of cases. **The majority of the patients who die have brain or liver metastases.**

Suggested Reading

Berkowitz RS, ImSS, Bernstein MR, Goldstein DP: Gestational trophoblastic disease: Subsequent pregnancy outcome including repeat molar pregnancy. J Reprod Med 43: 81, 1998.

Berkowitz RS, Goldstein DP: Presentation and management of molar pregnancy. *In* Hancock BW, Newlands ES, Berkowitz RS (eds): Gestational Trophoblastic Disease, London, Chapman and Hall, 1997, pp. 127–142.

Berkowitz RS, Goldstein DP: Chorionic tumors. N Engl J Med 335: 1740, 1996.

Homesly HD: Single-agent therapy for nonmetastatic and low-risk gestational trophoblastic disease. J Reprod Med 43: 69, 1998.

Newlands ES, Bower M, Fisher RA, et al: Management of placental site trophoblastic tumor. J Reprod Med 43: 53, 1998.

Index

Page numbers followed by *f* indicate figures, by *t* indicate tables, and by *b* indicate boxes.